ANNALS OF
THE NEW YORK ACADEMY
OF SCIENCES

Volume 880

EDITORIAL STAFF

Managing Editor
JUSTINE CULLINAN

Associate Editor
COOK KIMBALL

The New York Academy of Sciences
2 East 63rd Street
New York, New York 10021

THE NEW YORK ACADEMY OF SCIENCES
(Founded in 1817)

BOARD OF GOVERNORS, October 1998 – September 1999

ELEANOR BAUM, *Chairman of the Board*
BILL GREEN, *Vice Chairman of the Board*
RODNEY W. NICHOLS, *President and CEO* [ex officio]

Honorary Life Governors
WILLIAM T. GOLDEN   JOSHUA LEDERBERG

JOHN T. MORGAN, *Treasurer*

Governors

D. ALLAN BROMLEY	LAWRENCE B. BUTTENWIESER	PRAVEEN CHAUDHARI
JOHN H. GIBBONS	RONALD L. GRAHAM	HENRY M. GREENBERG
ROBERT G. LAHITA	MARTIN L. LEIBOWITZ	JACQUELINE LEO
WILLIAM J. McDONOUGH	KATHLEEN P. MULLINIX	SANDRA PANEM
CHARLES RAMOND	SARA LEE SCHUPF	JAMES H. SIMONS
	TORSTEN WIESEL	

RICHARD A. RIFKIND, *Past Chairman of the Board*
HELENE L. KAPLAN, *Counsel* [ex officio]   PETER KOHN, *Secretary* [ex officio]

CELL AND MOLECULAR BIOLOGY OF PANCREATIC CARCINOMA
RECENT DEVELOPMENTS IN RESEARCH AND EXPERIMENTAL THERAPY

ANNALS OF THE NEW YORK ACADEMY OF SCIENCES
Volume 880

CELL AND MOLECULAR BIOLOGY OF PANCREATIC CARCINOMA
RECENT DEVELOPMENTS IN RESEARCH AND EXPERIMENTAL THERAPY

Edited by J.-Matthias Löhr, David Colcher, Michael A. Hollingsworth, and Stefan Liebe

The New York Academy of Sciences
New York, New York
1999

Copyright © 1999 by the New York Academy of Sciences. All rights reserved. Under the provisions of the United States Copyright Act of 1976, individual readers of the Annals are permitted to make fair use of the material in them for teaching or research. Permission is granted to quote from the Annals provided that the customary acknowledgment is made of the source. Material in the Annals may be republished only by permission of the Academy. Address inquiries to the Executive Editor at the New York Academy of Sciences.

Copying fees: For each copy of an article made beyond the free copying permitted under Section 107 or 108 of the 1976 Copyright Act, a fee should be paid through the Copyright Clearance Center, Inc., 222 Rosewood Drive, Danvers, MA 01923. The fee for copying an article is $3.00 for nonacademic use; for use in the classroom it is $0.07 per page.

⊖The paper used in this publication meets the minimum requirements of the American National Standard for Information Sciences—Permanence of Paper for Printed Library Materials, ANSI Z39.48-1984.

Cover: Front—single-layer pancreatic duct epithelial lining (right) and the beginning of a ductal papillary hyperplasia (left). Back—full picture of this lesion on both epithelial linings of the duct representing a typical ductal papillary hyperplasia (H&E, 400×). (Courtesy Prof. Günter Klöppel, University of Kiel, Germany. See G. Klöppel & D.S. Longnecker, pp. 66–73.)

GYAT / PCP

Printed in the United States of America
ISBN 1-57331-219-3 (cloth)
ISBN 1-57331-220-7 (paper)
ISSN 0077-8923

ANNALS OF THE NEW YORK ACADEMY OF SCIENCES
Volume 880
June 30, 1999

CELL AND MOLECULAR BIOLOGY OF PANCREATIC CARCINOMA[a]
RECENT DEVELOPMENTS IN RESEARCH AND EXPERIMENTAL THERAPY

Editors and Conference Chairs
J.-MATTHIAS LÖHR, DAVID COLCHER, MICHAEL A. HOLLINGSWORTH, AND STEFAN LIEBE

CONTENTS

Preface. *By* THE EDITORS... xi

Part I. From the Precursor Cell to Carcinoma

Gene Expression in Pancreatic Adenocarcinoma. *By* MARSHA L. FRAZIER ... 1

Carbonic Anhydrase in Human Pancreas: Hypotheses for the Pathophysiological Roles of CA Isozymes. *By* ISAO NISHIMORI, KIYOMI FUJIKAWA-ADACHI, SABURO ONISHI, AND MICHAEL A. HOLLINGSWORTH 5

The Duct Cell in Cystic Fibrosis. *By* ANN HARRIS 17

Tumor Suppressor Gene Smad4/DPC4, Its Downstream Target Genes, and Regulation of Cell Cycle. *By* PAUL J. CHIAO, KELLY K. HUNT, ANA M. GRAU, ARAM ABRAMIAN, JASON FLEMING, WEI ZHANG, TARA BRESLIN, JAMES L. ABBRUZZESE, AND DOUGLAS B. EVANS...... 31

Proteins Expressed by Pancreatic Duct Cells and Their Relatives. *By* MICHAEL A. HOLLINGSWORTH 38

Immortalized Pancreatic Duct Cells *in Vitro* and *in Vivo*. *By* R. JESNOWSKI, P. MÜLLER, W. SCHARECK, S. LIEBE, AND M. LÖHR 50

Hyperplastic and Metaplastic Changes in Pancreatic Ducts: Nomenclature and Preneoplastic Potential. *By* GÜNTER KLÖPPEL AND DANIEL S. LONGNECKER... 66

Molecular Pathology of Invasive Carcinoma. *By* DANIEL S. LONGNECKER 74

Hollow-Spheres: A New Model for Analyses of Differentiation of Pancreatic Duct Epithelial Cells. *By* LASSE LEHNERT, HARTWIG TROST, WOLFF SCHMIEGEL, CHRISTIAN RÖDER, AND HOLGER KALTHOFF 83

---

[a]This volume contains the papers presented at a conference entitled *Baltic Pancreas Meeting on Pancreatic Carcinoma from Bench to Bedside* held on September 17–18, 1998 in Rostock-Warnemünde, Germany.

Part II. Cell and Molecular Biology

Sp1 and Its Likes: Biochemical and Functional Predictions for a Growing Family of Zinc Finger Transcription Factors. *By* TIFFANY COOK, BRIAN GEBELEIN, AND RAUL URRUTIA 94

Orthotopic Models of Human Pancreatic Cancer. *By* GABRIEL CAPELLÁ, LOURDES FARRÉ, ALBERTO VILLANUEVA, GERMÁN REYES, CARME GARCÍA, GEMMA TARAFA, AND FÈLIX LLUÍS 103

Growth Factors and Cytokines in Pancreatic Carcinogenesis. *By* HELMUT FRIESS, XIAO-ZHONG GUO, BI-CHENG NAN, ŐRG KLEEFF, AND MARKUS W. BÜCHLER 110

Strategies for the Detection of Disease Genes in Pancreatic Cancer. *By* C. WALLRAPP, F. MÜLLER-PILLASCH, A. MICHA, C. WENGER, M. GENG, S. SOLINAS-TOLDO, P. LICHTER, M. FROHME, J.D. HOHEISEL, G. ADLER, AND T.M. GRESS 122

p22/PRG1: A Novel Early Response Gene in Pancreatic Cancer Cells Regulated by p53 and NFκB. *By* WOLFGANG E. SCHMIDT, ALEXANDER ARLT, ANIA TRAUZOLD, AND HEINER SCHÄFER 147

Protein Tyrosine Dephosphorylation and the Maintenance of Cell Adhesions in the Pancreas. *By* J. SCHNEKENBURGER, J. MAYERLE, P. SIMON, W. DOMSCHKE, AND M.M. LERCH 157

Poster Papers

Differentially Expressed Genes in Normal and Tumor Pancreatic Tissue. *By* C. BACKHAUS, S. SCHNEUER, R. JESNOWSKI, S.LIEBE, AND M. LÖHR 166

Typing of Leukocytes in Pancreatic Tissue Surrounding Human Pancreatic Carcinoma. *By* JÖRG EMMRICH, GISELA SPARMANN, ULRICH HOPT, MATTHIAS LÖHR, AND STEFAN LIEBE 171

Apoptotic Molecules in Pancreatic Carcinoma Cell Lines. *By* B. RINGEL, S.M. IBRAHIM, H. KÖHLER, J. RINGEL, D. KOCZAN, S. LIEBE, M. LÖHR, AND H.-J. THIESEN 175

Part III. From Carcinogens to Carcinogenesis

Genomic Anomalies in Pancreatic Tumors Other Than Common Adenocarcinoma. *By* ALDO SCARPA AND GIUSEPPE ZAMBONI 179

Pancreatic Cancer: Development of a Unifying Etiologic Concept. *By* ALBERT B. LOWENFELS AND PATRICK MAISONNEUVE 191

Part IV. From Fibrosis to Carcinoma

Hereditary Pancreatitis and Pancreatic Carcinoma. *By* DAVID C. WHITCOMB, SUZANNE APPLEBAUM, AND STEPHEN P. MARTIN 201

Ki-Ras Oncogene Mutations in Chronic Pancreatitis: Which Discriminating Ability for Malignant Potential? *By* J.L. VAN LAETHEM 210

Acinar-Ductal-Carcinoma Sequence in Transforming Growth Factor-α Transgenic Mice. *By* ROLAND M. SCHMID, GÜNTHER KLÖPPEL, GUIDO ADLER, AND MARTIN WAGNER 219

Poster Papers

The Course of Pancreatic Fibrosis Induced by Dibutyltin Dichloride (DBTC). *By* J. MERKORD, H. WEBER, G. SPARMANN, L. JONAS, AND G. HENNIGHAUSEN 231

CD44, bFGF and Hyaluronan in Human Pancreatic Cancer Cell Lines. *By* JÖRG RINGEL, JOACHIM RYCHLY, BARBARA NEBE, CHRISTIAN SCHMIDT, PETRA MÜLLER, JENS RINGEL, JÖRG EMMRICH, STEFAN LIEBE, AND MATTHIAS LÖHR 238

Part V. From Experimental to Applied Therapeutic Strategies

Immunological Escape Mechanisms in Pancreatic Carcinoma. *By* HENDRIK UNGEFROREN, MARTINA VOSS, WOLFRAM V. BERNSTORFF, ANDREAS SCHMID, BERND KREMER, AND HOLGER KALTHOFF 243

The Novel Trk Receptor Tyrosine Kinase Inhibitor CEP-701 (KT-5555) Exhibits Antitumor Efficacy against Human Pancreatic Carcinoma (Panc1) Xenograft Growth and *In Vivo* Invasiveness. *By* SHEILA J. MIKNYOCZKI, CRAIG A. DIONNE, ANDRES J.P. KLEIN-SZANTO, AND BRUCE A. RUGGERI   252

Single-Chain Antibodies in Pancreatic Cancer. *By* DAVID COLCHER, GABRIELA PAVLINKOVA, GUY BERESFORD, BARBARA J.M. BOOTH, AND SURINDER K. BATRA 263

p53 in Relation to Therapeutic Outcome of Locoregional Chemotherapy in Pancreatic Cancer. *By* FRANK GANSAUGE, SUSANNE GANSAUGE, KARL H. LINK, AND HANS G. BEGER 281

The Matrix Metalloproteinases and Their Inhibitors in the Treatment of Pancreatic Cancer. *By* LUCIE JONES, PAULA GHANEH, MICHELLE HUMPHREYS, AND JOHN P. NEOPTOLEMOS 288

Exocrine Pancreatic Function following Pancreatectomy. *By* PAULA GHANEH AND JOHN P. NEOPTOLEMOS 308

Genetic Prodrug Activation Therapy for Pancreatic Cancer. *By* A.S. RIGG AND N.R. LEMOINE 319

Characterization of a Human Cell Clone Expressing Cytochrome P450 for Safe Use in Human Somatic Cell Therapy. *By* WALTER H. GÜNZBURG, PETER KARLE, RENATE RENZ, BRIAN SALMONS, AND MATTHIAS RENNER   326

Injection of Encapsulated Cells Producing an Ifosfamide-Activating Cytochrome P450 for Targeted Chemotherapy to Pancreatic Tumors. *By* PETRA MÜLLER, RALF JESNOWSKI, PETER KARLE, REGINA RENZ, ROBERT SALLER, HARTMUT STEIN, KATRIN PÜSCHEL, KERSTIN VON ROMBS, HORST NIZZE, STEFAN LIEBE, THOMAS WAGNER, WALTER H. GÜNZBURG, BRIAN SALMONS, AND MATTHIAS LÖHR 337

Discussion Paper

Ablation of Tumor Cells *In Vivo* by Direct Injection of HSV-Thymidine Kinase Retroviral Vector and Ganciclovir Therapy. *By* BRADLEY D. HOWARD, HOLGER KALTHOFF, AND TIMOTHY C. FONG 352

Poster Papers

Enhanced Retroviral Transduction Efficiency of Pancreatic Tumor Cell Lines Using Different Envelope Glycoproteins. *By* BRADLEY D. HOWARD, LARS BOENICKE, WULF SCHNEIDER-BRACHERT, AND HOLGER KALTHOFF   366

Construction of Recombinant Retroviruses Expressing Mutated k-ras or Mutated p53 Genes. *By* LILIAN KADAJA, RALF JESNOWSKI, TOIVO MAIMETS, STEFAN LIEBE, AND MATTHIAS LÖHR 371

Intraarterial Instillation of Microencapsulated Cells in the Pancreatic Arteries in Pig. *By* JENS C. KRÖGER, HELGA BERGMEISTER, ANNE HOFFMEYER, MANFRED CEIJNA, PETER KARLE, ROBERT SALLER, ILSE SCHWENDENWEIN, KERSTIN VON ROMBS, STEFAN LIEBE, WALTER H. GÜNZBURG, BRIAN SALMONS, KARLHEINZ HAUENSTEIN, UDO LOSERT, AND MATTHIAS LÖHR 374

Index of Contributors 379

Financial assistance was received from:
Principal Sponsor:
- SOLVAY PHARMACEUTICALS AG

Major Funders:
- BRITISH BIOTECH
- LILLY DEUTSCHLAND GmbH
- NOVARTIS

Contributors:
- ASTA MEDICA AG
- BAYER VITAL GmbH
- BOEHRINGER GmbH MANNHEIM
- BYK GULDEN GmbH
- CENTEON PHARMA GmbH
- GLAXO WELLCOME GmbH & CO
- KNOLL AG
- Q-ONE LTD.
- SCHEBOTECH GmbH

The New York Academy of Sciences believes it has a responsibility to provide an open forum for discussion of scientific questions. The positions taken by the participants in the reported conferences are their own and not necessarily those of the Academy. The Academy has no intent to influence legislation by providing such forums.

CELL AND MOLECULAR BIOLOGY OF PANCREATIC CARCINOMA
RECENT DEVELOPMENTS IN RESEARCH AND EXPERIMENTAL THERAPY

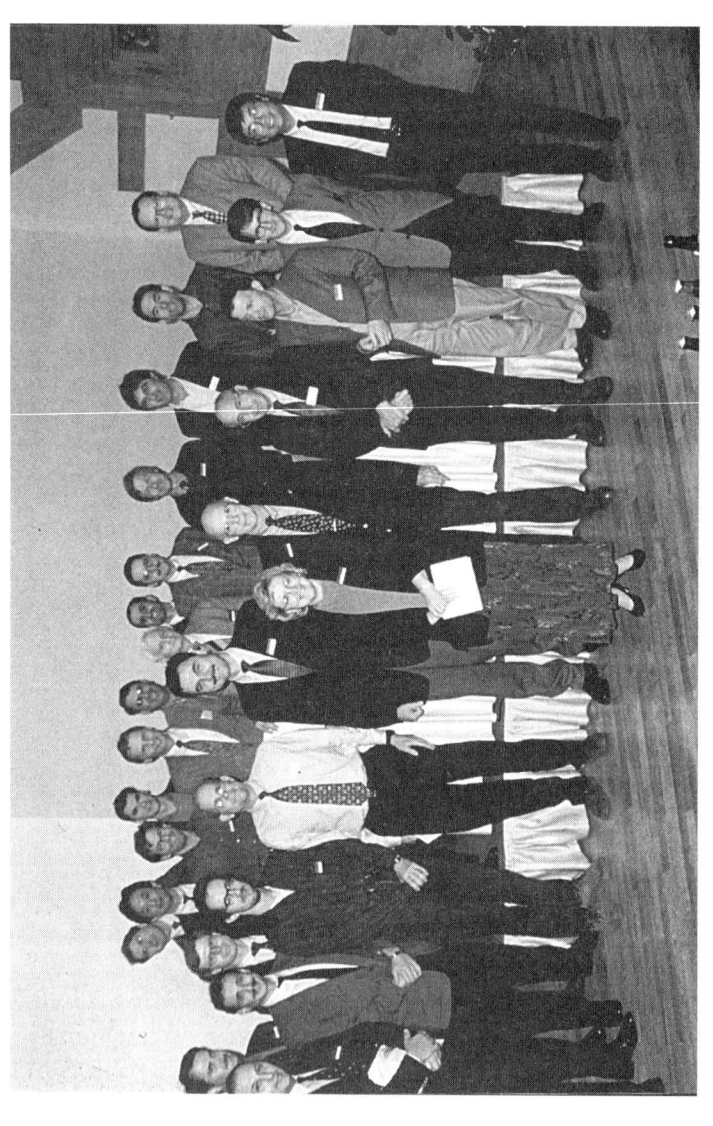

Contributing participants of the Baltic Pancreas Meeting on Pancreatic Carcinoma, Rostock-Warnemünde, Germany, September 17–18, 1998. *From left to right, starting in front*: J. Neoptolemos, R. Urrutia, R. Jesnowski, M.A. Hollingsworth, M.M. Lerch, M. Frazier, D.S. Longnecker, A.B. Lowenfels, H. Kalthoff, W.E. Schmidt, P. Chiao; T. Gress, H. Friess, R.M. Schmid, G. Klöppel, D. Colcher, S. Liebe, J. Emmrich, Å. Andrén-Sandberg, A. Scarpa, B.A. Ruggeri, M. Löhr; F. Gansauge, B. Wiedemann, I. Nishimori, L. van Laethem, G. Capella. *Not in picture*: A. Rigg, W.H. Günzburg, S.A. Hahn, A. Harris.

Preface

The idea for this workshop dates back to a small meeting held in 1992 at the Fondación Juan March in Madrid, Spain, where thirty scientists came together to exchange results, ideas and thoughts on the cell and molecular biology of pancreatic carcinoma.[1,2] Another meeting on this subject was organized in 1994. However, this meeting was larger and more formal.[3,4]

The advantage of such a small, single-topic meeting with speakers and a few contributing participants is obvious: intense exchange and open discussions. Several active collaborations resulted from the 1992 meeting that still continue and have resulted in a number of publications. Some of the participants of the 1992 Madrid meeting reunited for the 1998 Baltic Pancreas Meeting. Why hold the meeting in Rostock? The medical Faculty, together with the university hospital, carries a long tradition, dating back to the fifties, in pancreatic research. This tradition is firmly connected to the former Professor of Gastroenterology and Chairman, Martin Gülzow, who edited the first German book on the exocrine pancreas.[5]

This type of workshop should not be conducted every year. On the contrary, its value relates to the fact that these scientists do not meet that frequently and intensely during the normal annual meetings taking place throughout the year. Therefore, this meeting was planned for approximately thirty speakers. As hoped for, the meeting presented an excellent platform for discussions and exchange of ideas. Several investigators met in person for the first time.

Obviously, this format for a workshop can only take place with the help of generous sponsors. This support was provided by one principal sponsor and a group of additional sponsors. We thank all the sponsors for their generous support. In addition, we would like to acknowledge the professional help during the preparation of the meeting by Drs. Martin Rudmann, Thomas Wagner and Diethard Schwanitz from Solvay Pharmaceuticals. Their input was outstanding. We would also like to thank our local organizing committee, including Karin Otto, Burkhardt Arndt, Bärbel Brinkmann, Thomas Heller, Raimund Höft, Anne Hoffmeyer, Michael Johnson, Mario Kluth, Stefan Kurz, Anja Neuhaus, Katrin Püschel, Jörg Ringel, Christian Schmidt, and Heiko Wiesner.

The final thanks go to the participants: they made it happen! (See photo on facing page.)

Matthias Löhr
David Colcher
Michael A. Hollingsworth
Stefan Liebe

REFERENCES

1. LLUIS, F., G. CAPELLA & P. POUR, Eds. 1992. Cell and Molecular Biology of Pancreatic Cancer. Proceedings of the Fondación Juan March. Madrid, Spain. URL: http://www.march.es/NUEVO/IJM/CRIB/REUNIONES/1992_I.HTML
2. 1993. Meeting Summaries. Cell and Molecular Biology of Pancreatic Cancer. Int. J. Pancreatol. **14**: 47–93.

3. NEOPTOLEMOS, J.P. & N.R. LEMOINE, Eds. 1996. Pancreatic Cancer. Molecular and Clinical Advances. Blackwell Science. Oxford.
4. LÖHR, M. & H. FRIESS. 1996. Pancreatic cancer: molecular and clinical science. A meeting report. Eur. J. Gastroenterol. Hepatol. **8:** 89–91.
5. GÜLZOW, M., Ed. 1975. Erkrankung des exkretorischen Pankreas. VEB Gustav Fischer Verlag. Jena.

Gene Expression in Pancreatic Adenocarcinoma

MARSHA L. FRAZIER[a]

Department of Epidemiology, The University of Texas M.D. Anderson Cancer Center, Houston, Texas 77030-4095

> ABSTRACT: Both acinar and duct cell-specific gene products are expressed by pancreatic adenocarcinoma. In order to begin to understand the mechanisms by which genes of both cell types are expressed in pancreatic adenocarcinoma, an understanding of the underlying transcription factors is important. PDX1 plays an important role in the development of the pancreas and is also expressed in the adult pancreas; it is known to be involved in the regulation of expression of both acinar and islet cell-specific gene products. We have examined pancreatic adenocarcinoma cell lines and have determined that they also express PDX1, making it a candidate transcription factor for the abnormal regulation of these acinar and duc cell gene products.

INTRODUCTION

Most pancreatic adenocarcinomas are classified as ductal on the basis of their histological appearance.[4] In previous studies, we have demonstrated that five of six cell lines established from pancreatic adenocarcinomas expressed detectable levels of carbonic anhydrase II (CAII).[7] These findings therefore were consistent with a duct cell origin for these cell lines. We and others have also shown that the pancreatic acinar gene product ribonuclease is expressed by most pancreatic adenocarcinoma cell lines.[5,6] An understanding of the mechanisms of expression of both acinar and duct cell gene products in cell lines may provide new insights into the cellular origins of pancreatic adenocarcinoma. We have begun to examine transcription factors that modulate gene expression in the pancreas.

PDX1 is a homeodomain-containing transcription factor that plays an important role in the development of the pancreas. It is also known as IPF1,[16] STF1,[11] XIHbox8,[23] IDX1,[14] IUF-1,[12] and glucose-sensitive factor (GSF).[13] The major piece of evidence for its role in the development of the pancreas was the results of targeted disruption of this gene in mice, which results in pancreatic agenesis.[9,15] Fetuses that were homozygous for the targeted disruption developed a dorsal pancreatic bud, but this then regressed.[15] The pancreatic mesenchyme develops normally in the embryos that are homozygous for the targeted disruption, and is capable of supporting the growth of pancreatic epithelium from normal embryos *in vitro* in reconstitution studies.[1] These findings suggest that PDX1 is required by the epitheli-

---

[a]Address for correspondence: Marsha L. Frazier, Dept. of Epidemiology, The University of Texas M.D. Anderson Cancer Center, 1515 Holcombe Boulevard, Houston, TX 77030-4095. Phone, 713/792-3393; fax, 713/745-1163; e-mail, mfrazier@odin.mdacc.tmc.edu

um at this stage of pancreatogenesis to become responsive to signals from the mesenchyme.

In the adult pancreas, PDX1 is present selectively at a high level in cells of pancreatic islets, in a limited number of mucosal cells in the proximal duodenum and at lower levels yet in pancreatic acinar cells.[8,14,19]

DEVELOPMENT OF THE PANCREAS

During pancreatogenesis, the earliest event is the establishment of dorsal and ventral competent region in the gut endoderm from which the pancreatic buds arise. One early and distinctive property of these competent regions is the absence of the morphogen sonic hedgehog, otherwise distributed uniformly along the gut.[2] Next, signals from the notochord specify pancreatic fate and initiate pancreatogenesis in the dorsal competent region. The signaling process involves activin β (a member of the transforming growth factor β family) and basic fibroblast growth factor from the notochord.

The dorsal and then ventral site on the embryonic foregut become committed to pancreatic organ formation at about embryonic day 8–8.5 (10–13 somites), prior to midgestation in mice. When PDX1 first appears at 8.5 days, it is restricted to the ventral and dorsal walls of the primitive gut at the sites that give rise to the pancreatic buds a day later.[16] All three epithelial cell types of the mature pancreas, the islet, acinar and ductal cells arise from the nascent pancreatic buds.[8,10,18] First, branching ductules begin to form. As development of the buds proceeds, PDX1 is expressed in the cells of the pancreatic ducts, in the endocrine cells for each of the four principal islet hormones and in immature acinar cells containing amylase. Further endocrine development is distinguished by the appearance of single cells that separate from the ductal epithelium, cluster in small groups, and eventually form well-defined islets containing the different endocrine cell types, principally insulin-producing β-cells. The appearance of islets with mature morphology begins at about day 17.5 and continues after birth until weaning, after which no additional endocrine tissue appears. In the adult the ability to regenerate endocrine cells is minimal. Acinar cells form by the proliferation and differentiation of cells that remain within the ductal epithelium and develop into acinar structures. The distribution of PDX1 gradually becomes restricted, so that in the mature mammalian pancreas, PDX1 is readily detectable only in the nuclei of islet cells, principally in β-cells[8] and at lower levels in acinar cells.

PDX1 ROLE IN DIFFERENTIATION OF β- AND ACINAR CELLS

PDX-1 appears to bind to and help activate the promoters of several β-cell-specific genes that define the differentiate phenotype of mature β-cells, including *insulin*,[16] *Glut2*,[20] *glucokinase*,[22] and *IAPP*.[3,21]

In acinar cells, PDX1 participates in the activation of the promoter of at least one acinar-specific gene, *elastase I,* and therefore plays a role in defining mature acinar cell function as well.[19] In this case it does not act alone, but forms a trimeric complex with two additional homeodomain proteins, PBX1b and MRG1. PBX1b is one of five isoforms of a family of variant homeodomain proteins that form heterodimers with the Q50 class of HOX proteins, of which PDX1 is a member.[17] It has recently have shown that PDX1, PBX1b and MRG1 can form a novel trimeric complex *in vitro*. The trimeric complex of PDX1-PBX1b-MRG1 recognizes a bipartite site in the *elastase* promoter and is required for *elastase I* gene transcription.[19] The three PDX1 recognition sites in the *insulin* promoter are not associated with a PBX1 half site, and it is the monomeric form of PDX1 that binds the *insulin* promoter.[17] Moreover, β-cell lines do not have the trimeric form, because they express neither PBX1b nor MRG1.[19] Therefore, it appears that the complexed and uncomplexed forms of PDX1 contribute to the mechanisms that distinguish the endocrine and acinar cell lineage by binding to the activating different sets of PDX1-target genes.

REGULATION OF THE PANCREATIC RIBONUCLEASE GENE

Pancreatic ribonuclease is expressed by acinar cells in the adult pancreas. It is also expressed by pancreatic adenocarcinomas that are ductal in appearance.[6,5] We have examined the PDX1 gene expression in four pancreatic adenocarcinoma cell lines and could detect expression of PDX1 RNA using reverse transcribed-polymerase chain reaction, in all four cell lines (CAPAN-1, Panc-1, MDAPanc-3, and MDAPanc-28). Therefore expression of PDX1 does not correlate with ribonuclease gene expression, as Panc-1 does not elaborate ribonuclease.

CONCLUSION

In conclusion, our findings suggest that the combination of transcription factors necessary for expression of elastase and amylase are distinct from those required for ribonuclease gene expression, and while PDX1 may be involved in ribonuclease gene expression, it appears that other factors are needed, and that such factors are apparently absent from Panc-1.

REFERENCES

1. AHLGREN, U., J. JONSSON & H. EDLUND. 1996. The morphogenesis of the pancreatic mesenchyme is uncoupled from that of the pancreatic epithelium in IPF1/PDX1-deficient mice. Development **122:** 1409–1416.
2. APELQVIST, A., U. AHLGREN & H. EDLUND. 1997. Sonic hedgehog directs specialised mesoderm differentiation in the intestine and pancrase. Curr. Biol. **7:** 801–804.
3. CARTY, M.D., J.S. LILLQUIST, M. PESHAVARIA, R. STEIN & W.C. SOELLER. 1997. Identification of *cis*- and *trans*-active factors regulating human islet amyloid polypeptide gene expression in pancreatic beta-cells. J. Biol. Chem. **272:** 11986–11993.
4. CUBILLA, A.L. & P.J. FITZGERALD. Cancer of the pancreas (nonendocrine): a suggested morphologic classification. Semin Oncol **6:**285–297.
5. FERNANDEZ, E., M.J.M. FALLON, M.L. FRAZIER, R. DE LLORENS & C.M. CUCHILLO. 1994. Expression of acinar and ductal products in Capan-1 cells growing in synthetic serum and serum-free media. Cancer **73:** 2285–2295.
6. FRAZIER, M.L., E. FERNANDEZ, R. DE LLORENS, N.M. BROWN, S. PATHAK, K.R. CLEARY, J.L. ABBRUZZESE, K. BERRY, M. OLIVE, A. LE MAISTRE & D.B. EVANS.

1996. Pancreatic adenocarcinoma cell line, MDAPanc-28, with features of both acinar and ductal cells. Int. J. Pancreatol.. **19:** 31–38.
7. FRAZIER, M.L., B.J. LILLY, E.F. WU, T. OTA & D. HEWETT-EMMETT. 1990. Carbonic anhydrase II gene expression in cell lines from human pancreatic adenocarcinoma. Pancreas **5:** 507–514.
8. GUZ, Y., M.R. MONTMINY, R. STEIN, J. LEONARD, L.W. GAMER, C.V.E. WRIGHT & G. TEITELMAN. 1995. Expression of murine STF-1, a putative insulin gene transcription factor, in β cells of pancreas, duodenal epithelium and pancreatic exocrine and endocrine progenitors during ontogeny. Development **121:** 11–18.
9. JONSSON, J., L. CARLSSON, T. EDLUND & H. EDLUND. 1994. Insulin-promoter-factor 1 is required for pancreas development in mice. Nature **371:** 606–609.
10. LE DOUARIN, N.M. 1988. On the origin of pancreatic endocrine cells. Cell **53:** 169–171.
11. LEONARD, J., B. PEERS, T. JOHNSON, K. FERRERI, S. LEE & M.R. MONTMINY. 1993. Characterization of somatostatin transactivating factor-1, a novel homeobox factor that stimulates somatostatin expression in pancreatic islet cells. Mol. Endocrinol. **7:** 1275–1283.
12. MACFARLANE, W., M.L. READ, M. GILLIGAN, I. BUJALSKA & K. DOCHERTY. 1994. Glucose modulates the binding activity of the β cell transcription factor IUF-1 in a phorphorylation-dependent manner. Biochem. J. **303:** 625–631.
13. MARSAK, S., H. TOTARY, E. CERASI & D. MELLOUL. 1996. Purification of the β-cell glucose-sensitive factor that transactivates the insulin gene differentially in normal and transformed islet cells. Proc. Natl. Acad. Sci. USA **93:** 15057–15062.
14. MILLER, C.P., R.E. MCGEHEE & J. HABERER. 1994. IDX-1: a new homeodomain transcription factor expressed in rat pancreatic islets and duodenum that transactivates the somatostatin gene. EMBO J. **13:** 1145–1156.
15. OFFIELD, M.F., T.L. JETTON, P.A. LABOSKY et al. 1996. PDX-1 is required for pancreatic outgrowth and differentiation of the rostral duodenum. Development **122:** 983–995.
16. Ohlsson, H., K. Karlsson &. T. Edlund. 1993. IPF1, a homeodomain-containing transactivator of the insulin gene. EMBO J. **12:** 4251–4259.
17. PEERS, B., S. SHARMA, T. JOHNSON, M. KAMPS & M.R. MONTMINY. 1995. The pancreatic islet factor, STF-1 binds cooperatively with Pbx to a regulatory element in the somatostatin promoter: importance of the FPWMK motif and the homeodomain.. Mol. Cell. Biol. **15:** 7091–7097.
18. PICTET, R. & W.J. RUTTER. 1972. Development of the embryonic endocrine pancreas. *In* Handbook of Physiology: The Endocrine Pancreas. Vol. 1: 25–66. D.F. Steiner & N. Freinkel, Eds. Williams and Wilkins. Baltimore, MD.
19. SWIFT, G. H., Y. LIU, S.D. ROSE, L. BISCHOF, S. STEELMAN, A.M. BUCHBERG, C.V.E. WRIGHT & R.J. MACDONALD. 1998. A context dependent switch in the activity of the pancreatic homeodomain protein PDX1 through formation of a trimeric complex with Pbx1b and MRG1. Mol. Cell. Biol. **18:** 5109–5120.
20. WAEBER, G., N. THOMPSON, P. NICOD & C. BONNY. 1996. Transcriptional activation of the GLUT2 gene by the IPF-1/STF-1/IDX-1 homeobox factor. Mol. Endocrinol. **10:** 1327–1334.
21. WATADA, H., Y. KAJIMOTO, H. KANETO, T. MATSUOKA, Y. FUJITANI, J. MIYAZAKI & Y. YAMASAKI. 1996. Involvement of the homeodomain-containg transcription factor PDX1 in islet amyloid polypeptide gene transcription. Biochem. Biophys. Res. Commun. **229:** 746–751.
22. WATADA, H., Y. KAJIMOTO, Y. UMAYAHARA, T. MATSUOKA, H. KANETO, Y. FUJITANI, T. KAMADA, R. KAWAMORI & Y. YAMASAKI. 1996. The human glucokinase gene beta-cell-type promoter: an essential role of insulin promoter factor 1/PDX-1 in its activation in HIT-T15 cells. Diabetes **45:** 1478–1488.
23. WRIGHT, C.V., E.P. SCHNEGELSBERG & E.M. DE ROBERTIS. 1988. XIHbox 8: a novel *Xenopus* homeoprotein restricted to a narrow band of endoderm. Development **104:** 787–794.

Carbonic Anhydrase in Human Pancreas: Hypotheses for the Pathophysiological Roles of CA Isozymes

ISAO NISHIMORI,[a,c] KIYOMI FUJIKAWA-ADACHI,[a] SABURO ONISHI,[a] AND MICHAEL A. HOLLINGSWORTH[b]

[a]*First Department of Internal Medicine, Kochi Medical School, Kochi 783-8505, Japan*
[b]*Eppley Cancer Institute, University of Nebraska Medical Center, Omaha, Nebraska 68198, USA*

ABSTRACT: Among more than ten isozymes of the carbonic anhydrase (CA) family, only cytoplasmic CA II and membrane-bound CA IX have been reported to be expressed in human pancreas. To study the mRNA expression of CA isozymes in human pancreas, reverse transcriptase-polymerase chain reaction (RT-PCR)-Southern blot analysis and cDNA sequencing following RT-PCR were employed. CA II, IV, VI, IX, and XII were clearly identified in polyA+ RNA from normal human pancreas by RT-PCR-Southern blotting. Results with cultured pancreatic tumor cell lines suggest that CA II, IV, IX, and XII are expressed in the ductal cells, and CA VI is expressed in the acinar cells. We propose a hypothesis for the pathophysiological function of CA isozymes in human pancreas; (1) the intraluminal CA isozymes (CA IV, VI, and possibly XII) form a mutually complementary system with cytoplasmic CA II to regulate the luminal pH of the pancreatic duct system and work as a self-defense mechanism against pancreatitis; (2) CA II and other CA isozymes play a pathological role in the autoimmune process of idiopathic chronic pancreatitis.

OVERVIEW OF CARBONIC ANHYDRASE ISOZYMES

Carbonic anhydrase (CA) is a zinc metalloenzyme that catalyzes the reversible hydration-dehydration of CO_2 and HCO_3^-.[1] Among human CAs, several active isozymes, acatalytic isozymes, and CA-related proteins have been identified, and the CA gene family is still increasing.[2] The known enzymes differ in kinetic properties, susceptibility to different inhibitors, subcellular localization, and tissue-specific distribution.[1] It has been proposed that they contribute to diverse physiological and biological processes including respiration, acid-base balance, ion transport, bone absorption, renal acidification, gluconeogenesis, and ureagenesis.[1,3] To date, 14 members of CA gene family have been reported in humans; 12 were designated CA I–XII.[2,4,5] Two others were identified as a receptor-type protein tyrosine phosphatase (RPTP β and ζ) and shown to have a CA domain in their gene structure.[6,7] Complete cDNA sequences were reported for CA I–VI, VIII, IX, and XII, and RPTP β and ζ. CA VII was known conceptually from its gene. CA X and XI were reported

[c]Corresponding author: Isao Nishimori, M.D., Ph.D., First Department of Internal Medicine, Kochi Medical School, Nankoku, Kochi 783-8505, Japan. Phone and fax, +81 888-80-2338; e-mail, nisao@kochi-ms.ac.jp

as expressed sequence tags (EST; partial cDNA sequence) in databases. It has been shown that seven of the enzymes are catalytic CA activity (CA I–VI and XII). It is possible to theoretically presume catalytic activity of new CA isozymes by analyzing residues located in the active site including three zinc-binding histidine residues that are critical for CA activity.[8] These histidine residues are completely conserved at homologous positions in all seven active CA isozymes and also in CA VII and IX, which are presumed to have catalytic activity. Since CA VIII and RPTP β and ζ lack one of the three histidine residues, the CA activity of these isozymes is less certain.

CA I–III are cytoplasmic isozymes. CA II has the strongest activity and is widely expressed in different human organs and cell types including ductal epithelial cells of the human pancreas.[1] CA I and III have relatively low catalytic efficiencies and are primarily expressed in blood cells and skeletal muscle, respectively.[1] CA IV is a membrane-bound isozyme that attaches to the apical plasma membrane of epithelia by a glycosylphosphatidylinositol anchor and can be released from membranes by treatment with phosphatidylinositol-specific phospholipases.[9] CA IV has been shown to exist in several human tissues: colon, brain, lung, kidney, heart, and pancreas.[10–14] CA V is a mitochondrial isozyme that was cloned from a human liver cDNA library.[15] The distribution of CA V has not been established in human tissues. CA VI is a secreted isozyme that is highly expressed in salivary gland, but expression in other human tissues has not been reported.[16–22] CA IX and XII are transmembrane proteins.[5,23] CA IX was originally identified as a tumor-associated molecule (MN),[24–26] but its expression was recently reported in several normal human tissues including pancreas, liver, gallbladder, and gastrointestinal tracts.[27] CA XII is the most recently identified enzyme, and its mRNA expression was shown in human colon and kidney.[5]

The purpose of the present study is to determine the expression of CA isozymes in the human pancreas. We focused on five CA isozymes, CA II, IV, VI, IX, and XII, and studied mRNA expressions in the human pancreas and cultured pancreatic tumor cell lines by reverse transcription-polymerase chain reaction (RT-PCR), RT-PCR-Southern blot, and Northern blot analyses.

CA II IN HUMAN PANCREAS

CA II is a well-characterized isozyme in regard to its molecular nature, physiological role, and distribution in tissue and cell types.[1] A 1.7-kb transcript and a ~30 kD molecule for CA II have been reported in human pancreas by Northern and Western blot analyses, respectively.[28] Immunohistochemical studies showed an intense positive signal for CA II in the cytoplasm of the epithelial cells of intra- and interlobular pancreatic duct, but not in acinar cells.[29] FIGURE 1 demonstrates CA II localization in the human pancreas, which was shown immunohistochemically with a monoclonal antibody SP3-1.[30,31]

CA IV AND VI IN HUMAN PANCREAS

Only a few studies have reported the expression of CA IV and VI in the human pancreas. Carter *et al.* demonstrated CA IV expression in normal pancreas tissue ex-

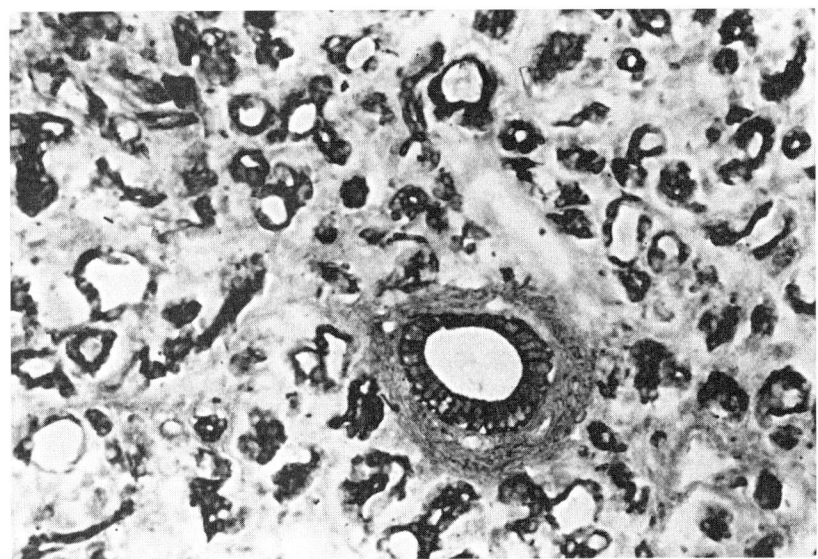

FIGURE 1. Immunohistochemical staining of CA II in human pancreas. A monoclonal antibody SP3-1 against CA II[30,31] showed an intense positive signal in pancreatic ducts.

tract by Western blotting.[11] They also reported that CA IV was detected in the apical plasma membrane of a pancreatic cancer cell line (Capan 1) by immunocytochemical analysis.[32] There are no reports of immunohistochemical studies for CA IV localization in normal pancreas. We recently studied mRNA expression for CA IV in the human pancreas.[33] Northern blot analysis clearly showed CA IV mRNA in polyA$^+$ RNA from normal pancreas. Interestingly, CA IV mRNA expression was also demonstrated in salivary glands but not in liver. In contrast, RT-PCR-Southern blotting showed CA IV message in liver, indicating low level expression of CA IV mRNA in human liver. A recent immunohistochemical study reported positive staining for CA IV in large bile ducts in human liver.[34] These results suggest that CA IV is commonly expressed in the ductal epithelial cells of these exocrine tissues.

CA VI was only reported in the salivary gland, but recently its presence in acinar cells of rat lacrimal glands was reported.[35] Immunohistochemical studies demonstrated no specific staining for CA VI in normal pancreas and pancreas cancer tissues.[22,36] Although Northern blotting failed to show a signal for CA VI, we successfully identified the CA VI mRNA expression in the human pancreas by RT-PCR-Southern blotting and cDNA sequencing of the RT-PCR product.[33]

It is still uncertain which cell types express CA IV and VI in the human pancreas; however, we obtained suggestive data related to this question. PCR-Southern blot analysis was employed with cDNA libraries from human pancreatic tumor cell lines that were derived from different cell types in exocrine pancreas: an acinar cell carcinoma (HPC-Y0) and a ductal cell carcinoma (HPC-Y3).[33] A significant signal for CA IV was detected in HPC-Y3, but not in HPC-Y0. Conversely, CA VI expression was detected in HPC-Y0, but not in HPC-Y3. We also detected CA IV mRNA expression in other pancreatic ductal tumor cell lines, PANC-1 and MIA PaCa-2, by RT-PCR-Southern blot analysis (unpublished data). Together with previous reports of the localization of CA IV and CA VI in other organs (CA IV in epithelial cells of renal tubule[10,11,13] and bile duct,[34] and CA VI in acinar cell in salivary and lacrimal glands[19,35]), these results suggest that ductal cells express CA IV and acinar cell express CA VI in human pancreas. These findings should be confirmed by further immunohistochemical analysis.

CA IX AND XII IN HUMAN PANCREAS

There are no reports of CA IX mRNA expression; however, an immunohistochemical analysis has shown faint staining for CA IX in the basolateral plasm membrane of the ductal epithelial cells in human pancreas.[27] Conversely, mRNA expression for CA XII has been reported in the pancreas,[37] but an immunohistochem-

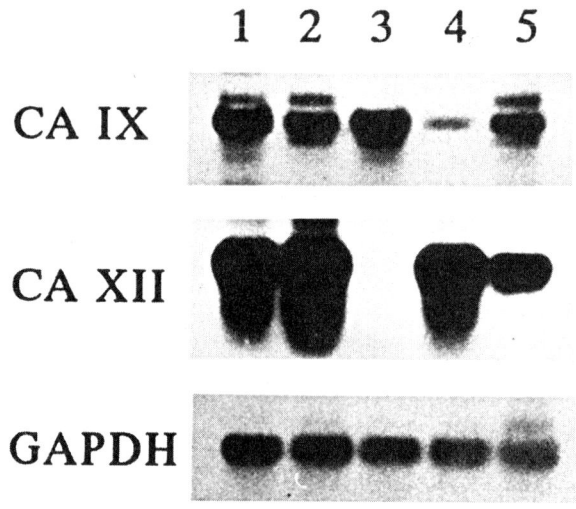

FIGURE 2. RT-PCR was employed to detect mRNA expression of CA IX and XII in normal human tissues, including pancreas (*lane 1*), kidney (*lane 2*), liver (*lane 3*) salivary glands (*lane 4*), and spinal cord (*lane 5*). RT-PCR was performed by using a commercial kit (TaKaRa, Kyoto, Japan). Primer DNA sequences used for PCR are as follows; 5'-caccgtttccctgccgagat-3' and 5'-agctgtagccgagagtcacc-3' for CA IX; 5'-ggacagcacttcgccgccga-3' and 5'-gtagcgg-taatattcagcgg-3' for CA XII, and 5'-cggatttggtcgtattgg-3' and 5'-tcctggaagatggtgatg-3' for glyceraldehyde-3-phosphate dehydrogenase (GAPDH). The RT reaction was performed using the manufacturers instructions with 0.1 µg PolyA$^+$ RNA from normal tissues that were obtained from Clontech (Palo Alto, CA), followed by PCR amplification with a hot-start (94°C, 2 min) and additional cycle programs (30 cycles) as described below: 94°C, 30 sec; 54°C, 30 sec; 72°C, 1.5 min for CA IX and XII; and 94°C, 30 sec; 51°C, 30 sec; 72°C, 1.5 min for GAPDH. Following RT-PCR, Southern blotting was performed as previously described (33). All tissues except liver showed specific signals for both CA IX and XII. A significant signal was seen for CA IX but none was detectable for CA XII in liver.

ical study has not been reported. We performed RT-PCR-Southern blotting to detect mRNA expression of CA IX and XII in human tissues, including pancreas, kidney, liver, salivary glands, and spinal cord (FIG. 2). All of these tissues except liver showed specific signals for both CA IX and XII. Interestingly, there was a significant signal for CA IX but no detectable signal for CA XII in liver. CA XII mRNA expression was also observed in cultured pancreatic tumor cell lines derived from ductal epithelia, PANC-1 and MIA PaCa-2, by RT-PCR-Southern blot analysis (unpublished data). Together with the evidence that CA XII is a membrane protein,[5] these results suggest that CA XII is present on the membrane of the epithelial cells of the pancreatic duct. However, it is still an open question regarding which side of the cell surface CA XII is expressed: apical, basolateral, or both.

PHYSIOLOGICAL ROLE OF CA ISOZYMES IN PANCREAS

The physiological roles of CA isozymes except CA II in the pancreas are uncertain. We propose a hypothesis that CA isozymes play an important role in regulating luminal pH in the pancreatic duct and work as a self-defense mechanism against acidification (FIG. 3). CA II, IV, VI, and possibly XII are predicted to be involved in this process. It has been well-documented that the pancreatic duct cells secrete a bicarbonate-rich isotonic fluid that serves as a vehicle for moving digestive enzymes down the ductal structure into the gut.[38] Bicarbonate plays a key role in maintaining a neutral or slightly basic pH for the secretions, since acidification (pH <6) would allow spontaneous autoactivation of trypsin and other proteases.[39] In the pancreas, ductal cells have an abundance of CA II in their cytoplasm to catalyze hydration of CO_2 and produce HCO_3^-.[38] It is widely believed that HCO_3^- is secreted by a Cl^--HCO_3^- exchanger that is coupled in parallel with a cAMP-regulated chloride channel.[40] In humans, a main functional chloride channel that contributes to this process is believed to be the cystic fibrosis transmembrane conductance regulator (CFTR), which plays a pivotal role in ductal bicarbonate secretion by recirculating the Cl^- imported into duct cells through Cl^--HCO_3^- exchanger (FIG. 3). In patients with cystic fibrosis, genetic dysfunction of a chloride channel (CFTR) results in a progressive acidification of the acinar and duct lumen, which leads to persistent aggregation of secretory enzymes released into the luminal space.[41]

A potential problem for pancreatic secretions would result from reflux of acidic duodenal juice via the sphincter of Oddi into the pancreatic ductal system. Acidic reflux may induce epithelial cell damage of the pancreatic duct and also cause reduced luminal pH, resulting in activation of pancreatic enzymes and aggregation of secretory proteins,[42] which may lead to pancreatitis or other pathological processes. We hypothesize that CA IV and XII on the luminal surface of the ductal cells and CA VI secreted from acinar cells would catalyze the reaction ($H^+ + HCO_3^- \rightarrow H_2O + CO_2$) under acidic conditions and thus eliminate excess acid from the ductal lumen. Carbon dioxide produced by this reaction would diffuse across the endothelial surface and pass into blood circulation or reenter the bicarbonate secretion pathway. The kinetics of this reaction would be driven by the fact that the duct secretions are rich in HCO_3^-. The uncatalyzed dehydration of HCO_3^- is relatively slow; in the presence of CA, balance of HCO_3^- and CO_2 will be maintained in equilibrium.[43] Thus,

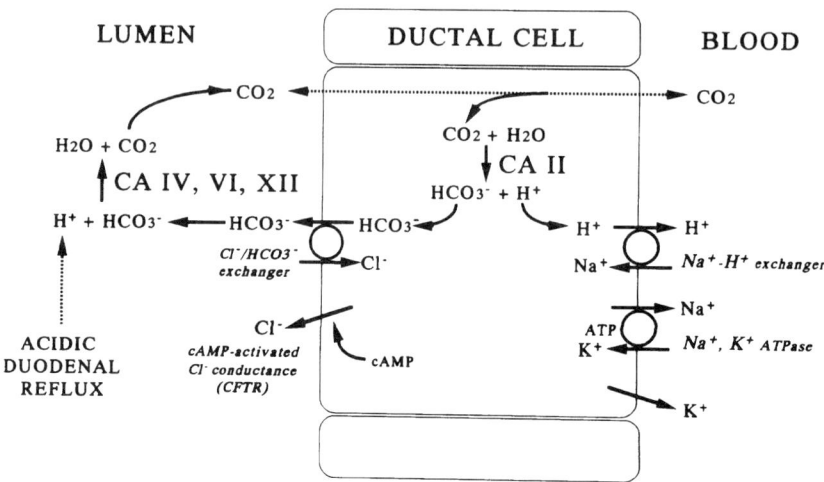

FIGURE 3. A hypothesis explaining the regulation of luminal pH in the pancreas. In the pancreas, ductal cells have a high cytoplasmic content of carbonic anhydrase II to catalyze hydration of CO_2 to produce HCO_3^-, and it is believed that HCO_3^- is secreted by the Cl^--HCO_3^- exchanger that is coupled in parallel with a cAMP-regulated chloride channel (CFTR). An acidic component is supplied from the reflux of the duodenal juice. It is hypothesized that CA IV and possibly CA XII on the luminal surface of the ductal cells and CA VI secreted from the acinar cells catalyze the reaction ($H^+ + HCO_3^- \rightarrow H_2O + CO_2$) and then remove an excessive acid in the form of carbon dioxide from the ductal lumen. It is possible that CA II and IV or VI display a mutually complementary system that maintains a balance of the luminal pH in the ductal system of the pancreas.

we predict that CA IV, VI, and XII are present in the ductal lumen for rapid neutralization of acid and maintenance of the luminal pH. These intraluminal CA isozymes would work at different levels of the pancreatic ducal system (FIG. 4). Since CA VI is secreted from acinar cells, it can function in the central lumens surrounded by acinar cells. It would not be surprising if CA VI passed through the duct system into the duodenum and hence functioned in the entire duct system. In contrast, CA IV and XII are expressed on the surface of the ductal cell and can regulate local pH in an ideal position. Under conditions of acidification of the lumen, CA IV is possibly cleaved by phosphatidylinositol-specific phospholipase and functions in a similar manner to CA VI.

A similar physiological function for CA IV in the lung has been proposed. CA IV exists on the luminal surface of pulmonary capillary endothelial cells, where it functions to catalyze the dehydration of HCO_3^- to CO_2.[44] Carbon dioxide produced by this reaction can readily diffuse across the capillary endothelial surface and be expired from the lung. The hypothesis presented herein may also be applied to pH regulation in salivary glands, since CA IV is also expressed in salivary glands along with a large quantity of secreted CA VI.[33] It has been suggested that CA VI secreted into saliva is responsible for accelerating the removal of excessive acid in the oral cavity and also in the upper alimentary tract.[45] CA II expressed in the salivary

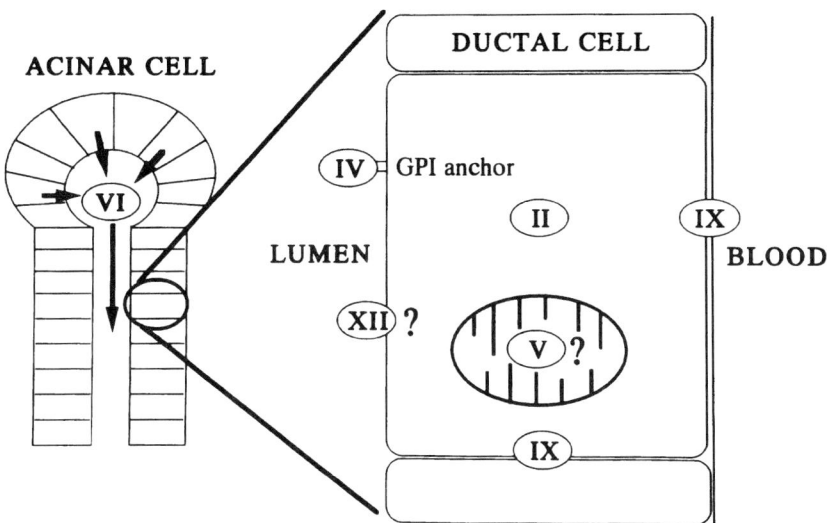

FIGURE 4. Prediction of subcellular localization of CA isozymes in human pancreas. CA II is well documented in the cytoplasm of the epithelial cells of human pancreas.[29] CA IV (membrane-bound CA) was shown to be present on the apical surface of cultured ductal cells by immunocytochemistry.[32] It is suggested that acinar cells secrete CA VI, from findings of specific expression in the acinar cells of salivary and lacrimal glands.[19,35] The positive mRNA signal was seen in pancreatic acinar cell tumors and no signal was detected in pancreatic ductal cell tumors by RT-PCR-Southern blotting.[33] CA IX (membrane protein) was reported to be present on the basolateral surface of the ductal cells.[27] CA XII (membrane protein) mRNA expression was identified in normal human pancreas (data presented herein) and cultured cell lines derived from pancreatic ductal cells (unpublished data), suggesting the localization of CA XII on the ductal epithelial cell membrane. The direction of CA XII expression on the membrane is uncertain. Possible localization of other CA isozyme include CA V in mitochondria, but there is no supporting data.

glands, esophagus, and stomach supplies bicarbonate to saliva and gastric juice. It has been suggested that CA II and CA VI form a mutually complementary system that functions to regulate acid-base balance in the upper alimentary canal.[46] Regarding known physiological roles of CA IV, it has been established that CA IV of some cell types in renal collecting tubules catalyze dehydration of HCO_3^- to CO_2.[10] However, this role is somewhat different from that in the lung and the pancreas. In the collecting duct system, the intercalated cells secrete H^+ to acidify urine and facilitate HCO_3^- reabsorption.[47] The same physiological role of CA IV for the luminal acidification is postulated for the epithelial cells in human gallbladder.[34]

Another physiological role is postulated for CA IX. Protein sequence prediction based on the cDNA sequence indicated that CA IX consists of 4 domains: a proteoglycan-like domain; a CA domain; a transmembrane anchor; and an intracytoplasmic tail.[23] The proteoglycan-like domain shows significant homology with a keratan sulfate attachment domain of a large proteoglycan, aggrecan. Interestingly, it has been postulated that one of another CA subfamily, RPTP β, is expressed as part of a proteoglycan (phosphacan) that modulates cell interaction.[48] Together with evidence on its localization to the basolateral surface of the pancreatic duct cells[27] and its upregulated expression during carcinogenesis of cervical mucosal cell of uterus,[25] CA IX is predicted to play a significant role in epithelial cell interaction in human pancreas.

PATHOLOGICAL ROLE OF CA ISOZYMES IN PANCREAS AND FUTURE DIRECTIONS

CAs have been implicated in the pathogenesis of human autoimmune diseases. Serum antibodies reactive with CA II have been reported in patients with several autoimmune diseases, including systemic lupus erythematosus (SLE), Sjögren's syndrome, and autoimmune cholangitis.[49–51] We previously reported that patients with idiopathic chronic pancreatitis have serum antibodies to CA II.[52] The presence of serum antibodies in patients with autoimmune disease to molecules such as CA, which is expressed by the ductal cells of multiple exocrine organs, has been cited as supporting the concept of a disease complex called "autoimmune exocrinopathy,"[53] "dry gland syndrome,"[54] or "autoimmune epithelitis."[55] It has been considered that a common antigen expressed by the ductal epithelial cells of exocrine organs is the target of autoimmune responses in the disease complex. Recently, autoimmune pancreatitis has been proposed as a new disease entity in a part of patients with idiopathic chronic pancreatitis, and serum anti-CA II antibody has been considered as a candidate for a disease-associated marker.[56] Our previous study showed serum antibody against not only CA II but also CA I in patients with idiopathic chronic pancreatitis and Sjögren's syndrome.[52] Interestingly, both antibodies independently occur in these patients, which was shown by a mutual inhibition study; anti-CA I antibody was absorbed with CA I but not with CA II, and conversely, anti-CA II antibody was absorbed with CA II but not with CA I. CA II is widely expressed in human cell types; however, CA I is expressed mainly in erythrocytes.[1] One possible explanation for this finding is that serum antibody primarily induced to another CA isozyme may have cross-reacted to CA I and CA II in these patients. This third CA isozyme may include CA IV, IX, and XII. A study for immune response to these CA isozymes in patients with various autoimmune diseases is currently underway.

Another possible role for CA isozymes in pathological processes is altered regulation of expression during carcinogenesis of the epithelial cells in human pancreatic duct. CA IX and CA XII may be involved in this process. Upregulated protein expression of CA IX has been reported in cervical cancer of uterus[25] and overexpression of CA XII mRNA was reported in renal cell carcinoma.[5] Moreover, it has been proposed that CA XII expression is downregulated by VHL tumor suppressor gene.[5] Studies of the involvement of the CA family in carcinogenesis have begun, and careful analysis of the expression of CA isozymes in pancreatic cancer is warranted.

Although congenital CA deficiency is a potential problem for human pancreas and other organs, only CA II deficiency syndrome has been clinically recognized and, to date, no clinical findings have been reported for human pancreas.[1] In mutant mice lacking CA II (Car-2^n/Car-2^n), a histochemical study showed only small calcium deposits in artery walls in the periphery of the pancreas.[57] Understanding the physiological roles of CA isozymes will allow us to discover whether diseases are caused by deficiencies of other CA isozymes.

CONCLUSION

We have demonstrated the expression of CA II, IV, VI, IX, and XII mRNA in human pancreas and have proposed hypotheses related to the physiological and pathological roles of these CA isozymes in the human pancreas. The hypotheses include a mutually complementary catalytic system that includes CA II, IV, VI, and probably CA XII and functions to maintain the luminal pH in the ductal system of the pancreas. The system is proposed to work as a self-defense mechanism to avoid pancreatitis. The participation of CA II and other CA isozymes as target antigen in the autoimmune process of chronic pancreatitis is also proposed. Overexpression of CA IX and XII is predicated during carcinogenesis of the epithelial cells in human pancreatic duct. Future studies into these hypotheses should include electrophysiology, immunohistochemistry, immunology, genetics, and molecular biology of these molecules.

ACKNOWLEDGMENTS

This work was supported in part by grants from the Japanese Ministry of Health and Welfare for study of intractable pancreatic disease and the Japan Rheumatism Foundation, by a grant-in-aid for scientific research (09770363) from the Japanese Ministry of Education, Science, Sports and Culture, and by grants from the NIH (R01DK46589, R01CA57362, P30CA37627).

REFERENCES

1. SLY, W.S. & P.Y. HU. 1995. Human carbonic anhydrases and carbonic anhydrase deficiencies. Annu. Rev. Biochem. **64:** 375–401.
2. HEWETT-EMMETT, D. & R.E. TASHIAN. 1996. Functional diversity, conservation, and convergence in the evolution of the α-, β-, and γ-carbonic anhydrase gene families. Mol. Phylogenet. Evol. **5:** 50–77.
3. HENRY, R.P. 1996. Multiple roles of carbonic anhydrase in cellular transport and metabolism. Annu. Rev. Physiol. **58:** 523–538.
4. LOVEJOY, D.A., D. HEWETT-EMMETT, C.A. PORTER et al. 1998. Novel 'acatalytic' carbonic anhydrase-related protein XI (CA-RP XI) contains a sequence motif present in the neuropeptide sauvagine. Genebank accession number; AF050106.
5. TÜRECI, Ö., U. SAHIN, E. VOLLMAR et al. 1998. Human carbonic anhydrase XII: cDNA cloning, expression, and chromosomal localization of a carbonic anhydrase gene that is overexpressed in some renal cell cancers. Proc. Natl. Acad. Sci. USA **95:** 7608–7613.
6. KRUEGER, N.X. & H. SAITO. 1992. A human transmembrane protein-tyrosine-phosphatase, PTP ζ, is expressed in brain and has an N-terminal receptor domain homologous to carbonic anhydrases. Proc. Natl. Acad. Sci. USA **89:** 7417–7421.
7. BARNEA, G., O. SILVENNOINEN, B. SHAANAN et al. 1993. Identification of a carbonic anhydrase-like domain in the extracellular region of RPTP γ defines a new subfamily of receptor tyrosine phosphatases. Mol. Cell. Biol. **13:** 1497–1506.
8. TASHIAN, R.E. 1989. The carbonic anhydrases: widening perspectives on their evolution, expression and function. BioEssays **10:** 186–192.
9. ZHU, X.L. & W.S. SLY. 1990. Carbonic anhydrase IV from human lung. J. Biol. Chem. **265:** 8795–8801.

10. BROWN, D., X.L. ZHU & W.S. SLY. 1990. Localization of membrane-associated carbonic anhydrase type IV in kidney epithelial cells. Proc. Natl. Acad. Sci. USA **87:** 7457–7461.
11. CARTER, N.D., A. FRYER, A.G. GRANT *et al.* 1990. Membrane specific carbonic anhydrase (CA IV) expression in human tissues. Biochim. Biophys. Acta **1026:** 113–116.
12. GHANDOUR, M.S., O.K. LANGLEY, X.L. ZHU *et al.* 1992. Carbonic anhydrase IV on brain capillary endothelial cells: a marker associated with the blood-brain barrier. Proc. Natl. Acad. Sci. USA **89:** 6823–6827.
13. WAHEED, A., X.L. ZHU & W.S. SLY. 1992. Membrane-associated carbonic anhydrase from rat lung. J. Biol. Chem. **267:** 3308–3311.
14. FLEMING, R.E., S. PARKKILA, A. PARKKILA *et al.* 1995. Carbonic anhydrase IV expression in rat and human gastrointestinal tract regional, cellular, and subcellular localization. J. Clin. Invest. **96:** 2907–2913.
15. NAGAO, Y., J.S. PLATERO, A. WAHEED *et al.* 1993. Human mitochondrial carbonic anhydrase: cDNA cloning, expression, subcellular localization, and mapping to chromosome 16. Proc. Natl. Acad. Sci. USA. **90:** 7623–7627.
16. FELDSTEIN, J.B. & D.N. SILVERMAN. 1984. Purification and characterization of carbonic anhydrase from the saliva of the rat. J. Biol. Chem. **259:** 5447–5453.
17. MURAKAMI, H. & W.S. SLY. 1987. Purification and characterization of human salivary carbonic anhydrase. J. Biol. Chem. **262:** 1382–1388.
18. FERNLEY, R.T., P. DARLING, P. ALDREDE *et al.* 1989. Tissue and species distribution of the secreted carbonic anhydrase isoenzyme. Biochem. J. **259:** 91–96.
19. PARKKILA, S., K. KAUNISTO, L. RAJANIEMI *et al.* 1990. Immunohistochemical localization of carbonic anhydrase isoenzymes VI, II, and I in human parotid and submandibular glands. J. Histochem. Cytochem. **38:** 941–947.
20. FERNLEY, R.T., R.D. WRIGHT & J.P. COGHLAN. 1991. Radioimmunoassay of carbonic anhydrase VI in saliva and sheep tissues. Biochem. J. **274:** 313–316.
21. ALDRED, P., P. FU, G. BARRETT *et al.* 1991. Human secreted carbonic anhydrase: cDNA cloning, nucleotide sequence, and hybridization histochemistry. Biochemistry. **30:** 569–575.
22. PARKKILA, S., A. PARKKILA, T. JUVONEN *et al.* 1994. Distribution of the carbonic anhydrase isoenzymes I, II, and VI in the human alimentary tract. Gut **35:** 646–650.
23. OPAVSKY, R., S. PASTOREKOVÁ, V. ZELNÍK *et al.* 1996. Human MN/CA9 gene, a novel member of the carbonic anhydrase family: structure and exon to protein domain relationships. Genomics. **33:** 480–487.
24. ZÁVADA, J., Z. ZÁVADOVÁ, S. PASTOREKOVÁ *et al.* 1991. Expression of MaTu-MN protein in human tumor cultures and in clinical specimens. Int. J. Cancer **54:** 268–274.
25. LIAO, S.Y., C. BREWER, J. ZÁVADA *et al.* 1994. Identification of the MN antigen as a diagnostic biomarker of cervical intraepithelial squamous and glandular neoplasia and cervical carcinomas. Am. J. Pathol. **145:** 598–609.
26. PASTOREK, J., S. PASTOREKOVÁ, I. CALLEBAUT *et al.* 1994. Cloning and characterization of MN, a human tumor-associated protein with a domain homologous to carbonic anhydrase and a putative helix-loop-helix DNA binding segment. Oncogene. **9:** 2877–2888.
27. PASTOREKOVÁ, S., S. PARKKILA, A. PARKKILA *et al.* 1997. Carbonic anhydrase IX, MN/CA IX: analysis of stomach complementary DNA sequence and expression in human and rat alimentary tracts. Gastroenterology **112:** 398–408.
28. FRAZIER, M.L., B.J. LILLY, E.F. WU. *et al.* 1990. Carbonic anhydrase II gene expression in cell lines from human pancreatic adenocarcinoma. Pancreas **5:** 507–514.
29. KUMPULAINEN, T. & P. JALOVAARA. 1981. Immunohistochemical localization of carbonic anhydrase isoenzymes in the human pancreas. Gastroenterology **80:** 796–799.
30. OKAZAKI, K., S. TAMURA, M. MORITA *et al.* 1989. Interspecies crossreactive antigen of the pancreatic duct cell prepared by monoclonal antibody. Int. J. Pancreatol. **5:** 359–377.

31. NISHIMORI, I., T. BRATANOVA, I. TOSHKOV et al. 1995. Induction of experimental autoimmune sialoadenitis by immunization of PL/J mice with carbonic anhydrase II. J. Immunol. **154:** 4865–4873.
32. MAHIEU, I., F. BECQ, T. WOLFENSBERGER et al. 1994. The expression of carbonic anhydrase II and IV in the human pancreatic cancer cell line (Capan 1) is associated with bicarbonate ion channels. Biol. Cell **81:** 131–141.
33. FUJIKAWA-ADACHI, K., I. NISHIMORI, S. SAKAMOTO et al. 1998. Identification of carbonic anhydrase IV and VI mRNA expression in human pancreas and salivary glands. Pancreas. In press.
34. PARKKILA, S., A. PARKKILA, T. JUVONEN et al. 1996. Membrane-bound carbonic anhydrase IV is expressed in the luminal plasma membrane of the human gallbladder epithelium. Hepatology **24:** 1104–1108.
35. OGAWA, Y., S. TOYOSAWA, T. INAGAKI et al. 1995. Carbonic anhydrase isozyme VI in rat lacrimal gland. Histochemistry **103:** 387–394.
36. PARKKILA, S., A. PARKKILA, T. JUVONEN et al. 1995. Immunohistochemical demonstration of the carbonic anhydrase isoenzymes I and II in pancreatic tumors. Histochem. J. **27:** 133–138.
37. TORCZYNSKI, R.M. & A.P. BOLLON, inventors. 1996. U.S. Patent 5,589,579.
38. ARGENT, B.E. & M.A. GRAY. 1997. Regulation and formation of fluid and electrolyte secretions by pancreatic ductal epithelium. In Biliary and Pancreatic Ductal Epithelia. A.E. Sirica & D.S. Longnecker, Eds.: 349–377. Marcel Dekker. New York.
39. RINDERKNECHT, H. 1993. Pancreatic secretory enzymes. In The Pancreas. 2nd edit. V.L.W. Go, E.P. DiMagno, J.D. Gardner et al., Eds. :219–251. Raven Press. New York.
40. RÆDER, M.G. 1992. The origin of and subcellular mechanisms causing pancreatic bicarbonate secretion. Gastroenterology **103:** 1674–1684.
41. SCHEELE, G.A., S. FUKUOKA, H.F. KERN et al. 1996. Pancreatic dysfunction in cystic fibrosis occurs as a result of impairments in luminal pH, apical trafficking of Zymogen granule membranes, and solubilization of secretory enzymes. Pancreas **12:** 1–9.
42. FREEDMAN, S.D. & G.A. SCHEELE. 1994. Acid-base interactions during exocrine pancreatic secretion: primary role for ductal bicarbonate in acinar lumen function. Ann. N.Y. Acad. Sci. **713:** 199–206.
43. HENRY, R.P. 1996. Multiple roles of carbonic anhydrase in cellular transport and metabolism. Annu. Rev. Physiol. **58:** 523–538.
44. HEMING, T.A., E.K. STABENAU, C.G. VANOYE et al. 1994. Roles of intra- and extracellular carbonic anhydrase in alveolar-capillary CO_2 equilibration. J. Appl. Physiol. **77:** 697–705.
45. PARKKILA, S., A. PARKKILA, J. LEHTOLA et al. 1997. Salivary carbonic anhydrase protects gastroesophageal mucosa from acid injury. Dig. Dis. Sci. **42:** 1013–1019.
46. PARKKILA, S. & A. PARKKILA. 1996. Carbonic anhydrase in the alimentary tract. Scand. J. Gastroenterol. **31:** 305–317.
47. BASTANI, B. & S.L. GLUCK. 1996. New insights into the pathogenesis of distal renal tubular acidosis. Miner. Electrolyte Metab. **22:** 396–409.
48. MAUREL, P., U. RAUCH, M. FLAD et al. 1994. Phosphacan, a chondroitin sulfate proteoglycan of brain that interacts with neurons and neural cell-adhesion molecules, is an extracellular variant of a receptor-type protein tyrosine phosphatase. Proc. Natl. Acad. Sci. USA **91:** 2512–2516.
49. INAGAKI, Y., Y. JINNO-YOSHIDA, Y. HAMASAKI et al. 1991. A novel autoantibodies reactive with carbonic anhydrase in sera from patients with systemic lupus erythematosus and Sjögren's syndrome. J. Dermatol. Sci. **2:** 147–154.
50. ITOH, S. & M. REICHLIN. 1992. Antibodies to carbonic anhydrase in systemic lupus erythematosus and other rheumatic diseases. Arthritis Rheum. **35:** 73–82.
51. GORDON, S.C., T.M. QUATTROCIOCCHI-LONGE, B.A. KHAN et al. 1995. Antibodies to carbonic anhydrase in patients with immune cholangitis. Gastroenterology **108:** 1802–1809.

52. KINO-OHSAKI, J., I. NISHIMORI, M. MORITA et al. 1996. Serum antibodies to carbonic anhydrase I and II in patients with idiopathic chronic pancreatitis and Sjögren's syndrome. Gastroenterology **110:** 1579–1586.
53. STRAND, V. & N. TALAL. 1980. Advances in the diagnosis and concept of Sjögren's syndrome (autoimmune exocrinopathy). Bull. Rheum. Dis. **30:** 1046–1052.
54. EPSTEIN, O., R.W.G. CHAPMAN, G. LAKE-BAKAAR et al. 1982. The pancreas in primary biliary cirrhosis and primary sclerosing cholangitis. Gastroenterology **83:** 1177–1182.
55. MOUTSOPULOS, H.M. 1994. Sjögren's syndrome: autoimmune epithelitis. Clin. Immunol. Immunopathol. **72:** 162–165.
56. ITO, T., I. NAKANO, S. KOYANAGI et al. 1997. Autoimmune pancreatitis as a new clinical entity. Dig. Dis. Sci. **42:** 1458–1468.
57. SPICER, S.S., S.E. LEWIS, R.E. TASHIAN et al. 1989. Mice carrying a Car-2 null allele lack carbonic anhydrase II immunohistochemically and show vascular calcification. Am. J. Pathol. **134:** 947–954.

The Duct Cell in Cystic Fibrosis

ANN HARRIS[a]

Paediatric Molecular Genetics, Institute of Molecular Medicine, Oxford University, John Radcliffe Hospital, Oxford OX3 9DS, UK

ABSTRACT: The pancreatic duct cell is central to the etiology of cystic fibrosis (CF) and is the site where pathology commences *in utero*. We have evaluated expression of the cystic fibrosis transmembrane conductance regulator gene (*CFTR*) through human development and shown it to be expressed from the early mid-trimester, with highest levels in the most distal portion of the developing duct system and in centroacinar cells. The precise cause of pancreatic destruction in CF is thought to be the obstruction of pancreatic ducts with inspissated secretions. We have shown that the MUC6 mucin is a significant component of the material that obstructs the ducts and that the *MUC6* gene shows a very similar pattern of expression to that of *CFTR* in the developing pancreas. These observations provide a starting point for investigating how mutations in CFTR lead to obstruction of the pancreatic ducts in CF.

INTRODUCTION

Cystic fibrosis (CF) is the result of mutations in the cystic fibrosis transmembrane conductance regulator (CFTR) protein, a small conductance cAMP-activated chloride ion channel. The protein is expressed in epithelial cells within the serous portion of the submucosal glands of the lung, intestinal crypts, sweat gland ducts, male genital ducts, bile and pancreatic ducts, among other sites.[1–4] A primary function of CFTR is chloride secretion and failure of a cAMP-mediated chloride secretion is a feature of CF epithelial cells. The involvement of CFTR in the pancreatic duct is more complex as the primary role of this epithelium is in bicarbonate secretion.[5] The bicarbonate concentration in pancreatic duct secretions from CF patients is markedly reduced.[6,7]

The exocrine portion of the pancreas is comprised of enzyme-secreting acini and ducts lined by epithelial cells that secrete a bicarbonate-rich fluid. The ductal tree extends from centroacinar cells within the acini, through intralobular and interlobular ducts into the main pancreatic duct. Pancreatic pathology is one of the earliest features of CF, and deposition of material within the pancreatic ducts can be observed by the mid-trimester of human gestation.[8] 85% of CF patients are pancreatic insufficient from birth and all show some pancreatic pathology. Obstruction of pancreatic ducts in the mid-trimester of development is followed by acinar autolysis as the acini differentiate and produce pancreatic enzymes by about 24 weeks of gestation. We have been particularly interested in dissecting the molecular basis of the early pathology of CF pancreatic disease.

---

[a]Phone, +44 1865 222341; fax, +44 1865 222626; e-mail, aharris@molbiol.ox.ac.uk

CFTR EXPRESSION IN THE DEVELOPMENT OF THE PANCREATIC DUCT

The ductal and acinar epithelial cells within the pancreas share a common developmental precursor. In the mid-trimester human pancreas, *CFTR* mRNA and protein are present in the ductal epithelium from the 12th week of gestation.[9–12] There is a clear gradient of expression of CFTR with increasing levels of mRNA moving distally through the duct system, with lowest levels in large interlobular ducts and highest levels in the distal intralobular ducts. Throughout this paper we refer to the proximal part of the pancreatic duct system as being closest to the main duct and the distal part being in the centroacinar cells. The pattern of distribution of *CFTR* mRNA during gestation led us to examine whether *CFTR* might be a useful marker of pancreatic duct cell development and differentiation. A number of studies with different anti-CFTR antibodies have shown the expression of CFTR protein in the epithelium of intralobular ducts in adult human pancreas and in centroacinar cells.[1,2,13] However, most anti-CFTR antibodies have limited usefulness in immunocytochemistry since they cross-react with other cellular proteins. In addition one study has examined *CFTR* expression in the adult human gastrointestinal tract by mRNA *in situ* hybridization.[4] We have examined CFTR expression by mRNA *in situ* hybridization in human pancreas samples from 13 weeks gestation through to 33 years of age.[12]

In situ hybridization was carried out as described previously.[11] Antisense (HCF-3) and sense (HCF-4) ^{35}S-labeled cRNA probes were generated from an *Eco*R1/*Xba*1 fragment (exons 1–5, bases 62–645) of the 10-1 *CFTR* cDNA clone.[14] The cell-specific expression of *CFTR* mRNA in the pancreas was examined by *in situ* localization in mid-trimester fetal tissue at 13, 15, 16.5, 18, 18.5, 19, 23, 24.5, and 32 weeks and postnatal tissue at 2, 7, 17, and 26 years. Data from the 18.5-week pancreas are shown in FIGURE 1, and results on postnatal tissues are shown in FIGURE 2. The first panel in each figure shows a brightfield image of the section, stained with hematoxylin and eosin, and hybridized with a single-stranded, ^{35}S-labeled RNA probe complementary to the *CFTR* mRNA (the antisense probe). The second panel shows a darkfield image of the same section. The silver grains, that appear as black dots on the brightfield image and white dots on the darkfield image, indicate expression of *CFTR*. In FIGURE 2, panels C and D show a section from the same 2-year-old pancreas that is shown in panels A and B, hybridized with the negative control sense probe. The 18.5-week-old fetus in FIGURE 1 illustrates well the pattern of *CFTR* mRNA expression throughout the mid-trimester of gestation, high levels of *CFTR* mRNA were detected in the epithelium lining the small inter- and intralobular ducts (indicated by the solid arrows) and in the developing acini (indicated by the squares). Higher magnification (×20 obj.) panels (FIG. 1C,D) illustrate the specific epithelial location of *CFTR* mRNA and tissue morphology in greater detail. Analysis of *CFTR* mRNA expression in postnatal tissue of all the ages examined (2, 7, 17, and 26 years) show high levels not only in interlobular and intralobular ducts (FIG. 2E,F, indicated by the solid arrows) and in the centroacinar cells (FIG. 2G,H, indicated by the squares) but also within the acini themselves (FIG. 2I,J, indicated by the squares). The islets of Langerhans shown by circles in FIGURE 2, panels A,B and I,J, showed no detectable CFTR mRNA expression. We have examined the expression of *CFTR*

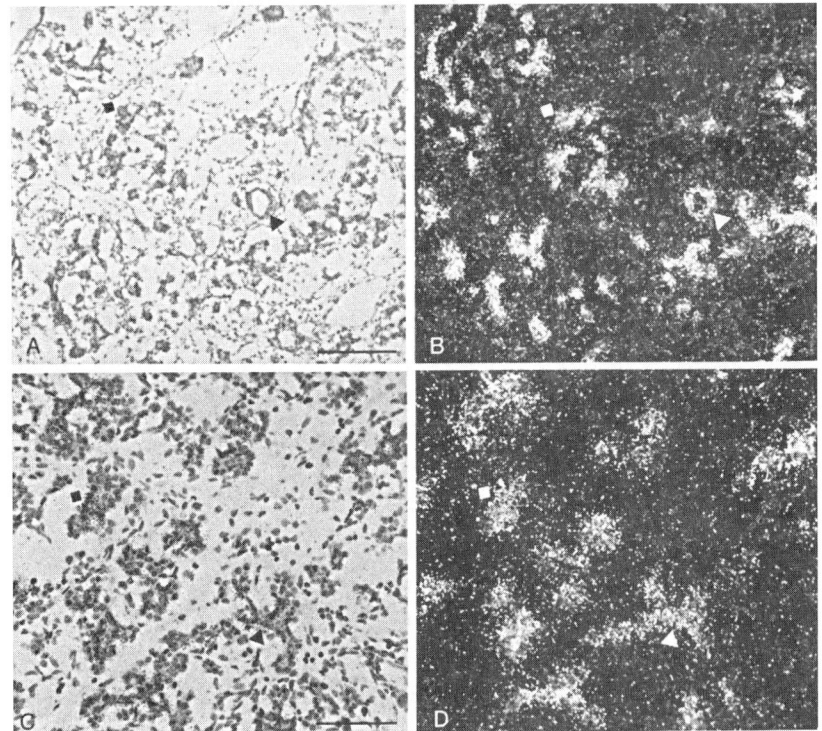

FIGURE 1. Expression of *CFTR* mRNA in 18.5-week fetal pancreas. Sections show expression of *CFTR* mRNA as detected by the HCF-3 (antisense) probe. Panels A and C show brightfield sections; and panels B and D show darkfield images of the same sections. Specific localization of *CFTR* mRNA is indicated in the epithelial lining of interlobular ducts (*solid arrows*), intralobular ducts (*open arrows*, panels A and B) and developing acini (*squares*). Size bar: panels A,B = 200 μm; panels C,D = 100 μm. (From Hyde *et al.*[12] Reprinted by permission from *Gastroenterology*.)

in a ΔF508 CF homozygote[15] at 32 weeks by *in situ* hybridization and have shown it to be similar to that of a normal pancreas.

CFTR protein expression was evaluated by immunocytochemistry with the M3A7 anti-CFTR (kindly donated by N. Kartner[16]), and a control for acinar tissue human pancreatic amylase was detected by monoclonal antibody 099(M) (Biogenex). Immunocytochemical studies of fetal (14.5-week) and adult pancreas tissue (FIG. 3) show the localization of CFTR to the apical membrane of cells within the ductal epithelium. A gradient of expression of CFTR protein is observed within the ducts with the highest levels seen in centroacinar cells and small intralobular ducts (FIG. 3A) and decreasing levels through interlobular ducts. The identity of the acinar cells was confirmed with a monoclonal antibody to human pancreatic amylase (FIG. 3B). At this level of resolution it is impossible to determine whether there is CFTR protein in other acinar cells, though other groups have now provided data to support this.[17,18]

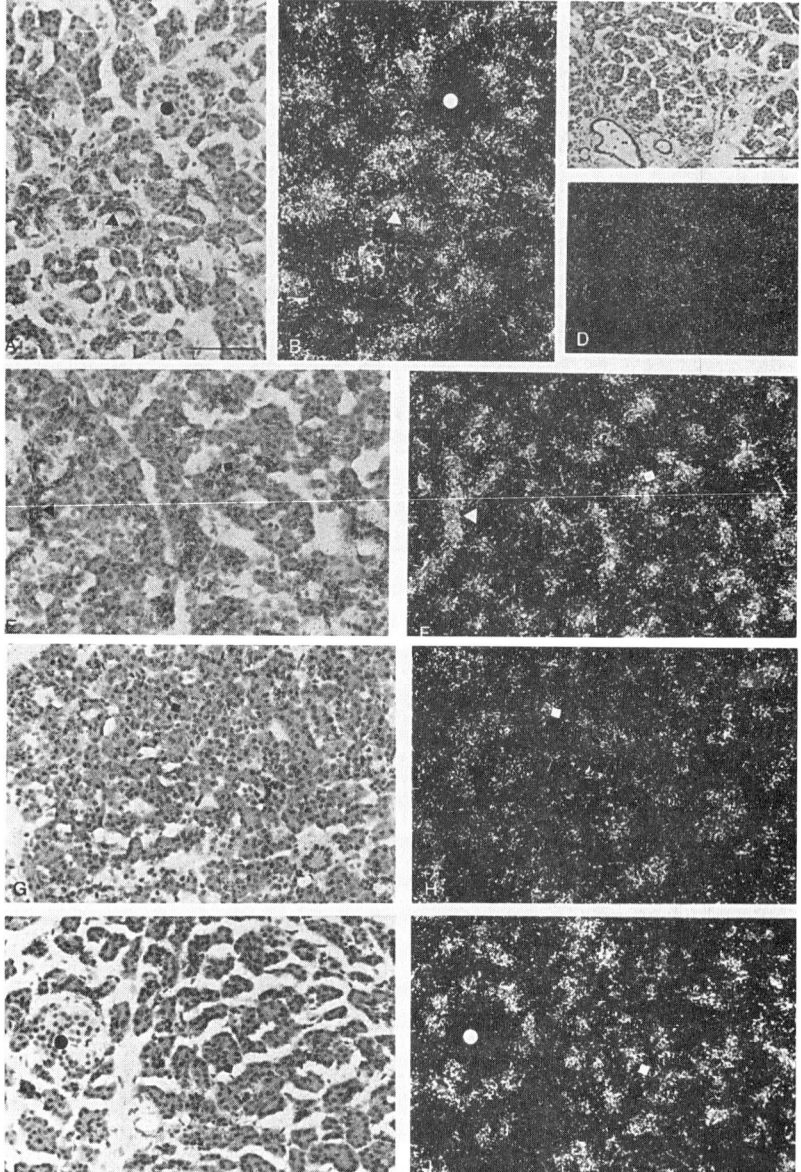

FIGURE 2. Expression of *CFTR* mRNA in postnatal pancreas. Sections through a 2-year (A–D); 7-year (E,F); 17-year (G,H) and 26-year (I,J) pancreas. Panels A, E, G, and I show brightfield sections hybridized with the HCF-3 (antisense) probe; and panels B, F, H, and J show darkfield images of the same sections. Panels C and D (2-year) show a brightfield view (of a consecutive section to panels A and B) and a darkfield image of the same section hybridized with the HCF-4 (sense) negative control probe. Specific localization of CFTR mRNA is indicated in the epithelium lining of interlobular ducts (A,B and E,F, *solid arrows*), intralobular ducts (E,F, *open arrows*) in centroacinar cells (G,H, *squares*) and in acinar cells (I-J, *squares*). In pancreatic islets there is no expression of CFTR mRNA (A,B and I,J,*circles*). Size bar: panels A,B and E–J = 100 µm; panels C,D = 200 µm. (From Hyde *et al.*[12] Reprinted by permission from *Gastroenterology*.)

The functional significance of this evolution of distribution of CFTR expression is of interest. CFTR is known to be a cAMP-activated chloride ion channel; our data suggest that the most active sites of secretin-activated chloride secretion in the pancreas are in the most distal portion of the ducts and within centroacinar cells. The distribution of CFTR in the fetal pancreas is important, since it has been suggested that as well as being a cAMP-activated chloride ion channel CFTR may have additional roles in epithelial development.[11]

The evolution in the pattern of expression of CFTR in the pancreatic duct system through human development into adult life may be of relevance to the pathology of CF. About 15% of CF patients are born pancreas sufficient, this usually being associated with "mild mutations" in the CFTR gene. It is possible that age-related changes in the pattern of expression of CFTR in the pancreas may be important in the disease progression. As pancreatic sufficiency in CF is often maintained for many

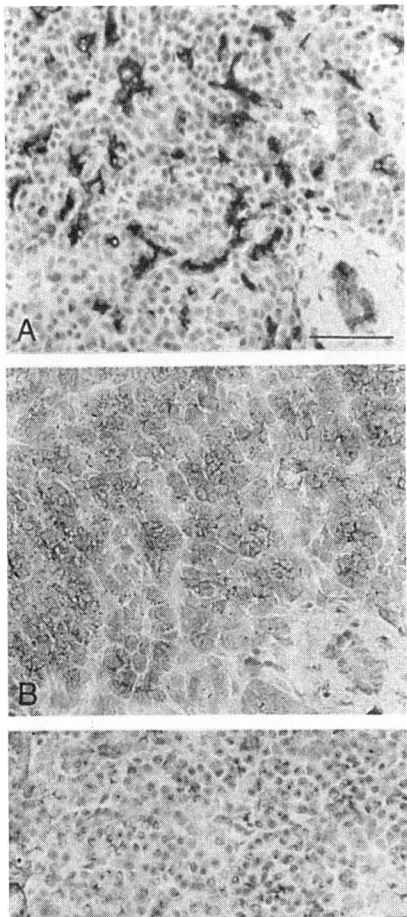

FIGURE 3. Expression of CFTR protein and amylase in adult pancreas. Panel A, CFTR protein detected by the anti-CFTR antibody M3A7; panel B, amylase detected by the 099M antibody; panel C secondary antibody alone. In panel A, CFTR is seen in interlobular and intralobular duct cells and centroacinar cells; in panel B, amylase is seen in acinar cells. Size bar: all panels = 100 μm. (From Hyde et al.[12] Reprinted by permission from *Gastroenterology*.)

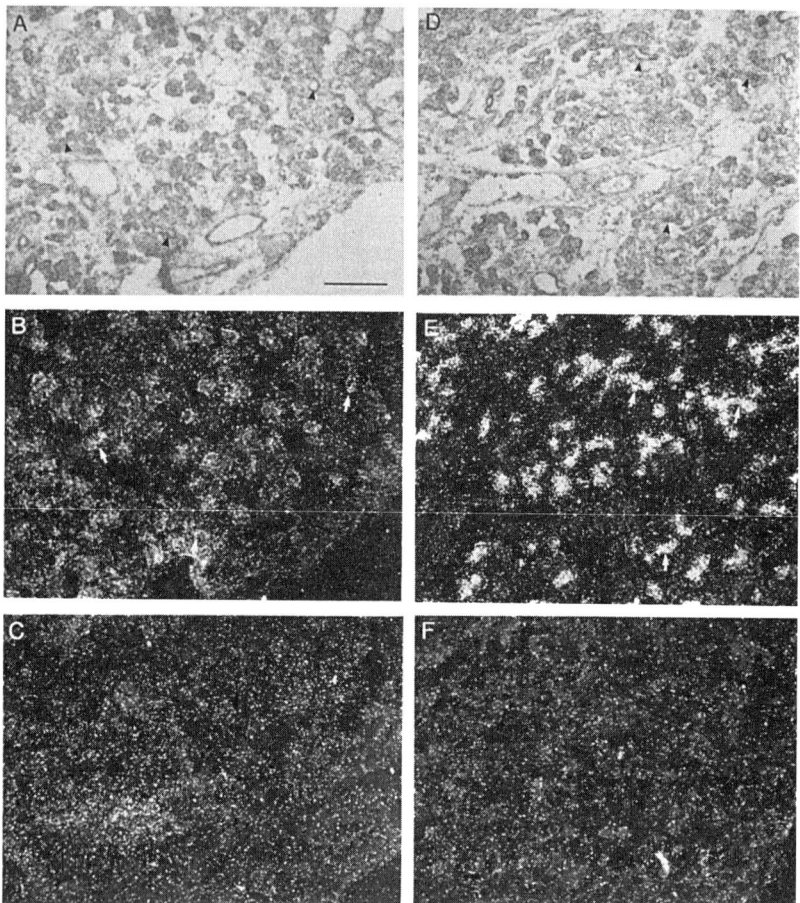

FIGURE 4. Expression of *MUC6* and *CFTR* mRNA in 13-week pancreas. Expression of MUC6 mRNA (panels A–C) and CFTR (panels D–F) in 13-week fetal pancreas. Panels A and D show brightfield views of pancreas sections hybridized with the *MUC6* and *CFTR* antisense probes, respectively, and panel B and E show darkfield images of the same sections. Panels C and F show darkfield views of consecutive sections hybridized with the *MUC6* and *CFTR* sense negative control probes, respectively. Size bar: all panels = 200 μm. *Arrows* show ductal epithelium. (From Reid et al.[15] Reprinted by permission from *Molecular Medicine*.)

decades of postnatal life, it is probable that the extent of *in utero* tissue damage is fundamental to pancreatic function in this disease.

MUCINS IN THE PANCREATIC DUCT IN CF

The precise cause of the pancreatic destruction characteristic of CF is thought to be obstruction of the pancreatic ducts by inspissated secretions. These secretions

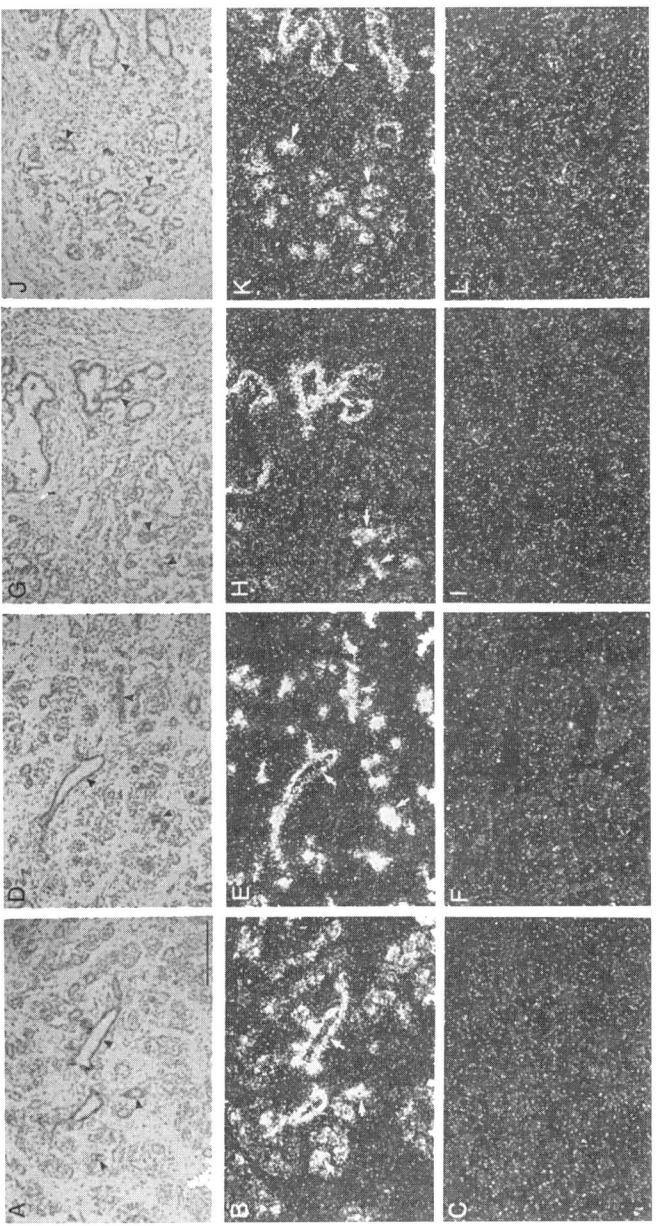

FIGURE 5. Expression of *MUC6* and *CFTR* mRNA in 23-week pancreas and in 28 + 3-week CF pancreas. Panels A–F, expression of *MUC6* mRNA (panels A–C) and *CFTR* (panels D–F) in 23-week fetal pancreas. Panels A and D show brightfield views of pancreas sections hybridized with the *MUC6* and *CFTR* antisense probes, respectively, and panel B and E show darkfield images of the same sections. Panels C and F show darkfield views of consecutive sections hybridized with the *MUC6* and *CFTR* sense negative control probes, respectively. Panels G–L show expression of *MUC6* mRNA (panels G–I) and CFTR (panels J–L) in 28 + 3-week CF fetal pancreas. Panels G and J show a brightfield views of pancreas sections hybridized with the *MUC6* and *CFTR* antisense probes, respectively, and panel H and K show darkfield images of the same sections. Panels I and L show darkfield views of consecutive sections hybridized with the *MUC6* and *CFTR* sense negative control probes respectively. Size bar: all panels = 200 μm. *Arrows* show ductal epithelium. (From Reid *et al.*[15] Reprinted by permission from *Molecular Medicine*.)

23

may include mucous glycoproteins and other proteins; however, the composition of the secretions has not been defined. As already mentioned, one of the earliest pathological manifestations of CF *in utero* is the deposition of periodic-acid Schiff-positive material in the fetal pancreatic ducts at about 12 weeks of gestation,[8,19] suggesting a contribution of mucins to these deposits. We have examined the developmental expression of 9 human mucin genes in the pancreas by mRNA *in situ* hybridization.[20,21] MUC 6 was identified as a major pancreatic mucin that is expressed by 13 weeks of gestation and shows a pattern of distribution that is very similar to that of CFTR from this age through to adult life.[15] *MUC1* was the only other mucin mRNA shown to be expressed in the mid-trimester pancreatic duct,[22,23] and this was evident later in gestation in the epithelium of larger pancreatic ducts.[20] However, the MUC1 mucin-like core protein is not gel-forming, and it is in part cell surface-associated via an integral transmembrane domain. MUC1 is not known to be a major component of the inspissated secretions that are found in CF pancreas, and its temporal and spatial patterns of expression are distinct from CFTR. Hence, MUC1 is unlikely to be involved in the initial pathobiochemical events that lead to ductal obstruction in CF. The *MUC6* cDNA was isolated by expression cloning from a human stomach cDNA library.[24,25] The cDNA has not been fully characterized but appears to be at least 15–16 kb long.[26] Similar to other mucins, MUC6 contains a serine and threonine rich tandem repeat sequence with an individual repeat unit of 507 bp and 169 amino acids. The probe used for MUC6 *in situ* hybridization was a 74 bp double-stranded oligonucleotide GGTCCACACACACAGCCCCACCAGT-GACGCCGACCACCAGTGGGACGAGCCAAG CCGCGAGCTCATTCAGCACA (bases 308–381 EMBL Accession number L07517) cloned into the Bam HI and Hind III sites of pBluescript. Antisense and sense MUC6 ^{35}S-labeled riboprobes were generated from the T7 and T3 promoters, respectively. Abundant MUC6 mRNA expression was detected throughout the pancreatic duct epithelia and the developing acini at or by 13 weeks of gestation, the earliest fetal age examined (FIG. 4A–C). A similar pattern of expression was seen at 23 weeks (FIG. 5A–C). Two CF pancreases were analyzed. One was from a male ΔF508 homozygote who was born prematurely at 28 weeks gestation and died 21 days later from respiratory failure, at an age equivalent to 31 weeks gestation (28 + 3 weeks). The second was a 29-week intrauterine death due to intestinal rupture. This fetus was diagnosed on the basis of pathology consistent with CF and was heterozygous for ΔF508 and an undefined mutation. *MUC6* mRNA expression patterns in both CF pancreases appeared normal (FIG. 5G–I shows the 28 + 3-week pancreas). In postnatal pancreas (FIG. 6A–D) *MUC6* expression was seen in interlobular and intralobular duct epithelial cells, centroacinar cells and possibly acinar cells (the *in situ* technique might not enable discrimination between centroacinar cells and acini). There was substantially less *MUC6* mRNA in larger pancreatic duct structures and no detectable expression in islets. A comparison between the *MUC6* and *CFTR* expression patterns in the same pancreatic sections is provided by the data presented in FIGURE 4D–F and FIGURE 5D–F, which show *CFTR* expression using the same probes described above at the relevant developmental stages. *CFTR* and *MUC6* transcripts have nearly identical expression patterns in the 13- and 23-week fetal pancreas. A similar pattern of colocalization of *MUC6* (panels A–D) and *CFTR* mRNA (panels E–H) is seen in postnatal pancreas (FIG. 6).

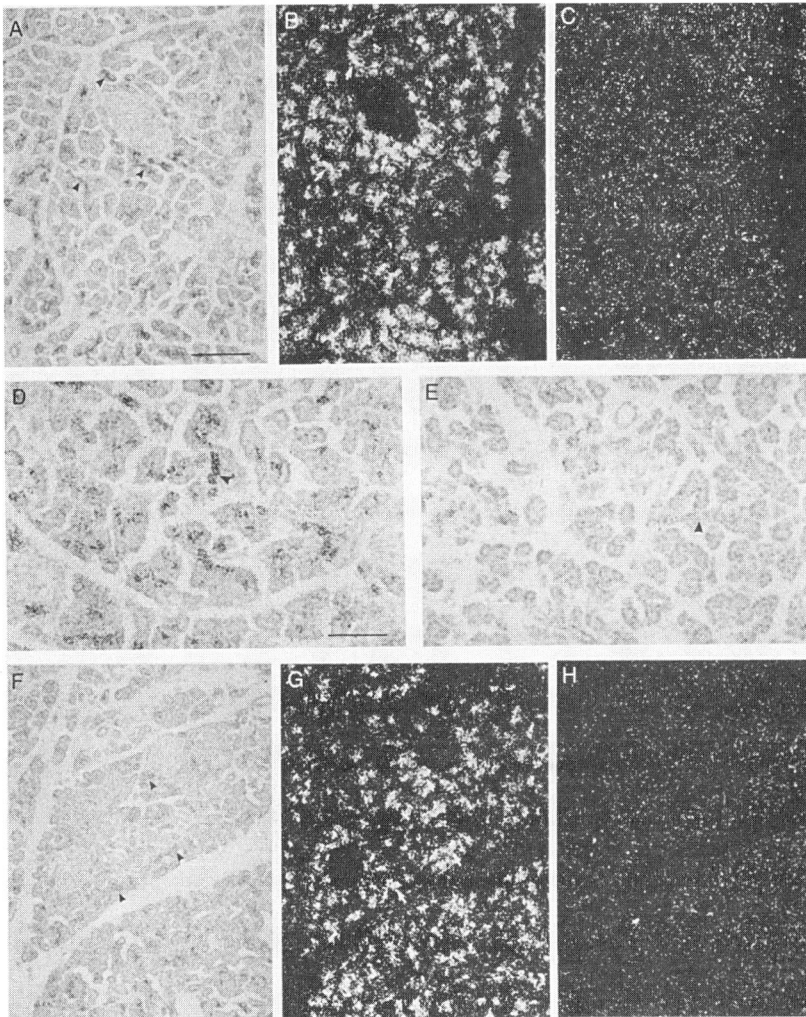

FIGURE 6. Expression of *MUC6* and *CFTR* mRNA in 2-year-old pancreas. Expression of MUC6 mRNA (panels A–D) and CFTR (panels E–H) in 2-year-old pancreas. Panels A and D show brightfield views of pancreas sections hybridized with the *MUC6* antisense probe; panels E and F show brightfield views of pancreas sections hybridized with the *CFTR* antisense probe. Panels B and G show darkfield images of the same sections shown in panels A and F. Panels C and H show darkfield views of consecutive sections hybridized with the *MUC6* and *CFTR* sense negative control probes, respectively. Size bar: panels A–C and F–H = 200 μm; panels D,E = 100 μm. *Arrows* show ductal epithelium. (From Reid et al.[15] Reprinted by permission from *Molecular Medicine*.)

The localization of *MUC6* expression by mRNA *in situ* hybridization was confirmed by immunocytochemistry. The M6P antibody, a chicken polyclonal antibody that was raised against a MUC6 tandem repeat peptide (kindly donated by Sam Ho), was used to localize the MUC6 glycoprotein in normal and CF pancreas (FIG. 7). Panels A–D show hematoxylin and eosin-stained sections of normal 32-week-gestation fetal pancreas (panels A,B) and the 28 + 3 week CF pancreas (panels C,D). An abnormal histology is apparent in the CF pancreas with material obstructing dilated ducts (see arrow in panel D). MUC6 protein expression is seen in 23-week pancreas in developing pancreatic ducts and acini (panels E–G: E, preimmune serum; F and G, M6P). The arrow in panel G identifies MUC6 expression in developing acini/centroacinar cells. MUC6 protein expression in a 2-year-old normal pancreas is illustrated in panels K–M (K, preimmune serum; L and M, M6P). The arrow in panel M shows acinar expression of MUC6, which is also seen in the epithelial cells lining

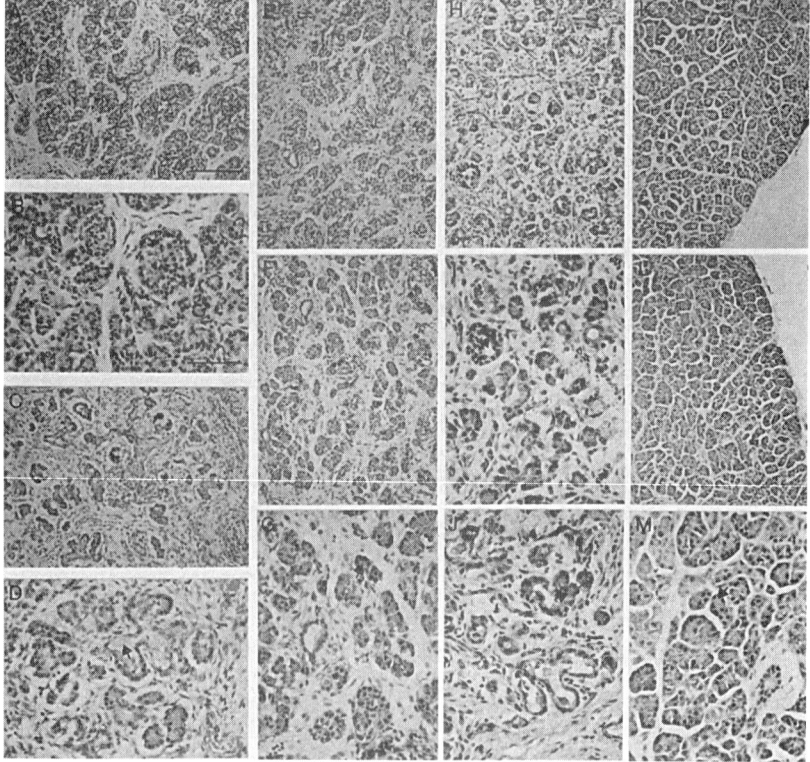

FIGURE 7. Expression of MUC6 protein in 32-week and 2-year-old normal pancreas and 28 + 3-week CF pancreas. Immunoperoxidase detection of MUC6 protein in the pancreas. Panels A–D, hematoxylin and eosin-stained pancreatic tissue, A and B, normal 32-week pancreas; C and D, 28 + 3-week CF fetal pancreas. Panels E–G show MUC6 protein expression, detected with the M6P antibody, in 23 week pancreas, E, preimmune serum, F and G, M6P. Panels H–J show MUC6 protein expression in 28 + 3-week CF fetal pancreas. Panels K–M show MUC6 protein expression in 2-year normal pancreas, K, preimmune serum, L and M, M6P. Size bars: panels A,C,E,F,I,H,K and L = 200 μm; panels B,D,G,I,J and M = 100 μm. (From Reid et al.[15] Reprinted by permission from *Molecular Medicine*.)

small ducts and in centroacinar cells. Panels H–J show MUC6 protein expression in 28 + 3-week CF fetal pancreas detected by the M6P antibody. The arrows in panels I and J show MUC6 to be a significant component of the material obstructing the small intralobular ducts in this CF pancreas. Similar results were obtained on a 29-week CF fetal pancreas, in which the histology was less abnormal, but there was also evidence of MUC6 in inspissated secretions within the intralobular ducts (not shown).

It is of particular interest in the context of CF that the localization of expression of the *CFTR* gene coincides with that of *MUC6* in the pancreas. The temporal and spatial distribution of *MUC6* and *CFTR* transcripts shows complete concordance in the pancreas (FIGS. 4–6). These results suggest that *MUC6* and *CFTR* are expressed in the same cell types within the pancreas. These observations may be of considerable importance to our understanding of the disease process in the CF pancreas. As already stated, the CFTR gene encodes a small conductance cAMP-activated chloride ion channel[27] that is expressed at high levels in the pancreatic duct epithelium *in utero* and postnatally.[28] A principal physiological defect in the CF pancreas is the failure to secrete bicarbonate ions that are essential for the normal flow of pancreatic duct secretions. One model that would explain the pathophysiology of CF in the pancreas, for which there is some physiological evidence, proposes that chloride ion efflux through CFTR is coupled to bicarbonate ion secretion via a chloride/bicarbonate exchanger in the apical membrane of the pancreatic duct cell.[5] The CF pancreatic duct fluid has reduced water and bicarbonate content[7] and this is believed to contribute to the deposition of material in the small intralobular ducts. The composition of these deposits has not been characterized, though it has been suggested that they may contain secreted proteins and/or mucus glycoproteins. We have now identified MUC6 as a significant constituent of these ductal deposits. Future experiments will determine the relationship between altered CFTR functioning and the solubility of MUC6.

HOW DO MUTATIONS IN CFTR LEAD TO OBSTRUCTION OF PANCREATIC DUCTS IN CF?

The cause of the mucus clearance problems in CF remains poorly understood. Several hypotheses to explain the mucus abnormalities have been put forward, including: mucin hypersecretion; dehydration of mucins due to ion transport defects that result from mutations in the CFTR cAMP-activated chloride ion channel; and biochemical abnormalities in the glycosylation of mucins in CF epithelial cells including increased sulphation and fucosylation, and reduced sialylation. However, there is currently no conclusive evidence to provide support for any one of these hypotheses.

Since the biochemical and biophysical properties of a mucin are dependent on O-glycosylation, this aspect of mucin biology has been investigated in CF. Reports of increased glycosylation and sulphation of mucins from CF airway tissue[29–31] and intestine[32] are complicated by the potential for secondary modifications in mucins secreted by diseased epithelia. Increased sulphation of glycoconjugates secreted by CF nasal epithelial cells in culture[33] or CF bronchial epithelial cells in a xenograft model[34] have also been observed. The cause of mucin abnormalities in the pancreas has not been studied extensively.

All the experiments in which CF mucins have been analyzed to date, regardless of the experimental model, have analyzed a mixture of glycoproteins secreted from epithelial cells, rather than evaluated the biochemistry of individual mucins. Our observation that MUC6 is a significant component of the material that obstructs the pancreatic ducts in CF provides a handle on investigating the molecular basis of mucin abnormalities in the CF pancreas. Our aim is to evaluate the O-glycosylation of MUC6 alone in matched pairs of pancreatic duct cells that differ with respect to CFTR expression status, for example, one cell line carrying mutations in both CFTR genes, and a derivative line in which normal CFTR expression has been restored by the introduction of a wild-type transgene. Examples of these cell lines exist, for example, the CFPAC line and its corrected pair that carries a retroviral vector expressing wild-type CFTR.[35] We will exploit an epitope-tagged MUC1 mucin cDNA[36] that, when stably expressed in cell lines, can be purified with an antibody specific for the epitope. This approach detected variation in mucin glycosylation (expression of blood group antigens) in different cell lines[36] including pancreatic and colon carcinoma cell lines. We have extended these studies to examine the expression of blood group antigens on MUC1F mucin in matched pairs of Caco2 cell lines that either express wild-type CFTR or have spontaneously switched off CFTR expression and so may be considered equivalent to CFTR null mutants.[37] Further, metabolic labeling experiments were then carried out to estimate the gross levels of glycosylation and sulphation of MUC1F mucin in these matched pairs of cell lines. Expression of CFTR in this experimental system did not affect the gross levels of glycosylation or sulphation of the MUC1F mucin or the antigenicity of the carbohydrates structures attached to the MUC1F protein. Similar experiments with MUC6 need to be performed in pancreatic duct cells. Given the size of the MUC6 cDNA it will be difficult to generate a full length epitope-tagged MUC6F cDNA construct. Hence we are using the MUC1F backbone in a tandem repeat-deleted form (Burdick *et al.*, submitted) as a vehicle for the tandem repeats of other mucins. The tandem repeats of mucin are rich in serine and threonine and they provide most of the sites for the O-glycosylation that is characteristic of these glycoproteins. We have generated a hybrid mucin carrying tandem repeat sequences from MUC5AC in a tandem repeat-deleted construct of the epitope-tagged MUC1 (MUC1/5ACF) and shown it to carry different carbohydrate structures from the native MUC1F construct when transfected in to the same cell line (unpublished data). This suggests that a hybrid MUC1/6TRF mucin will provide a powerful tool for investigating the glycosylation of the MUC6 mucin tandem repeats in differentiated pancreatic duct cells. These experiments should establish whether a primary defect in mucin processing is responsible for the obstruction of CF pancreatic ducts or whether the cause is dehydration of the epithelium, mucin hypersecretion or some other mechanism.

ACKNOWLEDGMENTS

This work was supported by Grant DK46589 from the National Institutes of Health and by the Cystic Fibrosis Research Trust UK. Karen Hyde, Colm Reid, Scott Tebbutt and Deborah Harrison contributed data described in this paper. I am grateful to N. Kartner for the M3A7 antibody, and to S. Ho for the M6P antibody. We thank W. B. Saunders Co. for permission to reproduce FIGURES 1–3 and *Molecular Medicine*, a joint publication of the Picower Institute Press and Springer-Verlag, NY, Inc. for permission to reproduce FIGURES 4–7.

REFERENCES

1. CRAWFORD, I.C., P.C. MALONEY, P.L. ZEITLIN, W.B. GUGGINO, S.C. HYDE, H. TURLEY, K.C. GATTER, A. HARRIS & C.F. HIGGINS. 1991. Immuno-cytochemical localization of the cystic fibrosis gene product CFTR. Proc. Natl. Acad. Sci. USA **88:** 9262–9266.
2. DENNING, G.M., L.S. OSTEDGAARD, S.H. CHENG, A.E. SMITH & M.J. WELSH. 1992. Localization of the cystic fibrosis transmembrane conductance regulator in chloride secretory epithelia. J. Clin. Invest. **89:** 339–349.
3. ENGELHARDT, J.F., J.R. YANKASKAS, S.A. ERNST, Y. YANG, C.R. MARINO, R.C. BOUCHER, J.A. COHN & J.M. WILSON. 1993. Submucosal glands are the predominant site of CFTR expression in the human bronchus. Nature Genet. **2:** 240–247.
4. STRONG, T.V., K. BOEHM & F.S. COLLINS. 1994. Localization of cystic fibrosis transmembrane conductance regulator mRNA in the human gastrointestinal tract by *in situ* hybridization. J. Clin. Invest. **93:** 347–354.
5. GRAY, M.A., C.E. POLLARD, A. HARRIS, L. COLEMAN, J.R. GREENWELL & B.E. ARGENT. 1990. Anion selectivity and block of the small-conductance chloride channel on pancreatic duct cells. Am. J. Physiol. **259:** C752–761.
6. GASKIN, K.J., P.R. DURIE, M. COREY, P. WEI & G.G. FORSTNER. 1982. Evidence for a primary defect of pancreatic HCO_3^- secretion in cystic fibrosis. Pediatr. Res. **16:** 554–557.
7. KOPELMAN, H., P.R. DURIE, K. GASKIN, Z. WEISMAN & G. FORSTNER. 1985. Pancreatic fluid secretion and protein hyperconcentration in cystic fibrosis. N. Engl. J. Med. **312:** 329–334.
8. HARRIS, A.& L. COLEMAN. 1987. Establishment of a tissue culture system for epithelial cells derived from human pancreas: a model for the study of cystic fibrosis. J. Cell Sci. **87:** 695–703.
9. FOULKES, A.G. & A. HARRIS. 1993. Localization of expression of the cystic fibrosis gene in human pancreatic development. Pancreas **8:** 3–6.
10. HARRIS, A., G. CHALKLEY, S. GOODMAN & L. COLEMAN. 1991. Expression of the cystic fibrosis gene in human development. Development **113:** 305–310.
11. TREZISE, A.E.O., J.A. CHAMBERS, C.J. WARDLE, S. GOULD & A. HARRIS. 1993. Expression of the cystic fibrosis gene in human fetal tissues. Hum. Mol. Genet. **2:** 213–218.
12. HYDE, K., C.J. REID, S.J. TEBBUTT, L. WEIDE, M.A. HOLLINGSWORTH & A. HARRIS. 1997. The cystic fibrosis transmembrane conductance regulator as a marker of human pancreatic duct development and differentiation. Gastroenterology **113:** 914–919.
13. MARINO, C.R., L.M. MATOVCIK, F.S. GORELICK & J.A. COHN. 1991. Localization of the cystic fibrosis transmembrane conductance regulator in pancreas. J. Clin. Invest. **88:** 712–716.
14. RIORDAN, J.R., J.M. ROMMENS, B.-S. KEREM, N. ALON, R. ROZMAHEL, G. GRZELCZAK, S. LOK, N. PLAVSIC, J.-L. CHOU, M.L. DRUMM, M.C. IANNUZZI, F.S. COLLINS & L.-C. TSUI. 1989. Identification of the cystic fibrosis gene: cloning and characterisation of complementary DNA. Science **245:** 1066–1073.
15. REID, C.J., K. HYDE, S.B. HO & A, HARRIS. 1997. Cystic fibrosis of the pancreas: involvement of MUC6 mucin in obstruction of pancreatic ducts. Mol. Med. **3:** 403–411.
16. KARTNER, N., O. AUGUSTINAS, T.J. JENSEN, A.L. NAISMITH & J.R. RIORDAN. 1992. Mislocalization of ΔF508 CFTR in cystic fibrosis sweat gland. Nature Genet. **1:** 321–327.

17. KOPELMAN, H., E. FERRETTI, C. GAUTHIER & P.R. GOODYER. 1995. Rabbit pancreatic acini express CFTR as a cAMP-activated chloride efflux pathway. Am. J. Physiol. **269:** C626–C631.
18. ZENG, W., M.G. LEE, M. YAN, J. DIAZ, I. BENJAMIN, C.R. MARINO, R. KOPITO, S. FREEDMAN, C. COTTON, S. MUALLEM & P. THOMAS. 1997. Immuno and functional characterization of CFTR in submandibular and pancreatic acinar and duct cells. Am. J. Physiol. **273:** C442-C455.
19. BOUE, A., F. MULLER, C. NEZELOF et al. 1986. Prenatal diagnosis in 200 pregnancies with a 1-in-4 risk of cystic fibrosis. Hum. Genet. **74:** 288–297.
20. CHAMBERS, J.A., M.A. HOLLINGSWORTH, A. TREZISE & A. HARRIS. 1994. Developmental expression of mucin genes MUC1 and MUC2. J. Cell Sci. **107:** 413–424.
21. REID, C.J. & A. HARRIS. 1998. Developmental expression of mucin genes in the human digestive system. Gut **42:** 220–226.
22. LAN, M.S., S.K. BATRA, W.-N. QI, R.S. METZGAR & M.A. HOLLINGSWORTH. 1990. Cloning and sequencing of a human pancreatic tumor cDNA. J. Biol. Chem. **265:** 15294–15299.
23. BATRA, S., R.S. METZGAR & M.A. HOLLINGSWORTH. 1992. Human MUC1 mucin gene expression in fetal pancreas. Pancreas **7:** 391–393.
24. HO, S., A.M. ROBERTSON, L.L. SHEKELS, C.T. LYFTOGT, G.A. NIEHANS & N.W. TORIBARA. 1995. Expression cloning of gastric mucin complementary cDNA and localization of mucin gene expression. Gastroenterology **109:** 735–747.
25. TORIBARA, N.W., A.M. ROBERTSON, S. HO et al. 1993. Human gastric mucin. J. Biol. Chem. **268:** 5879–5885.
26. TORIBARA, N.W., S.B. HO, E. GUM, J.R. GUM, P. LAU & Y.S. KIM. 1997. The carboxyl-terminal sequence of the human secretory mucin, MUC6. Analysis of the primary amino acid sequence. J. Biol. Chem. **272:** 16398-16403
27. ANDERSON, M.P., D.P. RICH, R.J. GREGORY, A.E. SMITH & M.J. WELSH. 1991. Generation of cAMP-activated chloride currents by expression of CFTR. Science **251:** 679–682.
28. GRAY, M.A., C.E. POLLARD, A. HARRIS, L. COLEMAN, J.R. GREENWELL & B.E. ARGENT. 1990. Anion selectivity and block of the small-conductance chloride channel on pancreatic duct cells. Am. J. Physiol. **259:** C752–761.
29. BOAT, T. F., P.W. CHENG, R.N. LYER, D.M. CARLSON & I. POLONY. 1976. Human respiratory tract secretions: mucous glycoproteins of nonpurulent tracheobronchial secretions, and sputum of patients with bronchitis and cystic fibrosis. Arch. Biochem. Biophys. **177:** 95–104.
30. FRATES, R.C., T.T. KAIZU & J.A. LAST. 1983. Mucus glycoproteins secreted by respiratory epithelial tissue from cystic fibrosis patients. Paediatr. Res. **17:** 30–34.
31. LO-GUIDICE, J., J. WIERUSZESKI, J. LEMOINE, A. VERBERT, P. ROUSSEL & G. LAMBLIN. 1994. Sialylation and sulfation of the carbohydrate chains in respiratory mucins from a patient with cystic fibrosis. J. Biol. Chem. **269:** 18794–18813.
32. WESLEY, A., J. FORSTNER, R. QURESHI, M. MANTLE & G. FORSTNER. 1983. Human intestinal mucin in cystic fibrosis. Paediatr. Res. **17:** 65–69.
33. CHENG, P.W., T.F. BOAT, K. CRANFILL, J.R. YANKASKAS & R.C. BOUCHER. 1989. Increased sulphation of glycoconjugates by cultured nasal epithelial cells from patients with cystic fibrosis. J. Clin. Invest. **84:** 68–72.
34. ZHANG, Y., B. DORANZ, J.R. YANKASKAS & J.F. ENGELHARDT. 1995. Genotypic analysis of respiratory mucus sulfation defects in cystic fibrosis. J. Clin. Invest. **96:** 2997–3004.
35. CLIFF, W.H., R.A. SCHOUMACHER & R.A. FRIZZELL. 1992. cAMP-activated Cl channels in CFTR-transfected cystic fibrosis pancreatic epithelial cells. Am. J. Physiol. **262:** C1154 -C1160.
36. BURDICK, M.D., A. HARRIS, C.J. REID, T. IWAMURA & M.A. HOLLINGSWORTH. 1997. Oligosaccharides expressed on MUC1 produced by pancreatic and colon tumor cell lines. J. Biol. Chem. **272:**24198–24202.
37. REID, C.J., M.D. BURDICK, M.A. HOLLINGSWORTH & A. HARRIS. 1998. CFTR expression does not influence glycosylation of an epitope-tagged MUC1 mucin in colon carcinoma cell lines. Glycobiology. In press.

Tumor Suppressor Gene Smad4/DPC4, Its Downstream Target Genes, and Regulation of Cell Cycle[a]

PAUL J. CHIAO,[b,c,g] KELLY K. HUNT,[b] ANA M. GRAU,[f] ARAM ABRAMIAN,[b] JASON FLEMING,[b] WEI ZHANG,[c,e] TARA BRESLIN, JAMES L. ABBRUZZESE,[d] AND DOUGLAS B. EVANS[b]

Departments of [b]Surgical Oncology, [c]Cancer Biology, [d]Gastrointestinal Medical Oncology and Digestive Diseases, and [e]Neuro-oncology, The University of Texas, M. D. Anderson Cancer Center, Houston, Texas 77030, USA
[f]Department of Surgery, The University of Arizona, Tucson, Arizona 85724, USA

> ABSTRACT: The tumor suppressor gene deleted in pancreatic cancer locus 4 (Smad4/DPC4) is inactivated in about 50% of pancreatic adenocarcinomas. The role of DPC4 in the transforming growth factor-β (TGF–β) receptor-mediated signal transduction cascade in human pancreatic, colon, and breast carcinoma cell lines has been investigated by a number of laboratories. The results demonstrate that Smad4/DPC4 protein functions as a key transcription factor required in regulation of TGF-β inducible gene expression and subsequent growth inhibition. Many transcription regulators that are involved in cell growth, differentiation, and oncogenesis have been identified and cloned. Yet paradoxically, it is much more difficult to identify the important downstream target genes responsible for the biological effects elicited by these transcription factors. Although numerous attempts have been made and different approaches have been used to identify the target genes, only limited success has been achieved. Our data show that p21waf1 is one of the Smad4/DPC4-regulated downstream target genes and suggest that overexpression of the Smad4/DPC4 gene can bypass TGF-β receptor activation and reestablish one of the key regulatory controls of cell proliferation. Identification of the Smad-regulated downstream target genes responsible for diverse biological processes that they control will extend our understanding of the mechanism for cell cycle regulation and cell differentiation.

INTRODUCTION

Pancreatic adenocarcinoma is the fifth leading cause of adult cancer mortality in the United States.[1] However, the epidemiology of pancreatic cancer provides few clues about its etiology and pathogenesis. Strategies for early detection of pancreatic adenocarcinoma have not yet been developed, and most pancreatic adenocarcinomas present with metastatic or locally advanced disease at the time of diagnosis.[2] Ther-

---

[g]To whom requests for reprints should be addressed: Department of Surgical Oncology and Cancer Biology, Box 107, The University of Texas M. D. Anderson Cancer Center, 1515 Holcombe Blvd. Houston, TX 77030. Phone, 713/794-1030; fax, 713/794-4830; e-mail, pchiao@notes.mdacc.tmc.edu

apeutic options for patients with advanced disease are few, as chemotherapy and irradiation are largely ineffective.[2,3] Metastatic disease often develops after potentially curative surgery.[3] Nonetheless, recent findings have improved our understanding of the biology of pancreatic cancer and have demonstrated that genetic and molecular alterations in adenocarcinomas of the pancreas involve activation of specific oncogenes and inactivation of specific tumor suppressor genes.[2,4]

The tumor suppressor gene Smad4/DPC4 was recently identified and found to be deleted or mutated in about 50% of pancreatic adenocarcinomas. A functional role for Smad4/DPC4 was suggested by the sequence of the peptide it encodes, which is similar to that of the *Drosphila melanogaster* Mad protein and the *Caenorhabditis elegans* Mad homologues sma-2, sma-3, and sma-4.[4] Mad proteins have been linked to the transforming growth factor-β (TGF-β) superfamily of cytokines that regulate cell differentiation and are potent inhibitors of cellular proliferation for most normal cells.[5] Many cancer cells have been shown to lose responsiveness to TGF–β-induced growth inhibition,[5,6] suggesting that a defect in the TGF–β receptor-mediated signal transduction cascade may eliminate a critical negative control for cell proliferation.

Recently, we demonstrated that deletion or mutational inactivation of the Smad4/DPC4 gene correlates with the loss of responsiveness to TGF–β-induced growth inhibition and abrogation of TGF–β-inducible p21waf1 expression in human pancreatic adenocarcinoma cells.[7] Others have shown that Smad4/DPC4 is required for TGF–β and activin signaling in colorectal cancer cells.[8] Several Smad proteins are phosphorylated by the cognate type I serine/threonine kinase receptor in response to ligand binding.[9,10] Once phosphorylated, Smad proteins translocate to the nucleus where they function as transactivators to regulate expression of the downstream target genes.[9,10] The *Drosophila* Mad protein binds to a specific DNA sequence,[11] while other Smad protein complex with DNA binding partners, such as FAST1, to function as transcriptional regulators.[12–14] Furthermore, both Smad3 and Smad4/DPC4 proteins in humans have been shown to recognize an 8-base-pair palindromic sequence (5'-GTCTAGAC-3') called the Smad binding element (SBE) and to act as sequence-specific transcriptional activators.[15] The current model for Smad function suggests that signal-dependent phosphorylation and nuclear translocation are the key regulatory steps in the TGF-β signaling pathway.[9] However, it remains unclear how growth inhibition is induced by transient overexpression of Smad4/DPC4.[14–18]

Smad4/DPC4 protein mediates transactivation of the TGF-β-inducible plasminogen activator inhibitor (PAI) promoter (3TP-lux reporter), which shares similarities with SBE within the PAI-1 promoter region of the 3TP-lux reporter.[9,15] This suggests that Smad4/DPC4 binds to the SBE-like sequence in the PAI-1 promoter to activate transcription. There are also SBEs within the regulatory region of the TGF-β-regulated gene p15 and p21waf1, suggesting that Smad4/DPC4 may regulate TGF-β-inducible p15 and p21waf1 expression.[15] Moreover, it has also been demonstrated that TGF-β-induced cell cycle arrest can partially be attributed to the regulatory effects of TGF-β on both the expression and the activity of cyclin-dependent kinase inhibitors such as p21waf1, and the binding of these inhibitors to specific cyclin-dependent kinase complexes blocks their activity and causes cell cycle arrest.[19,20] So, Smad4/DPC4 is the key transactivator that regulates TGF-β-inducible gene expression. However, before now, direct evidence for the downstream target genes regulated by Smad4/DPC4 have been lacking. Therefore, we initiated the current study to understand the role of Smad4/DPC4 in TGF-β signaling and the mechanism of TGF-β-mediated growth inhibition.

RESULTS AND DISCUSSION

To determine the effects of TGF-β on human pancreatic adenocarcinoma cell lines, standard cell proliferation assays were performed using five well-characterized cell lines (Panc-1, MDAPanc-28, HS766T, Capan-1, and MIaPaCa-2) in the presence and absence of TGF-β.[7] The results show statistically significant growth inhibition by TGF-β on Panc-1 cells after 48 and 72 hr of treatment. The other four cell lines did not demonstrate any TGF–β–induced growth inhibition in the assays, indicating that the TGF–β receptor-mediated signal cascade for growth inhibition is functional in Panc-1 cells but defective in the other four cell lines. This finding is consistent with earlier reports that many malignancies have lost responsiveness to TGF–β–induced growth inhibition, suggesting that inactivation of the components of TGF–β signaling may abolish one of the key negative controls of cell proliferation.

To determine whether the loss of TGF–β–mediated growth inhibition in human pancreatic tumor cell lines correlates with the inactivation of the tumor suppressor gene Smad4/DPC4, we analyzed five human pancreatic cancer cell lines using northern and southern blot analysis. Our results show that Smad4/DPC4 mRNA was expressed in a TGF–β-responsive cell line, Panc-1, but was absent from TGF–β-unresponsive cells lines HS766T and Capan-1. Previously published work shows that Panc-1 and HS766T share a subtype of the TGF–β type I receptor SKRI as well as a similarly low expression level of ALK5, the major type I receptor; the work also shows that HS766T cells express relatively high levels of the TGF–β type II and III receptors, whereas Panc-1 cells express low levels of these receptors.[18] Therefore, we believe that the differential response to TGF–β observed between these two cell lines cannot be explained on the basis of their TGF–β receptor status but is most probably caused by the lack of the Smad4/DPC4 gene in the HS766T cells. A truncated form of Smad4/DPC4 mRNA was detected in TGF–β-unresponsive MDA-Panc-28 cells. The unresponsiveness to TGF–β-induced growth inhibition in MiaPaCa-2 cells can be explained by the lack of TGF–β type II receptors in this cell line.[19] Southern blot analyses confirmed that the loss of expression of Smad4/DPC4 in Hs766T cells is caused by the homozygous deletion of the Smad4/DPC4 gene, whereas no deletion in the gene was detected in the other four cell lines studied.[7,20] These results suggest that the inactivation or loss of expression of Smad4/DPC4 or TGF–β type II receptor in the TGF–β signal transduction pathway abolished one of the critical negative controls for cell proliferation.

It has been demonstrated that TGF–β induces the expression of p21waf1 and induction of p21waf1 and subsequent G1 cell cycle arrest could account for at least one of the mechanisms of growth inhibition mediated by TGF–β.[21] Our results showed that p21waf1 expression was induced by TGF–β in Panc-1 cell and the induction is dose- and time-dependent. Our data also show that the increase in mRNA stability is not the mechanism of the TGF–β-mediated induction of p21waf1, suggesting that TGF–β regulates p21waf1 transcription. TGF–β failed to induce p21waf1 expression in the other four pancreatic cancer cell lines studied. Thus, our data show that the loss of TGF–β–inducible p21waf1 expression in all these pancreatic tumor cell lines can be explained by the absence of functional Smad4/DPC4 protein. However, Hs766T and Capan-1 cells express a high basal levels of p21 waf1 mRNA, and our finding is further supported by the report that some pancreatic adenocarcinomas express high levels of p21 protein as compared with the adjacent normal pancreatic tissues.[22] What leads to the high basal expression levels of the p21waf1 gene in HS766T and Capan-1 cells, which appear to be independent of p53 and DPC4 proteins, remains unknown.

To determine whether Smad4/DPC4 can restore the TGF–β signal transduction cascade in Hs766T, pancreatic tumor cells with homozygous deletion of this gene, we analyzed the activation of 3TP-lux, a TGF–β-inducible reporter gene containing a PAI promoter, by TGF–β in the presence and absence of the Smad4/DPC4 expression plasmid, TGF–β activated 3TP-lux in Panc-1, suggesting that this cell line has a functional TGF–β receptor signal transduction pathway, but failed to activate 3TP-lux in Hs766T cells. Cotransfection of 3TP-lux with an Smad4/DPC4 expression vector is effective in restoring the response to TGF–β in Hs766T cells, suggesting that the DPC4 tumor suppressor gene is a key element in the TGF–β signal transduction cascade.

To investigate whether reintroduction of a functional Smad4/DPC4 gene could inhibit tumor cell growth and to achieve more efficient gene transfer into various cell lines of interest, we constructed a replication-defective adenovirus expressing Smad4/DPC4 cDNA. Using adenovirus-mediated gene transfer, we demonstrated that (i) overexpression of Smad4/DPC4 induces p21waf1 expression in the presence and absence of TGF–β in Smad4/DPC4 null cells; (ii) Smad4/DPC4 proteins specifically bind to an Smad binding element in the p21waf1 promoter; (iii) Smad4/DPC4 activates the reporter gene 3TP-lux and SBE4-luc, which contains four SBEs in its promoter, in the presence or absence of TGF–β; (iv) overexpression of Smad4/DPC4 activates expression of the p21waf1 gene and induces the activity of the 3TP-lux reporter gene in the human pancreatic adenocarcinoma cell line, MiaPaCa-2, which does not express type II TGF–β receptor; (v) overexpression of Smad4/DPC4 induces similar levels of p21waf1 expression in TGF–β-responsive human pancreatic adenocarcinoma cells with or without TGF–β-stimulation; and (vi) overexpression of Smad4/DPC4 inhibits cell growth in MDA-MB-468 breast cancer cells, in which Smad4/DPC4 is homozygously deleted. Taken together, our data show that p21waf1 is one of the downstream target genes regulated by Smad4/DPC4. Furthermore, they suggest that Smad4/DPC4-inducible p21waf1 expression could be in part responsible for the effect of overexpression of Smad4/DPC4 gene on cell growth inhibition. When Smad4/DPC4 nuclear localization is forced by transient overexpression, we believe that Smad4/DPC4 may bypass TGF–β receptor activation and signal-dependent nuclear translocation, the key regulatory steps in TGF–β signaling pathways.

We previously reported that a series of p21waf1 promoter studies failed to demonstrate TGF–β-induced p21waf1 promoter reporter gene activity in transient transfections using Panc-1, a pancreatic tumor cell line in which endogenous p21waf1 expression is induced by TGF–β.[7] Yet, a wild-type p53 tumor suppressor gene activate this same p21waf1 reporter gene.[23] Overexpression of Smad4/DPC4 by adenovirus did not induce p21waf1 promoter reporter gene activity, and this finding was confirmed by the results reported by Moustakas and Kardassis.[24] Interestingly, overexpression of both Smad3 and Smad4 activated the 2.4-kb p21 promoter.[24] Taken together, our data suggest that the binding of Smad4/DPC4 to this p21 SBE alone in the p21waf1 promoter was not sufficient for transcriptional activation and the additional SBE sites to mediate Smad4/DPC4 transactivation were absent in the 2.4-kb p21 promoter. These conclusions are supported by the recent report that a reporter gene construct containing two copies of the SBE was relatively unresponsive to TGF–β, whereas one containing four copies of the SBE was highly responsive.[15]

Smad4 is recognized as a central mediator of TGF–β signaling. The current model suggests that when overexpressed by transfection, Smad1 and Smad2 proteins are mostly cytoplasmic.[25] Once Smad1 and Smad2 proteins are phosphorylated by the type I serine/threonine kinase receptor upon ligand binding, these phosphorylated Smad proteins complex with Smad4 and translocate to the nucleus where they function as transactivators.[9,10,25] Our data show that transient overexpression of Smad4-induced p21waf1 expression and SBE4-luc promoter reporter activity in a Smad4/DPC4 null cell line, MDA-MB-468 cells; in MiaCaPa-2 cells, which have lost expression of the type II TGF–β receptor; and in TGF–β responsive Panc-1 cells with or without TGF–β stimulation. Furthermore, TGF–β stimulation did not enhance p21waf1 expression and reporter gene activation. This would indicate that transiently overexpressed Smad4/DPC4 can bypass TGF–β receptor activation and translocate into the nucleus to provide an essential transcriptional activation function for TGF–β signaling. One possibility is that Smad4 with Smad1 or Smad2 forms constitutive heterodimeric complexes that might be regulated by the high basal level of Smad1 or Smad2 phosphorylation in these tumor cells used in our study. This is supported by the recent report by Wisotzkey *et al.* that Medea (*Drosophila* Smad4) and MAD are physically associated and that this interaction is induced by the high basal phosphorylation of MAD in COS cells but is not augmented by cotransfection with activated DPP receptors.[26]

In summary, our findings demonstrate that p21waf1 is one of the downstream target genes regulated by Smad4/DPC4 and support the role of Smad4/DPC4 as a tumor suppressor gene in human adenocarcinoma cells. Furthermore, they suggest that overexpression of a wild-type Smad4/DPC4 gene may override TGF–β receptor activation to reestablish one of the key negative controls of cellular proliferation and provide a basis for cancer gene therapy strategies that can restore the signal transduction pathways of TGF–β-mediated growth suppression.

ACKNOWLEDGMENTS

We are grateful to Dr. Bert Vogelstein for the SBE and p21waf1 promoter-luciferase reporter gene and to Dr. Scott Kern for the DPC4 cDNA plasmid. We thank members of the Chiao laboratory for helpful discussions and Jude Richard and Pat Thomas for editorial assistance. This work was supported in part by a grant from the University Cancer Foundation at M. D. Anderson Cancer Center and the Advanced Technology/Research Program of the Texas Higher Education Coordinating Board.

REFERENCES

1. PARKER, S.L., T. TONG, S. BOLDEN & P.A. WINGO. 1997. Cancer Statistics, 1997. CA-Cancer J. Clin. **47:** 5-27.
2. DIGIUSEPPE, J.A., C.J. YEO & R.H. HRUBAN. 1996. Molecular biology and the diagnosis and treatment of adenocarcinoma of the pancreas. Adv. Anat. Pathol. **3:** 139-155.
3. STALEY, C.A., J.E. LEE, K.A. CLEARY, J.L. ABBRUZZESE, F.C. AMES, C. FENOGLIO & D.B. EVANS. 1996. Preoperative chemoradiation, pancreaticoduodenectomy, and intraoperative radiation therapy for adenocarcinoma of the pancreatic head: Patient survival and patterns of treatment failure. Am. J. Surg. **171:** 118-124.
4. HAHN, S.A., M. SCHUTTE, A.T.M. SHAMSUL HOQUE, C.A. MOSKALUK, L.T. DACOSTA, E. ROZENBLUM, C.L. WEINSTEIN, A. FISCHER, C.J. YEO, R.H. HRUBAN & S.E. KERN. 1996. DPC4, a candidate tumor suppressor gene at human chromosome 18q21.1. Science **271:** 350-353.
5. MASSAGUE, J. 1996. TGF-b signaling: Receptors, transducers, and mad proteins. Cell **85:** 947-950.
6. FYNAN, T.M. & M. REISS. 1993. Resistance to inhibition of cell growth by transforming growth factor-b and its role in oncogenesis. Crit. Rev. Oncog. **4:** 493-540.
7. GRAU, A.M., L. ZHANG, W. WANG, S. RUAN, D.B. EVANS, A.L. ABBRUZZESE, W. ZHANG & P.J. CHIAO. 1997. Induction of p21waf1 expression and growth inhibition by transforming growth factor-b involve the tumor suppressor gene DPC4 in human pancreatic adenocarcinoma cells. Cancer Res. **57:** 3929-3934.
8. ZHOU, S., P. BUCKHAULTS, L. ZAWEL, Z. F. BUN, G. RIGGINS, J. LE DAI, S.E. KERN, K.W. KINZLER & B. VOGELSTEIN. 1998. Targeted deletion of Smad4 shows it is required for transforming growth factor beta and activin signaling in colorectal cancer cells. Proc. Natl. Acad. Sci. **95:** 2412-2416.
9. KRETZSCHMAR, M. & J. MASSAGUE. 1998. SMADs: Mediators and regulators of TGF-b signaling. Curr. Opin. Genet. Dev. **8:** 103-111.
10. ZHANG, Y., T. MUSCI & R. DERYNCK. 1997. The tumor suppressor Smad4/DPC4 as a central mediator of Smad function. Curr. Biol. **7:** 270-276.
11. KIM, J., K. JOHNSON, H. J. CHEN, S. CARROLL & A. LAUGHON. 1997. *Drosophila* Mad binds to DNA and directly mediates activation of vestigial by Decapentaplegic. Nature **388:** 304-308.
12. CHEN, X., M.J. ROBOCK & M. WHITMAN. 1996. A transcriptional partner for MAD proteins in TGF-b signaling. Nature **383:** 691-696.
13. CHEN, X., E. WEISBERG, V. FRIDMACHER, M. WATANABE, G. Naco & M. Whitman. 1997. Smad4 and FAST-1 in the assembly of activin-responsive factor. Nature **389:** 85-69.
14. CHEN, Y.G., A. HATA, R.S. LO, D. WOTTON, Y. SHI, N. PAVLETICH & J. MASSAGUE. 1998. Determinants of specificity in TGF-beta signal transduction. Genes Dev. **12:** 2144-2152.
15. ZAWEL, L., J.L. DAI, P. BUCKHAULTS, S. ZHOU, K.W. KINZLER, B. BOGELSTEIN & S.E. KERN. 1998. Human Smad3 and Smad4 are sequence-specific transcription activators. Mol. Cell **1:** 611-617.
16. ZHANG, Y., X. FENG, R. WE & R. DERYNCK. 1996. Receptor-associated Mad homologues synergize as effectors of the TGF-beta response. Nature **383:** 168-172.
17. YINGLING, J.M., P. DAS, C. SAVAGE, M. ZHANG, R.W. PADGETT & X.F. WANG. 1996. Mammalian dwarfins are phosphorylated in response to transforming growth factor beta and are implicated in control of cell growth. Proc. Natl. Acad. Sci. USA **93:** 8940-8944.
18. LAGNA, G., A. HATA, A. HEMMATI-BRIVANLOU & J. MASSAGUE. 1996. Partnership between DPC4 and SMAD proteins in TGF-b signalling pathways Nature **383:** 832-836.
19. FREEMAN, J.W., C.A. MATTINGLY & W.E. STRODEL. 1995. Increased tumorigenicity in the human pancreatic cell line MIA PaCa-2 is associated with an aberrant regulation of an IGF-1 autocrine loop and lack of expression of the TGF-b type RII receptor. J. Cell Physiol. **165:** 155-163.

20. HAHN, S.A., A.T. HOQUE, C.A. MOSKALUK, L.T. DA COSTA, M. SCHUTTE, E. ROZENBLUM, A.B. SEYMOUR, C.L. WEINSTEIN, C.J. YEO, R.H. HRUBAN & S.E. KERN. 1996. Homozygous deletion map at 18q21.1 in pancreatic cancer. Cancer Res. **56:** 490-494.
21. XIONG, Y., G.J. HAMNON, H. ZHANG, D. CASSO, R. KOBAYAASHI & D. BEACH. 1993. p21 is a universal inhibitor of cyclin kinases. Nature **366:** 701-704.
22. DIGIUSEPPE, J.A., M.S. REDSTON, C.J. YEO, S.E. KERN & R.H. HRUBAN. 1995. p53-independent expression of the cyclin-dependent kinase inhibitor p21 in pancreatic carcinoma. Am. J. Pathol. **147:** 884-888.
23. EL-DEIRY, W.S., T. TOKINO, V.E. VELCULESCU, D.B. LEVY, R. PARSONS, J. M. TRENT, D. LIN, W.E. MERCER, K.W. KINZLER & B. VOGELSTEIN. 1993. WAF1, a potential mediator of p53 tumor suppression. Cell **75:** 817-825.
24. MOUSTAKAS, A. & D. KARDASSIS. 1998. Regulation of the human p21/WAF1/Cip1 promoter in hepatic cells by functional interactions between Sp1 and Smad family members. Proc. Natl. Acad. Sci. USA **95:** 6733-6738.
25. LIU, F., C. POUPONNOT & J. MASSAGUE. 1997. Dual role of the Smad4/DPC4 tumor suppressor in TGFb-inducible transcriptional complexes. Genes & Dev. **11:** 5157-3167.
26. WISTZKEY, R.G., A. MEHRA, D.J. SUTHERLAND, L.L. DOBENS, X. LIU, C. DOHRMANN, L. ATTISANO & L.A. RAFTERY. 1998. Medea is a *Drosophila* Smad4 homolog that is differentially required to potentiate DPP responses. Development 125:1433-1445.

Proteins Expressed by Pancreatic Duct Cells and Their Relatives

MICHAEL A. HOLLINGSWORTH[a]

Eppley Institute for Research in Cancer and Allied Diseases, University of Nebraska Medical Center, 600 South 42nd Street, Omaha, Nebraska 68198-6805, USA

> ABSTRACT: Significant progress has been made in the characterization of the structure and function of pancreatic ductal cells. Our understanding at this point in time extends to knowledge of specific molecules that provide for the structural composition of the ductal cells, their interactions with the local environment, and the regulation of their growth and properties of differentiation. Knowledge of the molecular composition and structure of the secretory products of epithelial cells in the pancreas also has increased so that we now understand the individual contributions of several secretory products to the overall function of pancreatic juice. Further study of these parameters will give us important insight into the normal function of the ductal cells and into how these processes are altered during the development and progression of diseases of the pancreas such as pancreatitis and cancer.

STRUCTURE AND FUNCTION OF PANCREATIC DUCTS

The pancreatic ductal system connects secretory cells of the exocrine pancreas (acinar cells) to the duodenum. Ducts arise at the acinar unit of the pancreas and function by adding secretions that finalize the composition of pancreatic juice and facilitate the transport of secretions of the acinar cells to the duodenum.

A schematic of the general structure and function of the ductal system is presented in FIGURE 1. The acinar unit of the pancreas is comprised of a group of acinar cells arranged in a three-dimensional cul-de-sac around the lumen of the acinus. Acinar cells are polarized with a basolateral surface that is larger than the apical surface. The cells contain extensive Golgi apparatuses and numerous secretory granules containing zymogen components that lie near the apical surface. Acinar cells produce a number of products related to the digestive process (FIG. 1), including α-amylase, lipase, trypsinogen, chymotrypsinogen, α1-antitrypsin, pancreatic ribonuclease, elastase, and procarboxypeptidases A and B (pancreas-specific protein).[1–12] Secretion from the acinar cells is primarily by exocytic discharge of zymogen granules from the apical surface, which release highly concentrated aggregates of proteins into the luminal space.

Near the junction of the acinus is the centroacinar cell, whose nature and lineage remain controversial. Some pathologists claim that it represents a distinct cell type and others argue that it is either a ductal cell or an acinar cell.

---

[a]Address for correspondence: Michael A. Hollingsworth, Eppley Cancer Institute, University of Nebraska Medical Center, 600 South 42nd Street, Omaha, NE 68198-6805. Phone, 402/559-8343; fax, 402/559-4651; e-mail, mahollin@unmc.edu

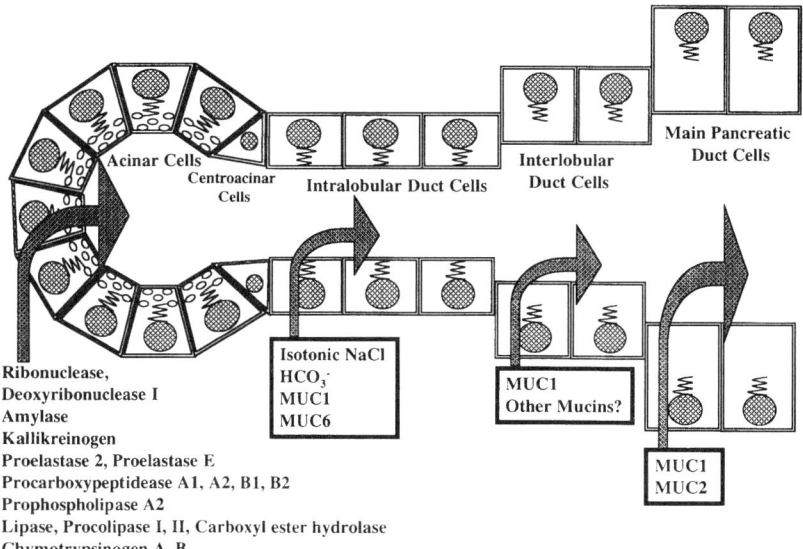

FIGURE 1. Schematic of the general structure of the ductal system showing important secretory products and the relative location of production.

Intercalated ducts form the initial part of the intralobular ductal system and are comprised of short cuboidal polarized epithelial cells. These cells function to secrete large amounts of bicarbonate-rich isotonic fluid that dissolves and dilutes the proteinaceous aggregates produced by the acinar cells.[13] The cells also express the MUC1 and MUC6 mucins. It is notable that many small duct cells contain a single kinocilia that may be involved in mixing the fluid and protein in this region of the ductal system.[13] The morphology of the ductal cells changes in moving away from the acinar unit towards the duodenum. The duct cells generally become taller when approaching the stage of the interlobular ducts. These cells continue to add glycoproteins to the pancreatic juice including MUC1 and perhaps other mucins; however, it is uncommon to see classic goblet cells at this level of cellular organization. The cells of the main pancreatic duct are taller than the intralobular ductal cells and retain the appearance of a simple columnar epithelial layer. Near the duodenum occasional goblet cells can be seen, and the secretion of additional mucins including MUC2 can be detected.

PROTEINS EXPRESSED ON THE BASOLATERAL ASPECT OF PANCREATIC EPITHELIAL CELLS

Several important proteins that are expressed on the basolateral aspect of pancreatic ductal epithelial cells are listed in the schematic shown in FIGURE 2. Included are integrins, intermediate filaments, extracellular matrix components, growth factors and their receptors, transport proteins, and other markers of differentiation.

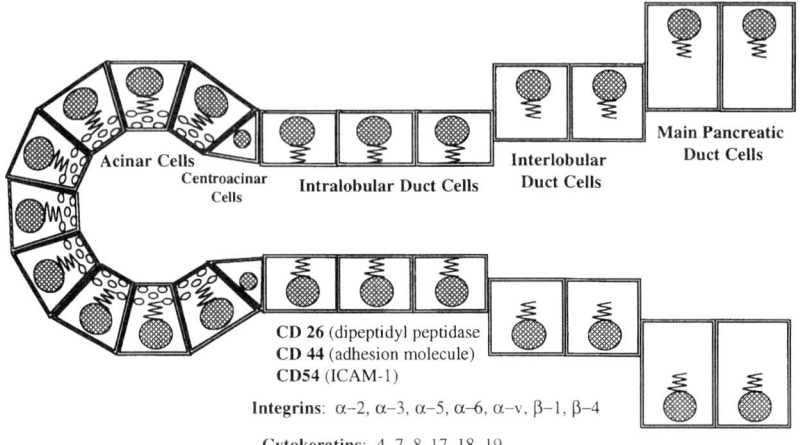

FIGURE 2. Schematic listing several important proteins that are expressed on the basolateral aspect of pancreatic ductal epithelial cells.

Integrins are a large family of cell surface proteins that share some sequence similarity and a heterodimeric structure (single α and β chains are complexed to form the functional integrin)[14] and are involved in cell surface adhesion events. Recent data have shown that integrins can mediate signal transduction events through their transmembrane and cytoplasmic tail domains.[15] One function of cell surface adhesion and signal transduction is to establish and maintain the differentiation status of epithelial cells. Thus, integrins may function to provide structural integrity to epithelial cells and to communicate loss of structural integrity and morphological status to the nucleus. Loss of regulation of these properties may contribute to the metastatic capacity of some pancreatic tumors.

Expression patterns of the VLA receptor family of integrins (α1-6 complexed with β1 subunits) have been well characterized in the pancreas.[16–18] Normal acinar cells and ductal cells express high levels of α2 and α5 at the basal surfaces. Normal centroacinar cells express α3 and α5 at the basal surface. During the pathogenesis of pancreatitis, types of VLA receptors expressed on pancreatic epithelia are not altered as compared to the normal pancreas; however, their levels of expression are often increased and the surface localization properties can become more diffuse. In pancreatic adenocarcinoma, different combinations of α2, α3, α5, and α6 have been reported, and their cell surface distribution is generally diffuse, consistent with their hypothesized adherence functions in invasion and metastasis. In addition, expression of other integrins has been reported in normal pancreatic ductal cells and in adenocarcinomas, including αv, β4, β5, and β6.[14–19]

Human pancreatic adenocarcinomas[20] produce laminin, fibronectin, vitronectin, and types I and III collagen. These proteins are constituents of extracellular matrices that comprise the connective tissues that help maintain general cell and organ structure. Their expression by pancreatic tumor cells is significant in that it may partly contribute to the desmoplastic response seen in many primary pancreatic tumors. Moreover, these molecules play an important role in attachment and migration of cells and thereby contribute to their metastatic behavior. Although these molecules are found in the normal pancreas, the extent of their production by normal pancreatic ductal cells or the surrounding stromal cells has not been well described.

Expression patterns of several intermediate filament proteins have been reported for normal pancreas and pancreatic tumors.[21-25] Virtually all normal adult and fetal pancreatic ductal cells express cytokeratins 7, 8, 18, and 19. Occasional cells in normal adult pancreas express cytokeratins 4, 5, 14, and 17. Cytokeratin 4 is also seen in the fetal pancreatic ductal cells. Virtually all pancreatic tumors express cytokeratins 7, 8, 18, and 19. Many pancreatic tumors have been found to express cytokeratins 14, 15, 16, or 17, and a few have been shown to express cytokeratins 4, 5, 13, or 14. Identification of cytokeratin expression patterns has been useful in the diagnosis of pancreatic tumor metastases in lymph nodes and liver.[25]

Normal pancreatic ductal cells express a variety of growth factors and their receptors. Growth factors produced by normal pancreatic ductal cells include TGFα, TGFβ-1, TGFβ-2, TGFβ-3, amphiregulin, Cripto, and EGF.[26-33] Many cells in the normal pancreas express low levels of TGFβ-1, TGFβ-2, and TGFβ-3; however, these may play unique roles in the regulation of differentiation of these cell types.[26] Normal acinar cells express high levels of TGFβ-1, whereas most ductal cells and islet cells express low levels of all three of these growth factors, as detected in the cytoplasm by immunocytochemistry. A proportion of the insulin-producing islet cells express high levels of TGFβ-2 and TGFβ-3.[26] Normal ductal cells also express the EGF receptor,[20] and fetal endocrine and ductal cells express the growth hormone receptor.[28] Expression of TGFα, Cripto, and EGF is increased (sometimes more than 10-fold) in pancreatic adenocarcinomas and, to a lesser extent, in chronic pancreatitis (up to fourfold).[26-33] Many cases of pancreatic adenocarcinoma and chronic pancreatitis show increased levels of surface EGF receptor and related receptors such as HER-2/neu.[34-43] In addition, there is a report of 10-fold overexpression of hepatocyte growth factor and one of its receptors, the c-*met* protooncogene, in pancreatic tumors compared to normal ductal cells.[44]

Normal pancreatic ductal cells and pancreatic adenocarcinomas express fibroblast growth factors (FGF) and their receptors (FGFR). Normal pancreatic ductal cells express FGF-1, FGF-2, and FGFR-1, and some adenocarcinomas and derived tumor cell lines overexpress these.[45,46] In addition, FGF-3, FGF-4, FGFR-3, and FGFR-4 have been detected in some pancreatic tumor cell lines.[45]

Steroid hormone receptor expression has been detected in the pancreas. The mineralocorticoid receptor is present in the intercalated and interlobular ducts but not in acini or islets.[46] A gradient of expression of glucocorticoid receptor mRNA has been detected in the rat pancreas by using *in situ* hybridization, in which endocrine cells > acinar cells > ductal cells.[47]

Several cell surface markers of differentiation of hematopoietic cells have been found to be expressed by pancreatic ductal epithelia. CD26 is a cell surface associated serine protease, dipeptidyl peptidase, and is expressed on ductal epithelial cells and islet cells.[49] CD44 is a cell surface adhesion molecule for leukocytes that is also expressed on normal acinar cells and ductal epithelial cells but not on islets in the pancreas. Different splice variants of CD44 are expressed by pancreatic adenocarcinomas and gastrinomas but not by other endocrine pancreatic tumors.[50] CD66, which belongs to the NCA subgroup of the CEA family, was shown to be identical to the biliary glycoprotein BGP-1 and is highly expressed on pancreatic ductal cells. CD66 is also found on acini and islets.[51] The antigen Leu-M1, originally described as a marker of myelomonocytic cells but later found to be widely expressed on epithelial tissues, is found on pancreatic acini and ductal cells.[52]

There is experimental evidence for a number of transport elements on the basolateral membrane of pancreatic ductal cells.[53] These include the Na^+/K^+ ATPase, K^+ channels, Na^+/H^+ exchanger, proton pump, and the $Na(HCO_3^-)$ cotransporter. These transporters regulate pH and ion concentrations in the local cellular environment and move CO_2 across the basolateral membrane to the cytoplasm where it can be converted into bicarbonate for secretion into the pancreatic duct.

TRANSPORT ELEMENTS AND MUCIN-LIKE PROTEINS EXPRESSED ON THE APICAL ASPECT OF PANCREATIC EPITHELIAL CELLS

Several important proteins that are expressed on the apical aspect of pancreatic ductal epithelial cells are listed in the schematic shown in FIGURE 3. Included are transport elements and mucin-like glycoproteins and oligosaccharide structures associated with them.

Transport elements expressed on the apical surface of pancreatic ductal cells include several chloride channels (CFTR, the Ca^{2+}-activated Cl^- channel, and a CLC channel) and the Cl^-/HCO_3^- exchanger.[53] These channels are believed to function in concert to secrete isotonic bicarbonate-rich fluid into the pancreatic duct to aid in the emulsification of acinar cell products.

Different epithelial cell types in different organs produce different types of mucin core proteins, and many of these cells can produce more than one type of mucin core protein.[54] The extent to which different differentiated cell types of different organs express the different mucins and associated oligosaccharide structures[54–57] has not been clearly established; however, it is under active investigation.

One mucin produced by the pancreas is MUC1, which is produced and secreted constitutively by most epithelial cell types of the adult pancreas other than goblet cells. The expression of MUC1 in human fetal pancreas of 14–26 weeks' gestation was examined by northern blotting, and it was found that significant levels of MUC1 mRNA were not detectable until 19 weeks' gestation[58] and higher levels of expression were found at later gestational ages. The developmental expression of the mRAs for MUC1 and MUC2 has been characterized in a number of tissues using *in situ* hybridization.[59] Significant expression of MUC1 in the human pancreas was not detected until sometime between 19 weeks and term when MUC1 mRNA was seen in the epithelia of large intralobular pancreatic ducts. MUC2 mRNA was not detected within the fetal pancreas at any gestational age evaluated in this study. Cultured cells from mid-trimester fetal pancreatic ducts do express MUC1.[60]

The expression of several other mucin mRNAs or core proteins in adult human pancreas has been examined by *in situ* hybridization and immunohistochemical techniques.[61] Normal pancreatic epithelial cells express predominantly MUC1 and

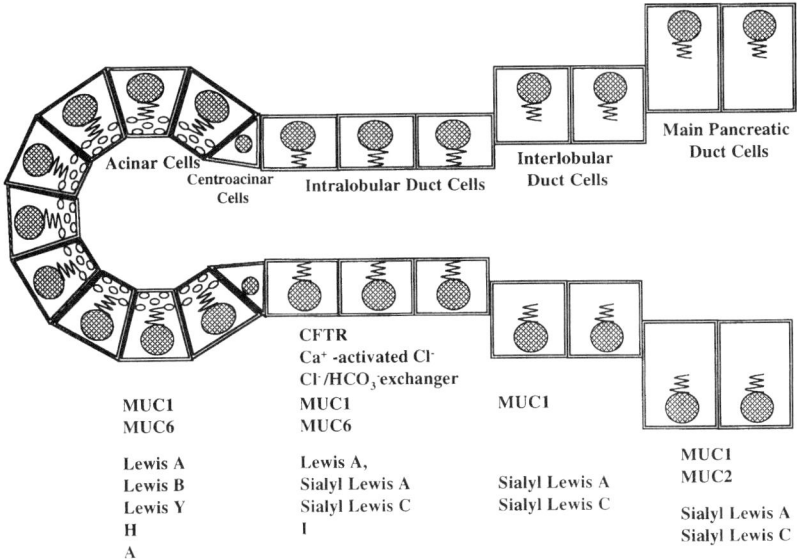

FIGURE 3. Schematic listing several important proteins that are expressed on the apical aspect of pancreatic ductal epithelial cells.

MUC6.[61,62] MUC3, MUC4, MUC5ac, and MUC5b are not expressed at detectable levels in the normal adult pancreas.[61,62]

Blood group antigens that are associated with mucin core proteins such as MUC1[63] show differential expression among fetal pancreas, normal ductal epithelial cells, and tumors. Several type I oligosaccharides are widely expressed on pancreatic epithelial cells. This group of antigens includes several well characterized tumor markers for pancreatic adenocarcinoma (CA19-9, CA50, DUPAN2, and others). Antigens on the precursor structure for Type I chains, Lec (MAb K21), and Leb epitopes are only reported to be expressed in fetal acinar cells.[64,65] Sialylated Lec (also called LSTa, identified by MAb DUPAN2), Lea (MAb CA3-F4), sialyl Lea (MAb CA19-9), and disialyl Lea (MAb FH7) are broadly expressed on fetal and adult ductal epithelial cells but are not found on acinar or islet cells.[64–66]

Most Type II chains, including NLac, H, A, Lex, sialyl Lex, disialyl Lex, and Ley, are not widely expressed on fetal or adult pancreatic ductal epithelia. These antigens are found in some normal fetal acini, on some pancreatic adenocarcinomas, and in the ductal epithelia during pancreatitis episodes.[67] One Type II chain broadly distributed on normal pancreatic ductal epithelia and tumors is the I structure.[64,65]

MOLECULAR FEATURES OF MUC1

MUC1 exists on the surface of most cells as a heterodimer that results from a proteolytic cleavage of the full-length protein and results in two associated fragments: a large extracellular domain that can be released from the cell surface and includes the tandem repeat domain, and a shorter domain that exists as an integral membrane protein and includes a short extracellular domain, a transmembrane domain, and a cytoplasmic tail.[63,68] The relative contributions of these domains to the full biological function of MUC1 are not known at this time; however, these are active areas of investigation. Some forms of MUC1 may be membrane bound and other forms are secreted or released from cells by the proteolytic cleavage event.[55,63,68]

There is great diversity in the post-translational processing of MUC1 by different epithelial cells. In the pancreas, evidence indicates that acinar and ductal cells attach different oligosaccharide structures to MUC1; many of the carbohydrate epitopes (DUPAN2 and CA19-9) found on MUC1 produced by ductal cells are not found on acinar cells. This finding is consistent with the fact that MUC1 produced by other epithelia (e.g., mammary gland, kidney, lung) are often distinct.[55–57]

MUC1 AS AN ANTI-ADHESION OR ADHESION MOLECULE

Several lines of evidence, including properties of subcellular localization and molecular characteristics, suggest that MUC1 may function as an anti-adhesion molecule. One line of supporting evidence comes from the normal cellular expression pattern: MUC1 is found on the apical surface of secretory ductal epithelial cells of many organs, including the pancreas. This localization places MUC1 on surfaces of secretory epithelia that are not in contact with other cells and in a location that is in stark contrast to that of adhesion molecules found on the basal and lateral aspects of these cells, which exist in tight contact with other cells or stromal elements. It may be that MUC1 plays a role in establishing and maintaining the zone of cell surface that is exposed to the lumen and not in contact with adjoining cells. Such a role is supported by findings demonstrating that the cell density and distance between cells expressing high levels of MUC1 are significantly greater than those of control cells not expressing MUC1.[69,70] Studies suggesting that MUC1 exists as a rigid elongated glycoprotein structure that extends over 100 nm above the cell surface (in some allelic forms with long tandem repeats) further support this hypothesis.

There is also evidence that post-translational processing of MUC1 by transformed epithelial cells (tumors) is distinct from that produced by normal epithelia. With the appearance of aberrant oligosaccharide structures (as compared to normal epithelia), it is possible that MUC1 acquires new properties of adhesion that may contribute to the ability of tumor cells to metastasize.[71] Thus, in the case of tumor cells, dysregulated expression of MUC1 (a loss of localized apical expression and acquisition of full cell surface expression) may lead to anti-adhesive effects that allow tumor cells to release from a primary location. The expression of novel oligosaccharide structures (such as sialyl Lex) may confer new adhesive properties on the tumor cell surface (for different sites). As such, MUC1 may play a role in both adhesion and anti-adhesion of normal epithelial cells and tumor cells that arise at these sites.

OTHER POTENTIAL FUNCTIONS FOR MUC1

It has been proposed that MUC1 may also function to protect epithelial cell surfaces from potentially harsh conditions of the ducts in which it is expressed.[72] In the case of the pancreas, it is predicted that MUC1 would lubricate the epithelial cell surfaces to facilitate passage of secreted components from acinar cells and protect epithelial cells from potentially toxic effects of secreted enzymes and cellular products. For example, the fully glycosylated tandem repeat of MUC1 is highly resistant to protease digestion, a seemingly necessary prerequisite for functioning in an environment in which several proteases may be active.

Another possibility is that structures (oligosaccharides, sulfate, or other undescribed modifications) on MUC1 interact specifically with proteins or compounds in the ducts. Thus, MUC1 may form specific molecular interactions with other secreted compounds in the ductal lumen. Forms of MUC1 released from the cell surface may aid in solubilizing proteins in the pancreatic juice or may associate with the acinar proteins and serve as extracellular chaperones during their passage through the ductal cell network.

Alternatively, forms of MUC1 associated with the cell surface may serve as molecular discriminators that attract some compounds towards the cell surface, repel other compounds from the cell surface, and, based on molecular properties, regulate the rate of passage of some molecules between the lumen and the cell surface. According to this hypothesized function, MUC1 glycoforms that extend above the cell surface would mediate a form of molecular column chromatograpy with respect to the cell surface. MUC1 exists on the cell surface as an extended molecule protruding up to 100 nm above the membrane with numerous attached oligosaccharide chains that may have charged residues attached (sialic acid or sulfate). Fully glycosylated and modified forms of MUC1 may have masses of greater than 1×10^6 daltons that would have significant capacity for a number of molecular interactions based on charge, hydrophilicity, Van der Waals forces, molecular size exclusion and inclusion, hydrogen bonding, or other forces.

REFERENCES

1. Arias, A.E. & M. Bendayan. 1993. Differentiation of pancreatic acinar cell into duct-like cells in vitro. Lab. Invest. **69:** 518.
2. Fernandez, E., J.M. Fallon, M.L. Frazier, R. de Llorens & C.M. Cuchillo. 1994. Expression of acinar and ductal products in Capan-1 cells growing in synthetic serum and serum-free media. Cancer **73:** 2285–2295.
3. Franz, M.G., B.C. Winkler, J.G. Norman, P.J. Fabri & W.R. Gower, Jr. 1994. Tumor necrosis factor-α induces the expression of carbonic anhydrase II in pancreatic adenocarcinoma cells. Biochem. Biophys. Res. Commun. **205:** 1815–1821.
4. Iovanna, J.L., P. Lechene de la Porte & J.-C. Dagorn. 1992. Expression of genes associated with dedifferentiation and cell proliferation during pancreatic regeneration following acute pancreatitis. Pancreas **7:** 712–718.
5. Kornek, G., T. Schenk, M. Raderer, M. Djavarnmad & W. Scheithauer. 1995. Tissue polypeptide-specific antigen (TPS) in monitoring palliative treatment response of patients with gastrointestinal tumours. Br. J. Cancer **71:** 182–185.
6. Li, L., J. Wang & M.D. Cooper. 1993. cDNA cloning and expression of human glutamyl aminopeptidase (aminopeptidase A). Genomics **17:** 657–664.
7. Li, L., Q. Wu, J. Wang, R.P. Bucy & M.D. Cooper. 1993. Widespread tissue distribution of aminopeptidase A, an evolutionarily conserved ectoenzyme recognized by the BP-1 antibody. Tissue Antigens **42:** 488–496.
8. Ohta, T., T. Terada, T. Nagakawa, H. Itoh, H. Tajima & I. Miyazaki. 1994. Presence of pancreatic α-amylase, trypsinogen, and lipase immunoreactivity in normal human pancreatic ducts. Pancreas **9:** 382–386.

9. ORELLE, B., V. KEIM, L. MASCIOTRA, J.-C. DAGORN & J.-L. IOVANNA. 1992. Human pancreatitis-associated protein. Messenger RNA cloning and expression in pancreatic diseases. J. Clin. Invest. **90:** 2284–2291.
10. PEZZILLI, R., P. BILLI, L. PLATE, F. BONGIOVANNI, A. M. MORSELLI LABATE & M. MIGLIOLI. 1994. Human pancreas-specific protein/procarboxypeptidase B: A useful serum marker of acute pancreatitis. Digestion **55:** 73–77.
11. VILA, M.R., J. LLORETA & F.X. REAL. 1994. Normal human pancreas cultures display functional ductal characteristics. Lab. Invest. **71:** 423–431.
12. YAMAMOTO, K.K., A. POUSETTE, P. CHOW, H. WILSON, S. EL SHAMI & C.K. FRENCH. 1992. Isolation of a cDNA encoding a human serum marker for acute pancreatitis. J. Biol. Chem. **267:** 2575–2581.
13. KERN, H. 1993. Fine structure of the human exocrine pancreas. Chapter 2. *In* The Pancreas, 2nd ed. V.L. Go, E. Dimagno, J. Gardner, I. Lebenthal, H. Reber & G. Scheele, Eds. :9–19. Raven Press. New York.
14. HENLER, M.E. 1990. VLA proteins in the integrin family: Structures, functions, and their roles on leukocytes. Ann. Rev. Immunol. **8:** 365–400
15. HYNES, R.O. 1992. Integrins: Versatility modulation and signalling in cell adhesion. Cell **69:** 11–25.
16. HALL, P.A., P. COATES, N.R. LEMOINE & M.A. HORTON. 1991. Characterization of integrin chains in normal and neoplastic human pancreas. J. Pathol. **165:** 33–41.
17. WEINEL, R.J., A. ROSENDAHL, K. NEUMANN, B. CHALOUPKA, D. ERB, M. ROTHMUND & S. SANTOSO. 1992. Expression and function of VLA a2, a3, a5 and a6 integrin receptors in pancreatic carcinoma. Int. J. Canc. **52**: 827–833.
18. ROSENDAHL, A., K. NEUMANN, B. CHALOUPKA, M. ROTHMUND & R.J. WEINEL. 1993. Expression and distribution of VLA receptors in the pancreas: An immunohistochemical study. Pancreas **8:** 711–718.
19. KAJIJI, S., R.N. TAMURA & V.A. QUARANTA. 1989. A novel integrin aE b4 from human epithelial cells suggests a fourth family of integrin adhesion receptors. EMBO J. **8**: 673–680.
20. LÖHR, M., B. TRAUTMANN, M. GOTTLER, S. PETERS, I. ZAUNER, B. MAILLET & G. KLOPPEL. 1994. Human ductal adenocarcinomas of the pancreas express extracellular matrix proteins. Br. J. Canc. **69:** 144–150.
21. KASPER, M., H. HAHN VON DORSCHE & P. STOSIEK. 1991. Changes in the distribution of intermediate filament proteins and collagen IV in fetal and adult human pancreas. Histochemistry **96:** 271–277.
22. SHÜSSLER, M.H., A. SKOUDY, F. RAEMAKERS, F.X. REAL. 1992. Intermediate filaments as differentiation markers of normal pancreas and pancreas cancer. Am. J. Pathol. **140:** 559–568.
23. RAFIEE, P., S.B. HO, R.S. BRESALIER, E.J. BLOOM, J.H. KIM & Y.S. KIM. 1992. Characterization of cytokeratins of human colonic, pancreatic, and gastrointestinal adenocarcinoma cell lines. Pancreas **7:** 123–131.
24. REAL, F.X., M.R. VILÁ, A. SKOUDY, F.C.S. RAEMAKERS & J.M. COROMINAS. 1993. Intermediate filaments as differentiation markers of exocrine pancreas. II. Expression of cytokeratins of complex and stratified epithelia in normal pancreas and pancreas cancer. Int. J. Canc. **54:** 720–727.
25. HERZIG, K.-H., M. ALTMANNSBERGER & U.R. Fölsch. 1994. Intermediate filaments in rat pancreatic acinar tumors, uman ductal carcinomas, and other gastrointestinal malignancies. Gastroenterology **106:** 1326–1332.
26. YAMANAKA, Y., H. FRIESS, M. BUCHLER, H.G. BEGER, L.I. GOLD & M. KORC. 1993. Synthesis and expression of transforming growth factor β-1, β-2, and β-3 in the endocrine and exocrine pancreas. Diabetes **42:** 746–756.
27. KORC, M., H. FRIESS, Y. YAMANAKA, M.S. KOBRIN, M. BUCHLER & H.G. BEGER. 1994. Chronic pancreatitis is associated with increased concentrations of epidermal growth factor receptor, transforming growth factor a, and phospholipase Cg. Gut **35**: 1468–1473.
28. HILL, D.J., S.C. RILEY, N.S. BASSETT & M.J. WATERS. 1992. Localization of the growth hormone receptor, identified by immunocytochemistry, in second trimester

human fetal tissues and in placenta throughout gestation. J. Clin. Endocrinol. Metab. **75:** 646–650.
29. FRIESS, H., Y. YAMANAKA, M. BUCHLER, H.G. BEGER, D.A. DO, M.S. KOBRIN & M. KORC. 1994. Increased expression of acidic and basic fibroblast growth factors in chronic pancreatitis. Am. J. Pathol. **144:** 117–128.
30. FRIESS, H., Y. YAMANAKA, M. BUCHLER, M.S. KOBRIN, E. TAHARA & M. Korc. 1994. Cripto, a member of the epidermal growth factor family, is over-expressed in human pancreatic cancer and chronic pancreatitis. Int. J. Cancer **56:** 668–674.
31. EBERT, M., M. YOKOYAMA, M.S. KOBRIN, H. FRIESS, M.E. LOPEZ, M.W. BUCHLER, G.R. JOHNSON & M. KORC. 1994. Induction and expression of amphiregulin in human pancreatic cancer. Cancer Res. **54:** 3959–3962.
32. SMITH, J.J., R. DERYNCK & M. KORC. 1987. Production of transforming growth factor a in human pancreatic cancer cells: Evidence for a superagonist autocrine cycle. Proc. Natl. Acad. Sci. USA **84:** 7657–7570.
33. BARTON, C.M., P.A. HALL, C.M. HUGHES, W.J. GULLICK & N.R. LEMOINE. 1991. Transforming growth factor alpha and epidermal growth factor in human pancreatic cancer. J. Pathol. **163:** 111–116.
34. KOBRIN, M.S., H. FUNATOMI, H. FRIESS, M.W. BUCHLER, P. STATHIS & M. KORC. 1994. Induction and expression of heparin-binding EGF-like growth factor in human pancreatic cancer. Biochem. Biophys. Res. Commun. **202:** 1705–1709.
35. LEMOINE, N.R., C.M. HUGHES, C.M. BARTON & R.A. POULSOM. 1992. Growth factor receptor in human pancreatic cancer. J. Pathol. **166:** 7–12.
36. WILLIAMS, T.M., D.B. WINER, M.I. GREENE & H.C. MAGUIRE. 1991. Expression of c-erbB-2 in human pancreatic adenocarcinomas. Pathobiology **59:** 46–52.
37. LEMOINE, N.R., M. LOBRESCO, H.Y. LEUNG, C.M. BARTON, S.A. PRIGENT, W.J. GULLICK & G. KLOPPEL. 1992. The erbB3 gene in human pancreatic cancer. J. Pathol. **168:** 269–273.
38. FRIESS, H., Y. YAMANAKA, M. BUCHLER, K. HAMMER, M.S. KOBRIN, H.G. BEGER & M. KORC. 1994. A subgroup of patients with chronic pancreatitis overexpress the c- erb B-2 protooncogene. Ann. Surg. **220:** 183–192.
39. KORC, M., B. CHANDRASEKAR, Y. YAMANAKA, H. FRIESS, M. BUCHLER & G. BEGER. 1992. Overexpression of epidermal growth factor receptor in human pancreatic cancer is associated with concomitant increases in the levels of epidermal growth factor and transforming growth factor alpha. J. Clin. Invest. **90:** 1352–1360.
40. HALL, P.A., C.M. HUGHES, S.L. STADDON, P.I. RICHMAN, W.J. Gullick & N.R. LEMOINE. 1990. The c-erbB-2 proto-oncogene in human pancreatic cancer. J. Pathol. **161:** 195–200.
41. KORC, M., B. CHANDRASEKAR & G.N. SHAH. 1991. Differential binding and biological activities of epidermal growth factor and transforming growth factor a in a human pancreatic cancer cell line. Cancer Res. 51: 6243–6249.
42. SATOH, K., H. SASANO, T. SHIMOSEGAWA, M. KOIZUMI, T. YAMAZAKI, F. MOCHIZUKI, N. KOBAYASH, T. OKANO, T. TOYOTA & T. SAWAI. 1993. An immunohistochemical study of the c-erbB-2 oncogene product in intraductal mucin-hypersecreting neoplasms and in ductal cell carcinomas of the pancreas. Cancer **72:** 51–56.
43. YAMANAKA, Y., H. FRIESS, M.S. KOBRIN, M. BUCHLER, J. KUNZ, H.G. BEGER & M. KORC. 1993. Overexpression of HER2/neu oncogene in human pancreatic carcinoma. Human Pathol. **24:** 1127–1134.
44. EBERT, M., M. YOKOYAMA, H. FRIESS, M.W. BUCHLER & M. KORC. 1994. Coexpression of the c-met to-oncogene and hepatocyte growth factor in human pancreatic cancer. Cancer Res. **54:** 5775–5778.
45. LEUNG, H.Y., W.J. GULLICK & N.R. LEMOINE. 1994. Expression and functional activity of fibroblast growth factors and their receptors in human pancreatic cancer. Int. J. Cancer **59:** 667–675.
46. YAMANAKA, Y., H. FRIES, M. BUCHLER, H.G. BEGER, E. UCHIDA, M. ONDA, M.S. KOBRIN & M. KORC. 1993. Overexpression of acidic and basic fibroblast growth factors in human pancreatic cancer correlates with advanced tumor stage. Cancer Res. **53:** 5289–5296.

47. SASANO, H., K. FUKUSHIMA, I. SASAKI, S. MATSUNO, H. NAGURA & Z.S. KROZOWSKI. 1992. Immunolocalization of mineralocorticoid receptor in human kidney, pancreas, salivary, mammary and sweat glands: A light and electron microscopic immunohistochemical study. J. Endocrinol. **132:** 305–310.
48. MATTHES, H., A. KAISER, U. STIER, E.-O. RIECKEN & S. ROSEWICZ. 1994. Glucocorticoid receptor gene expression in the exocrine and endocrine rat pancreas. Endocrinology **135:** 476–479.
49. ABBOTT, C.A., E. BAKER, G.R. SUTHERLAND & G.W. McCaughan. 1994. Genomic organization, exact localization, and tissue expression of the human CD26 (dipeptidyl peptidase IV) gene. Immunogenetics **40:** 331–338.
50. CHAUDHRY, A., A. GOBL, B. ERIKSSON, B. SKOGSEID & K. OBERG. 1994. Different splice variants of CD44 are expressed in gastrinomas but not in other subtypes of endocrine pancreatic tumors. Cancer Res. **54:** 981–986.
51. MAYNE, K.M., K. PULFORD, M. JONES, K. MICKLEM, G. NAGEL, C.E. VAN DER SCHOOT & D.Y. MASON. 1993. Antibody By114 is selective for the 90kD PI-linked component of the CD66 antigen: A new reagent for the study of paroxysmal nocturnal haemoglobinuria. Br. J. Haematol. **83:** 30–38.
52. SWEDERLOW, S.H. & S.A. WRIGHT. 1986. The spectrum of Leu-M1 staining in lymphoid and hematopoietic proliferations. Am. J. Clin. Pathol. **85:** 283–288.
53. ARGENT, B.E. & M.G. GRAY. 1996. Regulation and formation of fluid and electrolyte secretions by pancreatic duct epithelium. Chapt. 11. In Biliary and Pancreatic Ductal Epithelia: Pathobiology and Pathophysiology. :349–377. Marcel Dekker. New York.
54. LESUFFLEUR, T., N. PORCHET, J.-P. AUBERT, D. SWALLOW, J.R. GUM, Y.S. KIM, F.X. REAL, & A. ZWEIBAUM. 1993. Differential expression of the human mucin genes MUC1 to MUC5 in relation to growth and differentiation of different mucus–secreting HT-29 cell subpopulations. J. Cell Sci. **106:** 771–783.
55. BAECKSTROM, D., G.C. HANSSON, O. NILSSON, C. JOHANSSON, S.J. GENDLER & L. LINDHOLM. 1991. Purification and characterization of a membrane–bound and a secreted mucin–type glycoprotein carrying the carcinoma–associated sialyl–LeA epitope on distinct core proteins. J. Biol. Chem. **266:** 21537–21547.
56. KIM, Y.S. 1992. Altered glycosylation of mucin glycoproteins in colonic neoplasia. J. Cell. Biochem. **16G:** 91–96.
57. BARA, J., A. IMBERTY, S. PEREZ, K. IMAI, A. YACHI & R. ORIOL. 1993. A fucose residue can mask the MUC–1 epitopes in normal and cancerous gastric mucosae. Int. J. Cancer **54:** 607–613.
58. BATRA, S.K., R.S. METZGAR & M.A. HOLLINGSWORTH. 1992. Human MUC1 mucin gene expression in the fetal pancreas. Pancreas **7:** 391–393.
59. CHAMBERS, J.A., M.A. HOLLINGSWORTH, A.E.O. TREZISE & A. HARRIS. 1994. Developmental expression of mucins MUC1 and MUC2. J. Cell Sci. **107:** 413–424.
60. HARRIS, A. & L. COLEMAN. 1988. Cultured epithelial cells derived from human fetal pancreas as a model for the study of cystic fibrosis: Further analysis on the origins and nature of the cell types. J. Cell Sci. **90:** 73–77.
61. BALAGUE, C., G. GAMBUS, C. CARRATO, N. PORCHET, J.P. AUBERT, Y.S. KIM & F. REAL. 1994. Altered expression of MUC2, MUC4, and MUC5 mucin genes in pancreas tissues and cancer cell lines. Gastroenterology **106:** 1054–1061.
62. REID. C.J., K. HYDE, S.B. HO & A. HARRIS. 1997. Cystic fibrosis of the pancreas: Involvement of MUC6 mucin in obstruction of pancreatic ducts. Mol. Med. **3:** 403–411.
63. BURDICK, M.D., A. HARRIS, C.J. REID, T. IWAMURA & M.A. HOLLINGSWORTH. 1997. Oligosaccharides expressed on MUC1 produced by pancreatic and colon tumor cell lines. J. Biol. Chem. **272:** 24198–24202.
64. PHILIPSEN, E.K., H. CLAUSEN, E. DABELSTEEN & N. GRAEM. 1988. Blood group related carbohydrate antigens in human fetal pancreas. Apmis **96:** 1109–1117.
65. TUO X.-H., S. ITAI, J. NISHIKATA, T. MORI, O. TANAKA & R. KANNAGI. 1992. Stage-specific expression of cancer-associated type 1 and type 2 chain polylactosamine antigens in the developing pancreas of human embryos. Cancer Res. **52:** 5744–5751.

66. HOLLINGSWORTH, M.A. & R.S. METZGAR. 1985. Antigens of normal and malignant human exocrine pancreatic cells. *In* Monoclonal Antibodies in Cancer.: 279–308. Marcel Dekker. New York.
67. POUR, P.M., H. TAKAHASHI & M. BUCHLER. 1980. Immunologic aspects of pancreatitis. Chapt. 19. *In* The Pancreas in Connection with the Epigastric Unit. U. Becker & K. Hübner, Eds. :170–180. Gustav Fischer Verlag. New York.
68. LIGTENBERG, M.J.L., L. KRUIJSHAAR, F. BUIJS, M. VAN MEIJER, S.V. LITVINOV & J. HILKENS. 1992. Cell–associated episialin is a complex containing two proteins derived from a common precursor. J. Biol. Chem. **267:** 6171–6177.
69. Wesseling, J., van der Valk, S.W. and Hilkens, J. 1996. A mechanism for inhibition of E-cadherin-mediated cell-cell adhesion by the membrane-associated mucin episialin/MUC1. Mol. Biol. Cell **7:** 565–577.
70. WESSELING, J., S.W. VAN DER VALK, H.L. VOS, A. SONNENBERG & J. HILKENS. 1995. Episialin (MUC1) overexpression inhibits integrin-mediated cell adhesion to extracellular matrix components. J. Cell Biol. **129:** 255–265.
71. SPICER, A., G. ROWSE, T. LIDNER & S. GENDLER. 1995. Delayed mammary tumor progression in *Muc-1* null mice. J. Biol. Chem. **270:** 30093–30101.
72. LAN, M.S., S.K. BATRA, W.N. QI, R.S. METZGAR & M.A. HOLLINGSWORTH. 1990. Cloning and sequencing of a human pancreatic tumor mucin cDNA. J. Biol. Chem. **265:** 15294–15299.

Immortalized Pancreatic Duct Cells *in Vitro* and *in Vivo*

R. JESNOWSKI, P. MÜLLER, W. SCHARECK,[a] S. LIEBE, AND M. LÖHR[b]

Department of Medicine, Division of Gastroenterology and [a]Surgery, University of Rostock, Rostock, Germany

> ABSTRACT: Although pancreatic adenocarcinoma has become one of the best characterized malignant diseases, severe diagnostic and therapeutic problems are still associated with this disease. The establishment of a molecular model of pancreatic carcinogenesis may provide tools that could result in earlier diagnosis of this disease and, in turn, improves prognosis. Since pancreatic adenocarcinoma seems to originate in epithelial cells in the pancreatic ducts, cultivation of native pancreatic duct epithelial cells (PDEC) is the initial step in the establishment of an *in vitro* model of pancreatic carcinogenesis. As these native cells survive only a short period in culture, the aim of this study was to establish a stable pancreatic duct cell line by immortalization with the SV40 large T antigen. Furthermore, initial steps in pancreatic carcinogenesis should possibly be imitated by additional transfections of mutated ki-ras and/or mutated p53 genes. By optimization of the isolation protocol and the culture medium, yield as well as proliferative activity of isolated PDEC was increased considerably. Transfection of SV40 large T antigen resulted in an increase in the proliferative lifetime of the isolated cells, but no real immortal phenotype was obtained. Moreover, one step in the transformation from the normal to the malignant phenotype was imitated successfully by additional transfection of mutated ki-ras.

INTRODUCTION

Although not explicit in the title, pancreatic carcinoma was the starting point of this work. Pancreatic carcinoma is the fourth leading cause of cancer death in western countries, and the incidence has been constant or even slightly increasing over the last decades.[1-4] At the time of diagnosis, up to 80% of pancreatic adenocarcinomas already are metastatic (regional lymph nodes, liver),[2] and so prognosis of this disease is very poor, with 5-year survival rates between 0.4%[4,5] and 10%.[2] The mean survival time after diagnosis is 4-6 months.[4, 5]

Based on microscopic and immunohistological criteria, about 90% of malignant tumors of the pancreas are classified as ductal adenocarcinoma. Ductal markers carboanhydrase type II,[6] muc2,[7] cytokeratins types 7, 8, 18, and 19,[8-10] and CEA[6] are expressed by the vast majority of these tumors. Besides the ductal cells, acinar cells[11] and islet cells[12,13] are discussed as potential origins of pancreatic carcinoma.

---

[b]Corresponding author: M. Löhr, MD, Department of Medicine, Division of Gastroenterology, University of Rostock, Ernst-Heydemann-Str. 6, 18057 Rostock, Germany. Phone, +49 381 494-7497; fax: +49 381 494-7348; e-mail, loehr@med.uni-rostock.de

In this way a transdifferentiation from acinar to ductal cells was observable *in vitro*.[14,15] In rat, pancreatic cells developed into functional hepatocytes after transplantation into the liver.[16] After chemically induced destruction of islet cells in mice, new formation of functional islet cells from epithelial "stem cells" could be demonstrated.[17-19] Furthermore, in rat acinar tumor cell line AR42J it is possible to direct transdifferentiation. Thus, incubation of AR42J cells with HGF and/or activin A results in a neuroendocrine phenotype.[20,21] Consequently a final, irrevocable differentiation into the different types of pancreatic cells has been discussed intensively in the last years.

Morphologically most pancreatic adenocarcinomas are well to moderately differentiated,[2] and these tumors are characterized by the intense proliferation of connective tissue.[22,23] Over the last years several genetic alterations associated with pancreatic carcinoma have been identified. Up to 90% of pancreatic tumors harbor activating mutations of the ki-ras gene.[24-27] In contrast to other carcinomas, in pancreatic adenocarcinoma these mutations nearly exclusively lie within codon 12 of the ki-ras gene; very rarely are codons 13, 59, and 61 mutated.[26,28] Loss of heterozygosity of tumor suppressor gene p53 is detectable in about 80% of pancreatic tumors,[29,30] accompanied by inactivating mutations, deletions, and microinsertions. Furthermore, inactivation of genes DPC4[31,32] and p16/MTS1[33,34] is frequently associated with pancreatic carcinogenesis. Also, complex rearrangements of the genome, for example, tri- to tetraploidy, loss of chromosomes, or more frequently gain of additional chromosomes, are common in pancreatic carcinoma.[35,36]

Besides these direct genetic alterations, pancreatic carcinoma is characterized by deregulation of the expression of growth factors and their respective receptors. These potential autocrine loops could be demonstrated for the EGF receptor and its ligands EGF and TGFα,[37,38] for aFGF and bFGF and their receptors,[39,40] as well as for PDGF-A/B and their receptors.[41,42] In a paracrine way these growth factors could result in induction of fibroblast proliferation, which finally could lead to the desmoplasia seen in many pancreatic tumors.[38]

Pancreatic tumor cells themselves can express extracellular matrix (ECM) proteins,[43] contributing to the stromal component of the desmoplastic tissue. Furthermore, the expression of functional receptors for these ECM proteins could be demonstrated in pancreatic tumor cells.[44] Therefore, in a manner analogous to the aforementioned situation, autocrine and paracrine growth stimulation may be possible by this expression of extracellular matrix proteins and their receptors.[38] Binding of the integrins to the ECM proteins may induce signal transduction via cytoskeleton and matrix proteins to the nucleus, resulting in alteration of gene expression.[38]

MATERIALS AND METHODS

Pancreatic duct cells were isolated from transplant organs that could not be used for transplantation for several reasons such as HLA-mismatch. For optimization, resected pancreatic tissues and bovine pancreatic tissue were used. Controls included pancreatic tumor cell lines, an immortalized bovine PDEC line (V-A), established by our group previously, and a human PDEC line (M540) provided by F. Real from Barcelona.

TABLE 1. Techniques for PDEC isolation

Method	Execution	Advantages	Disadvantages
0	digestion of duct pieces with collagenase and chymotrypsin		time consuming, practicable only with large specimens, fibroblast contamination
1	seeding of small duct pieces	fast, economic method, practicable with small specimens, cells grow well, tissues grow out repeatedly	fibroblast contamination
2	trypsin digest of duct pieces	fast	practicable only with large specimens, fibroblast contamination
3	seeding of scraped cells, short trysination	fast, nearly no fibroblast contamination	practicable only with large specimens
4	cells isolated from ERCP	fast	fibroblast contamination cells do not grow very well
5	digest of pancreatic tissue with collagenase, DNase and hyaluronidase; seeding of isolated cells into a collagen gel	practicable with small specimens, pure epithelial cells	cumbersome, very time consuming

At first, PDEC were isolated according to a method established by our group previously[45] (method 0 in TABLE 1). Because the yield of isolated cells was not satisfactory with this method, several isolation techniques (summarized in TABLE 1) to improve the output were tested and optimized.

Contaminating fibroblasts were either removed mechanically or labeled with a complement activating fibroblast-specific antibody (anti-fibroblast surface protein, clone 1B10, mouse monoclonal IgM, 1:500 in serum-free culture medium; 30 min, 37°C). After washing the cells three times with phosphate-buffered saline solution (PBS) to remove unbound antibody, the fibroblasts were lysed by subsequent incubation in rabbit complement (1:10 in serum-free medium). Cells were washed again with PBS and refed with fresh culture medium.

Several culture media were tested to improve the growth of the isolated epithelial cells. Primary bovine pancreatic duct epithelial cells were seeded in culture dishes and incubated overnight. Non- adhering cells were removed by washing with PBS and the cells were refed with the different culture media (TABLE 2). Media were changed every 3 days, and the growth of epithelial colonies and contaminating fibroblasts was monitored for a 10-day period.

For immortalization the isolated cells were transfected with plasmids pSV3neo or pLXSN/large T. Besides the large T antigen, these vectors expressed the neo resistance gene, enabling selection with the antibiotic G418. To optimize the transfections both HEPES and BES-buffered calcium phosphate coprecipitation and the lipid-mediated transfection systems DOTAP (Boehringer, Mannheim), Lipo-

TABLE 2. Optimization of culture medium

Medium	Growth epithelial cells	Growth fibroblasts
DMEM, 5% FCS	+	+
DMEM, 10% FCS	+	++
DMEM, 20% FCS	++	+++
RPMI 1640, 5% FCS	+	+
RPMI 1640, 10% FCS	+	++
RPMI 1640, 20%FCS	++	+++
CMRL1066, 5% FCS, plus supplements 1[a]	+++	+
Keratinocyte Medium, 5% FCS, plus supplements 2[b]	+++	+

[a]Supplements 1: bovine pituitary extract 50 µg/ml, cholera toxin 50 ng/ml, EGF 10 ng/ml, glutamine 4 mM, hydrocortison 1 µg/ml, insulin 0,2 IU/ml, selenium 5 ng/ml, transferrin 5 µg/ml.
[b]Supplements 2: bovine pituitary extract 50 µg/ml, EGF 5 ng/ml.

fectamin (Life Technologies), Transfectam (Promega), and Maxifectin (Dr. Sourovoi, Germany) were tested.[46] Coprecipitation was performed according to standard procedures[47]; within the lipid-mediated transfections the manufacturer's recommendations were followed. In two cases the isolated cells were infected using a recombinant retrovirus, based on the pLXSN vector (Clontech), additionally coding for the SV40 large T antigen. Furthermore, we tried to imitate the initial steps in pancreatic carcinogenesis by transfection with plasmids pCMVki-ras(mut) and/or pCMV273H(p53mut).

To determine the growth characteristics of the individual clones the cells were counted every 2 days over a period of 14 days. Soft agar cloning was performed as described previously.[38] In brief, 2×10^6 cells in 2 ml soft agar (0.3% agar in culture medium) were seeded onto a layer of polymerized soft agar in 6-well plates. Colony building was monitored for 3 weeks.

To check the ability of tumor induction the isolated cells were injected orthotopically into athymic nude mice. For that the abdominal cavity of anesthetized nude mice was opened, pancreas and spleen were pulled out carefully, and 1 or 5×10^6 cells were injected into the pancreas. Organs were put back and the incision was sutured. Nude mice were checked twice a week until a solid tumor mass was palpable or for 12 weeks at the longest. At this time the pancreas was removed and fixed in 5% formaldehyde.

For cultivation on matrigel 1×10^5 cells were seeded onto a layer of solidified matrigel. Cultivation was performed by mixing cells (2×10^5/ml) with the same volume of cold matrigel. This mixture was pipetted into each well of a 12-well tissue culture dish (0.5 ml/well) and polymerized by incubation for 30 min at 37°C. The gel was overlayed with 0.5 ml culture medium, which was changed every 2 days. Growth was monitored for 14 days. Conditioned media of the isolated cell clones were tested for their ability to induce fibroblast proliferation by the use of the BrdU labeling and detection kit III (Boehringer, Mannheim) according to the manufacturer's recommendations. The mitogenic effect of the conditioned media should be blocked by preincubation with neutralizing antibodies against bFGF, PDGF, or

TABLE 3. Antibodies used for immunocytochemistry

Antigen	Species	Subtype	Source of supply
Cytokeratin 7	mouse	IgG1	Sigma
Cytokeratin 8/18	mouse	IgG1	Sigma
Cytokeratin 19	mouse	IgG1	Sigma
Cytokeratin pan	mouse	IgG1, IgG2a	Sigma
Muc 1 Core Protein	mouse	IgG1	Novocastra
Ca 19-9	mouse	IgG1	Novocastra
CA II	sheep	IgG	Pan System
Epithelial Specific Antigen	mouse	IgG1	Novocastra
CEA	mouse	IgG1	Novocastra
CD 44st	mouse	IgG	Bender
CD 44v5	mouse	IgG	Bender
CD 44v6	mouse	IgG	Bender
Laminin	rabbit	IgG	Heyl Chemie
Fibronektin	mouse	IgG	Boehringer
Collagen Type III	rabbit	IgG	Chemicon
Collagen Type IV	rabbit	IgG	Heyl Chemie
bFGF	rabbit	IgG	Santa Cruz
TGFβ1	rabbit	IgG	Santa Cruz
PDGF-A	rabbit	IgG	Santa Cruz
Tissue Factor	mouse	IgG	Dr. Ruf
Amylase	rabbit	IgG	Prof. Klöppel
Insulin	mouse	IgG	Biogenex/Camon
Fibroblast (AS 02)	mouse	IgG	Dianova
SV 40 T-Antigen	mouse	IgG2a	Oncogene Science
p53 Mut (Pab 240)	mouse	IgG1	Santa Cruz

TGFβ1 (R&D, 7.5 µg/ml conditioned medium) for 24 hr at 4°C. Thereafter, the media were subjected to proliferation assays as described above.

Immunocytochemistry was performed using the three-step method with HRP-conjugated secondary and tertiary antibodies as described previously. First antibodies are summarized in TABLE 3.

Western blotting of conditioned media and cell lysates was performed by standard procedures (Ausubel). Antibodies used were as follows: bFGF, PDGF-A, TGFβ1 (Santa Cruz, 1:500 in blocking buffer), and SV40 large T antigen (Oncogene Science, 1:1000 in blocking buffer). Detection of the first antibodies was performed with the chemoluminescent Western-Light Plus Kit (Tropix) according to the manufacturer's recommendations.

Growth factors bFGF, PDGF, and TGFβ1 in the conditioned media of the isolated cells were quantified by ELISA (R&D, Germany).

Expression of several oncogenes, tumor suppressor genes, and genes for differentiated duct cells (summarized in TABLE 4) was investigated by reverse slot blot.

TABLE 4. cDNAs used for reverse slot blot

Plasmid	Gene	Size (in kb)	Source of supply
pHCAL1U	Collagen I	0,37	E. Vuorio, Finnland
pHFS3	Collagen III	0,70	E. Vuorio, Finnland
FN711	Fibronektin	1,4	R.O. Hynes, Cambridge, MA
VNCDNA	Vitronektin	1,6	J.W. Smith, La Jolla, CA
pCA 38.8	CA II	1,5	M. Frazier
pJJ11-1	FGF2	1,4	J.A. Abraham, Washington DC
int2d	FGF3 (int 2)	1,1	N. Lemoine, London
phEGF15#3	EGF	1,9	ATCC
pPDGF-A	PDGF-A	0,4	H. Kalthoff, Kiel
pPDGF-B	PDGF-B	0,4	H. Kalthoff, Kiel
pBS/TGFb	TGFβ1	1,4	M. Gruschwitz, Erlangen
pSW11-1	ki-ras	1,1	Pharmacia
pLTRp53cG	p53	2,0	M. Oren, Haifa
RPN 1314	fos	3,1	Pharmacia
p627	raf	2,9	ATCC
S6	S6	0,8	J. Kruppa, Hamburg

For that, plasmid DNA corresponding to 1 µg of cDNA insert was blotted onto a nylon membrane (Qiagen) by the use of a slot blot apparatus (Schleicher & Schuell). Hybridization was performed according to standard procedures with a probe obtained by Dig-labeling (Boehringer, Mannheim) of 7.5 µg total RNA in a reverse transcription reaction. Hybrids were detected using the chemoluminescent Dig detection system (Boehringer, Mannheim).

Expression of growth factors bFGF, PDGF, and TGFβ1 was verified by northern blotting of 10 µg total RNA by standard procedures.[47]

DNA uptake of the transfected ki-ras gene was proven by RE-mismatch polymerase chain reaction (PCR) as described previously.[48] This method utilizes a mod-

---

ki-ras sequence (wildtype, codon 12 underlined):

5´..T AAA CTT GTG GTA GTT GGA GC**T** GGT GGC ..

PCR-primer (modification in bold letter):

5´   AAA CTT GTG GTA GTT GGA GC**C**

PCR-produkt containing artificial Msp I site (underlined):

5´..   AAA CTT GTG GTA GTT GGA GCC G][GT GGC ..

FIGURE 1. Principle of the RE (restriction enzyme) = mismatch PCR (from Ref. 38).

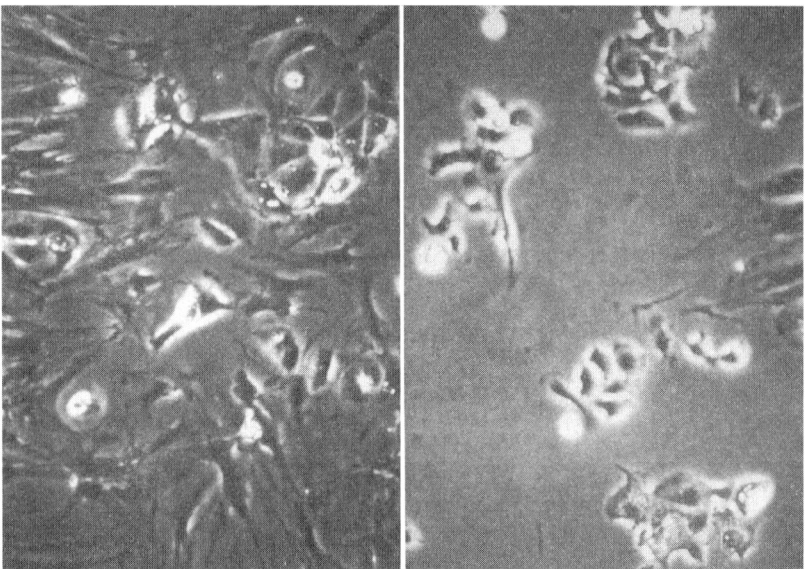

FIGURE 2. Complement lysis of contaminating fibroblasts. Before (*left*) and after (*right*) complement treatment.

ified 5´-primer, thus creating an artificial Msp1 restriction site in case of a wild-type ki-ras gene (FIG. 1); therefore, Msp1 digest of the PCR product results in two fragments. In case one of the two first bases of ki-ras codon 12 is mutated, the PCR product will be undigested. Chromosome analysis of the SV40 transfected clones was done by standard procedures as described previously.[38]

RESULTS

Optimization of the isolation technique demonstrated that two methods were superior to the others. Scraping the epithelial cell layer is the fastest and most elegant method for isolating PDEC. The output clearly was increased compared to that of the method used first. Moreover, the number of cells seeded in parallel can be approximated, a mandatory prerequisite for physiological assays. Contamination with fibroblasts, a problem associated with the other methods, was avoided with this technique. A drawback of this method is that it is not reliable with all pancreases. Whereas it worked well with most of the organs, in some cases the output dropped and was comparable to that of the first isolation technique.

Seeding small duct pieces, simply cut down with scissors, combined several advantages. The cells isolated with this method had a high proliferative index during the first weeks of cultivation, a fact needed for efficient transfections and for retroviral gene transfer. Furthermore, the tissue clumps grew out repeatedly after transfer to a fresh culture dish, improving the yield dramatically. Contaminating fibroblasts

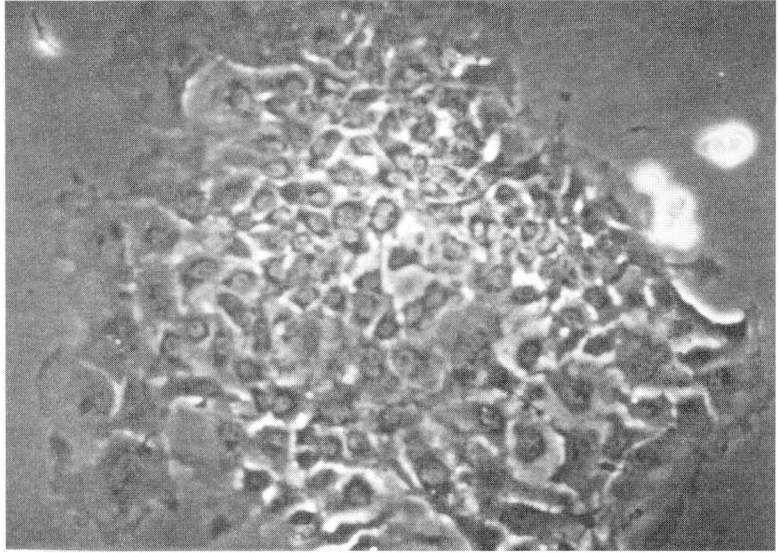

FIGURE 3. Phase contrast microscopy of isolated PDEC.

were removed either mechanically or by using a complement activating fibroblast-specific antibody and subsequent incubation in rabbit complement (FIG. 2).

Cells isolated with these methods exhibited morphological and functional markers of differentiated epithelial cells. By phase contrast microscopy, abundantly granulated monolayers were visible, as expected for secretory epithelial cells (FIG. 3).

The isolated cells expressed cytokeratins types 7 and 19, typical for PDEC, as well as marker antigens CA19-9, MUC1, and carboanhydrase type II. Cells were negative for amylase and for insulin, markers for acinar cells and endocrine cells, respectively.

Subculturing of the cells was possible only with restriction. After trypsinization or dispase treatment, only a small percentage of cells attached to the new culture dish.

Keratinocyte SFM supplemented with EGF and BPE and CMRL1066 plus supplements performed best in this test by simultaneously supporting the growth of epithelial cells and retarding the growth of fibroblasts. Since the keratinocyte medium was easier to handle, it was used as culture medium in the following study.

Different culture substrates, such as collagen or matrigel, did not induce an increase in proliferation rate, as was reported for several other primary cells such as prostatic epithelial cells.

Optimization of the transfection parameters revealed that the BBS buffered calcium phosphate coprecipitation technique[46] was the method of choice for these cells. The transfections resulted in three, infections in two G418-resistant epithelial clones. Whereas four of these clones died within the first 5 months of cultivation, the clone E4, obtained by transfection with the plasmid pSV3neo, survived over 14 months before reaching terminal crisis and extinction. Within this period the clone

58 ANNALS NEW YORK ACADEMY OF SCIENCES

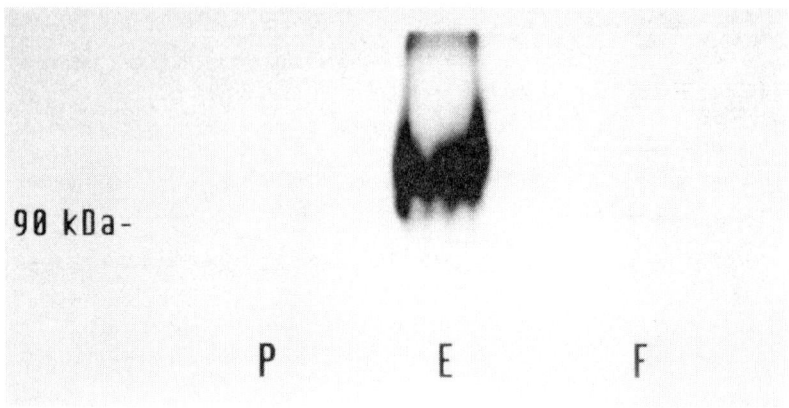

FIGURE 4. Expression of the large T antigen demonstrated in Western Blot: E, epithelial clone E4; F, fibroblast; P, panel.

was characterized in detail. Expression of the transfected gene was verified by western blotting (FIG. 4) and immunocytochemistry.

Within the transfections of mutated ki-ras and p53 genes, two clones expressing the mutated ki-ras gene were established, human clone M540/ki-ras and bovine clone V-A/ki-ras. DNA uptake was proven by RE-mismatch PCR. FIGURE 5 illustrates the result of such a digest.

No signs of malignancy or invasiveness were detectable in the clones merely transfected with the SV40 large T antigen. They were able neither to grow in colonies in soft agar-cloning assays nor to induce tumor growth in nude mice.

In contrast, the additionally ki-ras transfected bovine cells built colonies in soft agar, and orthotopic application into nude mice resulted in formation of pancreatic tumors. Mutation of the ki-ras gene was verified by RE-mismatch PCR, thus proving that the applied cells were the origin of tumor development.

Differentiation of the SV40 transfected cells was triggered by cultivation on or in matrigel. Cultivation on matrigel resulted in formation of cell heaps within several

FIGURE 5. Restriction enzyme mismatch PCR for the ki-ras gene of the clones M540 (*lanes 1 and 2*) and M540/ki-ras (*lanes 3–8*): u, undigested; d, Msp1 digested.

TABLE 5. Results immunocytochemistry

	Native PDEC	Immortalized PDEC	ki-ras transfected PDEC	tumor cell line Panc1
Cytokeratin 7	3	2	2	3
Cytokeratin 8/18	2	1	1	2
Cytokeratin 19	3	1	1	3
Cytokeratin pan	3	2	2	3
Muc 1 Core Protein	1	1	n.d.	1
Ca 19-9	2	1	1	2
CA II	1	3	3	3
Epithelial Specific Antigen	1	1	n.d.	2
CEA	1, some	1, some	1, some	1, some cells 2
CD 44st	n.d.	1	1	1
CD 44v5	n.d., 0^a	1	1	1
CD 44v6	n.d., 0^a	1	1	1
Laminin	n.d., 0–1^a	2, punctiform	2, punctiform	n.d., 2^a
Fibronektin	n.d., 0^a	2	2	n.d., 2^a
Collagen Type III	n.d., 0–1^a	1, punctiform	1, punctiform	n.d., 1–2^a
Collagen Type IV	n.d., 0–1^a	1, punctiform	1, punctiform	n.d., 2^a
bFGF	0, CP 1	2	2	2
TGFβ1	0, CP 1	1	1	1
Tissue Factor	0, CP 2	2	2	2
Amylase	0	0	0	0
Insulin	0	0	0	0
Fibroblast (AS 02)	0	0, 2^b	0	0
SV 40 T-Antigen	0	3, nuclear	3, nuclear	0
p53 Mut (Pab 240)	0	0	0	2, nuclear

NOTATION: semiquantitative scoring: 0, negative; 1, weak positive; 2, positive; 3, strong positive. n.d., not done; CP, OP-material from chron. pancreatitis; ^{a}, data from Ref. 38; ^{b}, some cells positive after 17 weeks of cultivation.

hours, branching out in the course of cultivation. Cultivation in matrigel induced formation of ramified ductular structures.

The results of immunocytochemistry are summarized in TABLE 5. The native PDEC and all transfected clones expressed the markers of differentiated pancreatic duct cells as CA II, cytokeratins, the carbohydrate epitops CA19-9 and Du-Pan2, and Muc1 core protein. Expression of the ECM proteins laminin, collagen types III and IV, and fibronectin was more prominent in the transfected clones; expression was verified by reverse slot blot (FIG. 6). In contrast to the native PDECs, the transfected clones expressed CD44 variants 5 and 6, growth factors bFGF and TGFβ1 as well as tissue factor, a cofactor of the coagulation cascade. Expression of these growth factors as well as of PDGF was confirmed by northern blot and reverse slot blot (FIG. 6).

Using ELISA these growth factors were detectable in conditioned media from the SV40 transfected clones.

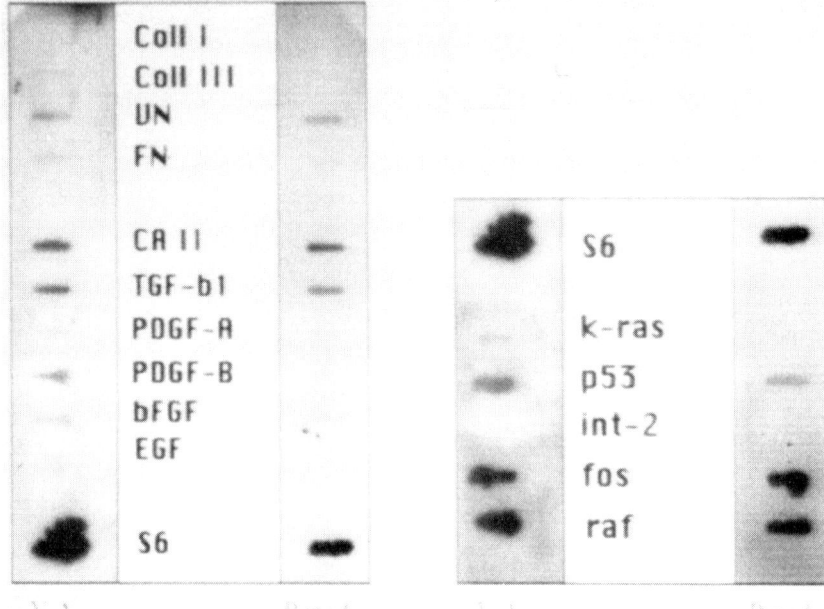

FIGURE 6. Expression of oncongenes, tumorsuppressorgenes and genes for differentiation markers in bovine clone V-A and tumor cell line Panc1 demonstrated in a reverse slot blot.

Chromosome analysis of the SV40 transfected clones revealed structural as well as numerical aberrations (FIG. 7). The mean chromosome number in bovine clone V-A was 96 instead of the normal 60; in the human clone the number was raised to 72. This complex alteration in the genome is the major drawback of SV40-induced immortalization.

DISCUSSION

Proceeding from an established protocol the output of viable PDEC was clearly increased by optimization of the isolation technique. In this seeding of duct pieces, simply cutting down with scissors turned out to be the method of choice for our aims. First, the cells isolated by this method had a high proliferative index during the first time of cultivation, a prerequisite for the subsequent transfection and transduction experiments. Second, the tissue clumps grew out repeatedly when transferred to fresh culture dishes, thus increasing the output dramatically.

Furthermore, adaptation of the culture medium resulted in an increase in the rate and period of proliferation of the isolated cells. In this keratinocyte medium plus supplements and CMRL 1066 plus supplements performed best by simultaneously increasing the proliferation of epithelial cells and retarding the growth of contami-

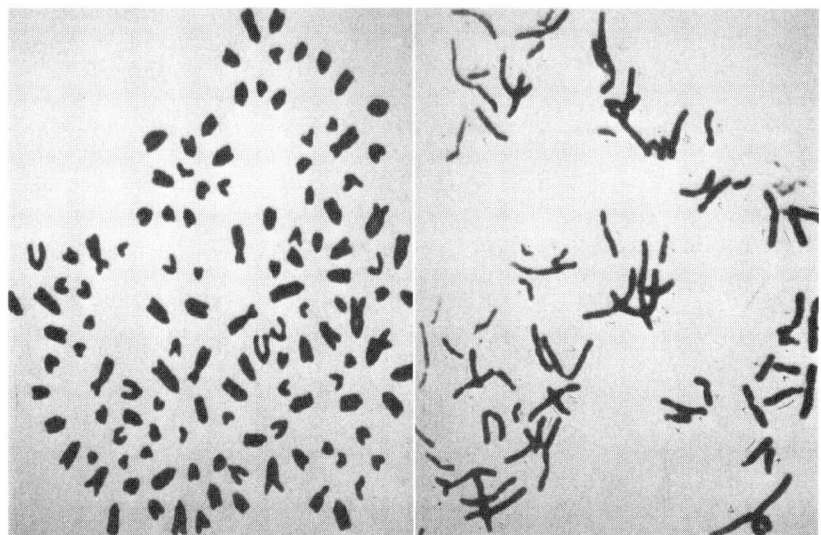

FIGURE 7. Chromosome analysis of the bovine clone V-A (*left*) and the human clone M540 (*right*).

nating fibroblasts. With CMRL1066 this effect may be due to the presence of cholera toxin in the medium, which by activation of the adenylate cyclase leads to inhibition of fibroblast growth[49,50] and promotes the growth of epithelial cells.[51] How these cAMP effects are mediated has not yet been solved conclusively.[52,53]

Cultivation on collagen or matrigel should result in an increased growth rate of primary cells.[54,55] This could not be confirmed in our experiments. The different culture substrates tested had no positive effect on the proliferative index of the isolated PDEC.

Even though the parameters had been optimized thoroughly, transfection efficiency was quite low, reaching 6% transient expression in the immortalized bovine clone.[46] Also, transduction by retroviral vectors, though using viruses, which can enter cells by the amphotrophic retroviral receptor and the GALV receptor, did not solve this problem completely. The parameters, however, were not optimized due to lack of time. Optimization may increase transduction efficiency.

Transfection of the plasmid pSV3neo resulted in epithelial clone E4, which could be cultivated for over 14 months, before reaching terminal crisis and extinction. By additional transfection of mutated ki-ras gene, two clones, human clone M540/ki-ras and bovine clone V-A/ki-ras, were established. DNA uptake was verified by RE-mismatch PCR.

All clones were characterized intensively. Transfection of the SV40 large T antigen at least resulted in prolongation of the life span of clone E4, also demonstrated in literature.[56,57] The way by which the large T finally leads to immortalization has not yet been solved completely. It is known that large T complexes p53, thus perturbing transactivation of subsequent elements of the cell cyclus control (e.g., p21/WAF1).[58] Furthermore, large T interferes with RB1 protein,[58] potentially resulting in additional disturbance of the cell cyclus control. On the other hand, it could be demonstrated that mutated large T protein, though not capable of binding p53, induced immortalization.[58,59] Moreover, it was shown that large T did lead to a decrease in chromosome stability,[60] and this alteration of the genome may finally cause immortalization by activation of growth stimulatory genes and inactivation of genes that control the cell cyclus or cellular senescence.[60]

The cells merely transfected with the large T antigen could neither grow in soft agar nor induce tumor growth in athymic nude mice. Thus, expression of large T alone is not sufficient to cause malignant transformation in our cells, a fact also demonstrated in other cell types.[61,62] In contrast, cells additionally transfected with a mutated ki-ras gene did induce tumor growth when injected orthotopically into nude mice. Consequently the cooperation of mutated ki-ras and large T did cause a malignant transformation, as was shown for other cells.[62,63]

All transfected cells exhibited the markers of differentiated PDEC such as cytokeratins, MUC1 CA 19-9, and carboanhydrase type II. In addition, the cells expressed growth factors bFGF, TGFβ1, and PDGF normally expressed only in pancreatic cancer or pancreatitis,[34,64] thus demonstrating the altered phenotype of transfected cells.

This alteration also could be demonstrated at the genetic level by chromosome analysis. Here the cells exhibited a markedly altered genome. The bovine clone had a mean chromosomal number of 96 instead of the normal 60, whereas in the human clone the number was raised to 72. This marked alteration in the genome is the major drawback of SV40-induced immortalization. Results obtained with such cells have to be judged very critically when transferred to native cells. This problem may be solved by transfection of the human telomerase cDNA. The introduction of telomerase into normal human foreskin fibroblasts and retinal pigment epithelial cells resulted in an extension of the life span beyond the normal life span of these cells without any visible chromosomal alterations.[65]

REFERENCES

1. BORING, C. *et al.* 1991. Cancer statistics, 1991. Cancer **41:** 19–36.
2. BÜCHLER, M. *et al.* 1996. Pankreaserkrankungen. S. Karger GmbH. Freiburg.
3. Gordis, L. & E.B. GOLD. 1993. Epidemiology and etiology of pancreatic cancer. *In* The Pancreas: Biology, Pathobiology and Disease, 2nd Ed. V.L.W. Go *et al.*, Eds.: 837–855. Raven Press. New York.
4. MURR M.M. *et al.* 1994. Pancreatic cancer. CA Cancer J. Clin. **44:** 304–318.
5. SEARLE, P.F. *et al.* 1996. Gene-transfer therapy and pancreatic cancer. *In* Pancreatic Cancer. Molecular and Clinical Advances. J.P. Neoptolemos & N.R. Lemoine, Eds. Blackwell Science Ltd. Oxford.
6. KIM, J.H. *et al.* 1990. Cell lineage markers in human pancreatic cancer. Cancer **66:** 2134–2143.
7. BALAGUÉ, C. *et al.* 1994. Altered expression of MUC2, MUC4, and MUC5 mucin genes in pancreas tissue and cancer cell lines. Gastroenterology **106:** 1054–1061.
8. BOUWENS, L. *et al.* 1994. Cytokeratins as markers of ductal cell differentiation and islet neogenesis in the neonatal rat pancreas. Diabetes **43:** 1279–1283.
9. OSBORN, M. *et al.* 1986. Methods in laboratory investigation. Differential diagnosis of gastrointestinal carcinomas by using monoclonal antibodies specific for individual keratin polypeptides. Lab. Invest. **55:** 497–504.
10. SCHÜSSLER, M.H. *et al.* 1992. Intermediate filaments as differentiation markers of normal pancreas and pancreas cancer. Am. J. Pathol. **140:** 559–568.

11. SCARPELLI, D.G. et al. 1991. Are acinar cells involved in the pathogenesis of ductal adenocarcinoma of the pancreas? Cancer Cells **3:** 275–277.
12. POUR, P.M. 1997. The role of Langerhans islets in pancreatic ductal adenocarcinoma. Front Biosci. **2:** D271–D282.
13. POUR, P.M. et al. 1997. Experimental evidence for the origin of ductal-type adenocarcinoma from the islets of Langerhans. Am. J. Pathol. **150:** 2167–2180.
14. HALL, P.A. et al. 1992. Rapid acinar to ductal transdifferentiation in cultured human exocrine pancreas. J. Pathol. **166:** 97–103.
15. VILÁ, M.R. et al. 1994. Normal human pancreas cultures display functional ductal characteristics. Lab. Invest. **71:** 423–431.
16. DABEVA M.D. et al. 1997. Differentiation of pancreatic epithelial progenitor cells into hepatocytes following transplantation into rat liver. Proc. Natl. Acad. Sci. USA **94:** 7356–7361.
17. CORNELIUS, J.G. et al. 1997. In vitro-generation of islets in long-term cultures of pluripotent stem cells from adult mouse pancreas. Horm. Metab. Res. **29:** 271–277.
18. FERNANDES, A. et al. 1997. Differentiation of new insulin-producing cells is induced by injury in adult pancreatic islets. Endocrinology **138:** 1750–1762.
19. ROSENBERG, L. 1995. In vivo cell transformation: Neogenesis of beta cells from pancreatic ductal cells. Cell Transplant. **4:** 371–383.
20. MASHIMA, H. et al. 1996. Formation of insulin-producing cells from pancreatic acinar AR42J cells by hepatocyte growth factor. Endocrinology **137:** 3969–3976.
21. OHNISHI, H. et al. 1995. Conversion of amylase-secreting rat pancreatic AR42J cells to neuronlike cells by activin A. J. Clin. Invest. **95:** 2304–2314.
22. KLÖPPEL, G. 1984. Pancreatic non-endocrine tumors. In Pancreatic Pathology. G. Klöppel & P.U. Heitz, Eds.: 79–113. Churchill Livingstone. Edinburgh.
23. KLÖPPEL, G. 1993. Pathology of nonendocrine pancreatic tumors. In The Pancreas: Biology, Pathobiology, and Disease. 2nd Ed. V.L.W. Go et al., Eds.: 871–897. Raven Press. New York.
24. ALMOGUERA, C. et al. 1988. Most human carcinomas of exocrine pancreas contain mutant c-K-ras genes. Cell **53:** 549–554.
25. BOS. J.L. 1989. Ras oncogenes in human cancer: A review. Cancer Res. **49:** 4682–4689.
26. CAPELL, G. et al. 1996. Molecular epidemiology of protooncogene and tumour-suppressor gene mutations. In Pancreatic Cancer. Molecular and Clinical Advances. J. Neoptolemos & N. Lemoine, Eds.: 169–180. Blackwell Science Ltd. Oxford.
27. LEMOINE, N.R. 1997. Molecular pathology of pancreatic neoplasms. In Biliary and Pancreatic Ductal Epithelia. Pathobiology and Pathophysiology. A.E. Sirica & D.S. Longnecker, Eds.: 505–525. Marcel Dekker. New York.
28. RALL, C. et al. 1996. Ki-ras and p53 mutations in pancreatic ductal adenocarcinoma. Pancreas **12:** 10–17.
29. BAKER, S.J. et al. 1989. Chromosome 17 deletions and p53 gene mutations in colorectal carcinomas. Science **244:** 217–221.
30. KALTHOFF, H. et al. 1993. p53 and k-ras alterations in pancreatic epithelial cell lesions. Oncogene **8:** 289–298.
31. MOSKALUK, C.A. et al. 1997. Genomic sequencing of DPC4 in the analysis of familial pancreatic carcinoma. Diagn. Mol. Pathol. **6:** 85–90
32. SCHUTTE, M. et al. 1996. DPC4 gene in various tumor types. Cancer Res. **56:** 2527–2530.
33. CALDAS, C. et al. 1994. Frequent somatic mutations and homozygous deletions of the p16 (MTS1) gene in pancreatic adenocarcinoma. Nature Genet. **8:** 27–31.
34. HAHN, S. et al. 1997. Neue molekularbiologische Erkenntnisse aus der Pankreaskarzinomforschung. Deutsches fRzteblatt. **94:** C 2440–C 2446.
35. BARDI, G. et al. 1993. Karyotypic abnormalities in tumours of the pancreas. Br. J. Cancer **67:** 1106–1112.
36. GRIFFIN, C. et al. 1994. Chromosome abnormalities in pancreatic adenocarcinoma. Genes Chromosomes Cancer **9:** 93–100.
37. KALTHOFF, H. et al. 1993. Cytokine-mediated regulation of growth factor receptors (EGF-R and erb-B2) in pancreatic tumors. In Molecular Diagnostics of Cancer. C.

Wagener & S. Neumann, Eds.: 175–186. Springer Verlag. Berlin.
38. LÖHR, M. 1996. Zell- und Molekularbiologie der Bindegewebsreaktion bei Pankreatitis und Pankreaskarzinom. Die Gastroenterologische Reihe, Band 32, Solvay, Hannover.
39. FRIESS, H. et al. 1992. Acidic and basic fibroblast growth factors and their receptors are expressed in the human pancreas. Pancreas **7:** 737 (abstr.).
40. LEUNG, H.Y. et al. 1994. Expression and functional activity of fibroblast growth factors and their receptors in human pancreatic cancer. Int. J. Cancer **59:** 667–675.
41. KALTHOFF, H. et al. 1991. Modulation of platelet-derived growth factor A- and B-chain/c-sis mRNA by tumor necrosis factor and other agents in adenocarcinoma cells. Oncogene **6:** 1015–1021.
42. KORC, M. 1991. Growth factors and pancreatic cancer. Int. J. Pancreatol. **9:** 87–91.
43. LÖHR, M., B. TRAUTMANN, M. GÖTTLER, S. PETERS, I. ZAUNER, B. MAILLET & G. KLÖPPEL. 1994. Human ductal adenocarcinomas of the pancreas express extracellular matrix proteins. Br. J. Cancer **69:** 144–151.
44. LÖHR, M., B.TRAUTMANN, M. GÖTTLER, S.PETERS, I. ZAUNER, A. MEIER, G. KLÖPPELG, S. LIEBE & E.D. KREUSER. 1996. Expression and function of receptors for extracellular matrix proteins in human ductal adenocarcinomas of the pancreas. Pancreas **12:** 248–259.
45. TRAUTMANN, B. et al. 1993. Isolation, culture, and characterization of human pancreatic duct cells. Pancreas **8:** 248–254.
46. JESNOWSKI, R. et al. 1998. Increasing the transfection efficacy of resting pancreatic duct epithelial cells and long term culture of human pancreatic duct epithelial cells. Panreas. In press.
47. AUSUBEL, F.M., R. BRENT, R.E. KINGSTON, J.G. SEIDMAN, J.A. SMITH & K. STRUHL. 1990. Current Protocols in Molecular Biology. Greene Publisher Assoc. Brooklyn, NY. 1994th ed.
48. HELLER, T., B. TRAUTMANN, I. ZÖLLER-UTZ, H.J. KÖNIG, C. ELL, S. LIEBE & M. LÖHR. 1995. Restriktionsenzym-Mismatch-Polymerase-Kettenreaktion zum Nachweis von ki-ras-Onkogen-Mutationen beim Pankreaskarzinom. Dtsche. Med. Wchnschr. **120:** 826–830.
49. CHEN, J.K. et al. 1993. Cyclic AMP-induced inhibition of collagen lattice contraction by fibroblasts may be attenuated by both cyclic AMP dependent and independent mechanisms. J. Cell Physiol. **155:** 8–13.
50. MAGNALDO, I. et al. 1989. Cyclic AMP inhibits mitogen-induced DNA synthesis in hamster fibroblasts, regardless of the signalling pathway involved. FEBS Lett. **245:** 65–69.
51. TAYLOR-PAPADIMITRIOU, J. et al. 1980. Cholera toxin and analogues of cyclic AMP stimulate the growth of cultured human mammary epithelial cells. J. Cell Physiol. **102:** 317–321.
52. HORDIJK, P.L. et al. 1994. cAMP abrogates the p21 ras-mitogen-activated protein kinase pathway in fibroblasts. J. Biol. Chem. **269:** 3534–3538.
53. MCKENZIE, F.R. et al. 1996. cAMP-mediated growth inhibition in fibroblasts is not mediated via mitogen-activated protein (MAP) kinase (ERK) inhibition. cAMP-dependent protein kinase induces a temporal shift in growth factor-stimulated MAP kinases. J. Biol. Chem. **271:** 13476–13483.
54. MCGUIRE, P.G. et al. 1987. Isolation of rat aortic endothelial cells by primary explant techniques and their phenotypic modulation by defined substrata. Lab. Invest. **57:** 94–105.
55. TSAO, M.-S. et al. 1987. Establishment of propagable epithelial cell lines from normal adult rat pancreas. Exp. Cell Res. **168:** 365–375.
56. CHENG, R.Z. et al. 1997. Expression of SV40 large T antigen stimulates reversion of a chromosomal gene duplication in human cells. Exp. Cell Res. **234**(2): 300–312.
57. GIRARDI, A. et al. 1965. SV40-induced transformation of human diploid cells: crisis and recovery. J. Cell Comp. Physiol. **65:** 69–84.
58. TRUCKENMILLER, M.E. et al. 1998. A truncated SV40 large T antigen lacking the p53 binding domain overcomes p53-induced growth arrest and immortalizes primary mesencephalic cells. Cell Tissue Res. **291**(2): 175–189.

59. MICHAEL-MICHALOVITZ, D. *et al.* 1991. Simian virus 40 can overcome the antiproliferative effect of wild-type p53 in the absence of stable large T antigen-p53 binding. J. Virol. **65:** 4160–4168.
60. RAY, F.A. *et al.* 1990. SV40 T antigen alone drives karyotype instability that precedes neoplastic transformation of human diploid fibroblasts. J. Cell Biochem. **42(1):** 13–31.
61. REDDEL, R.R. *et al.* 1995. SV40-induced immortalization and ras-transformation of human bronchial epithelial cells. Int. J. Cancer **61:** 199–205.
62. RHIM, J.S. *et al.* 1994. Stepwise immortalization and transformation of adult human prostate epithelial cells by a combination of HPV-18 and v-Ki-ras. Proc. Natl. Acad. Sci. USA **91:** 11874–11878.
63. CAVENDER, J.F. *et al.* 1995. Simian virus 40 large T antigen contains two independent activities that cooperate with a ras oncogene to transform rat embryo fibroblasts. J. Virol. **69:** 923–934.
64. KORC, M. 1998. Role of growth factors in pancreatic cancer. S. Oncol. Clin. N. Am. **7:** 25–41.
65. BODNAR, A. *et al.* 1998. Extension of life-span by introduction of telomerase into normal human cells. Science **279:** 349–352.

Hyperplastic and Metaplastic Changes in Pancreatic Ducts: Nomenclature and Preneoplastic Potential

GÜNTER KLÖPPEL[a,c] AND DANIEL S. LONGNECKER[b]

[a]*Department of Pathology, University of Kiel, Michaelisstrasse 11, D-24105 Kiel, Germany*

[b]*Department of Pathology, Dartmouth-Hitchcock Medical Center, One Medical Center Drive, Lebanon, New Hampshire 03756, USA*

INTRODUCTION

Changes in the duct epithelium were first described by Priesel in 1922,[1] and Sommers *et al.* in 1954.[2] Sommers distinguished a papillary hyperplasia from an adenomatous ductular proliferation. Currently recognized ductal epithelial lesions include ulceration, squamous, mucous and pyloric gland metaplasia, and a continuum of hyperplastic and dysplastic changes. TABLE 1 lists recommended terms as well as others that have been used previously to designate the lesions. There is a need for standardization of nomenclature for these lesions, and we recommend the adoption of simple, descriptive designations.

SQUAMOUS METAPLASIA

Squamous metaplasia is the process and the diagnostic term used when ductal epithelium is replaced by squamous epithelium. Typically, only a segment of the main duct or a branch is involved. This lesion is found in 8 to 47 percent of the nontumorous pancreases as well as in chronically inflamed pancreases.[3] Extensive squamous metaplasia may occur in the main pancreatic duct after prolonged stenting, or secondary to infestation with *Clonorchis sinensis*.[4] Although the incidence of squamous metaplasia increases with age,[5] no association with pancreatic cancer has been noted.[3]

Changes described as focal epithelial hyperplasia[3,6] and basal cell metaplasia[7] exhibit an increase in number of epithelial layers with incomplete squamous metaplasia. These can be regarded as an immature variant of squamous metaplasia. The surface layer in immature squamous metaplasia may retain mucus cells.

---

[c]Corresponding author: Günter Klöppel, MD, Department of Pathology, University of Kiel, Michaelisstr. 11, D-24105 Kiel, Germany. Phone, +49 431–597–3400; fax, +49 431–597–3462; e-mail, gkloeppel@path.uni-kiel.de

TABLE 1. List of recommended terms with synonyms for focal proliferative and metaplastic lesions in the human exocrine pancreas[a]

Recommended term	WHO classification[21]	Other synonyms
squamous metaplasia	same	epidermoid metaplasia, multilayered metaplasia
incomplete squamous metaplasia	same	focal epithelial hyperplasia, focal atypical epithelial hyperplasia, multilayered metaplasia
ductal nonpapillary hyperplasia	mucinous cell hypertrophy	mucinous cell hyperplasia, mucoid transformation, simple hyperplasia, flat ductal hyperplasia, mucous hypertrophy, hyperplasia with pyloric gland metaplasia, ductal hyperplasia grade 1, non-papillary epithelial hypertrophy
ductal papillary hyperplasia	same	papillary ductal hyperplasia, ductal hyperplasia grade 2
adenomatoid ductal hyperplasia	same	adenomatous hyperplasia, ductular cell hyperplasia
severe ductal dysplasia	same	ductal hyperplasia grade 3, atypical hyperplasia,
tubular complex	tubular hyperplasia	ductal complex, ductular hyperplasia, ductal metaplasia

[a]References 3, 6, 8, 10, 11, 13, 17, 20, 21.

DUCTAL NONPAPILLARY HYPERPLASIA

Ductal nonpapillary hyperplasia (mucinous cell hypertrophy, see TABLE 1) indicates the replacement of the ductal epithelium by tall columnar cells with elongated basal nuclei and considerable supranuclear mucin (FIG. 1). These cells appear crowded, and their elongated nuclei are arranged perpendicularly to the basement membrane. The change may occur in ducts of any size. Neutral mucin and sialomucin are found in these cells, while sulphated mucin that is normally produced in the ducts is markedly reduced.[8] Occasionally there are also pyloric type gland cells that stain intensely with periodic acid-Schiff.[9] These are particularly seen in small glands surrounding a large- or medium-sized duct with nonpapillary hyperplasia.

This change has also been called mucinous cell hypertrophy. However, the number of cells is increased, and the designation of hyperplasia seems more appropriate even though mitoses are seldom seen. Conversion of ductal epithelium into tall mucin-containing columnar cells of the intestinal or goblet type should also be regarded as metaplasia, since these are not normal duct cell phenotypes.[10]

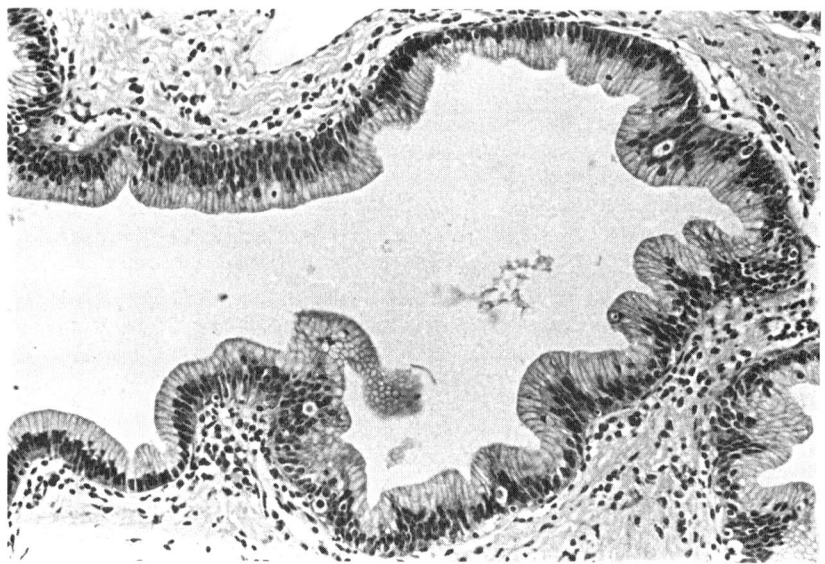

FIGURE 1. Medium-sized pancreatic duct showing ductal nonpapillary hyperplasia in association with beginning papillary hyperplasia. The epithelium is well differentiated and contains large amounts of mucin in the apical part of the cell. Hemotoxylin and eosin (H&E) stain, ×240.

This is the most frequent epithelial change in the pancreatic ducts. Changes of this type were present in 55% of one series.[11] It was found in 86% of nontumorous pancreases in another autopsy series.[12]

Ductal nonpapillary hyperplasia is particularly prevalent in association with moderate obstruction and chronic pancreatitis. It occurred in about the same percentage of patients with pancreatic cancer as in a matched control group of patients with other types of nonpancreatic cancer.[3,13]

DUCTAL PAPILLARY HYPERPLASIA

Ductal papillary hyperplasia is characterized by the formation of papillary folds of hyperplastic ductal cells similar to those seen in nonpapillary hyperplasia. Papillary hyperplasia occurs in large and medium ducts. The papillary epithelial folds characteristically contain a vascular tissue stalk (FIG. 2). In general, the epithelium has the same characteristics as are seen in nonpapillary hyperplasia, but pseudostratification is more likely to be seen.

The incidence of ductal papillary hyperplasia increases with age and is higher in patients with pancreatic cancer than in control autopsy patients without pancreatic cancer (50 vs 12%).[3,13,8] Kozuka detected no ductal hyperplasia in infants and children.[10]

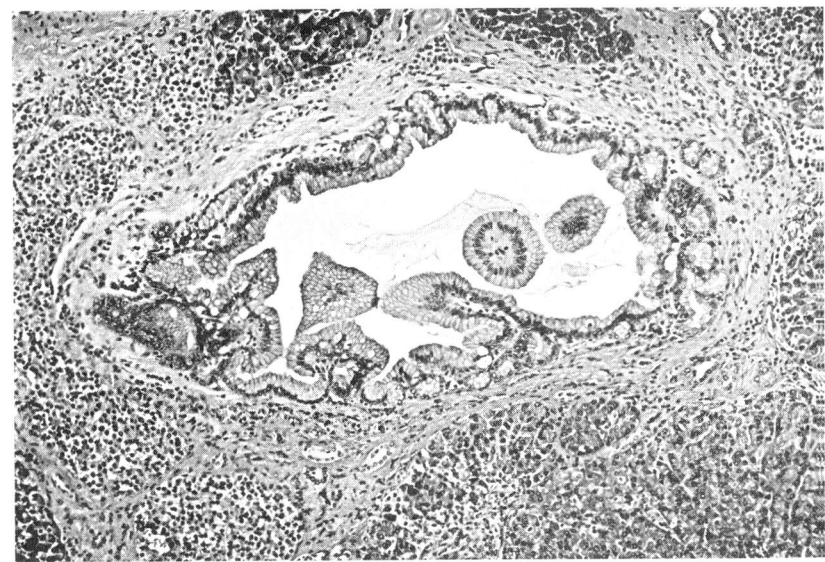

FIGURE 2. Pancreatic duct showing ductal papillary hyperplasia (*left lower part*) in association with nonpapillary hyperplasia. H&E, ×120.

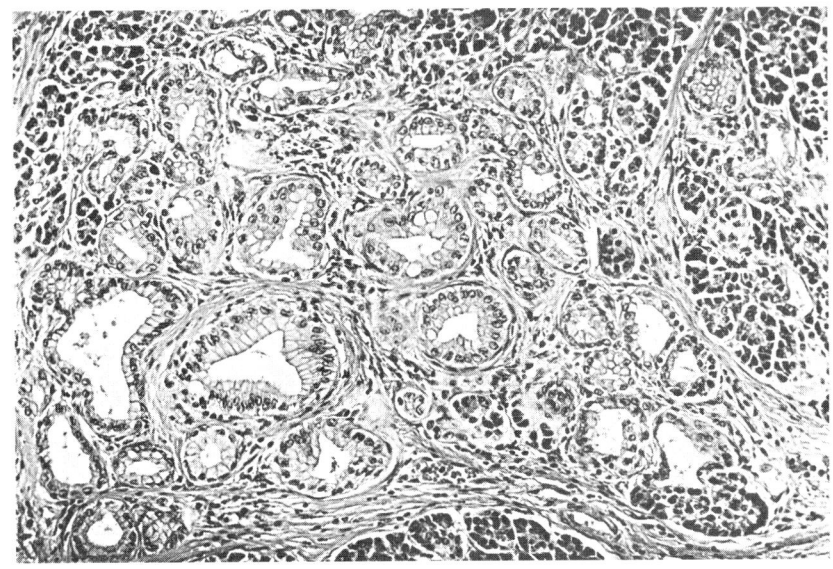

FIGURE 3. Adenomatoid ductal hyperplasia composed of small ducts lined by mucin containing columnar cells. H&E, ×240.

ADENOMATOID DUCTAL HYPERPLASIA

Adenomatoid ductal hyperplasia is characterized by aggregation of small ducts or acini lined by mucus-containing epithelial cells that commonly exhibit pyloric gland metaplasia (FIG. 3). Occasionally this lesion forms small adenoma-like nodules,[14] but the lesion is not regarded as a neoplasm.

Ductal nonpapillary and papillary hyperplasia may be found adjacent to one another in the same duct, and both are often closely associated with focal adenomatoid ductal hyperplasia.[2,15] Ductal hyperplasia is commonly multifocal within a pancreas, and all three patterns are commonly present in the same pancreas. These changes can usually easily be distinguished from the much rarer tubular complexes that are discussed below.

SEVERE DUCTAL DYSPLASIA

Severe ductal dysplasia defines a severe cellular atypia of the duct epithelium, with or without papillary proliferation. The cells of this unequivocally neoplastic lesion show enlarged nuclei, reduced or no mucin and an increased nuclear cytoplasmic ratio. Mitotic figures may be seen. Papillary structures usually lack stromal cores. Some authors distinguish between ductal papillary hyperplasia with severe atypia (dyplasia) and carcinoma *in situ*, but morphometric evaluation of this distinction has suggested that it is clinically meaningless.[16] Severe ductal dysplasia or atypical hyperplasia, as it is also called (see TABLE 1), is usually found in close proximity to well-differentiated ductal adenocarcinoma (FIG. 4). In this condition, the lesion

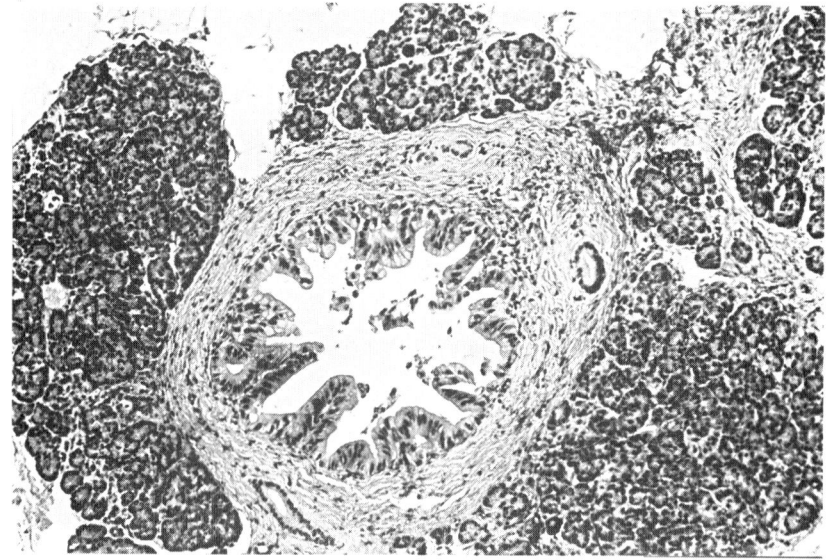

FIGURE 4. Severe ductal dysplasia-carcinoma *in situ* lesion in close proximity to an invasive ductal adenocarcinoma. H&E, ×120.

may therefore represent intraductal extension from an established invasive carcinoma rather than a multicentric tumor focus.

TUBULAR COMPLEX

Tubular complex denotes the replacement of acinar tissue focally or in entire lobules by tubular or ductular structures. The lumens remain small in the size range of acini or small ductules. The cells lining these structures most often have characteristics of centroacinar or ductal cells, but acinar cells may be interspersed.

The origin of these lesions is felt to involve metaplasia of acinar cells to assume a ductal phenotype. Loss of apical cytoplasm appears to be the initial step in this process.[17] This lesion has also been called focal acinar dilation.[11]

A form of tubular complexes is seen in chronic pancreatitis.[17] In the context of chronic pancreatitis, they seem to reflect atrophic or regressive changes, and these lesions typically have a conspicuous fibrous stroma. A similar change has been described in uremia,[11] and cachexia. In both chronic pancreatitis and uremia, the change may be widespread, patchy or diffuse, rather than focal.

Tubular complexes may also occur in apparently normal pancreases, and in this setting may represent a different category of lesion. These lesions have also been called ductular hyperplasia[5] and ductal metaplasia,[18] reflecting the uncertainty as to whether they arise as a result of proliferation of ductular cells to replace acinar cells or metaplasia of acinar cells to a ductal phenotype. The cells lining these structures do not appear atrophic, and may contain mucin, although they usually do not show mucous metaplasia as discussed above. Such lesions have minimal stroma between the ductular units. Lesions with high mucus content may represent variants of adenomatoid ductal hyperplasia. Similarity to those induced in rodents by pancreatic carcinogens has been noted.[19,3] In animal models, it is clear that some of these lesions give rise to acinar cell carcinomas.

PHENOTYPIC INTERRELATIONSHIPS AND PRENEOPLASTIC POTENTIAL

The three categories of focal epithelial lesions that are described as ductal nonpapillary hyperplasia, ductal papillary hyperplasia, and adenomatoid ductal hyperplasia appear to be closely related. They are usually closely associated, suggesting that these three patterns of ductal change may have a common etiology[20,21] and represent a biologic continuum.[10] It seems intuitive that nonpapillary hyperplasia precedes papillary hyperplasia in ducts. Adenomatoid ductal hyperplasia seems to represent extension of metaplasia and hyperplasia into small branch ducts and intralobular ductules or coincident development in these sites.

Dysplastic changes suggesting neoplastic progression in ducts are usually seen in papillary lesions, but severe dysplasia has also been observed in nonpapillary hyperplastic ductal epithelium. A sequence of ductal hyperplasia, dysplasia and carcinoma is therefore assumed to occur.[10] However, it has to be emphasized that a transition from a ductal papillary hyperplasia to carcinoma *in situ* and invasive ductal adenocarcinoma is usually only seen in the vicinity of an already invasive carcinoma, while the same finding in a pancreas without a grossly visible invasive carcinoma has yet to be established.

It is widely assumed that some of the focal lesions in ducts are precursors in the development of exocrine pancreatic neoplasms, i.e., preneoplastic lesions. The basis for this assumption is that some of these lesions, notably ductal nonpapillary and papillary hyperplasia, are found in increased incidence in pancreases with ductal adenocarcinoma, often in close proximity to the primary tumor. There are several key studies based on this approach.[3,10,13] A second reason for the assumption of preneoplastic significance is the similarity of some of these lesions to severe ductal dysplasia-carcinoma *in situ* changes in the human pancreas and focal lesions induced in animal models of pancreatic carcinogenesis.[13] In these models it is possible to follow the evolution of some of the lesions sequentially through stages of increasing dysplasia to frank malignancy. Refined molecular technology allows a third approach that is beginning to contribute data bearing on the preneoplastic significance of focal lesions. Immunostaining and microdissection of samples for polymerase chain reaction (PCR)-based analyses of individual lesions allows evaluation of the expression of some oncogenes and tumor suppressor genes in these focal lesions. This new information is beginning to alter assessment of the significance of some lesions. It has been found that hyperplastic duct lesions commonly exhibit mutations of the K-ras gene at codon 12, a mutation that occurs in 80–95% of pancreatic ductal adenocarcinomas (for further details see contributions by Longnecker and others in this volume). Hyperplastic duct lesions with codon 12 K-ras mutations were not only detected in the pancreas with an invasive carcinoma but also in non-neoplastic pancreases with or without inflammation.[12,23]

REFERENCES

1. PRIESEL, A. 1922. Beiträge zur Pathologie der Bauchspeicheldrüse. Frankf. Z. Pathol. **26:** 453–518.
2. SOMMERS, S.C., S.A. MURPHY & S. WARREN. 1954. Pancreatic duct hyperplasia and cancer. Gastroenterology **27:** 629–640.
3. CUBILLA, A.L. & P.J. FITZGERALD. 1976. Morphological lesions associated with human primary invasive nonendocrine pancreas cancer. Cancer Res. **36:** 2690–2698.
4. CHAN, P. & T.B. TEOH. 1967. The pathology of *Clonorchis sinensis* infestation of the pancreas. J. Pathol. **93:** 185–189.
5. POUR, P.M., S. SAYED & G. SAYED. 1982. Hyperplastic, preneoplastic and neoplastic lesions found in 83 human pancreases. Am. J. Clin. Pathol. **77:** 137–152.
6. OERTEL, J.E. 1989. The pancreas. Non-neoplastic alterations. Am. J. Surg. Pathol. **13:** 50–65.
7. KORPASSY, B. 1939. Die Basalzellmetaplasie der Ausführungsgänge des Pankreas. Virchows Arch. Pathol. Anat. **303:** 359–378.
8. CHEN, J., S.I. BAITHUN & M.A. RAMSAY. 1985. Histogenesis of pancreatic carcinoma: a study based on 248 cases. J. Pathol. **146:** 65–76.
9. SESSA, F., M. BONATO, B. FRIGERIO *et al.* 1990. Ductal cancers of the pancreas frequently express markers of gastrointestinal epithelial cells. Gastroenterology **98:** 1655–1665.
10. KOZUKA, S., R. SASSA, T. TAKI *et al.* 1979. Relation of pancreatic duct hyperplasia to carcinoma. Cancer **43:** 1418–1428.
11. STAMM, B.H. 1984. Incidence and diagnostic significance of minor pathologic changes in the adult pancreas at autopsy: a systematic study of 112 autopsies in patients with known pancreatic disease. Hum. Pathol. **15:** 677–683.

12. TADA, M., M. OHASHI, Y. SHIRATORI et al. 1996. Analysis of K-ras gene mutation in hyperplastic duct cells of the pancreas without pancreatic disease. Gastroenterology **110:** 227–231.
13. KLÖPPEL, G., G. BOMMER, K. RÜCKERT et al. 1980. Intraductal proliferation in the pancreas and its relationship to human and experimental carcinogenesis. Virchows Arch. A **387:** 221–233.
14. KLÖPPEL, G. 1993. Pathology of nonendocrine pancreatic tumors. *In* The Pancreas: Biology, Pathobiology, and Disease. V.L.W. Go, E.P. DiMagno, J.D. Gardner et al., Eds.: 871–897. Raven Press. New York.
15. TERHUNE, P.G., D.M. PHIFER, T.D. TOSTESON et al. 1998. K-ras mutation in focal proliferative lesions of human pancreas. Cancer Epidemiol. Biomarkers Prevention **7:** 515–521.
16. FURUKAWA, T., R. CHIBA, M. KOBAIN et al. 1994. Varying grades of epithelial atypia in the pancreatic ducts of humans: classification based on morphometry and multivariate analysis and corrlated with positive reactions of carcinoembryonic antigen. Arch. Pathol. Lab. Med. **118:** 227–234.
17. BOCKMANN, D.E. 1981. Cells of origin of pancreatic cancer. Experimental animal tumors related to human pancreas. Cancer. **47:** 1528–1534.
18. PARSA, I., D.S. LONGNECKER, D.G. SCARPELLI et al. 1985. Ductal metaplasia of human exocrine pancreas and its association with carcinoma. Cancer Res. **45:** 1285–1290.
19. LONGNECKER, D.S., Y. HASHIDA & H. SHINOZUKA. 1980. Relationship of age to prevalence of focal acinar cell dysplasia in the human pancreas. J. Natl. Cancer Inst. **65:** 63–66.
20. POUR, P.M., Y. KONISHI, G. KLÖPPEL et al. 1994. Atlas of Exocrine Pancreatic Tumours: Morphology, Biology, and Diagnosis with an International Guide for Tumour Classification. Springer. Tokyo.
21. KLÖPPEL, G., E. SOLCIA, D.S. LONGNECKER et al. 1996. Histological Typing of Tumours of the Exocrine Pancreas. 2nd edit. WHO International Histological Classification of Tumours. Springer. Berlin.
22. YANAGISAWA, A., K. OHTAKE, K. OHASHI et al. 1993. Frequent c-Ki-ras oncogene activation in mucous cell hyperplasias of pancreas suffering from chronic inflammation. Cancer Res. **53:** 953–956.
23. KLÖPPEL, G., A. REINECKE-LÜTHGE, B. MÖLLMANN et al. 1999. Duct changes and K-ras mutation in the disease-free pancreas: an analysis of type, age relation and spatial distribution. Langenbecks Arch. Surg. **384:** 111.

Molecular Pathology of Invasive Carcinoma

DANIEL S. LONGNECKER[a]

Department of Pathology, Dartmouth Medical School, Lebanon, New Hampshire 03756, USA

> ABSTRACT: Abnormalities of several oncogenes and tumor suppressor genes have been identified in carcinomas of the pancreas during the last decade, and multiple genetic changes have been demonstrated in individual carcinomas. The variety of genetic changes suggests that multiple etiologic factors contribute to carcinogenesis in the pancreas. Several of these changes are characteristically found in specific types of tumors, suggesting that different causes and molecular mechanisms are involved. One example is the loss of heterozygosity at the von Hippel-Lindau (VHL) gene locus in both wild type and hereditary serous cystadenomas, and another is the virtual absence of K-*ras* mutation and *p53* abnormalities in acinar cell carcinomas, whereas both are frequently found in ductal adenocarcinomas. Multiple lines of evidence place *K-ras* mutation very early and loss of *p53* and *p16* as late events during ductal cell carcinogenesis. The timing and order of other genetic changes such as loss of the *DPC4* tumor suppressor function is less certain.

INTRODUCTION

Knowledge of the specific gene targets in carcinogenesis is relatively new and was initially based mainly on the study of neoplasms other than those of the pancreas. During the past 10 years, a great deal has been learned about the genetic abnormalities that are found in pancreatic ductal adenocarcinomas, the most prevalent type of pancreatic cancer. Several excellent reviews of this topic are available, and should be consulted for additional details and perspectives.[1-8] This review will briefly summarize the current status of the field and explore some issues that these new data have raised.

The view that neoplasms are caused by genetic changes in cells had gained a high level of acceptance in the field of carcinogenesis research during the several decades preceeding the first identification of a specific oncogene in the mid-1980s. The study of neoplasms by new molecular techniques since that time has firmly established the concept that several mutations or other functional genetic abnormalities are required to convert a normal cell to a neoplastic cell. The identification of tumor suppressor genes beginning in 1987 strengthened the logical basis for a synergy of multiple genetic abnormalities in establishing neoplastic growth potential. The idea that defects in DNA repair would predispose to the development of neoplasms also antedated the identification of specific genes for DNA repair pathways. This concept has also been supported by new molecular data.

---

[a]Address for correspondence: Daniel S. Longnecker, MD, Department of Pathology, Dartmouth-Hitchcock Medical Center, One Medical Center Drive, Lebanon, NH 03756. Phone, 603/650-7899; fax, 603/650-6120; e-mail, daniel.s.longnecker@dartmouth.edu

TABLE 1. Oncogenes and oncogene products reported to be mutated, amplified, or overexpressed in pancreatic cancer

Class	Examples
Growth factors	TGF-α, EGF, TGF-β, PDGF, FGFs
Growth factor receptors	EGFR, *c-erb B-2, c-erb B-3, c-erb B-4, c-met*
Intracellular signal transducers	
protein-serine/threonine kinases	AKT2
guanine nucleotide-binding proteins	*K-ras*
Nuclear transcription factors	*c-myc, c-fos*

MOLECULAR ABNORMALITIES IN DUCTAL ADENOCARCINOMAS OF THE PANCREAS

Loss or gain of function of five general categories of gene activity can contribute to the development of a neoplastic phenotype, and even that list is a simplification. These categories are:
(1) Oncogenes
(2) Tumor suppressor genes
(3) DNA repair genes
(4) Longevity genes that control apoptosis
(5) Immortalizing genes

Structural or functional abnormalities of genes or gene products in four of these groups have been reported in pancreatic neoplasms, usually in ductal adenocarcinomas. TABLE 1 lists genes that fall into the protooncogene/oncogene group of growth promoting genes, and TABLE 2 lists the major growth-inhibiting tumor suppressor genes associated with pancreatic neoplasms. Some authorities would classify DNA repair genes as a subset of tumor suppressors.

Carcinoma of the pancreas has the highest rate of mutational activation of the *K-ras* oncogene demonstrated in any cancer. The rate is commonly said to be in the range of 75–100 percent, and many reports cite the higher end of this range.[9–13] Several published series of pancreatic carcinomas report *K-ras* mutation rates of less than 70 percent,[14–19] and we conclude that a more accurate statement of the rate,

TABLE 2. Tumor suppressor genes reported to be inactivated in pancreatic cancer

Gene	Overall rate
p16	~30–80%
DPC4	~50%
p53	~30–50%
BRCA2	low
Rb	low
Others (APC)	controversial

even for series consisting entirely of ductal adenocarcinomas and its subtypes, should clearly use an upper limit of less than 100 percent.[20] As is indicated below, K-ras mutation is absent or rare in several other histologic types of pancreatic carcinomas, so the overall rate of K-ras mutaton in pancreatic neoplasms is even lower, perhaps 75–85 percent. It is striking that nearly all the K-ras mutations reported in pancreatic carcinomas are in codon 12, whereas mutations in codons 13 or 61 are more common in carcinomas from other sites.[4,21] Within codon 12, a variety of specific mutations have been identified. Mutations of the normal GGT sequence to GAT are most frequent in Western series.[4]

Although overexpression of transforming growth factor-α (TGF-α) and several other growth factors and receptors is common in ductal adenocarcinomas,[8,22] mutation, amplification or overexpression of oncogenes other than K-ras that are part of intracellular signal transduction pathways are reported in a smaller fraction of pancreatic carcinomas, e.g., AKT2,[3] or have been evaluated only in small series or a few cell lines, e.g., c-myc and c-fos.[23, 24] AKT2 is reported to be amplified in 7–10 percent of ductal adenocarcinomas.[6] The data for c-myc and c-fos are too few to establish a rate of abnormal expression. Similarly, growth factor receptors that are reported in limited series include c-met, the receptor for hepatocyte growth factor.[25]

The increased risk of carcinoma of the pancreas that is reported in families with the hereditary nonpolyposis colorectal cancer (HNPCC) syndrome[26] establishes the potential importance of defective DNA repair in pancreatic carcinogenesis. This is further supported by reports of microsatellite instability, an indicator of defective repair, in four percent of one sizable series of pancreatic carcinomas.[27] All hereditary syndromes that predispose to development of carcinoma of the pancreas have been estimated to contribute about five percent of cases.[28] These numbers suggest that defects in DNA repair play a role in the genesis of less than five percent of pancreatic carcinomas.

The genes underlying the hereditary syndromes that predispose to pancreatic cancers are dominated by tumor suppressor genes, which function in a recessive manner (TABLE 3). The affected individual typically inherits one defective and one normal copy of the critical gene, and then the good gene is mutated or deleted in somatic cells so that function is lost. In sporadic (nonfamilial) cancers, both alleles of the tumor suppressor gene must be mutated or lost.

TABLE 3. Hereditary cancer syndromes affecting the pancreas

Syndrome (acronym)	Gene Defect or Comment
Hereditary nonpolyposis colon cancer (HNPCC)	Defective DNA mismatch repair enzymes
Familial atypical multiple mole melanoma (FAMMM)	p16
Familial breast cancer	BRCA2
Ataxia-telangectasia	ATM
von Hippel-Lindau disease	VHL
Familial pancreatitis	cationic trypsin
Peutz-Jeghers	unknown

TABLE 4. Incidence of single and multiple mutations in 42 pancreatic adenocarcinomas that were evaluated for genetic alterations in *p16*, *p53*, and *DPC4*, and for *K-ras* mutation[28]

Number of Abnormal Genes	Percent
4	38
3	38
2	15
1	8

There is no report of abnormalities of apoptosis genes that prolong the lifespan of individual cells, unless one assigns defective *p53* function to this group in addition to classifying it as a tumor suppressor gene. It is not clear if genes such as BCL2 have been evaluated in pancreatic neoplasms. (For new information on this topic, see H. Kalthoff, this volume.)

Recent reports of increased telomerase activity in high fractions of two series of pancreatic carcinomas provides a mechanism that can contribute to immortalization of a cell lineage.[18,29] The structural basis for the increased activity of telomerase has not been defined.

The information summarized in TABLE 2 suggests that more than one tumor suppressor gene must be inactivated in a considerable fraction of pancreatic carcinomas because of the high prevalence of several of the abnormalities. A recent report documents that most ductal adenocarcinomas have genetic abnormalities in two or more of the four most commonly involved genes (TABLE 4).[30] These data directly support the concept that multiple genetic changes are required to establish a malignant phenotype. *K-ras* mutation was the one abnormality present in all of this series. This is consistent with many other studies suggesting that *K-ras* mutation is an early event in the genesis of most pancreatic ductal adenocarcinomas. Murakami[3] has speculated on the timing and order of occurrence of the common mutations found in pancreatic adenocarcinoma. He concludes that *K-ras* mutation occurs early and that *p16* and *p53* inactivation occur late in carcinogenesis, leaving *DPC4* in limbo for the present.

MOLECULAR CHANGES IN OTHER TYPES OF CARCINOMA

Several histologic types of carcinoma of the pancreas seem rarely or never to harbor *K-ras* mutation. Thirty-two of 33 acinar cell carcinomas are reported to have wild-type *K-ras*.[31–33] Acinar cell carcinomas also seem consistently to lack abnormalities of the *p53* gene.[34] Pancreaticoblastoma,[35] solid pseudopapillary tumors,[32,36] serous cystadenomas, and one serous cystadenocarcinoma[37] are all reported to have only wild-type *K-ras* in the cases that have been studied. Composite series of intraductal papillary mucinous carcinomas and mucinous cystic tumors are reported to have a mutational rate (54 percent)[38] that is lower than the average for ductal adenocarcinomas. Inclusion of types of carcinomas other than ductal in any series should influence the observed rate of *K-ras* mutation, so it is important to carefully specify the types of tumors that are included when abnormality of *K-ras* or any other gene is evaluated.

Serous cystadenomas have occurred in some patients with von Hippel-Lindau (VHL) disease. Loss of heterozygosity at the VHL gene locus was demonstrated in both of two such tumors from patients with VHL disease.[39] Furthermore, loss of heterozygosity was present in seven of 10 sporadic cases of serous cystadenoma, suggesting that abnormalities of the VHL gene are associated with the genesis of these tumors.

CLINICAL APPLICATIONS OF MOLECULAR DATA

Beyond gaining an understanding of the molecular mechanisms of carcinogenesis, researchers are making numerous attempts to apply new molecular data to solve clinical problems in the diagnosis and treatment of pancreatic cancer.

The simplest application is correlation of survival with the presence or absence of specific changes in oncogenes and tumor suppressor genes. In general there has been no consistent correlation of prognosis with the presence of mutant vs wild-type *K-ras*, although one report indicates that survival is poorer for patients whose cancers have two mutations, and is poorer for patients with GAT compared with other mutations in codon 12.[40] On the other hand, the loss of *p53*, expression of c-erbB-3, and the coexpression of epidermal growth factor receptor (EGFR) and either EGF or TGF-α in carcinomas have all been associated with shorter survival (Korc, quoted in Ref. 41).[8] While this type of information has limited utility at present, it might become more important when the range of therapeutic options for carcinoma of the pancreas is expanded.

Knowledge of the genetic abnormalities may have potential therapeutic implications, either for selection of specific chemotherapeutic agents, or for application of "gene therapy." A straightforward and relevant example of the former is the potential use of farnesyl transferase inhibitors for treatment of patients with carcinomas that harbor mutant *K-ras*.[42] Such agents would obviously find application in many patients with ductal adenocarcinomas of the pancreas. Therapeutic strategies classed as gene therapy are so diverse that no discussion will be attempted here. Other reviews should be consulted for an introduction to this field.[4]

Application of molecular approaches to the diagnosis of pancreatic cancer is the focus of considerable effort currently. Most studies have focussed on detection of mutant codon 12 *K-ras* sequences because of the high prevalence of these mutations in pancreatic cancers, and because assays based on the polymerase chain reaction (PCR) are sensitive and specific in detection of the mutations. Such assays have been applied to DNA harvested from pancreatic juice,[43–45] bile[46] pancreatic duct brushings obtained by endoscopic retrograde cholangiopancreatography (ERCP),[47] duodenal aspirates[19] and lavage samples, fecal specimens,[48] blood,[49,50] plasma,[49] and fine needle aspiration biopsy.[52,53] Mutant *K-ras* has been demonstrated in samples from each of these sources. The rate of detection of *K-ras* mutation is clearly higher among samples obtained from patients with ductal carcinomas than from patients with other pancreatic diseases, usually chronic pancreatitis, and the specific mutation has been the same as that demonstrated in the primary neoplasms in numerous instances. There is no question that the assays can detect mutations in DNA that was apparently shed from pancreatic neoplasms. However, issues of both sensitivity and specificity arise. Series based on pancreatic juice[44] and duodenal fluid specimens[54] have yielded positive results in the absence of clinically detected pancreatic carcinoma.

A number of reports now support the finding that mutation of the *K-ras* gene is a common event in pancreatic ductal epithelium.[55] *K-ras* mutations have been demonstrated in foci of hyperplasia of pancreatic duct cells in pancreases without a carcinoma, and in foci of flat, papillary, or adenomatoid ductal hyperplasia that lack dysplastic cellular changes associated with preneoplastic change. We have found mutant *K-ras* in about half of such foci, and have calculated the probability that any one such focus with mutant *K-ras* will progress to become a carcinoma is less than 1 percent.[55] This finding predicts that application of sensitive PCR-based methods for detection of *K-ras* mutations to pancreatic juice, duct brushings, or duodenal lavage specimens has the potential to yield a significant rate of positive results in the absence of a carcinoma, or even carcinoma *in situ*. Mutant *K-ras* has been reported in a pancreatic juice sample when ductal hyperplasia but no carcinoma was present.[43] To a lesser extent, this concern extends to samples obtained by fine needle aspiration (FNA) biopsy. Several investigators have questioned the diagnostic significance of the finding of *K-ras* mutation in such specimens.[3,6,7,55] It appears that assays for additional or alternate abnormalities will be required to avoid an unacceptable false positive rate.

Detection of the *K-ras* mutations in either cellular or soluble DNA[51] in the blood would seem to require the presence of an invasive carcinoma that harbored the mutation in the pancreas or elsewhere. This approach seems free of the hazard of a false positive arising from a ductal hyperplasia with mutant *K-ras,* but questions of sensitivity for detection of small carcinomas and specificity for pancreatic carcinoma remain.

Since *K-ras* mutations do not occur in all ductal adenocarcinomas, even less often in intraductal papillary-mucinous neoplasms and mucinous cystic neoplasms, and perhaps never in several rare types of pancreatic neoplasms, all methods for diagnosis or screening based on detection of such mutations seem likely to yield false negative results in 15–25 percent of patients with a pancreatic neoplasm.

Alternate molecular parameters that have been evaluated in the context of diagnosis of carcinomas include assays for telomerase activity, staining cytologic samples for *p53*, and staining for tumor markers such as CEA and CA19-9.

COMMENTS

The data reviewed above provide an overall picture of the genetic basis of ductal adenocarcinoma of the pancreas; however, many details are missing. Thus, further progress will require filling in details that pertain to minor fractions of ductal adenocarcinomas, and establishing the genetic basis for less common and rare pancreatic neoplasms. Several examples of such detail can easily be identified.

Hruban[7] lists several chromosomal loci that are deleted in small but significant fractions of pancreatic carcinomas, and suggests that they might be the site of additional tumor suppressor genes that have not yet been identified. These are located on as many as 10 different chromosomes, especially including 1, 6 and 7, i.e., chromosomes other than those on which *p16* (on 9p), *p53* (on 17p) and *DPC4* (on 18q) are located. If such new tumor suppressor genes are identified, they become candidates for a role in sporadic pancreatic cancers, as is the case for *p16, p53* and *BRCA2*, and also become candidates for assessment in familial groups of pancreatic cancers for which no predisposing germline mutation is known.

We need to know if another oncogene is activated or overexpressed in pancreatic ductal adenocarcinomas that lack a mutation in *K-ras,* or is the ras protein overexpressed in such tumors? The *AKT2* gene is a candidate for such a role.

We need to know more about the genetic basis of the less common histologic types of pancreatic neoplasms. We have several clues indicating that they will have different genetic abnormalities, for example, the occurrence of serous cystadenomas in patients with VHL disease and the presence of abnormalities of the VHL locus in sporadic cases.[39]

Filling in these and other details presents a challenge, because the study of rare events requires larger numbers of tumors; assembling an adequate number of rare tumors such as solid pseudopapillary tumors is difficult or impossible in a single center; and study of minor subsets of common tumors will present a similar problem, e.g., assembly of a sizable group of ductal adenocarcinomas with wild-type *K-ras*. The devil is in the details.

REFERENCES

1. CALDAS, C. & S.E. KERN. 1995. K-ras mutation and pancreatic adenocarcinoma: state-of-the-art. Int. J. Pancreatol. **18:** 1–6.
2. HAHN, S.A. & S.E. KERN. 1995. Molecular genetics of exocrine pancreatic neoplasms. Surg. Clin. North Am. **75:** 857–869.
3. MURAKAMI, Y. 1997. Genetic alterations in human pancreatic cancer. J. Hep. Bil. Pancr. Surg. **4:** 283–290.
4. LEMOINE, N.R. 1997. Molecular pathology of pancreatic duct neoplasms. *In* Biliary and Pancreatic Ductal Epithelia. Pathobiology and Pathophysiology. A.E. Sirica & D.S. Longnecker, Eds.: 505–525. Marcel Dekker. New York.
5. HOWE, J.R. & K.C. CONLON.1997. The molecular genetics of pancreatic cancer. Surg. Oncol. **6:** 1–18.
6. SLEBOS, R.J.C., H.M. CEHA, S.E. KERN *et al.* 1998. Molecular genetics of pancreatic cancer. *In* Pancreatic Cancer: Advances in Molecular Pathology, Diagnosis & Clinical Management. F.H. Sarkar & M.C. Dugan, Eds.: 65–82. BioTechniques Books. Natick, MA.
7. HRUBAN, R.H., G.M. PETERSEN & S.E. KERN. 1998. Genetics of pancretic cancer. From genes to families. Surg. Oncol. Clin. North Am. **7:** 1–23.
8. KORC, M. 1998. Role of growth factors in pancreatic cancer. Surg. Oncol. Clin. North Am. **7:** 25–41.
9. BANERJEE, S.K., W.F. MAKDISI, A.P. WESTON *et al.* 1997. A two-step enriched-nested PCR technique enhances sensitivity for detection of codon 12 K-ras mutations in pancreatic adenocarcinoma. Pancreas **15:** 16–24.
10. BERROZPE, G., J. SCHAEFFER, M.A. PEINADO *et al.* 1994. Comparative analysis of mutations in p53 and K-ras genes in pancreatic cancer. Int. J. Cancer **58:** 185–191.
11. BRAT, D.J., K.D. LILLEMOE, C. YEO *et al.* 1998. Progression of pancreatic intraductal neoplasias to infiltrating adenocarcinoma of the pancreas. Am. J. Surg. Pathol. **22:** 163–169.
12. TADA, M., M. OMATA, & M. OHTO. 1991. Clinical application of ras gene mutation for diagnosis of pancreatic adenocarcinoma. Gastroenterology **100:** 233–238.

13. URBAN, T., S. RICCI, J.-D. GRANGE et al. 1993. Detection of c-Ki-ras mutation by PCR/RFLP analysis and diagnosis of pancreatic adenocarcinomas. J. Natl. Cancer Inst. **85:** 2008–2012.
14. MALATS, N., M. PORTA, J.M. COROMINAS et al. 1997. Ki-ras mutations in exocrine pancreatic cancer: association with clinico-pathological characteristics and with tobacco and alcohol consumption. PANK-ras I Project Investigators. Int. J. Cancer **70:** 661–667.
15. SUGIO, K., K. MOLBERG, J. ALBORES-SAAVEDRA et al. 1997. K-ras mutations and allelic loss at 5q and 18q in the development of human pancreatic cancers. Int. J. Pancreatol. **21:** 205–217.
16. RALL, C.J., Y.X. YAN, F. GRAEME-COOK et al. 1996. Ki-ras and p53 mutations in pancreatic ductal adenocarcinoma. Pancreas **12:** 10–17.
17. TABATA, T., T. FUJIMORI, S. MAEDA et al. 1993. The role of ras mutation in pancreatic cancer, precancerous lesions, and chronic pancreatitis. Int. J. Pancreatol. **14:** 237–244.
18. TSUTSUMI, M., T.TSUJIUCHI, O. ISHIKAWA et al. 1997. Increased telomerase activities in human pancreatic duct adenocarcinomas. Jpn. J. Cancer Res. **88:** 971–976.
19. WILENTZ, R.E., C.H. CHUNG, P.D.J. STURM et al. 1998. K-ras mutations in the duodenal fluid of patients with pancreatic carcinoma. Cancer **82:** 96–103.
20. LONGNECKER, D.S. & P.G. TERHUNE. 1998. What is the true rate of KRAS mutation in carcinoma of the pancreas? Pancreas **17:** 323–324.
21. Bos, J.L. 1989. ras Oncogenes in human cancer: a review. Cancer Res. **49:** 4682–4689.
22. KORNMANN, M., H.G. BEGER & M. KORC. 1998. Role of fibroblast growth factors and their receptors in pancreatic cancer and chronic pancreatitis. Pancreas **17:** 169–175.
23. WAKITA, K., H. OHYANAGI, K. YAMAMOTO, T. TOKUHISA & Y. SAITOH. 1992. Overexpression of c-Ki-ras and c-fos in human pancreatic carcinomas. Int. J. Pancreatol. **11:** 43–47.
24. LI, D.C. & T.H. LIU. 1992. Oncogene expression and point mutation in human pancreatic adenocarcinomas. Chung-hua Ping LiHsueh Tsa Chih (China) **21:** 152–155.
25. KIEHNE, K., K.H. HERZIG & U.R. FOLSCH. 1997. c-met expression in pancreatic cancer and effects of hepatocyte growth factor on pancreatic cancer cell growth. Pancreas **15:** 35–40.
26. LYNCH, H.T. & T. SMYRK. 1996. Hereditary nonpolyposis colorectal cancer (Lynch syndrome). An updated review. Cancer **78:** 1149–1167.
27. GOGGINS, M., C.A. GRIFFIN, K. TURNACIOGLU et al. 1998. Pancreatic adenocarcinomas with DNA replication errors (RER+) are associated with wild/type K-ras and characteristic histopathology: poor differentiation, a syncytial growth pattern, and pushing borders suggest RER+. Am. J. Pathol. **152:** 1501–1507.
28. LYNCH, H.T., T. SMYRK, S.E. KERN et al. 1996. Familial pancreatic cancer: a review. Semin. Oncol. **23:** 251–275.
29. HIYAMA, E., T. KODAMA, K. SHINBARA et al. 1997. Telomerase activity is detected in pancreatic cancer but not in benign tumors. Cancer Res. **57:** 326–331.
30. ROZENBLUM, E., M. SCHUTTE, M. GOGGINS et al. 1997. Tumor-suppressive pathways in pancreatic carcinoma. Cancer Res. **57:** 1731–1734.
31. TERHUNE, P.G., C. HEFFESS & D.S. LONGNECKER. 1994. Human pancreatic acinar cell carcinomas contain only wild-type c-K-ras codons 12, 13 and 61. Mol. Carcinog. **10:** 110–114.
32. PELLEGATA, N.S., F. SESSA, B. RENAULT et al. 1994. K-ras and p53 gene mutations in pancreatic cancer: ductal and nonductal tumors progress through different genetic lesions. Cancer Res. **54:** 1556–1560.
33. HOORENS, A., N.R. LEMOINE & E. MCLELLAN. 1993. Pancreatic acinar cell carcinoma: an analysis of cell lineage markers, p53 expression, and Ki-ras mutation. Am. J. Pathol. **143:** 685–698.
34. TERHUNE, P.G., V.A. MEMOLI & D.S. LONGNECKER. 1998. Evaluation of p53 mutation in pancreatic acinar cell carcinomas of humans and transgenic mice. Pancreas **16:** 6–12.

35. DUNN, J.L. & D.S. LONGNECKER. 1995. Pancreatoblastoma in an older adult. Arch. Pathol. Lab. Med. **119:** 547–551.
36. LEE, W.-Y., C.-C. TZENG, R.M.-Y. CHEN et al. 1997. Papillary cystic tumors of the pancreas: assessment of malignant potential by analysis of progesterone receptor, flow cytometry, and ras oncogene mutation. Anticancer Res. **17:** 2587–2592.
37. ISHIKAWA, T., A. NAKAO, S. NOMOTO et al. 1998. Immunohistochemical and molecular biological studies of serous cystadenoma of the pancreas. Pancreas **16:** 40–44.
38. TERHUNE, P.G. & D.S. LONGNECKER. 1995. Do oncogene and tumor suppressor gene abnormalities vary with type of carcinoma of the pancreas? J. Hep. Bil. Pancr. Surg. **2:** 1–7.
39. VORTMEYER, A., I. LUBENSKI, F. FOGT et al. 1997. Allelic deletion and mutation of the von Hippel-Lindau (VHL) tumor suppressor gene in pancreatic microcystic adenomas. Am. J. Pathol. **151:** 951–956.
40. SONG, M., Y. NIO, Y. SATO et al. 1996. Clinicopathological significance of Ki-ras point mutation and p21 expression in benign and malignant exocrine tumors of the human pancreas. Int. J. Pancreatol. **20:** 85–93.
41. KONISHI, Y., M. TSUTSUMI & D.S. LONGNECKER. 1998. Mechanistic analysis and chemoprevention of pancreatic carcinogenesis. Pancreas **17:** 334–340.
42. URA, H., T. OBARA, R. SHUDO et al. 1998. Selective cytotoxicity of farnesylamine to pancreatic carcinoma cells and ki-ras-transformed fibroblasts. Mol. Carcinog. **21:** 93–99.
43. TRUMPER, L.H., B. BURGER, F. VON BONIN et al. 1994. Diagnosis of pancreatic adenocarcinomoa by polymerase chain reaction from pancreatic secretions. Br. J. Cancer **70:** 278–284.
44. UEHARA, H., A. NAZAIZUMI, M. BABA et al. 1996. Diagnosis of pancreatic cancer by K-ras point mutation and cytology of pancreatic juice. Am. J. Gastroenterol. **91:** 1616–1621.
45. TADA, M., T. TERATANI, Y. KOMATSU et al. 1998. Quantitative analysis of ras gene mutation in pancreatic juice for diagnosis of pancreatic adenocarcinoma. Dis. Dis. Sci. **43:** 15–20.
46. ABBRUZZESE, J.L., D.B. EVANS, I. RAIJMAN et al. 1997. Detection of mutated c-Ki-ras in the bile of patients with pancreatic cancer. Anticancer Res. **17:** 795–801.
47. VAN LAETHEM, J.L., P. VERTONGEN, J. DEVIERE et al. 1995. Detection of c-Ki-ras gene condon 12 mutations from pancreatic duct brushings in the diagnosis of pancreatic tumours. Gut **36:** 781–787.
48. CALDAS, C., S.A. HAHN, R.H. HRUBAN et al. 1994. Detection of K-ras mutations in the stool of patients with pancreatic adenocarcinoma and pancreatic ductal hyperplasia. Cancer Res. **54:** 3568–3573.
49. SORENSON, G.D., D.M. PRIBISH, F.H. VALONE et al. 1994. Soluble normal and mutated DNA sequences from single-copy genes in human blood. Cancer Epid. Biomarkers Prev. **3:** 67–71.
50. NOMOOTO, S., A. NAKAO, Y. KASAI et al. 1996. Detection of ras gene mutations in perioperative peripheral blood with pancreatic adenocarcinoma. Jpn. J. Cancer Res. **87:** 793–797.
51. MULCAHY, H.E., J. LYAUTEY, C. LEDERREY et al. 1998. A prospective study of K-ras mutations in the plasma of pancreatic cancer patients. Clin. Cancer Res. **4:** 271–275.
52. APPLE, S.K., J.R. HECHT, J.M. NOVAK et al. 1996. Polymerase chain reaction-based K-ras mutation detection of pancreatic adenocarcinoma in routine cytology smears. Am. J. Clin. Pathol. **105:** 321–326.
53. PINTO, M.M. J.R. EMANUEL, V. CHATURVEDI et al. 1997. Ki-ras mutations and the carcinembryonic antigen level in fine needle aspirates of the pancreas. Acta Cytol. **41:** 427–434.
54. FURUYA, N. S. KAWA, T. AKATMATSU et al. 1997. Long-term follow-up of patients with chronic pancreatitis and K-ras gene mutation detected in pancreatic juice. Gastroenterology **113:** 593–598.
55. TERHUNE, P.G., D.M. PHIFER, T.D. TOSTESON et al. 1998. K-ras mutation in focal proliferative lesions of human pancreas. Cancer Epid. Biomarkers Prev. **7:** 515–521.

Hollow-Spheres: A New Model for Analyses of Differentiation of Pancreatic Duct Epithelial Cells

LASSE LEHNERT,[a] HARTWIG TROST,[b] WOLFF SCHMIEGEL,[c]
CHRISTIAN RÖDER,[a] AND HOLGER KALTHOFF[a,d]

[a]*Department of Molecular Oncology, Clinic for General Surgery and Thoracic Surgery, Christian Albrechts University of Kiel, Germany*
[b]*Kreiskrankenhaus Buchholz, Nordheide, Germany*
[c]*Medical Clinic, Knappschaftskrankenhaus, Ruhr-University of Bochum, Germany*

ABSTRACT: We discovered a unique feature of a subclone of the pancreatic carcinoma cell line A818. A818-1-derived hollow-spheres developed under three-dimensional growth conditions. Hollow-spheres consist of a single layer of 50–200 epithelial cells surrounding an inner lumen. In contrast to A818-1, the subclone A818-4 and all other pancreatic tumor cell lines tested ($n = 5$), formed spheroids as the only three-dimensional phenotype. A dramatically reduced proliferation rate compared to the corresponding monolayer was observed in hollow-spheres when bromodeoxyuridine (BrdU) incorporation was measured. This finding was confirmed by immunostaining using the MIB-1 antibody. Mechanically disrupted hollow-spheres not only attached but also grew as monolayer with the same doubling time as the founder cells. Hollow-spheres developed in fetal calf serum (FCS) containing RPMI 1640 medium without additionally added cytokines. A818-1 hollow-sphere formation and integrity was influenced by interferon-γ. Tumor necrosis factor-α (TNF-α) led to cell death. Exogenously added hepatocyte growth factor (HGF) showed no effect neither on hollow-sphere formation nor on the integrity of completely developed hollow-spheres. Moreover, no changes were observed when cells were treated with a neutralizing antibody for HGF. Interestingly, hollow-spheres showed intensive immunoreactivity for the HGF-receptor (c-met) and its ligand (HGF). Immunostaining for the biliary glycoprotein (BGP), the non-specific cross-reacting antigen 95 (NCA95) and β-catenin revealed a polar organization of hollow-spheres. Immunhistochemically, hollow-spheres were negative for the carcinoembryonic antigen (CEA). When hollow-spheres were embedded into matrigel, duct-like tubes grew out. Taken together, A818-1 hollow-spheres resemble normally differentiated duct-like structures and will serve as an excellent model to study differentation of human pancreatic epithelial cells.

[d]Address for correspondence: Prof. Holger Kalthoff, Dept. of Molecular Oncology, Clinic for General Surgery and Thoracic Surgery, Christian-Albrechts-University, Arnold-Heller-Strasse 7, 24105 Kiel, FRG. Phone, +49 431-597-1938; fax, +49 431-597-1939; e-mail, hkalthoff@email.uni-kiel.de

INTRODUCTION

Cancer of the pancreas is a highly aggressive tumor that currently represents the fourth cause of cancer death in the United States. The majority of tumors arise in the exocrine component and are classified as ductal adenocarcinomas on the basis of their microscopic appearance.[1] Despite the fact that a number of molecular alterations have been reported that are associated with pancreatic cancer, including mutations in the K-*ras*, p53, and MTS-1 genes,[2] there are few clues about the aggressive nature of its biological behavior. Epigenetic alterations also contribute to tumor progression. Overexpression of growth factor receptors and their ligands such as c-*met*/hepatocyte growth factor (HGF), can lead to the activation of autocrine and paracrine loops enhancing tumor cell motility, protease secretion, and invasiveness *in vitro* and in animal models.[3] The biological relevance of these alterations is suggested by their association with a worse prognosis.[4] An autocrine effect of transforming growth factor-α (TGF-α) was reported[5] as well as the upregulation of the epidermal growth factor (EGF)-receptor and TGF-α after tumor necrosis factor-α (TNF-α) stimulation.[6,7] Members of the carcinoembryonic antigen (CEA) family like the nonspecific cross-reacting antigen 95 (NCA95) or the biliary glycoprotein (BGP) were found to be downregulated in colorectal adenocacinomas,[8] which may be similar in pancreatic adenocarcinomas. Increasing malignancy or a lower differentiation of pancreatic carcinoma cell lines correlates with the loss of or changes in expression of several molecules involved in cell adhesion, like E-cadherin or β-catenin.[9] β-Catenin is further known to complex the adenomatous polyposis coli (APC) gene product for degradation in proteosomes. Mutations in the APC gene lead to an accumulation of cytosolic β-catenin followed by an increase in transcription of unknown genes due to the association of β-catenin with Tcf-4 forming a transcription factor complex.[10] Eighty percent of colorectal carcinomas bear mutations in the APC gene, whereas the frequency of APC mutations in the pancreas seems to be lower.[11]

In contrast to colorectal diseases with easy accessible precursor lesions, the rapid development of pancreatic cancer limits the ability to isolate early forms of pancreatic lesions. This hampers the correlation of genetic alterations with the morphology in pancreatic malignant diseases. An *in vitro* model that allows the investigation of early lesions and malignant progression is warranted. We have established several subclones of a highly differentiated pancreatic ductal adenocarcinoma cell line that we investigated under three-dimensional growth conditions without supplying any semisolid three-dimensional environment. Other systems were described that use matrigel or collagen-gel to generate a three-dimensional environment for cells derived from the mammary gland, prostate, digestive system and lung.[12] Additionally, an artificial *in vitro* tumor model was described.[13] Here we present data on a three-dimensional, reversibly differentiated *in vitro* system that in many parts reflects the situation found in normal human pancreatic epithelial duct cells.

MATERIALS AND METHODS

Chemicals

All plastic ware was obtained from Nunc (Wiesbaden, Germany). The agarose was from Difco (Augsburg, Germany). Bovine serum albumine (BSA) was from

Dulbecco. Diamino-Benzidine was obtained from Polyscience (England), and hemalaun was bought from Merck (Darmstadt, Germany). The bromdesoxyuridine (BrdU) labeling and staining kit was obtained by Boehringer Ingelheim (Ingelheim, Germany).

Cells

The pancreatic cell line A818 was isolated from the ascites of a 75-year-old female patient suffering from a differentiated pancreatic head carcinoma. By limiting dilution technique, the subclones A818-1 and A818-4 and were obtained. All cell lines were cultured in RPMI 1640 supplemented with 10% fetal calf serum (FCS), 2 mM glutamine, 1 mM sodium pyruvate, 100 units penicillin/ml, 100 μg streptomycin/ml. Cells were trypsinized with 0.25% trypsin and 0.01% ethylenediaminetetraacetic acid (EDTA) (all obtained from Gibco-BRL, Wiesbaden, Germany).

For standard experiments, cells were seeded in plastic 6-well plates at a density of $1-5 \times 10^5$ cells. For three-dimensional growth cells were seeded in precoated 6-well plates at the same density. The coating solution contained agarose at 31 mg/ml mixed with nonsupplemented RPMI 1640 (preheated to 37°C) at a ratio of 1:3. One ml was poored into each well. This coating prevented adherence of cells.

Antibodies And Rekombinant Proteins

The following antibodies were obtained from Dianova (Hamburg, Germany): p53(ab2), CD67, KL1, collagen receptor, CDw49bVLA2, p21/waf, MIB-1 as well as all secondary antibodies. The following antibodies were received as a generous gift from C. Wagener and M. Neumaier (Institute of Clinical Chemistry of the University Clinic of Eppendorf, Hamburg): T84-66, T84-1 and 4D1/C2. The following antibodies were previously established and purified in the laboratory of Schmiegel/Kalthoff in Hamburg: Ra 96, C54-1, C1N3, Ca19-9 and C1P83. The antibody 225 was from J. Mendelson, Memorial Sloan Kettering Cancer Center, New York. The antibody against L-Cam was obtained from Bissendorf Biochemicals GmbH, Germany.

Recombinant HGF and neutralizing antibody against HGF were obtained by R&D-Systems (Wiesbaden, Germany). The antibody against c-Met was from NovoCastra, and the antibody against vimentin was obtained from Boehringer Mannheim (Mannheim, Germany). The antibody against β-catenin was obtained from Transduction Laboratories (Lexington, KY).

Immunohistochemistry

For immunohistochemistry, cells were harvested by means of trypsination and cytocentrifugation onto coverslips. Completely developed hollow-spheres were centrifuged onto protein-precoated coverslips from Marienfeld (Darmstadt, Germany) without previous trypsination or stained in phosphate-buffered saline (PBS) containing 0.05% sodium azide for one hour.

The Vectastain Elite Kit (horse-anti-mouse immunoglobulin G (IgG)) from Vector Laboratories (Burlingame, CA) was used for the detection of peroxidase staining. The immunofluorescence experiments were detected via a Cy3-conjugated goat-anti-mouse IgG + IgM secondary antibody from Dianova (Hamburg, Germany). All primary antibodies were used in dilutions ranging from 1:10–1:100. Primary antibodies were diluted in PBS/1% BSA. The secondary antibodies were used in dilutions ranging from 1:500–1:2000 and were diluted in PBS containing 1% human serum. Unspecific binding of the biotinylated secondary antibody was blocked with an A/B-blocking kit from Vector Laboratories (Burlingame, CA).

All immunohistochemical experiments were carried out for 1–3 hours at room temperature or overnight at 4°C. Sections or spins were than washed with PBS 3–5 times and incubated for 1–2 hours with the secondary antibodies. For Cy3-detection, the cells were incubated for 1–1.5 hours with the primary antibody and 30 minutes with the secondary antibody. Specificity of the immunoreactivity was assessed by replacing the primary antibody by PBS/1% BSA. For all kits used we strictly followed the user's manual.

Cytokine-Treatment of A818-1 Cells

The following cytokines were added a) to freshly seeded A818-1 cells or b) to completely developed hollow-spheres: γ-interferon, TNF-α, TGF-α, EGF and HGF. The concentrations are given in TABLE 1. In a second attempt, an HGF-neutralizing antibody was used a) to neutralize exogenously added HGF and b) to block intrinsic HGF produced by the cells. A concentration of 10 µg/ml was used. All cytokines and the antibody were freshly added on day 2, 5 and 7 after seeding. The cultures were checked daily via microscope.

Proliferation-Assay of A818-1 Cells

To determine the differences in proliferation ratios between A818-1 monolayer cells and A818-1 cells cultured under three-dimensional conditions, we seeded cells into ten precoated 6-well plates and harvested as described.

Every day one well was incubated with BrdU (10 µM/l) for 3.5 hours. Cells were washed with PBS and allowed to grow in normal RPMI for additional 2.5 hours. Finally, the cells were washed with PBS and trypsinized followed by cytocentrifugation and fixation in 70% ethanol/50 mM glycin buffer for 30 minutes. The detection of BrdU incorporation was carried out as recommended by the manufacturers. The nuclei were counterstained with hemalaun and the number of positive cells was evaluated using an Olympus BH-2 microscope.

RESULTS

Hollow-Sphere Formation

A panel of 5 pancreatic carcinoma cell lines was tested under three-dimensional growth conditions. When cells were seeded under normal tissue culture conditions all cell lines grew as monolayers (FIG. 1a, A). One subclone of the cell line A818 called A818-1 was found to form hollow-spheres and spheroids. Hollow-spheres consist of a single layer of 50–200 epithelial cells (FIG. 1a, C). The mean time of hollow-sphere formation was 8–10 days. During this time a characteristic intermediate form was observed that looked like signet-ring cells (FIG. 1a, B). Spheroids differ from hollow-spheres by the lack of an inner lumen and consist of 50 up to several thousand cells. In contrast to the subclone A818-1, all other cell lines formed spheroids as the only three-dimensional phenotype (FIG. 1a, D).

Response to Cytokine Treatment

A818-1 cells were seeded and treated with different cytokines and growth factors. We found that hollow-sphere development was inhibited by interferon-γ in a concentration-dependent manner. At a concentration of 20 U/ml, hollow-spheres were able to develop but only in reduced numbers. 200 U/ml prevented hollow-sphere development.

TNF-α lead to cell death at a concentration of 1000 U/ml, whereas interferon-γ only prevented hollow-sphere development but left the cells alive. All other cytokines and growth factors tested showed no visible influence on hollow-sphere formation over a period of 8 days. Even with exogenously added HGF, no visible changes in hollow-sphere development occurred. A neutralizing antibody against HGF added to freshly seeded cells at a concentration of 1 µg/ml had no influence on hollow-sphere formation (TABLE 1).

In a second experimental setting we added cytokines and growth factors to fully developed hollow-spheres. We found corresponding results to the ones we achieved with the first experimental setting. TNF-α at a concentration of 1000 U/ml induced cell death and disaggregation of existing hollow-spheres. Interferon-γ at a concentration of 200 U/ml showed influence on fully developed hollow-spheres by means of leading to a more "condensed" form. The visible single cell layer appeared to be

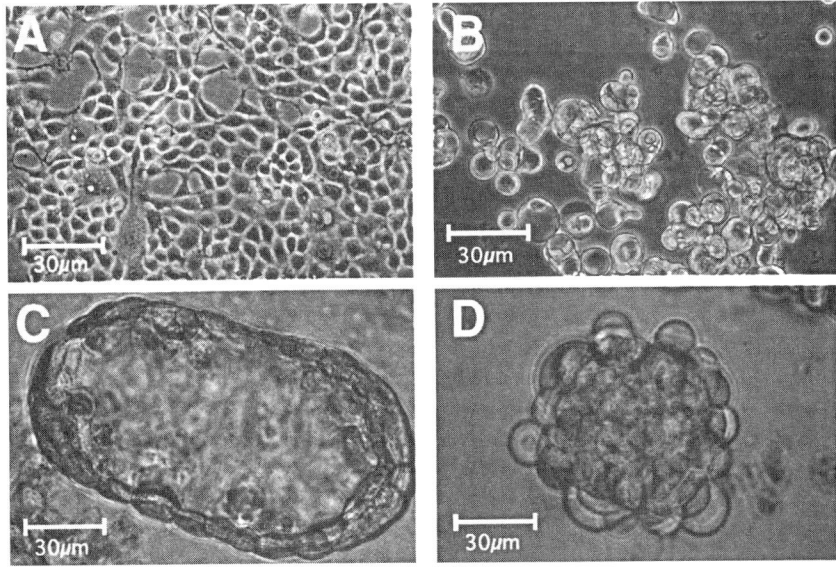

FIGURE 1a. Phenotypes of the pancreatic adenocarcinoma cell line A818-1 under different growth conditions. (**A**) Monolayer under normal tissue culture conditions. (**B**) Signet-ring-like cells after 2–3 days under three-dimensional growth conditions. (**C**) Hollow-sphere and (**D**) spheroid after 8–10 days under three-dimensional growth conditions.

TABLE 1. Influence of cytokines on hollow-sphere formation[a]

Cytokine	Concentration	Hollow-sphere formation	Integrity
No	∅	development within 6–10 days	standard
IFN-γ	0.2–20 U/ml	no influence	smaller
IFN-γ	200 U/ml	inhibition	no spheres
TGF-α	10 ng/ml	no influence	standard
EFG	10 ng/ml	no influence	standard
TNF-α	1000 U/ml	cell death	no spheres
HGF	100 ng/ml	no influence	standard

[a]Cytokine treatment was started under three-dimensional growth conditions following trypsinization of A818-1 cells prior to hollow-sphere formation. Medium was replaced on day 2, 5, and 7 after seeding.

TABLE 2. Influence of cytokines on fully developed hollow-spheres[a]

Cytokine	Concentration	Integrity of Hollow-spheres
No	∅	standard
IFN-γ	0.2–20 U/ml	smaller
IFN-γ	200 U/ml	no spheres
TGF-α	10 ng/ml	standard
EFG	10 ng/ml	standard
TNF-α	1000 U/ml	no spheres
HGF	100 ng/ml	standard

[a]Cytokine treatment was started after day ten of hollow-sphere formation. Fully developed hollow-spheres were washed twice with PBS and transferred to medium containing cytokines and growth factors. Medium was replaced on day 2, 5, and 7 after the transfer.

thicker, and the hollow-spheres were reduced in size. All other cytokines and growth factors tested did not show visible influences on shape or viability of hollow-spheres (TABLE 2). The antiproliferative effects of interferon-γ and TNF-α on monolayers of A818-1 was previously shown.[14] Interferon-γ caused a decrease of vitality of 67.1%. TNF-α caused a decrease of 37.2%. These data were obtained by ^{3}H-thymidine incorporation assays.

Proliferation of Hollow-Spheres

During hollow-sphere formation a dramatic decrease in proliferation was observed (TABLE 3). In comparison to the corresponding monolayer, which showed 42% of proliferating cells, 0.48% were detected for hollow-spheres. This finding was confirmed when fully developed hollow-spheres were stained for the Ki-67 antigen with the MIB-1 antibody.

Polarity of Hollow-Spheres

Immunostaining for antigens of the CEA-family revealed a reaction at the outer membrane of hollow-spheres, as it is typically observed in histological investiga-

TABLE 3. Decrease in proliferation of A818-1 cells cultured under three-dimensional growth conditions[a]

Day	Number of labeled cells	Percentage of proliferating cells
1	12 out of 104	11.5%
2	7 out of 247	2.8
4	5 out of 206	2.4
8	1 out of 205	0.48

[a]Decrease in proliferation was observed when A818-1 cells were grown under three-dimensional conditions. The proliferation was measured over a period of ten days. Every day BrdU at a final concentration of 10 µMol/l was added to one well. Cells were incubated for 3.5 hours, followed by 3 hours in fresh medium without BrdU. Cells were centrifuged onto coverslips and stained with an anti-BrdU antibody.

tions. The polarity of hollow-spheres with the basal membrane orientated towards the inner lumen, was further proved by staining for β-catenin, which exhibited a basolateral reaction. Immunohistochemically, hollow-spheres were negative for CEA-180 but positive for BGP and NCA95 (TABLE 4, FIG. 1b, E, F, H). Interestingly, CEA-180 mRNA was detected by reverse transcriptase polymerase chain reaction (RT-PCR, data not shown). Released protein was found in the supernatant: 1.9 ng CEA-180 per 1×10^5 cells was detected in the supernatant of hollow-spheres, where-

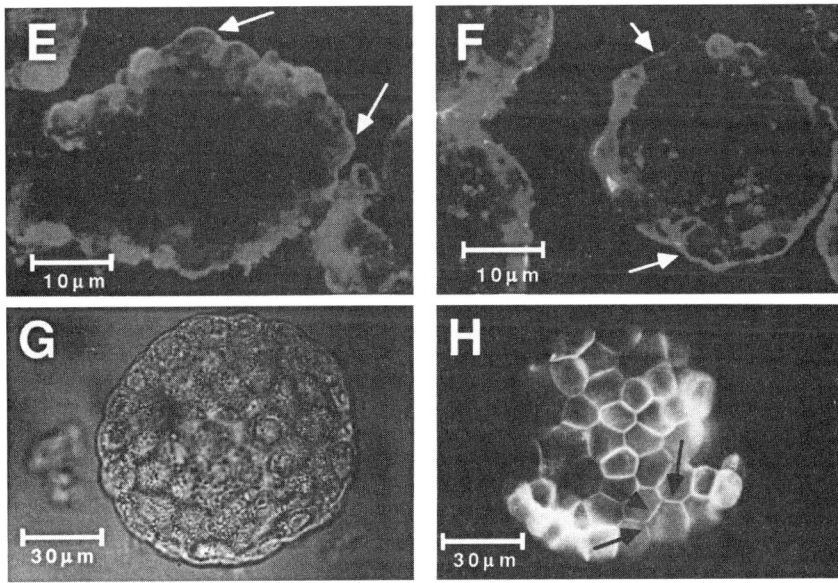

FIGURE 1b. Cryosections of A818-1 hollow-spheres (**E, F**) and native hollow-spheres (**H**), stained for BGP and NCA95 and β-catenin. The apical expression of both antigens BGP (E) and NCA95 (F) is indicated by *white arrows*. The basolateral expression of β-catenin (H) is marked by *black arrows*. The integrity of the hollow-sphere after staining and fixation (H) was controlled by light microscopy (**G**).

TABLE 4. Polarity of hollow-spheres indicated by epithlial marker antigens[a]

Antibody	Antigen	Hollow-sphere	Monolayer
C1N3	CEA family	apical membrane	membrane
C1P83	CEA	negative	cytoplasmic
CD67	NCA 95	apical membrane and total cells	cytoplasmic
CD66b	BGP	apical membrane	membrane
NCL c-met	c-met	apical membrane	cytoplasmic/membrane
Anti-β-catenin	β-catenin	basolateral membrane	membrane

[a]Polar expression of epithelial marker antigens detected via immunofluorescence. Cryosections of 6 μm were stained for members of the CEA-family CEA, NCA95 and BGP. Fully developed hollow-spheres were stained for the c-met receptor and β-catenin as described.

as the monolayer released 0.79 ng per 1×10^5 cells in 24 hours. This resembles the normal situation in gastrointestinal epithelial tissues. The polarity of intact hollow-spheres prevented attachment to plastic surfaces of normal tissue-culture flasks even when flasks were coated with collagen, fibronectin or laminin.

Reversibility

Mechanically disrupted hollow-spheres not only attached but also grew again as monolayer with the same doubling time as the founder cells. When these "remonolayers" were trypsinized and seeded under three-dimensional growth conditions, hollow-sphere formation was observed again (FIG. 2).

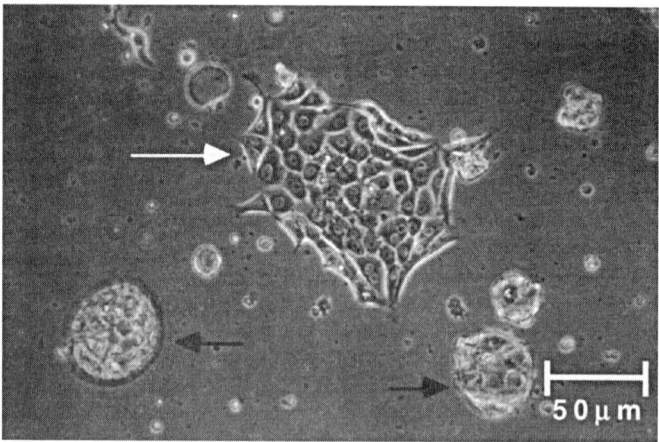

FIGURE 2. Regrowth of hollow-sphere cells as monolayer. After hollow-sphere formation was completed, hollow-spheres were retransferred to plastic tissue culture flasks. Mechanically disrupted hollow-spheres attached to the surface and grew as "remonolayers," as indicated by the *white arrow*. Intact hollow-spheres did not attach with their outer/apical (mucinous) surface.

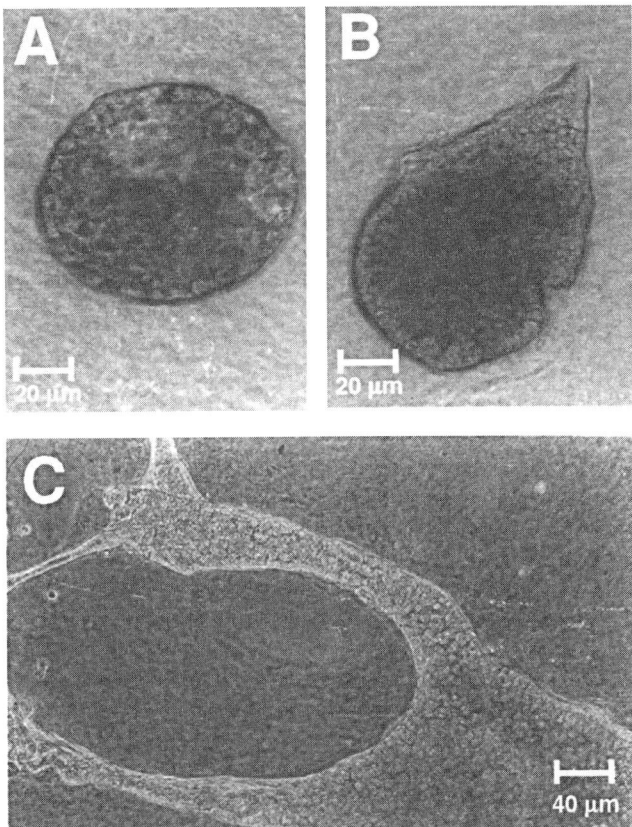

FIGURE 3. Tube formation. A818-1 hollow-spheres were embedded into matrigel (**A**). After 3 days they formed buds (**B**). These buds grew out to thin, duct-like tubes during the following days. These tubes enlarged, connected to others and developed a network (**C**).

Tube Formation

When embedded into matrigel, duct-like tubes were observed after 8–10 days. During the first days, hollow-spheres formed buds (FIG. 3B). These buds grew out, and thin duct-like tubes developed. These structures enlarged during the following days and built a network consisting of many connected duct-like tubes (FIG. 3C).

CONCLUSION

The loss of contact inhibition and polarity of cancer cells are major events in tumor development.[15] So far, all systems that were thought to resemble a situation comparable to normal tissues required an artificial three-dimensional environment. Some systems depended on exogenously added components like growth factors or other cytokines.[13] The A818-1 hollow-sphere system developed spontaneously. Neither an artificial matrix nor additional cytokines are required. A818-1 ductal adenocarcinoma cells are able to recover the ability to grow in a highly differentiated, three-dimensional manner only depending on a single stimulus: the prevention from adherence. Furthermore, they recovered a functional contact inhibition as indicated by a dramatic decrease in proliferation during and after hollow-sphere formation. The polarized expression of members of the CEA-family, BGP and NCA95 as well as β-catenin displays a situation found in normal pancreatic tissue. Polarity is underlined by secretion of CEA-180 into the supernatant of hollow-sphere cultures.[16] When hollow-spheres were disrupted or trypsinized and seeded into normal tissue culture flasks, cells grew as monolayers. When these cells were trypsinized again and seeded under three-dimensional growth conditions, hollow-sphere formation took place. This system is able to differentiate and dedifferentiate in a reversible manner. The ability to form duct-like tubes in matrigel and all indicated features demand this system for general investigations of differentiation, cell cycle and apoptosis in human pancreatic epithelial cells.

ACKNOWLEDGMENT

This work was supported by the Deutsche Forschungsgemeinschaft, Grant KA1346-1/1.

REFERENCES

1. FERNANDEZ-DEL CASTLLIO, C. *et al.* 1994. Curr. Opin. Gastroenterol. **10:** 507–512.
2. SCHUTTE, M. *et al.* 1996. The molecular genetics of pancreatic adenocarcinoma. *In* Pancreatic Cancer: Molecular and Clinical Advances. J.P. Neoptolemos & N.R. Lemoine, Eds.: 115–129. Blackwell Science, Ltd. London.
3. FRIESS, H. *et al.* 1996. Growth factors and growth factor receptors in pancreatic cancer. *In* Pancreatic Cancer: Molecular and Clinical Advances. J.P. Neoptolemos & N.R. Lemoine, Eds.: 51–60. Blackwell Science, Ltd. London.
4. KORC, M. *et al.* 1992. Overexpression of the epidermal growth factor receptor in human pancreatic cancer is associated with concomitant increases in the levels of epidermal growth factor and transforming growth factor alpha. J. Clin. Invest. **90:** 1352–1360.
5. KALTHOFF, H. *et al.* 1993. Tumor necrosis factor (TNF) up-regulates the expression of p75 but not p55 TNF receptors, and both receptors mediate, independently of each other, up-regulation of transforming growth factor alpha and epidermal growth factor receptor mRNA. J. Biol. Chem. **268:** 2762–2766.
6. BENTON, H.P. *et al.* 1991. Cytokines and their receptors. Curr. Opin. Cell Biol. **3:** 171–175.
7. KALTHOFF, H. *et al.* 1991. Modulation of platelet-derived growth factor A- and B-chain/c-sis mRNA by tumor necrosis factor and other agents in adenocarcinoma cells. Oncogene **6:** 1015–1021.
8. NEUMAIER, M. *et al.* 1993. Biliary glycoprotein, a potential human cell adhesion molecule, is down-regulated in colorectal carcinomas. Proc. Natl. Acad. Sci. USA **90:** 10744–10748.
9. SPARKS, A.B. *et al.* 1998. Mutational analysis of the APC/beta-catenin/Tcf pathway in colorectal cancer. Cancer Res. **58:** 1130–1134.

10. MANN, B. et al. 1998. β-Catenin overexpression in metastasized colorectal carcinomas: an important mechanism during the progression of the disease. Langenbecks Arch. Chir. I. Forumband 1998.
11. HORII, A. et al. 1992. Frequent somatic mutations of the APC gene in human pancreatic cancer. Cancer Res. **52:** 6696–6698.
12. BRINKMANN, V. et al. 1995. Hepatocyte growth factor/scatter factor induces a variety of tissue-specific morphogenic programs in epithelial cells. J. Cell Biol. **131:** 1573–1586.
13. KAMMERER, R. et al. 1995. Artificial tumor: a novel heterotypic, polymorphic, three-dimensional *in vitro* model of individual human solid tumors. Tumour Biol. **16:** 213–221.
14. HERINGSLAKE, T. 1991. Klonale Unterschiede der antiproliferativen und antigenmodulierenden Wirkung von rekombinanten humanen Zytokinen auf Pancreas-karzinomzellen. Ph.D. thesis, University of Hamburg, FRG.
15. BRACKE, M.E. et al. 1997. Functional downregulation of the E-cadherin/catenin complex leads to loss of contact inhibition of motility and of mitochondrial activity, but not of growth in confluent epithelial cell cultures. Eur. J. Cell Biol. **74:** 342–349.
16. BARANOV, V. et al. 1994. Expression of carcinoembryonic antigen and nonspecific cross-reacting 50-kDa antigen in human normal and cancerous colon mucosa: comparative ultrastructural study with monoclonal antibodies. Cancer Res. **54:** 3305–3314.

Sp1 and Its Likes: Biochemical and Functional Predictions for a Growing Family of Zinc Finger Transcription Factors

TIFFANY COOK,[a] BRIAN GEBELEIN,[b] AND RAUL URRUTIA[a,b,c,d]

[a]*Gastroenterology Research Unit,* [b]*Department of Molecular Neurosciences, and* [c]*Department of Biochemistry and Molecular Biology, Mayo Clinic, Rochester, Minnesota 55905, USA*

ABSTRACT: The discovery and functional characterization of Sp1 as a GC-rich binding zinc finger protein provided a useful paradigm for understanding mechanisms mediating transcriptional activation in eukaryotic cells. This early paradigm suggested that promoters carrying GC-rich sequences are activated by Sp1 through its interaction with proteins from the basal transcriptional machinery to upregulate gene expression. Since the time of this seminal work, studies from several laboratories have led to the discovery of many Sp1-like transcription factors containing highly homologous DNA binding motifs that bind to similar sequences. Consequently, this knowledge poses many important questions regarding whether these related proteins have similar or antagonistic biochemical and functional properties to Sp1. The goal of this article is to use available database information and recent experimental evidence to describe the current repertoire of Sp1-like zinc finger transcription factors in mammalian cells. Furthermore, we discuss structural and functional studies that reveal that these proteins may share a role in morphogenetic pathways. Altogether, this information is aimed at better understanding how this growing family of transcription factors work to regulate gene expression and morphogenesis.

INTRODUCTION

Sp1, the founding member of a growing family of highly related zinc finger proteins, was the first mammalian transcription factor for RNA polymerase II ever described.[1,2] This protein contains a DNA binding domain at the C-terminus composed of three zinc finger motifs. Structurally, these motifs belong to the C_2H_2-containing family of proteins that includes the well-characterized *Drosophila* protein, Krüppel, and the *Xenopus* transcription factor, TFIIIA. Biochemical characterization, structural analyses, and molecular modeling approaches have revealed that the zinc finger motifs of Sp1 bind to a GC-rich DNA core sequence.[1-4] On the other hand, the N-terminal domain of this protein contains several glutamine-rich sequences that activate transcription by recruiting the basal transcription apparatus onto target promoters through the binding to the dTAF$_{II}$110/hTAF$_{II}$130 proteins.[5-7] GC-rich binding

---

[d]Address for correspondence: Dr. Raul Urrutia, Gastroenterology Research Unit, 2-445A Alfred Building, 200 First Street SW, Rochester, MN 55905. Phone, 507/255-6028; fax, 507/255-6318; e-mail, urrutia.raul@mayo.edu

sites for Sp1 are found in more than one thousand promoters that drive the expression of genes involved in the regulation of many vital cellular functions, including cell proliferation, differentiation, apoptosis, metabolism, and secretion.[8] Consequently, mice carrying a homozygous deletion for Sp1 display severe embryonic malformations and die during development.[9] Thus, current data support an essential role for both GC-rich sequences and Sp1 in maintaining the homeostasis of mammalian cells. This paper describes the existence of a large family of Sp1-like transcription factors, some of which bind to the GC-rich binding sites originally thought to be specific for Sp1. We also use structural and biochemical information derived from studying Sp1 to predict functional properties for other members of this family. We are optimistic that the data discussed here will be useful in guiding further research on individual Sp1-like proteins.

IDENTIFICATION OF A GROWING FAMILY OF SP1-LIKE TRANSCRIPTION FACTORS IN MAMMALIAN CELLS

Immediately after the discovery of Sp1, other structurally and functionally related proteins such as Sp2, Sp3, Sp4, basic transcription element B1 (BTEB1), and BTEB2 were discovered in mammalian cells.[10–14] These proteins share a remarkable similarity with Sp1 within their zinc finger domains and also bind to GC-rich sequences to regulate gene expression. We have recently characterized two novel transforming growth factor-β (TGF-β)-inducible Sp1-like proteins, the transcription factors TIEG1 and TIEG2.[15,16] Interestingly, database comparisons and library screening performed as a part of our studies have revealed the existence of 14 different proteins containing an Sp1-like DNA binding domain composed of three C-terminal zinc finger motifs (FIG. 1). The major advantage of grouping these proteins into a family is the possibility of predicting important biochemical and functional features of newly described members based on previous data available on Sp1. For instance, using previous biochemical and structural data obtained from the zinc finger domain of Sp1 bound to its *cis*-regulatory DNA sequences, we predicted the DNA binding sequence for the TIEG proteins. The amino acid residues within the first (KHA), second (RER), and third (RHK) zinc finger domains of TIEG1 and TIEG2 that are predicted to make contact with DNA are identical to the corresponding regions within Sp1 that bind to the sequences GGG (ZF1), GCG (ZF2), and GGG (ZF3), respectively.[17] We next constructed a comparative structural model for the zinc finger domain of the TIEG2 and the Sp1 proteins using the SWISS-MODEL Automated Protein Modeling Server (www.expasy.ch/swissmod/SM_3DCrunch.html). As shown in FIGURE 2, these two proteins are predicted to form almost identical tertiary structures, a result that further supports the idea that they exhibit similar DNA binding properties. We and others have recently shown that both TIEG proteins bind to and regulate the function of promoters that contain Sp1-like sequences, supporting the validity of the predictions described above.[16,18,19] A similar predictive method has been applied to reveal the binding site for other Sp1-like proteins. In this regard, all the available biochemical data indicate that a shared functional property of Sp1-like transcription factors is their ability to bind to highly related GC-rich sequences (TABLE 1). Thus, sequence comparisons and comparative structural analy-

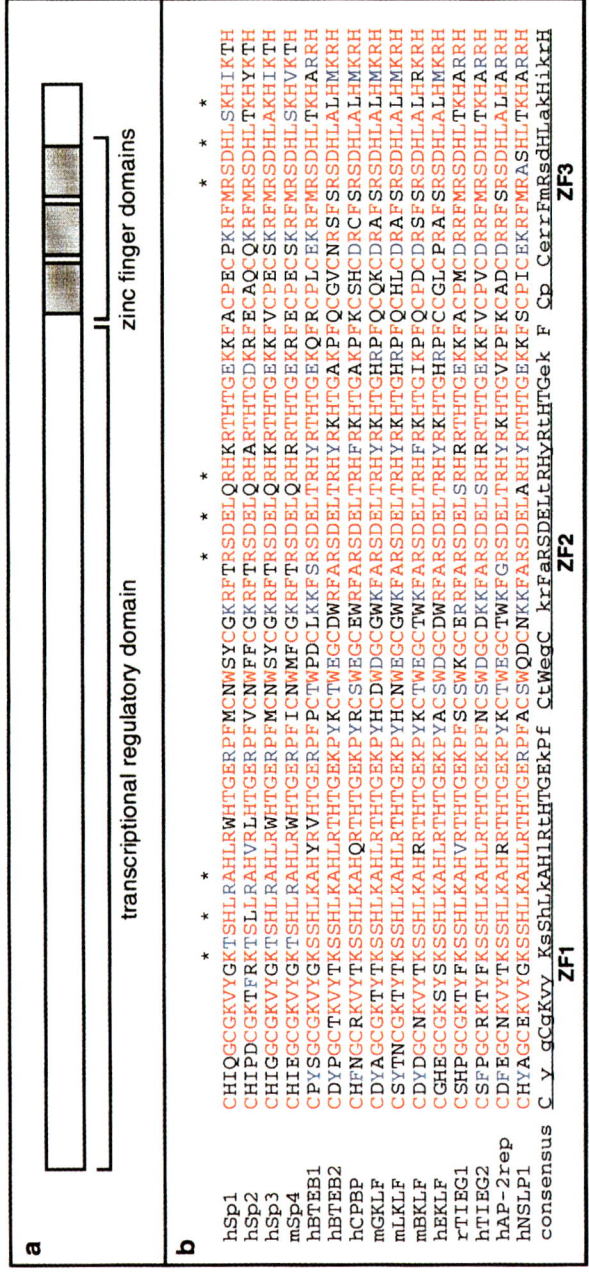

FIGURE 1. Comparison of the zinc finger motifs of Sp1-like proteins. (**a**) Structural diagram of members of the Sp1-like family of proteins. Three zinc finger motifs are located within the C-terminal region of the protein, while a transcriptional regulatory domain resides within the N-terminus. (**b**) Sequence alignment of the zinc finger region of Sp1 (A29635), Sp2 (M97190), Sp3 (M97191), Sp4 (U62522), BTEB1 (D31716), BTEB2 (D14520), CPBP (U44975), GKLF (U20344), LKLF (U25096), BKLF (U36340), and EKLF (U37106), TIEG1 (U88630), TIEG2 (AF028008), AP-2rep (Y14295), and NSLP1 (R.U., unpublished). Individual zinc finger motifs are *underlined*. Asterisks indicate residues predicted to interact with DNA according to the Klevit model.[17]

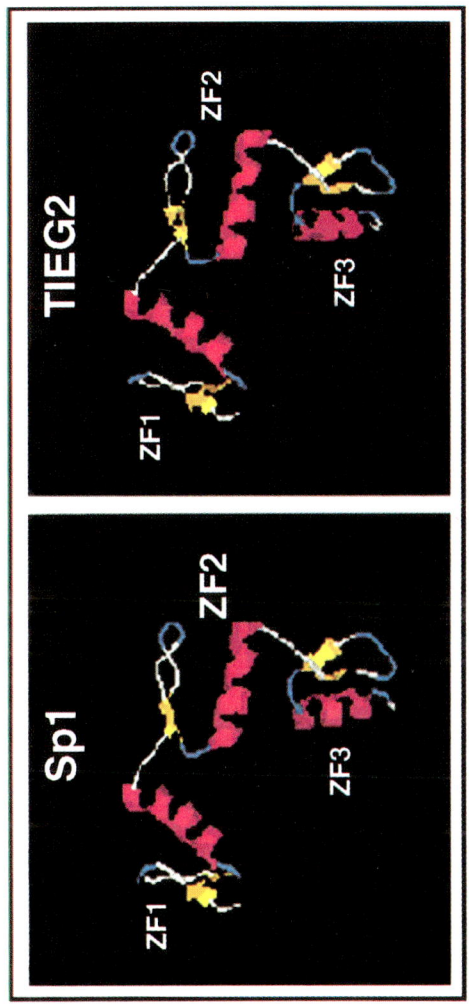

FIGURE 2. Comparative structural model for the zinc finger domains of Sp1 and TIEG2. The models were generated using the SWISS-MODEL Automated Protein Modeling Server (www.expasy.ch/swissmod/SM_3DCrunch.html). Comparison between these models reveals a remarkable structural similarity between these two proteins. This similarity is further supported by recent experimental evidence demonstrating that these two proteins indeed bind similar GC-rich sequences.[16]

TABLE 1. DNA binding activity, transcriptional regulatory function, expression, and physiological role of the current members of the Sp1-like family of proteins

Gene	DNA binding sites	Transcriptional regulation	Expression pattern	Cellular function	Refs
Sp1	GC box, CACCC	Activator	Ubiquitous	Embryogenesis	1, 5, 9, 20, 26
Sp2	GC/GT box	ND	ND	ND	11
Sp3	GC/GT box	Weak activator	Ubiquitous	ND	11, 14, 27, 28
Sp4	GC/GT box	Activator	Brain-enriched	Embryogenesis, male fertility	10, 25, 29
TIEG1	GC box	Repressor	Ubiquitous	Apoptosis, anti-proliferation	15, 18, 19, 30
TIEG2	GC box	Repressor	Ubiquitous	Anti-proliferation	16
BKLF	CACCC	Activator	Ubiquitous	ND	31
EKLF	CCACACCCT	Activator	Erythroid, mast cells	Erythropoiesis	21, 23, 24
GKLF	CACCC, (G/A)(G/A)GG(C/T)G(C/T)	Activator/repressor	Gut, Lung, Testis	Anti-proliferation	32, 33, 34
LKLF	CACCC	Activator	Lung, Spleen	T cell quiescence/survival	22, 35
CPBP	CCCCACCCA	Activator	Placenta, lung, pancreas, heart, liver, muscle	Proto-oncogene	36, 37
BTEB1	GC/GT box	Activator/repressor	Ubiquitous	ND	12
BTEB2	GC/GT box	Activator	Testis, Placenta	ND	13
AP-2rep	GGCGTGGCGG	Repressor	Kidney, liver, lung, embryonic brain	ND	38
NSLP1	ND	ND	ND	ND	

NOTE: Sp1-like proteins have been demonstrated to bind to similar GC-rich sequences. Some of these proteins are transcriptional activators, others repress gene expression, and in the case of BTEB, has either function depending upon promoter context. Note that most mammalian tissues thus far studied express a combination of Sp1-like proteins. The results of cellular studies and knockout experiments indicate that a unifying feature of these proteins is their participation in morphogenetic pathways. References to the source of information used in this table are found on the right. ND = not determined.

ses similar to those described here have been used for assembling the growing family of Sp1-like proteins shown in FIGURE 1b. One important implication of these data is that they may allow us to predict important biochemical functions for newly identified members of this group of proteins, e.g., DNA binding.

FUNCTIONAL PREDICTIONS FOR SP1-LIKE PROTEINS IN MAMMALIAN CELL PHYSIOLOGY

The existence of a family of Sp1-like proteins raises several important biological questions about their function. For example, do Sp1-like proteins: 1) have redundant or distinct roles in mammalian cell physiology; 2) form homo- and/or heterodimers; 3) work in a cell type-specific manner; 4) participate in a hierarchical cascade of gene expression; and/or 5) antagonize each other's functions to fine tune specific cellular processes? We and others have begun to address these questions with some promising results. For example, an answer to the question of whether Sp1-like proteins work in a more tissue-selective manner arises from analyzing the combined results of expression and gene knockout studies. The Sp1 gene, for instance, is ubiquitously expressed in murine cells,[20] suggesting that most, if not all, mammalian cells require Sp1 for proper function. Interestingly, the knockout of this gene leads to gross morphological defects in a large number of tissues, supporting the validity of this hypothesis.[9] In contrast, other members of the Sp1-like family, such as EKLF, LKLF, and Sp4, are expressed in a tissue-enriched manner.[11,21,22] This selective pattern of expression raises the possibility that these proteins have a cell-specific function. Indeed, this idea is supported by the results from knocking out these tissue-enriched genes. EKLF, for example, is expressed in erythroid cells and its knockout results in selective defects in erythropoiesis.[23,24] Thus, while some Sp1-like proteins play a ubiquitous role in mammalian cell physiology, others members of this family display more cell-restricted functions. Based upon these observations, we propose a unifying hypothesis that Sp1-like proteins participate in morphogenetic pathways. This idea is supported by the fact that GC-rich Sp1-like binding sites are required for the regulation of a large number of genes involved in cell growth regulation and development. We have tested the validity of this hypothesis by analyzing the function of the recently identified TIEG proteins. Our results demonstrate that both TIEG1 and TIEG2 are indeed negative regulators of cell growth in epithelial cell populations.[15,16] Thus, it is likely that other yet uncharacterized members of this family of proteins, such as AP-2rep (Genbank Accession No. Y14295)[38] and NSLP1 (Urrutia, unpublished), also play a role in morphogenesis.

Because several Sp1-like proteins that recognize identical DNA sequences can be coexpressed in a single mammalian cell, it becomes important to determine whether they have redundant or distinct transcriptional regulatory activity. In this regard, the biochemical comparison between Sp1, Sp4, the TIEG proteins, and BTEB1 can be utilized as a useful paradigm to begin understanding this type of question. Sp1, for instance, acts as a potent transcriptional activator on reporter plasmids carrying GC boxes, while the TIEG proteins act as transcriptional repressors.[5,16,18] Thus, it is likely that different Sp1-like proteins can function as "on" or "off" switches for similar promoters. In contrast, both Sp1 and Sp4 behave as transcriptional activators, and thus are likely to upregulate the expression of similar genes.[25] Interestingly, BTEB1 activates transcription on promoters containing multiple GC boxes but behaves as a repressor on promoters containing a single copy of this sequence, supporting the idea that the regulation of gene expression by Sp1-like proteins may also depend upon promoter context.[12] Altogether, these studies reveal that the regulation of promoters containing GC-rich sequences is exceedingly complex. Consequently, a defined understanding of the mechanisms underlying the regulation of these promoters will only arise from careful studies focused on defining the transcriptional regulatory activity of individual members of this family and their potential combinatorial effects.

CONCLUSION

The data summarized in this article demonstrate the use of structural data for assembling a family of Sp1-like zinc finger proteins. In addition, based upon these structural analyses and the functional data derived from the studies described here, we have two important generalizations: 1) Sp1-like proteins are likely to bind GC-rich sequences, and 2) Sp1-like proteins are likely to participate in the regulation of morphogenetic pathways. Furthermore, emerging data demonstrate that different members of this family of proteins are differentially expressed and can display either similar or antagonistic transcriptional regulatory functions. Thus, these analyses expand our understanding of the repertoire of Sp1-like proteins present in mammalian cells. More importantly, this knowledge can serve as a guide for characterizing the function of newly identified members of this family of transcription factors.

ACKNOWLEDGMENTS

The authors wish to thank Dr. Karen Hedin for critically reviewing the manuscript of this paper. This work was supported by the Mayo Cancer Center and NIH Grant DK52913 to R.U. T.C. was supported by NIH Training Grant DK07198.

REFERENCES

1. BRIGGS, M.R., J.T. KADONAGA, S.P. BELL & R. TJIAN. 1986. Purification and biochemical characterization of the promoter-specific transcription factor, Sp1. Science **234:** 47–52.
2. KADONAGA, J.T., K.R. CARNER, F.R. MASIARZ & R. TJIAN. 1987. Isolation of cDNA encoding transcription factor Sp1 and functional analysis of the DNA binding domain. Cell **51:** 1079–1090.
3. BUCHER, P. 1990. Weight matrix descriptions of four eukaryotic RNA polymerase II promoter elements derived from 502 unrelated promoter sequences. J. Mol. Biol. **212:** 563–578.
4. KRIWACKI, R.W., S.C. SCHULTZ, T.A. STEITZ & J.P. CARADONNA. 1992. Sequence-specific recognition of DNA by zinc-finger peptides derived from the transcription factor Sp1. Proc. Natl. Acad. Sci. USA **89:** 9759–9763.
5. COUREY, A.J. & R. TJIAN. 1988. Analysis of Sp1 in vivo reveals multiple transcriptional domains, including a novel glutamine-rich activation motif. Cell **55:** 887–898.
6. GILL, G., E. PASCAL, Z.H. TSENG & R. TJIAN. 1994. A glutamine-rich hydrophobic patch in transcription factor Sp1 contacts the dTAFII110 component of the *Drosophila* TFIID complex and mediates transcriptional activation. Proc. Natl. Acad. Sci. USA **91:** 192–196.
7. TANESE, N., D. SALUJA, M.F. VASSALLO, J.L. CHEN & A. ADMON. 1996. Molecular cloning and analysis of two subunits of the human TFIID complex: hTAFII130 and hTAFII100. Proc. Natl. Acad. Sci. USA **93:** 13611–13616.
8. LIU, C., A. CALOGERO, G. RAGONA, E. ADAMSON & D. MERCOLA. 1996. EGR-1, the reluctant suppression factor: EGR-1 is known to function in the regulation of growth, differentiation, and also has significant tumor suppressor activity and a mechanism involving the induction of TGF-beta1 is postulated to account for this suppressor activity. Crit. Rev. Oncog. **7:** 101–125.
9. MARIN, M., A. KARIS, P. VISSER, F. GROSVELD & S. PHILIPSEN. 1997. Transcription factor Sp1 is essential for early embryonic development but dispensable for cell growth and differentiation. Cell **89:** 619–628.

10. HAGEN, G., S. MULLER, M. BEATO & G. SUSKE. 1992. Cloning by recognition site screening of two novel GT box binding proteins: a family of Sp1 related genes. Nucleic Acids Res. **20:** 5519–5525.
11. KINGSLEY, C. & A. WINOTO. 1992. Cloning of GT box-binding proteins: a novel Sp1 multigene family regulating T-cell receptor gene expression. Mol. Cell. Biol. **12:** 4251–4261.
12. IMATAKA, H., K. SOGAWA, K.-I. YASUMOTO, Y. KIKUCHI, K. SASANO, A. KOBAYASHI, M. HAYAMI & Y. FUJII-KURIYAMA. 1992. Two regulatory proteins that bind to the basic transcription element (BTE), a GC box sequence in the promoter region of the rat P-4501A1 gene. EMBO J. **11:** 3663–3671.
13. SOGAWA, K., H. IMATAKA, Y. YAMASAKI, H. KUSUME, H. ABE & Y. FUJII-KURIYAMA. 1993. cDNA cloning and transcriptional properties of a novel GC box-binding protein, BTEB2. Nucleic Acids Res. **21:** 1527–1532.
14. LANIA, L., B. MAJELLO & P. DE LUCA. 1997. Transcriptional regulation by the Sp family proteins. Int. J. Biochem. Cell Biol. **29:** 1313–1323.
15. TACHIBANA, I., M. IMOTO, P.N. ADJEI, G.J. GORES, M. SUBRAMANIAM, T.C. SPELSBERG & R. URRUTIA. 1997. Overexpression of the TGFbeta-regulated zinc finger encoding gene, TIEG, induces apoptosis in pancreatic epithelial cells. J. Clin. Invest. **99:** 2365–2374.
16. COOK, T., B. GEBELEIN, K. MESA, A. MLADEK & R. URRUTIA. 1998. Molecular cloning and characterization of TIEG2 reveals a new subfamily of TGFβ-inducible Sp1-like zinc finger encoding genes involved in the regulation of cell growth. J. Biol. Chem. **273:** 25929–25936.
17. KLEVIT, R.E. 1993. Recognition of DNA by Cys2,His2 zinc fingers. Science **253:** 1367–1393
18. YAJIMA, S., C.H. LAMMERS, S.H. LEE, Y. HARA, K. MIZUNO & M.M. MOURADIAN. 1997. Cloning and characterization of murine glial cell-derived neurotrophic factor inducible transcription factor (MGIF). J. Neurosci. **17:** 8657–8666.
19. COOK, T., I. TACHIBANA, K. MESA, M. IMOTO, B. GEBELEIN, A. TUMA & R. URRUTIA. 1998. Characterization of a highly related family of Sp1-like transcriptional repressor proteins from pancreatic epithelial cell populations. Gastroenterology **114:** G2381.
20. SAFFER, J.D., S.P. JACKSON & M.B. ANNARELLA. 1991. Developmental expression of Sp1 in the mouse. Mol. Cell. Biol. **11:** 2189–2199.
21. MILLER, I.J. & J.J. BIEKER. 1993. A novel, erythroid cell-specific murine transcription factor that binds to the CACCC element and is related to the Kruppel family of nuclear proteins. Mol. Cell. Biol. **13:** 2776–2786.
22. ANDERSON, K.P., C.B. KERN, S.C. CRABLE & J.B. LINGREL. 1995. Isolation of a gene encoding a functional zinc finger protein homologous to erythroid Kruppel-like factor: identification of a new multigene family. Mol. Cell. Biol. **15:** 5957–5965.
23. NUEZ, B., D. MICHALOVICH, A. BYGRAVE, R. PLOEMACHER & F. GROSVELD. 1995. Defective haematopoiesis in fetal liver resulting from inactivation of the EKLF gene. Nature **375:** 316–318.
24. PERKINS, A.C., A.H. SHARPE & S.H. ORKIN. 1995. Lethal beta-thalassaemia in mice lacking the erythroid CACCC-transcription factor EKLF. Nature **375:** 318–322.
25. HAGEN, G., J. DENNIG, A. PREISS, M. BEATO & G. SUSKE. 1995. Functional analyses of the transcription factor Sp4 reveal properties distinct from Sp1 and Sp3. J. Biol. Chem. **270:** 24989–24994.
26. HARTZOG, G.A. & R.M. MYERS. 1993. Discrimination among potential activators of the beta-globin CACCC element by correlation of binding and transcriptional properties. Mol. Cell. Biol. **13:** 44–56.
27. HAGEN, G., S. MULLER, M. BEATO & G. SUSKE. 1994. Sp1-mediated transcriptional activation is repressed by Sp3. EMBO J. **13:** 3843–3851.
28. MAJELLO, B., P. DE LUCA & L. LANIA. 1997. Sp3 is a bifunctional transcription regulator with modular independent activation and repression domains. J. Biol. Chem. **272:** 4021–4026.

29. SUPP, D.M., D.P. WITTE, W.W.BRANFORD, E.P. SMITH & S.S. POTTER. 1996. Sp4, a member of the Sp1-family of zinc finger transcription factors, is required for normal murine growth, viability, and male fertility. Dev. Biol. **176:** 284–299.
30. TAU, K.R., T.E. HEFFERAN, K.M. WATERS, J.A. ROBINSON, M. SUBRAMANIAM, B.L. RIGGS & T.C. SPELSBERG. 1998. Estrogen regulation of a transforming growth factor-beta inducible early gene that inhibits deoxyribonucleic acid synthesis in human osteoblasts. Endocrinology **139:** 1346–1353.
31. CROSSLEY, M., E. WHITELAW, A. PERKINS, G. WILLIAMS, Y. FUJIWARA & S.H. ORKIN. 1996. Isolation and characterization of the cDNA encoding BKLF/TEF-2, a major CACCC-box-binding protein in erythroid cells and selected other cells. Mol. Cell. Biol. **16:** 1695–1705.
32. SHIELDS, J.M., R.J. CHRISTY & V.W. YANG. 1996. Identification and characterization of a gene encoding a gut-enriched Kruppel-like factor expressed during growth arrest. J. Biol. Chem. **271:** 20009–20017.
33. YET, S.F., M.M. MCA'NULTY, S.C. FOLTA, H.W. YEN, M. YOSHIZUMI, C.M. HSIEH, M.D. LAYNE, M.T. CHIN, H. WANG, M.A. PERRELLA, M.K. JAIN & M.E. LEE. 1998. Human EZF, a Kruppel-like zinc finger protein, is expressed in vascular endothelial cells and contains transcriptional activation and repression domains. J. Biol. Chem. **273:** 1026–1031.
34. SHIELDS, J.M. & V.W. YANG. 1998. Identification of the DNA sequence that interacts with the gut-enriched Kruppel-like factor. Nucleic Acids Res. **26:** 796–802.
35. KUO, C.T., M.L. VESELITS & J.M. LEIDEN. 1997. LKLF: a transcriptional regulator of single-positive T cell quiescence and survival. Science **277:** 1986–1990.
36. KORITSCHONER, N.P., J.L. BOCCO, G.M. PANZETTA-DUTARI, C.I. DUMUR, A. FLURY & L.C. PATRITO. 1997. A novel human zinc finger protein that interacts with the core promoter element of a TATA box-less gene. J. Biol. Chem. **272:** 9573–9580.
37. EL ROUBY, S. & E.W. NEWCOMB. 1996. Identification of Bcd, a novel proto-oncogene expressed in B-cells. Oncogene **13:** 2623–2630.
38. IMHOF, A., M. SCHUIERER, O. WERNER, M. MOSER, C. ROTH, R. BAUER & R. BUETTNER. 1999. Transcriptional regulation of the AP-2α promoter by BTEB-1 and AP-2rep, a novel wt-1/egr-related zinc finger repressor. Mol. Cell. Biol. **19:** 194–204.

Orthotopic Models of Human Pancreatic Cancer

GABRIEL CAPELLÁ,[a] LOURDES FARRÉ, ALBERTO VILLANUEVA, GERMÁN REYES, CARME GARCÍA, GEMMA TARAFA, AND FÈLIX LLUÍS

Laboratori d'Investigació Gastrointestinal, Institut de Recerca Hospital de Sant Pau, and Institut Català d'Oncologia, Barcelona, Spain

ABSTRACT: Orthotopic transplantation of solid tumor fragments of human tumors in nude mice reproduces their pattern of local growth and distal dissemination. While lymphatic, hepatic or peritoneal dissemination can be reproduced, perineural invasion is absent. Early passages (less than 3) of xenografts show a high degree of stability regarding K-*ras*, *p53* and *p16* gene status. On the other hand, advanced passages of tumors acquire additional alterations in the *p15* and *Smad4* genes. Mutations in K-*ras*, *p53*, *p15* and *Smad4* genes can be acquired, in this model system, in the more advanced stages of pancreatic tumor dissemination. Finally, it is also possible to standardize local growth of these tumors as well as its dissemination pattern giving us a preclinical tool to evaluate the anticancer activity of new drugs.

INTRODUCTION

Adenocarcinoma of the exocrine pancreas is the fourth leading cause of cancer death in Western countries.[1] Diagnosis of pancreatic cancer is often difficult, and in most patients the tumor is already disseminated when discovered. Median survival after diagnosis is 6 months, and it has not improved in the last 30 years.[2] Effective treatment is not available, and in most patients surgical resection is not feasible. Moreover, radio- and chemotherapy have shown limited effectiveness. A better knowledge of the molecular and cell biology of this tumor will eventually lead to a better management of patients. The aim of this review is to discuss some recent advances in the development of clinically relevant animal models for human pancreatic cancers.

CHEMICAL CARCINOGENESIS

In the hamster, administration of *N*-nitroso-bis(2-oxopropyl)amine (BOP) induces, preferentially, pancreatic ductal adenocarcinomas that closely resemble human tumors at the histological, biological and genetic level.[3,4] BOP-induced hamster pancreatic carcinoma has been considered to be a good model for the study of the

---

[a]Address for correspondence: Dr. Gabriel Capellá, Laboratori de Biologia Molecular, Institut Català d'Oncologia, Av. Gran Via s/n, km 2,7 08907 L'Hospitalet, Barcelona, Spain. Phone, +34 (93) 260-7822; fax, +34 (93) 260 7741; e-mail, gcapella@ico.scs.es

sequence of genetic alterations that underly pancreatic tumor induction and progression.

A number of cell lines and transplantable ductal hamster adenocarcinomas have been derived from chemically obtained tumors.[5,6] The majority (>90%) of BOP-induced tumors and cell lines contain an aspartic acid substitution at codon 12 of this gene.[6,7] In contrast, p53 gene alterations are restricted to cell lines where they are located at known hot spots of human neoplasia.[6] The discrepancy in the prevalence of p53 gene mutations between human pancreatic adenocarcinoma (60–80%) and chemically induced tumors is not surprising and has been previously reported for colon and lung tumors. In BOP-induced hamster pancreatic duct carcinogenesis, *p53* mutations are late events associated with tumor transplantation and cell culture establishment.[6,8] Altogether, hamster pancreatic cancer cells can be considered an acceptable model to study pancreatic carcinogenesis. Several approaches have been used to perform *in vivo* studies with these cells. Singenic injection in the cheek pouch has been used to test the growth effects of gastrointestinal peptides on hamster cancer cells.[9] Orthotopic implantation—in the corresponding organ of origin—in the hamster has been used to gain insight in the dissemination pattern of these tumor cells showing that these cells share with their corresponding humans the perineural and lymphatic dissemination routes.[10] Moreover, after intrapancreatic injection of hamster pancreatic cancer cells, it is possible to obtain metastases in distant organs such as lung, kidney and liver (N. Erill, *et al.*, unpublished observations). Metastasis-derived sublines of hamster pancreatic tumors may be also obtained (N. Erill, *et al.*, unpublished observations). While these models have been mainly used for biological or genetic study, they can also be of importance in the study of the immunological response elicited by tumor cells as well as in the evaluation of the efficacy of cancer vaccines.

IMPLANTATION OF HUMAN TUMOR CELLS IN THE IMMUNOSUPPRESSED ANIMALS

The implantation of human tumor cells or fragments in nude mice or rats has proved useful in the study of tumor growth *in vivo*.[11] Implantation of established tumor cell lines in the subcutaneous tissue has been used as a tumorigenicity test, as a tool for the study of tumor cell/host interaction and to evaluate *in vivo* the efficacy of new anticancer drugs. Subcutaneous implantation of solid tumor fragments has been used to perpetuate solid tumors. Recently, a high take rate has been reported using Matrigel soaking.[12] Injection of cells in other sites (i.e., intrasplenic or in the dorsal vein of the tail) has been used to obtain experimental metastases, to select distinct metastatic subpopulations and also to evaluate the efficacy of new drugs on the development of new metastases.[11]

ORTHOTOPIC IMPLANTATION IN THE NUDE MICE

Injection of tumor cell suspensions in the corresponding organ of the mice—orthotopic implantation—has shown a higher take rate with preservation of cell populations with metastatic potential.[13–15] However its technical difficulty—injection with a 30-G needle may result in disruption of the pancreatic capsule with significant intraabdominal tumor cell spilling—has precluded its widespread use. More recently, orthotopic implantation of human pancreatic tumor solid fragments xenografted in nude mice resulted in a high (66–100%) take rate.[16,17] Several weeks after anchoring a small solid tumor fragment, a big (2–3 cm in diameter) solid mass that extensively replaces the mouse pancreas can be evidenced. A perfect correlation is observed between the histological appearance of the primary and the perpetuated tumors in mice[16,17] as well as in the expression of tumor-associated antigens expression.[16] Therefore, by using this approach it is possible to obtain a library of perpetuated human pancreatic carcinomas in nude mice that includes all degrees of histological differentiation.[17] It is noteworthy that, in this model system, the reproduction of the desmoplastic host reaction is possible, including the appearance of pancreatic calcifications, so characteristic of pancreatic tumors.[17]

In contrast to subcutaneous implantation, where only local growth occurs, orthotopic implantation more closely reproduces the metastatic behavior of the tumor.[16,17] Dissemination is present in a high (up to 50%) proportion of cases of perpetuated tumors, is tumor specific, and keeps stable through a high number of passages.[17] The use of solid tumor fragments, where heterogeneity of tumor cell populations is high, in conjunction with the implantation in a favorable microenvironment, may account for this high percentage. Although lymphatic, blood-borne and peritoneal dissemination patterns were reproducible, limitations in the nude mouse model during dissemination became apparent. We did not observe perineural invasion, and lymph node invasion was evidenced at a relatively low frequency in our mouse model.[16] Lack of dissemination through these routes is in contrast with their prominent role in the dissemination of human pancreatic carcinoma.[18,19] This discrepancy may be due to incompatibility between the human and mouse proteins that participate in the modulation of normal cell-cell and/or cell-substrate interactions.

Scarcity of fresh human tumor has made difficult the establishment of a large bank of pancreatic cancer cell lines. Enrichment for the neoplastic cell population of pancreatic adenocarcinomas in xenografts provides an immortal tumor that facilitates the establishment of cell lines. Pancreatic cancer cell lines reported in the past were established from either primary tumor, ascitis or metastasis. Some cell lines have already been established using subcutaneous implantation in nude mice.[20] Four pancreatic cancer cell lines were established from two poorly differentiated metastatic (NP9, NP18) and two moderately differentiated primary (NP29, NP31) adenocarcinomas of the pancreas, which had been perpetuated as xenografts in nude mice with a high overall success rate of 57%.[17] In addition, a family of eight metastasis-derived sublines was established from tumoral tissue or malignant ascites obtained from nude mice bearing NP18 cells or NP18 tumor (C. García *et al.*, unpublished observations). Perpetuation and dissemination of human tumors in nude mice may increase the success rate because of enrichment and selection of human tumor cells and elimination of stromal human cells. It is of note that tumors generated by inoculation of cell lines are histologically similar to the original tumor and xenograft. Moreover, implantation of cells in the favorable pancreatic microenvironment allows the reproducibility of the tumor metastasic behavior and cellular heterogeneity.

GENETIC ANALYSIS

The enrichment of human tumor cells using the xenograft method has been shown to facilitate genetic analysis.[12] The lack of contamination by normal human cells has been shown to increase the sensitivity of detection of allelic losses and has enabled the identification of homozygous deletions that otherwise would have not been detected in primary tumors.[21,22] A previous report has shown that both the allelotype and the presence of point mutations in subcutaneous xenografts reproduces the pattern present in their corresponding human pancreatic primary tumors of origin.[12] A perfect match regarding K-*ras* mutations, *p53* gene aberrations as well as *DCC*, *RB* and *APC* allelic losses has been evidenced between the human tumor and orthotopic pancreatic xenografts.[17] Homozygous deletions at the *p16* and *Smad4* gene have been detected in perpetuated tumors. In the majority (40–80%) of perpetuated xenografts, *p16* homozygous deletions were detected,[17,21] while the incidence of homozygous deletions at the *Smad4* locus oscillates between 15 and 40%.[22,23] Finally, recently we have described a high (more than 50%) incidence of p15 homozygous deletions in the xenografts analyzed.[23] Both *p15* and *p16* genes are located in the 9p21 region, and losses of this region occur at high frequency in pancreatic carcinomas.[12,17] Codeletions of *p15* and *p16* genes have been previously reported in pancreatic cancer cell lines, and it was suggested that *p16* was more likely the target gene in this region.[24] Interestingly, the concurrent analyses of *p15* and *p16* genes in the xenografts have demonstrated that *p15* gene aberrations occur independently of *p16* status, and suggests that *p15* may also be an important target gene in the 9p21 region.[23]

The usefulness of xenografts for genetic analysis is high. However, caution should be added when trying to extrapolate the incidence of genetic alterations in xenografts and primaries. Tumor cell selection occurring during tumor implantation and perpetuation may introduce a bias for specific genetic alterations, similar to what has been reported in established cell lines.[25] *p53* gene mutations are overrepresented in our pancreatic xenografts. While six of our eight (75%) perpetuated tumors contained *p53* gene mutations, only 45% of the primary tumors were *p53* positive.[17] These findings suggest that *p53* abnormalities confer growth advantage to tumor cells during tumor implantation in nude mice. The recent description of a better cell hypoxia endurance of *p53*-deficient cells may be related to the higher take rate of *p53*-positive tumors perpetuated in nude mice.[26] Unfortunately, it cannot be ruled out that the incidence of homozygous deletions in *p16*, *p15* or *Smad4* genes detected in xenografts does not overestimate its presence in primaries.

On the other hand, subcutaneous xenografts of pancreatic carcinomas have shown a high degree of genetic integrity compared to the primary tumor.[12] In a previous report it has been shown that orthotopically implanted human pancreatic xenografts show a high degree of genetic stability regarding K-*ras*, *p53* and *p16* through several passages.[17] In contrast, additional *p15* and/or *Smad4* gene alterations have been shown to accumulate in advanced passages of xenografts[23] In fact, P15 protein is absent from all xenografts in their advanced passages.[23] Altogether, regarding genetic analysis, early passages (less than 3) of orthotopic xenografts should be considered to be close to their corresponding human pancreatic primary tumors.

ACCUMULATION DURING DISTAL DISSEMINATION

Orthotopic implantation of human pancreatic cancers in the nude mice facilitates the reproduction, in the experimental animal, of their distal dissemination patterns. While genotype of early passages of pancreatic xenografts is stable, additional genetic alterations can be detected during dissemination. We have observed that K-*ras* and *p53* mutations[17] as well as *p15* and *Smad4* gene aberrations[23] accumulate in metastases obtained from early passages of orthotopic xenografts, indicating that these alterations are selected for and confer selective growth advantage *in vivo*. It may be speculated that among the new cell clones arising in orthotopic xenografts, some contain additional genetic alterations. These clones eventually enter into the venous system, implant in a distal organ and grow as a new metastasis. Finally, it is of note that no additional genetic aberrations in *p16* gene were detected during dissemination,[17] supporting the notion that *p16* genes occur early in pancreatic tumorigenesis.[21]

ORTHOTOPIC IMPLANTATION AS A PRECLINICAL MODEL TO EVALUATE NEW ANTICANCER DRUGS

When trying to establish a preclinical model system to evaluate *in vivo* agents that might have a cytotoxic or cytostatic action, it is critical to obtain a model both close to the human situation and highly reproducible. Intrapancreatic injection of cell suspensions in the nude mice has been used,[13–15] although its technical difficulty has limited its usefulness. The orthotopic model, using solid tumor fragments, provides a unique and useful tool for preclinical evaluation of agents, which may be effective against local and distal dissemination. This approach has previously been used with pancreatic[27] and colorectal[28,29] cancer cells. By implanting tumor fragments of similar weight (approx. 10 mg), it has been possible to standardize the local tumor growth of two of our xenografts (NP9 and NP18) with a moderate variability that permits evaluation of the anticancer activity of novel substances (G. Reyes, *et al.*, manuscript in preparation). Time of sacrifice when evaluation of local tumor growth is performed must be adapted to the growth characteristics of each tumor. In addition, it has also been possible to standardize the timing of distal dissemination in order to evaluate its influence both in overall survival and in the distal dissemination pattern.

We have used this model to evaluate the action of tungstate,[30] an inhibitor of protein tyrosine phosphatases (PTPases) that can be orally administered,[31] on pancreatic cancer growth. PTPases have been suggested to function as tumor suppressor genes, which when activated, may inhibit tumor growth.[32] Recently, *in vitro* studies using somatostatinn analogs (RC-121, RC-160 and SMS 201-995), showed an increase in tyrosine phosphatase activity associated with tumor cell growth inhibition.[33]

According to previous reports, tungstate was expected to stimulate tumor growth. Paradoxically, local growth of human pancreatic tumors NP18 and NP9 was significantly diminished by the continuous administration of oral tungstate (2 mg/mL) during the whole period of study (NP18; 255 ± 143 mg vs 575.2 ± 246 mg; $p < 0.005$;

NP9, 348.3 ± 180.3 mg vs 894.7 ± 227.0 mg; p <0.0005). Opposite results were obtained when effects of long-term tungstate administration were evaluated. All animals were sacrificed when moribund, 13 to 16 weeks after tumor implantation, and no differences regarding survival rate and distal dissemination pattern between the two groups (G. Reyes *et al.*, manuscript in preparation). Moreover, local tumor growth was higher in tumors growing in animals treated with tungstate.

Our results confirm the utility of this model system to prelinically evaluate the action of candidate drugs on pancreatic cancer growth. The combined evaluation on local tumor growth and distal dissemination allows a more accurate evaluation of the putative activity of the tested drugs. As an example, our results suggest that, albeit unexpected, short-term oral administration of tungstate may play a role as an adjuvant treatment in pancreatic cancer patients.

ACKNOWLEDGMENTS

This work was supported in part by grants from CICYT (SAL91-0873; SAF 95-0873; SAF97-0214), FISS (94-0001), CDTI(93-0200), Laboratorios Dr. Esteve S.A. and Fundació Catalana de Gastroenterologia.

REFERENCES

1. BORING, C.C. *et al.* 1994. Cancer statistics, 1994. CA Cancer J. Clin. **44:** 7–26.
2. LILLEMOE, K.D. 1995. Current management of pancreatic carcinoma. Ann. Surg. **221:** 133–148.
3. POUR, P.M. 1989. Experimental pancreatic cancer. Am. J. Surg. Pathol. **13**(Suppl. 1): 96–103.
4. CHANG, K.W. *et al.* 1994. Multiple genetic alterations in hamster pancreatic ductal adenocarcinomas. Cancer Res. **55:** 2560–2568.
5. TOWNSEND, C.M. JR. *et al.* 1982. Development of a transplantable model of pancretic duct adenocarcinoma. Surgery **92:** 72–78.
6. ERILL, N. *et al.* 1996. K-ras and p53 mutations in hamster pancreatic ductal adenocarcinomas and cell lines. Am. J. Pathol. **149:** 1333–1339.
7. CERNY, W.L. *et al.* 1992. K-*ras* mutation is an early event in pancreatic duct carcinogenesis in the Syrian golden hamster. Cancer Res. **52:** 4507–4513
8. CHANG, K.W. *et al.* 1994. Genomic p53 mutation in a chemically-induced hamster pancreatic ductal adenocarcinoma. Cancer Res. **54:** 3878–3883.
9. FARRÉ, A. *et al.* 1994. Bombesin inhibits growth of pancreatic ductal adenocarcinoma (H2T) in nude mice. Pancreas **9:** 652–656.
10. POUR, P.M. *et al.* 1991. Patterns of growth and metastases of induced pancreatic cancer in relation to the prognosis and its clinical implications. Gastroenterology **100:** 529–536.
11. FIDLER, I. J. 1986. Rationale and methods for the use of nude mice to study the biology and therapy of human cancer metastasis. Cancer Metastasis Rev. **5:** 29–49.
12. HAHN, S.A. *et al.* 1995. Allelotype of pancreatic adenocarcinoma using xenograft enrichment. Cancer Res. **55:** 4670–4675.
13. MARINCOLA, F.M. *et al.* 1989. The nude mouse as a model for the study of human pancreatic cancer. J. Surg. Res. **47:** 520–529.
14. TAN, M.H., *et al.* 1985. Characterization of the tumorigenic and metastatic properties of a human pancreatic tumor cell line (AsPc-1) implanted orthotopically into nude mice. Tumour Biol. **6:** 89–98.

15. VEZERIDIS, M.P. et al. 1989. Invasion and metastasis following orthotopic transplantation of human pancreatic cancer in the nude mouse. J. Surg. Oncol. **40:** 261–265.
16. FU, X. et al. 1992. A metastatic nude-mouse model of human pancreatic cancer constructed orthotopically with histologically intact patient specimens. Proc. Natl. Acad. Sci. USA **89:** 5645–5649.
17. REYES, G. et al. 1996. Orthotopic implantation of human carcinomas of the exocrine pancreas in nude mice. Cancer Res. **56:** 5713–5719.
18. KAYAHARA, M. et al. 1991. Clinicopathological study of pancreatic carcinoma with particular reference to the invasion of the extrapancreatic neural plexus. Int. J. Pancreatol. **10:** 105-111.
19. NAGAKAWA, T. et al. 1993. The pattern of lymph node involvement in carcinoma of the head of the pancreas. A histological study of the surgical findings in patients undergoing extensive nodal dissections. Int. J. Pancreatol. **13:** 15–22.
20. YAMADA, H. et al. 1986. Establishment of a human pancreatic adenocarcinoma cell line (PSN-1) with amplifications of both c-*myc* and activated c-Ki-*ras* by a point mutation. Biochem. Biophys. Res. Commun. **140:** 167–173.
21. CALDAS, C. et al. 1994. Frequent somatic mutations and homozygous deletions of the *p16* (*MTS1*) gene in pancreatic adenocarcinoma. Nat. Genet. **8:** 27–32.
22. HAHN, S.A. et al. 1996. *DPC4*, a candidate tumor suppressor gene at human chromosome 18q21.1. Science **271:** 350–353.
23. VILLANUEVA, A. et al. 1998. Disruption of the antiproliferative TGF-beta signaling pathways in human pancreatic cancer cells. Oncogene. In press.
24. NAUMANN, M. et al. 1996. Frequent codeletion of *p16/MTS1* and *p16/MTS2* and genetic alterations in *p16/MTS1* in pancreatic tumors. Gastroenterology **110:** 1215–1224.
25. HUANG, L. et al. 1996. Deletion and mutation analysis of the *p16/MTS-1* tumor suppressor gene in human ductal pancreatic cancer reveals a higher frequency of abnormalities in tumor-derived cell lines than in primary ductal adenocacinomas. Cancer Res. **56:** 1137–1141.
26. GRAEBER, T.G. et al. 1996. Hypoxia-mediated selection of cells with diminished apoptotic potential in solid tumours. Nature **379:** 88–91.
27. FURUKAWA, T. et al. 1993. A novel "patient-like" treatment model of human pancreatic cancer constructed using orthotopic transplantation of histologically intact human tumor tissue in nude mice. Cancer Res. **53:** 3070 -3072.
28. WANG, X. et al. 1994. Matrix metalloproteinase inhibitor BB-94 (Batimastat) inhibits human colon tumor growth and spread in a patient-like orthotopic model in nude mice. Cancer Res. **54:** 4726–4728.
29. POTMESIL, M. et al. 1995. Growth inhibition of human cancer metastases by camptothecins in newly developed xenograft models. Cancer Res. **55:** 5637-5641.
30. STUCKEY, J.A. et al. 1994. Crystal structure of Yersinia protein tyrosine phosphatase at 2.5 Å and the complex with tungstate. Nature **370:** 571–575.
31. BARBERÀ, A. et al. 1994. Insulin-like actions of tungstate in diabetic rats. J. Biol. Chem. **269:** 20047–20053.
32. HUNTER, T. 1989. Protein tyrosine phosphatase: the other side of the coin. Cell **58:** 1013–1016.
33. BUSCAIL, L. et al. 1994. Stimulation of tyrosine phosphatase and inhibition of cell proliferation by somatostatin analogues: mediation by human somatostatin receptor subtypes SSTR1 and SSTR2. Proc. Natl. Acad. Sci. USA **91:** 2315–2319.

Growth Factors and Cytokines in Pancreatic Carcinogenesis

HELMUT FRIESS,[a] XIAO-ZHONG GUO, BI-CHENG NAN, ÖRG KLEEFF, AND MARKUS W. BÜCHLER

Department of Visceral and Transplantation Surgery, University of Bern, Inselspital, Switzerland

> ABSTRACT: Pancreatic cancer is a deadly disease challenging basic and clinical researchers alike in characterizing its pathobiology and finding better treatment options. A number of molecular alterations including gene mutations such as k-*ras*, p53, and Smad4 and aberrant expression of a variety of genes have been identified in recent years. This review focuses on two families of growth factors and growth factor receptors which are representative for the molecular alterations observed in pancreatic cancer: the transforming growth factor-β superfamily of serine-threonine kinase receptors and their ligands, which usually act as negative growth regulators, and the epidermal growth factor receptor family and their ligands, which have the potential to act as growth promoters in pancreatic cancer. In addition, we will discuss the role of the cytokines TNF-α, IFN-γ, and IL-6 and its effects on pancreatic cancer cell proliferation *in vitro* and *in vivo*. Pancreatic cancer cell biology consists of complex interactions of various factors, and a better understanding of the molecular pathogenesis of this disorder might lead to better treatment strategies in the near future.

INTRODUCTION

Pancreatic cancer is a devastating disease with a poor prognosis, an overall five-year survival rate of <1%, and a median survival after diagnosis of approximately 5–6 months.[1–3] At present, pancreatic cancer is the fourth or fifth leading cause of cancer-related death in Western industrialized countries.[4–6] The incidence of pancreatic cancer seems to have increased in recent decades,[1,2] although this may be due to better diagnostic options. At the time of diagnosis, between 75% and 85% of pancreatic cancer patients have unresectable tumors, and these patients can be offered only palliative surgical options such as biliary or enteral bypass operations.[5–8] Conservative oncological strategies such as chemotherapy and radiotherapy have failed to significantly improve the prognosis of advanced pancreatic cancers.[9–11] In addition, antihormonal modalities using tamoxifen or buserelin[12,13] or the systemic use of specific antipancreatic cancer cell monoclonal antibodies[14,15] have not led to a significant improvement in the survival of patients with pancreatic cancer. Furthermore, pancreatic cancer is a silently growing tumor, and one of its typical features is the presence of metastatic lesions at the time of diagnosis. Most patients who undergo

---

[a]Address for correspondence: Helmut Friess, M.D. Department of Visceral and Transplantation Surgery, University of Bern, Inselspital, CH-3010 Bern, Switzerland. Phone, +41 31-632-9722; fax, +41 31-632-9732; e-mail, helmut.friess@insel.ch

curative tumor resection die within the first two postoperative years due to local recurrence or distant metastases. In these patients no further effective therapy is presently available which offers cure or effective palliation.

The development of human cancer involves the clonal evolution of cell populations that gain competitive advantage over other cells through the alteration of at least two distinct classes of genes: (a) protooncogenes, through gene amplification, mutations, or overexpression; and (b) tumor suppressor genes, through alterations that inactivate the functions of both alleles.[16,17] A variety of regulatory mechanisms contribute to the development and growth of pancreatic carcinoma, and only a few of them are known so far. In order to establish an understanding of the multistage process that leads to carcinogenesis, numerous genetic and cellular alterations remain to be evaluated. Oncogene activation, loss of tumor suppressor gene function[18] and the overexpression of receptor ligand systems[19] show tumor-dependent variation. A high prevalence of K-ras oncogene mutations in pancreatic cancer has been described, and it has been suggested that these mutations are highly indicative of pancreatic malignancies.[20] K-ras activation evolves at an early stage in pancreatic carcinogenesis, and the fact that it is also present in chronic pancreatitis supports the assumption that chronic pancreatitis might be a premalignant condition for pancreatic cancer or that K-ras mutations play a limited role in tumor pathogenesis. Furthermore, pancreatic tissues contain a high degree of certain components of the so-called autocrine and paracrine growth regulation machinery, most noticeably the epidermal growth factor receptor (EGFR) and its ligands, transforming growth factor-α (TGF-α), EGF and amphiregulin.

In the present paper we can cover only a few aspects of growth factors and cytokines in pancreatic cancer. First, we will discuss the behavior of growth factors and growth factor receptors with normally negative influence on cell proliferation in pancreatic cancer. Next, we will evaluate growth-promoting factors and their function in pancreatic cancer pathogenesis. And last, we will assess the ability of pancreatic cancer cells to produce cytokines and thereby directly or indirectly affect tumor pathogenesis.

GROWTH FACTORS AND GROWTH FACTOR RECEPTORS WITH NEGATIVE INFLUENCE ON EPITHELIAL CELL PROLIFERATION

Mammalian cells express three isotypes of transforming growth factor-β (TGF-β1, TGF-β2 and TGF-β3) and three TGF-β receptors: type I (TβR-I), type II (TβR-II) and type III (TβR-III).[21,22] In contrast, TGF-β4 and TGF-β5 are only present in chickens and frogs, respectively.[22,23] The TGF-β isotypes exert pleiotrophic effects in a variety of cell types. TGF-βs inhibit growth in many epithelial cells, influence the structure of the extracellular matrix, regulate cell differentiation and angiogenesis, and have been described as immunosuppressive factors.[21–23] However, cell proliferation is not inhibited in all pancreatic cancer cell lines by TGF-β1, which represents the prototype protein in this growth factor family. Meanwhile, it has been shown that the influence of TGF-β on growth of tumor cell lines is dependent on the cell type, the culture conditions and the concentration of TGF-β.[23–25] Therefore, alterations in cell culture conditions can change the effect of TGF-β from inhibitory to neutral or to a stimulatory effect. However, in most cells of epithelial origin TGF-β isoforms generally act as potent growth inhibitors.[21–23,26,27]

The effect of TGF-βs in human pancreatic carcinoma has been characterized in a recent study. This study demonstrated that pancreatic cancer samples, in comparison with normal pancreatic samples, exhibited an 11-fold, 7-fold, and 9-fold increase in TGF-β1, TGF-β2 and TGF-β3 mRNA expression in Northern blot analysis, respectively.[28] By *in situ* hybridization, mRNA grains encoding TGF-β1, TGF-β2 and TGF-β3 mRNA moieties were present in great abundance in approximately 30% of the cancer cells. The remaining cells, as well as connective tissue, did not show any specific mRNA grains. Overexpression of the TGF-βs as determined by *in situ* hybridization and Northern blot analysis was associated with increased immunoreactivity of the peptides in the pancreatic cancer cells. Analysis of the survival data of 60 resected pancreatic cancer patients demonstrated that the presence of TGF-β1, TGF-β2 and TGF-β3 in the pancreatic tumor cells is associated with more aggressive growth and with significantly reduced postoperative survival periods. These findings suggest that TGF-βs may act as growth stimulators in human pancreatic cancer *in vivo*, or that growth-inhibiting effects of TGF-βs on pancreatic cancer cells are lost.[28] Alterations in TGF-ß receptors might be one reason for this.

TGF-β receptors consist of a small extracellular region, a single transmembrane segment, and a cytoplasmic region that possesses serine/threonine kinase activity. Cross-linking experiments with radiolabeled TGF-βs have identified three primary binding proteins of 53 kDa (type I TGF-β receptor, TβR-I), 70 kDa (type II TGF-β receptor, TβR-II) and 200–400 kDa (type III TGF-β receptor, TβR-III).[21,23,29–32] TGF-β causes a delayed but sustained increase in the protein levels of the cyclin-dependent kinase inhibitors p15(Ink4B), p21(Cip1), and p27(Kip1), and a sustained increase in type I and type II TGF-β receptor mRNA and protein levels. The protein synthesis inhibitor cycloheximide completely blocks the TGF-β-mediated increase in TβR-I and TβR-II expression.[33] Tumor suppressor gene DPC4 (deleted in pancreatic cancer locus 4), which is present in approximately 50% of pancreatic cancer samples, was found to be homologous to Smad4, which functions as a transcription factor in the TGF-β receptor-mediated signal transduction pathway.[34] Inactivation of the DPC4 gene and other components of the TGF-β signal cascades may abolish one of the key negative control elements of cell proliferation in pancreatic adenocarcinoma,[35] thereby allowing pancreatic cancer cells to escape physiological growth inhibition. Cloning and biochemical studies indicate that TβR-II has intrinsic serine/threonine kinase activity, which is dependent on the presence of TβR-I.[36,37] However, TβR-I is necessary for binding of TGF-β to TβR-II,[36] whereas TβR-III is a membrane proteoglycan that binds TGF-β isoforms but is not believed to have direct signal-transducing activity.[31,36,38] Several TβR-I subtypes have been described. However, only TβR-I$_{ALK5}$ seems to participate in TGF-β-mediated signal transduction.

All three TGF-β receptors have been found in the normal human pancreas.[29,32] Northern blot analysis of total RNA revealed low levels of TβR-I$_{ALK5}$ and TβR-II mRNA in all normal pancreatic tissues. In contrast, TβR-III mRNA expression was readily evident in the normal pancreas. In pancreatic cancer, TβR-I$_{ALK5}$ and R-II were markedly overexpressed in most samples, whereas the expression levels of TβR-III were unchanged in comparison with normal controls. *In situ* hybridization showed that both TβR-I$_{ALK5}$ and TβR-II mRNA were highly expressed in the majority of pancreatic cancer cells, forming duct-like structures within the tumor, whereas TβR-III mRNA grains were mainly expressed in the stroma of the tumors but not in the cancer cells.[32] Immunohistochemical analysis of TβR-I$_{ALK5}$ and TβR-II revealed positive immunostaining in 73% and 56% of the pancreatic cancer cells, respectively. Both receptors were concomitantly present in 54% of the pancreatic cancer samples.[29] The presence of TβR-I$_{ALK5}$ or TβR-II and the concomitant presence of TβR-I$_{ALK5}$ and TβR-II in the cancer cells was associated with advanced tumor stage {p <0.01}. These findings suggest that TGF-βs, via activation of their receptors, contribute to the neoplastic process in pancreatic cancer.[29,32] However, it is not clear by which mechanisms the growth-inhibiting functions of TGF-βs are lost in pancreatic cancers. This might be due to direct effects of TGF-β isoforms on the cancer cells, or by stimulating angiogenesis and/or suppressing immune function. Thus, TGF-β isoforms may influence tumorigenicity by stimulating angiogenesis, suppressing cancer-directed immune function[39] and increasing the expression adhesion molecules and extracellular matrix components, which subsequently might enhance the metastatic ability of the cancer cells. Inasmuch as approximately 50% of pancreatic tumors lose DPC4 (deleted in pancreatic cancer, also named SMAD4), an intracellular signaling protein that is required for signal transduction of TGF-β, it also seems to be possible that the negative effect of TGF-β on cell growth is no longer functioning in many pancreatic cancer cells.[34]

EPIDERMAL GROWTH FACTOR RECEPTOR (EGFR) AND ITS LIGANDS: FACTORS THAT STIMULATE EPITHELIAL CELL PROLIFERATION

The epidermal growth factor (EGF) receptor can be activated by EGF, TGF-α, heparin-binding EGF-like growth factor (HB-EGF), β–cellulin and amphiregulin.[40–44] All five growth factors have six cysteine residues in the same relative position as EGF, and are produced as precursor molecules, which are inserted into the cell membrane prior to undergoing proteolytic cleavage to yield the mature protein. In addition, β–cellulin, HB-EGF, and amphiregulin have heparin-binding characteristics.[45] Early studies on cancer cells showed that overexpression of the EGF receptor leads to malignant cell transformation, and that the presence of EGF and TGF-α additionally stimulates the proliferation of the transformed cells.[46–48] By immunohistochemical and *in situ* hybridization techniques, the presence of low levels of EGFR, EGF, and TGF-α in the normal human pancreas and the presence of increased levels of these moieties in pancreatic tumors have been described.[48] Many cancer cells show concomitant overexpression of the EGF receptor and EGF and/or TGF-α, indicating that autocrine and/or paracrine mechanisms of this receptor-ligand system play a crucial role in the pathogenesis of pancreatic cancer growth.[30,49,50] Correlation analysis of immunopositivity of EGFR, EGF and TGF-α in pancreatic cancer cells with clinicopathological parameters has revealed that the concomitant presence of the EGF receptor with either EGF and/or TGF-α is associated with more aggressive disease and a significantly shorter survival time postoperatively.[49,50]

These findings in human cancer samples are in accordance with *in vitro* experiments in which HB-EGF, EGF, TGF-α and amphiregulin enhance the proliferation of cultured human pancreatic cancer cell lines.[50–54] Interestingly, growth factors in pancreatic cancer can stimulate their own expression and enhance the production of other growth-promoting peptides. For example, HB-EGF mRNA levels are upregulated in cultured pancreatic cancer cells by HB-EGF, TGF-α and tissue plasminogen activator (TPA).[52] As in the case of EGF and TGF-α, amphiregulin and HB-EGF mRNA levels are increased in pancreatic cancer by comparison with the levels expressed in the normal pancreas.[49,50,54] These findings suggest that multiple members of the EGF growth factor family may participate in the aberrant autocrine and paracrine activation of the EGF receptor, thereby contributing to growth and proliferation of pancreatic cancer cells. Based on these findings, new treatment possibilities are presently being evaluated for pancreatic cancer. Amphiregulin antisense oligonucleotide (AR-AS) abolishes amphiregulin immunoreactivity in T3M4 pancreatic cancer cells, decreases amphiregulin release into the medium and inhibits cancer cell growth in a dose-dependent manner, whereas a random oligonucleotide did not alter either cell growth or cellular amphiregulin synthesis. Based on the observation that there is an important EGFR/amphiregulin autocrine loop in pancreatic cancer cells, which negatively influences survival in pancreatic cancer *in vivo*, a therapeutic approach aiming to abrogate amphiregulin action[55] or to block the EGF receptor may be possible.

The EGF receptor, also known as human EGF receptor 1 (HER-1), is closely related to several receptors including EGF receptor type 2 (HER-2 or c-erb-B2), HER-3 (c-erb-B3), and HER-4 (c-erb-B4), which has recently been cloned.[56,57] These four growth factor receptors contain an extracellular ligand-binding domain, a transmembrane domain, and an intracellular domain.[58,59] The intracellular domain possesses tyrosine kinase activity, and activation of the receptors by specific ligands leads to the phosphorylation of various intracellular substrates such as phospholipase C-gamma.[58,60] The c-erb-B2 gene encodes a transmembrane receptor with a molecular weight of 185 kDa.[60] Overexpression of c-erb-B2 leads to malignant cell transformation *in vitro*.[58,60,61] Approximately 40–50% of pancreatic cancers exhibit increased c-erb-2 immunoreactivity.[62,63] Northern blot analysis and/or *in situ* hybridization indicates that the increase in EGF receptor, c-erb-B2 and c-erb-B3 immunoreactivity is due to overexpression of the respective mRNA moieties.[62–64] The presence of c-erb-B2 is not associated with advanced tumor stage and shorter postoperative survival periods, whereas positive immunoreactivity for c-erb-3 has been associated with advanced tumor stage and significantly shorter postoperative survival.[64,65] Taking these findings together, we conclude that overexpression of the EGF receptor and/or c-erbB3 seems to play a role in pancreatic cancer progression and influences the prognosis after tumor resection negatively.[64]

CYTOKINES AND PANCREATIC CANCER

A variety of cytokines are expressed in pancreatic cancer, indicating that these molecules, which are important in immune response, also have a function in tumor pathogenesis and tumor progression. Cytokines are involved in the attraction of inflammatory cells, altering cell adhesion molecules and chemotaxis, and they mediate various interactions between tumor cells and the extracellular matrix. Tumor necrosis factor-α (TNF-α) is a cytokine that upregulates platelet-derived growth factor

(PDGF) expression in cultured pancreatic cancer cells, even in those cell lines that do not express PDGF without TNF-α exposure.[65] Inasmuch as PDGF strongly stimulates fibrogenesis, this leads to the possibility that TNF-α released initially from tumor-infiltrating macrophages initiates a cascade of events that finally results in a marked increase in extracellular matrix synthesis, thereby causing the strong desmoplastic reaction that is normally seen in pancreatic malignancies.

Besides having indirect influences on extracellular matrix composition, TNF-α also induces the expression of further cytokines, can exhibit cytotoxic effects on tumor cells, and modulates pancreatic cancer cell growth by growth factor and growth factor receptor upregulation. The cellular functions of TNF-α are mediated via well-characterized TNF-α receptors, which can be differentiated by their molecular weight into a type I (TNF-RI, 55 kDa) and a type II (TNF-RII, 75 kDa) TNF receptor. Both receptors show high-affinity binding of TNF-α and TNF-β. However, the cytotoxic effects of TNF-α have been assumed to be mediated via TNF-RI, whereas TNF-RII seems to be less important in TNF-αssociated cytotoxicity. TNF-RI mRNA expression is present in pancreatic cancer, and the application of TNF-α does not modulate the levels of TNF-RI.[66] Signal transduction of TNF-α leads to an intracellular increase of protein kinase C, phospholipase A2 and lipoxygenase,[67] which are considered mediators of TNF-α signaling. However, binding of TNF-α to TNF-RII also upregulates the EGF receptor and its activating ligand TGF-α, thereby contributing to cancer cell proliferation. Therefore, the balance between cytotoxic effects and stimulation of growth factor synthesis decides which biological effects will finally result from the presence of TNF-α. This critical balance between growth promotion influences and cell cytotoxicity might explain why TNF-α treatment has limited effectiveness in pancreatic cancer treatment and why pancreatic cancer cells might escape the antiproliferative effects of TNF-α. Besides TNF-α, pancreatic cancer cells also secrete granulocyte colony stimulating factor (G-CSF) and granulocyte macrophage colony-stimulating factor (GM-CSF).[68,69] The exact function of GM-CSF and G-CSF in pancreatic cancer is not known; however, the growth of malignant nonhematopoietic cell lines is strongly stimulated by GM-CSF. Furthermore, there exists a relationship between TNF-α and GM-CSF. In seven out of eight pancreatic cancer cell lines, TNF-α stimulates the production of GM-CSF, G-CSF and interleukin (IL)-1β.[69]

Another cytokine with potential effects on pancreatic cancer cell behavior is interferon-γ (IFN-γ), which, like TNF-α and IL-1, induces at least four adhesion molecules that subsequently modify the ability of pancreatic cancer cells to metastasize.[70,71] The intercellular adhesion molecule-1 (ICAM-1, also named CD4) is expressed to various degrees in pancreatic cancer cell lines[72] as well as in human pancreatic tumor samples.[73] Similarly, endothelial leukocyte adhesion molecule-1 (ELAM-1, also known as E selectin-1), is present in pancreatic carcinoma cell lines and mediates cell-to-cell adhesion, indicating that disturbances in cancer cell attachment molecules are involved in the risk of hematogenic metastasis formation.[72,74] These findings show the close relationship between cancer cell-produced cytokines and cell surface molecules, enlarging the biological influences of cytokines in cancer cell biology.

The clinical single use of TNF-α and IFN-γ in pancreatic cancer treatment has not resulted in prognosis improvement. In addition, the combination of both cytokines, when applied to patients, leads to serious side effects resulting from IFN-γ.[75,76] The problem of TNF-α-induced expression of the EGF receptor, which subsequently promotes growth of pancreatic cancer cells, can be overcome by the use of EGF receptor-binding monoclonal antibodies, which block EGF receptor activity.[77] Therefore, the combination therapy of TNF-α with anti-EGF receptor antibodies permits the exclusion of the indirect growth-promoting effects of TNF-α but maintains the TNF-α-associated antiproliferative effects.

Interleukin-6 (IL-6) is another cytokine with tumor-influencing effects. It has been reported to influence tumor-associated cachexia, and together with TNF-α it has an additive effect on the resting energy expenditure, which cannot only be attributed to an elevated serum concentration in these cytokines, but is linked to increased local cytokine production by mononuclear cells.[78] Approximately 55% of pancreatic cancer patients show increased IL-6 serum levels.[79] However, one normal control and two chronic pancreatitis patients exhibited high IL-6 serum levels, indicating that this increase can also occur in benign circumstances.[79] Experimental data indicate that IL-6 can influence the formation of cancer cell metastasis negatively.[80] Transfection experiments in pancreatic cancer cell lines revealed that IL-6 production has a negative effect on hematogenic tumor metastasis formation. However, in severe combined immunodeficiency (SCID) beige-mice, IL-6-producing cancer cells form palpable tumor lesions, which were not observed in nude mice, indicating a dual action of tumor-derived IL-6 on cancer cell growth.

In summary, based on the findings in cytokines we can conclude that they belong to a complex network in immunology but also potentially influence cancer cell proliferation behavior *in vitro* and *in vivo*.

CONCLUSION

Molecular research in the past years has significantly contributed to a better understanding of pathophysiological aspects in pancreatic cancer. Increased expression of a variety of growth-promoting factors and growth factor receptors enhance the malignant phenotype of pancreatic cancer cells. Together with gene mutations such as p53, k-ras, etc., these molecular alterations are important in pancreatic cancer pathogenesis. However, growth factors and their receptors are closely related to a variety of other tumor-related factors, such as cytokines, which influence their expression but also exhibit direct and indirect effects on pancreatic cancer cells. Cancer cell biology consists of complex interactions among both known and probably to a major extent unknown systems. Therefore, therapeutic approaches aimed at influencing one of these alterations in pancreatic cancer patients might fail to improve the prognosis of these patients substantially. As a result, the future of therapy for pancreatic cancer must apply our present molecular knowledge to the development of new innovative and more effective treatment protocols in this dismal disorder.

REFERENCES

1. PARKER, S.L., T. TONG, S. BOLDEN & P.A. WINGO. 1997. Cancer statistics, 1997. Ca. Cancer J. Clin. **47:** 5–27.

2. GUDJONSSON, B. 1987. Cancer of the pancreas. 50 years of surgery. Cancer **60:** 2284–2303.
3. FRIESS, H., M.W. BÜCHLER, M. EBERT, P. MALFERTHEINER, H.J. DENNLER & H.G. BEGER. 1993. Treatment of advanced pancreatic cancer with high dose octreotide. Int. J. Pancreatol. **14:** 290–291.
4. FRIESS, H., M. BÜCHLER, C. BEGLINGER, M. KRÜGER & H.G. BEGER. 1993. Low-dose octreotide treatment is not effective in patients with advanced pancreatic cancer. Pancreas **8:** 540–544.
5. WARSHAW, A.L. & C. FERNANDES-DEL CASTILLO. 1992. Pancreatic carcinoma. N. Engl. J. Med. **326:** 455–465.
6. National Cancer Institute. Annual cancer statistics review 1973–1998. NIH publication no. 91-2789. Department of Health and Human Services, Bethesda, MD, USA.
7. BÜCHLER, M., M. EBERT & H.G. BEGER. 1993. Grenzen chirurgischen Handelns beim Pankreaskarzinom. Langenbecks. Arch. Chir. Suppl. **378:** 460–464.
8. FRIESS, H., W. UHL, H.G. BEGER & M. BÜCHLER. 1994. Surgical treatment of pancreatic cancer. Dig. Surg. **11:** 378–386.
9. CULLINAN, S.A., C.G. MOERTEL, T.R. FLEMING, J.R. RUBIN, J.E. KROOK, L.K. EVERSON, H.E. WINDSCHITL, D.I. TWITO, R.F. MARSCHKE, J.F. FOLEY et. al. 1985. A comparison of three chemotherapeutic regimens in the treatment of advanced pancreatic and gastric carcinoma. Fluorouracil vs fluorouracil and doxorubicin vs fluorouracil, doxorubicin, and mitomycin. JAMA **253:** 2061–2067.
10. MOERTEL, C.G., S. FRYTAK, R.G. HAHN et al. 1981. Therapy of locally unresectable pancreatic carcinoma: a randomized comparison of high dose (6000 rads) radiation alone, moderate dose radiation (4000 rads) + 5-fluorouracil, and high dose radiation + 5-fluorouracil: the Gastrointestinal Tumor Study Group. Cancer **48:** 1705–1710.
11. NEOPTOLEMOS, J.P., Ed. 1990. Cancer of the pancreas. Baillierea Clin. Gastroenterol. London **4:** 4.
12. ANDREN-SANDBERG, A. 1990. Treatment with an LHRH analogue in patients with advanced pancreatic cancer. Acta Chir. Scand. **156:** 549–551.
13. FRIESS, H., M. BÜCHLER, M. KRUGER & H.G. BEGER. 1992. Treatment of duct carcinoma of the pancreas with the LH-RH analogue buserelin. Pancreas **7:** 516–521.
14. BÜCHLER, M., H. FRIESS, K.H. SCHULDTHEISS, C. GEBHARDT, R. KUBEL, K.H. MUHRER, M. WINKELMANN, T. WAGENER, R. KLAPDOR, M. KAUL, G. MÜLLER & H.G. SCHULZ. 1991. A randomized controlled trial of adjuvant immuno-therapy (murine monoclonal antibody; 494/32) in resectable pancreatic cancer. Cancer **68:** 1507–1512.
15. FRIESS, H., M. BÜCHLER, G. SCHULZ & H.G. BEGER. 1989. Therapie des Pankreaskarzinoms mit dem monoklonalen Antikorper BW 494/32: erste klinische Ergebnisse. Immun. Infekt. **17:** 24–26.
16. GUO, X., H. FRIESS, H.U. GRABER, M. KASHIWAGI, A. ZIMMERMANN, M. KORC & BÜCHLER. 1996. KAI 1 expression is up-regulated in early pancreatic cancer and decreased in the presence of metastases. Cancer Res. **56:** 4876–4880.
17. MARK, S.R., C. CARLOS, B.S. ALBERT, H.H. RALPH, D.C. LUIS, J.Y. CHARLES & E.K. SCOTTE. 1994. P53 mutations in pancreatic carcinoma and evidence of common involvement of homocopolymer tracts in DNA micro deletions. Cancer Res **54:** 3025–3033.
18. FEARON, E.R. & B. VOGELSTEIN. 1990. A genetic model for colorectal tumorigenesis. Cell **61:**759–767.
19. LEMOINE, N.R., C.M. HUGHES & C.M. BARTON. 1992. The epidermal growth factor receptor in human pancreatic cancer. J. Pathol. **166:** 7–12.
20. KALTHOFF, H., W. SCHMIEGEL, C. ROEDER et al. 1993. P53 and K-ras alteration in pancreatic cell lesions. Oncogene **8:** 289–298.
21. MASSAGUE, J. 1990. The transforming growth factor-β family. Annu. Rev. Cell. Biol. **6:** 597–641.
22. MASSAGUE, J., S. CHEIFETZ, M. LAIHO, D.A. RALPH, F.M. WEIS & A. ZENTELLA. 1992. Transforming growth factor-β. Cancer Surv. **12:** 81–103.

23. SPORN, M.B. & A.B. ROBERTS. 1992. Transforming growth factor-β: recent progress and new challenges. J. Cell Biol. **119**: 1017–1021.
24. HEBDA, P.A. 1988. Stimulatory effects of transforming growth factor-beta and epidermal growth factor on epidermal cell outgrowth from porcine skin explant cultures. J. Invest. Dermatol. **91**: 440–445.
25. STEINER, M.S. & E.R. BARRACK. 1992. Transforming growth factor-beta1 overproduction in prostate cancer: effects on growth *in vivo* and *in vitro*. Mol. Endocrinol. **6**: 15–25.
26. ROBERT, A.B. & M.B. SPORN. 1990. The transforming growth factor-β. *In* Peptide Growth Factors and Their Receptors. Handbook of Experimental Pharmacology. Vol. 95. M.B. Sporn & A.B. Robert, Eds. Vol. 119: 419–472. Springer. Heidelberg.
27. BALDWIN, R.L. & M. KORC. 1993. Growth inhibition of human pancreatic carcinoma cells by transforming growth factor beta-1. Growth Factors **8**: 23–34.
28. FRIESS, H., Y. YAMANAKA, M. BÜCHLER, M. EBERT, H.G. BEGER, L.I. GOLD & M. KORC. 1993. Enhanced expression of transforming growth factor beta isoforms in pancreatic cancer correlates with decreased survival. Gastroenterology **105**: 1846–1856.
29. LU, Z., H. FRIESS, H.U. GRABER, X. GUO, M. SCHILLING, A. ZIMMERMANN, M. KORC & M.W. BÜCHLER. 1997. Presence of two signaling TGF-β receptors in human pancreatic cancer correlates with advanced tumor stage. Dig. Dis. Sci. **42**: 2054–2063.
30. FRIESS, H., P. BERBERAT, M. SCHILLING, J. KUNZ, M. KORC & M.W. BÜCHLER. 1996. Pancreatic cancer: the potential clinical relevance of alterations in growth factors and their receptors J. Mol. Med. **74**: 35–42.
31. LOPEZ-CASILLAS, F., S. CHEIFETZ, J. DOODY, J.L. ANDRES, W.S. LANE & J. MASSAGUE. 1991. Structure and expression of the membrane proteoglycan betaglycan, a component of the TGF receptor system. Cell **67**: 785–795.
32. FRIESS, H., Y. YAMANAKA, M. BÜCHLER *et al.* 1993. Enhanced expression of the type II transforming growth factor beta receptor in human pancreatic cancer cells without alteration of type III receptor expression. Cancer Res. **53**: 2704–2707.
33. KLEEFF, J. & M. KORC. 1998. Up-regulation of transforming growth factor (TGF)-beta receptors by TGF-βeta in COLO-357 cells. J. Biol. Chem. **273**: 7495–7500.
34. HAHN, S.A., M. SCHUTTE, A.T. HOQUE, C.A. MOSKALUK, L.T. DA COSTA, E. ROZENBLUM, C.L. WEINSTEIN, A. FISCHER, C.J. YEO, R.H. HRUBAN & S.E. KERN. 1996. DPC4, a candidate tumor suppressor gene at human chromosome 18q21.1. Science **271**: 350–353.
35. GRAU, A.M., L. ZHANG, W. WANG, S. RUAN, D.B. EVANS, J.L. ABBRUZZESE, W. ZHANG & P.J. CHIAO. 1997. Induction of p21waf1 expression and growth inhibition by transforming growth factor beta involve the tumor suppressor gene DPC4 in human pancreatic adenocarcinoma cells. Cancer Res. **57**: 3929–3934.
36. WRANA, J.L., L. ATTISANO, J. CARCAMO *et al.* 1992. TGF beta signals through a heteromeric protein kinase receptor complex. Cell **71**: 1003–1014.
37. LIN, H.Y., X.F. WANG, E. NG-EATON, R.A. WEINBERG & H.F. LODISH. 1992. Expression cloning of the TGF-beta type II receptor, a functional transmembrane serine/threonine kinase. Cell **68**: 775–785.
38. WANG, X.F, H.Y. LIN, E. NG-EATON, J. DOWNWARD, H.F. LODISH & R.A. WEINBERG. 1991. Expression cloning and characterization of the TGF-beta type III receptor. Cell **67**: 797–805.
39. SPORN, M.B. & A.B. ROBERTS. 1990. TGF-β: problems and prospects. Cell Regul. **1**: 875–882.
40. ABRAHAM, J.A., D. DAMM, A. BAJARDI, J. MILLER, M. KLAGSBRUN & R.A. EZEKOWITZ. 1993. Heparin-binding EGF-like growth factor: characterization of rat and mouse cDNA clones, protein domain conservation across species, and transcript expression in tissues. Biochem. Biophys. Res. Commun. **190**: 125–133.
41. SHING, Y., G. CHRISTOFORI, D. HANAHAN *et al.* 1993. Betacellulin: a mitogen from pancreatic beta cell tumors. Science **259**: 1604–1607.

42. PLOWMAN, G.D., J.M. GREEN, V.L. MCDONALD et al. 1990. The amphiregulin gene encodes a novel epidermal growth factor-related protein with tumor-inhibitory activity. Mol. Cell. Biol. **10**: 1969–1981.
43. KORC, M. 1998. Role of growth factors in pancreatic cancer. Surg. Oncol. Clin. North Am. **7**: 25–41.
44. FUNATOMI, H., J. ITAKURA, T. ISHIWATA, I. PASTAN, S.A. THOMPSON, G.R. JOHNSON & M. KORC. 1997. Amphiregulin antisense oligonucleotide inhibits the growth of T3M4 human pancreatic cancer cells and sensitizes the cells to EGF receptor-targeted therapy. Int. J. Cancer **72**: 512–517.
45. MASSAGUE, J. & A. PANDIELLA. 1993. Membrane-anchored growth factors. Annu. Rev. Biochem. **62**: 515–541.
46. AARONSON, S.A. 1991. Growth factors and cancer. Science **254**: 1146–1153.
47. LIBERMANN, T.A., H.R. NUSBAUM, N. RAZON, R. KRIS, I. LAX, H. SOREQ, N. WHITTLE, M.D. WATERFIELD, A. ULLRICH & J. SCHLESSINGER. 1985. Amplification, enhanced expression, and possible rearrangement of the EGF receptor gene in primary human brain tumors of glial origin. Nature **313**: 144–147.
48. SAINSBURY, J.R., J.R. FARNDON, G.V. SHERBET & A.L. HARRIS. 1985. Epidermal-growth-factor receptor and oestrogen receptors in human breast cancer. Lancet **1**: 364–366.
49. YAMANAKA, Y., H. FRIESS, M.S. KOBRIN, M. BÜCHLER, H.G. BEGER & M. KORC. 1993. Coexpression of epidermal growth factor receptor and ligands in human pancreatic cancer is associated with enhanced tumor aggressiveness. Anticancer Res. **13**: 565–569.
50. KORC, M., B. CHANDRASEKAR, Y. YAMANAKA, H. FRIESS, M. BÜCHLER & H.G. BEGER. 1992. Overexpression of the epidermal growth factor receptor in human pancreatic cancer is association with concomitant increases in the levels of epidermal growth factor and transforming growth factor alpha. J. Clin. Invest. **90**: 1352–1360.
51. EBERT, M., M. YOKOYAMA, M.S. KOBRIN, H. FRIESS, M.E. LOPEZ, M.W. BÜCHLER, G.R. JOHNSON & M. KORC. 1994. Induction and expression of amphiregulin in human pancreatic cancer. Cancer Res. **54**: 3959–3962.
52. KOBRIN, M.S., H. FUNATOMI, H. FRIESS, M.W. BÜCHLER, P. STATHIS & M. KORC. 1994. Induction and expression of heparin-binding EGF-like growth factor in human pancreatic cancer. Biochem. Biophys. Res. Commun. **202**: 1705–1709.
53. YOKOYAMA, M., M. EBERT, H. FUNATOMI, H. FRIESS, M.W. BÜCHLER, G.R. JOHNSON & M. KORC. 1995. Amphiregulin is a potent mitogen in human pancreatic cancer cells: correlation with patient survival. Int. J. Oncol. **6**: 625–631.
54. LEMOINE, N.R., C.M. HUGHES, C.M. BARTON et al. 1992. The epidermal growth factor receptor in human pancreatic cancer. J. Pathol. **166**: 7–12.
55. FUNATOMI, H., J. ITAKURA, T. ISHIWATA, I. PASTAN, S.A. THOMPSON, G.R. JOHNSON & M. KORC. 1997. Amphiregulin antisense oligonucleotide inhibits the growth of T3M4 human pancreatic cancer cells and sensitizes the cells to EGF receptor-targeted therapy. Int. J. Cancer **72**: 512–517.
56. CARRAWAY, K.L. 3RD & L.C. CANTLEY. 1994. A neu acquaintance for erbB3 and erbB4: a role for receptor heterodimerization in growth signaling. Cell **78**: 5–8.
57. SOLTOFF, S.P., K.L. CARRAWAY 3RD, S.A. PRIGENT, W.G. GULLICK & L.C. CANTLEY. 1994. ErbB3 is involved in activation of phosphatidylinositol 3-kinase by epidermal growth factor. Mol. Cell. Biol. **14**: 3550–3558.
58. ULLRICH, A. & J. SCHLESSINGER. 1990. Signal transduction by receptors with tyrosine kinase activity. Cell **61**: 203–212.
59. SCHLESSINGER, J. & A. ULLRICH. 1992. Growth factor signaling by receptor tyrosine kinases. Neuron **9**: 383–391.
60. HOLMES, W.E., M.X. SLIWKOWSKI, R.W. AKITA et al. 1992. Identification of heregulin, a specific activator of p185erbB2. Science **256**: 1205–1210.
61. DI FIORE, P.P., J.H. PIERCE, M.H. KRAUS, O. SEGATTO, C.R. KING & S.A. AARONSON. 1987. erb-2 is a potent oncogene when overexpressed in NIH/3T3 cells. Science **237**: 178–182.

62. YAMANAKA, Y., H. FRIESS, M.S. KOBRIN, M. BÜCHLER, J. KUNZ, H.G. BEGER & M. KORC. 1993. Overexpression of HER2/neu oncogene in human pancreatic carcinoma. Hum. Pathol. **24:** 1127–1134.
63. LEMOINE, N.R., M. LOBRESCO, H. LEUNG, C. BARTON, C.M. HUGHES, S.A. PRIGENT, W.J. GULLICK & G. KLOPPEL. 1992. The erb-3 gene in human pancreatic cancer. J. Pathol. **168:** 269–273.
64. FRIESS, H., Y. YAMANAKA, M.S. KOBRIN, M.W. BÜCHLER & M. KORC. 1995. Enhanced erbB3 expression in human pancreatic cancer correlates with tumor progression. Clin. Cancer Res. **1:** 1413–1420.
65. KALTHOFF, H., C. ROEDER, I. HUMBURG, H.G. THIELE, H. GRETEN & W. SCHMIEGEL. 1991. Modulation of platelet-derived growth factor A- and B-chain/c-sis mRNA by tumor necrosis factor and other agents in adenocarcinoma cells. Oncogene. **6:** 1015–1021.
66. KALTHOFF, H., C. ROEDER, M. BROCKHAUS, H.-G.THIELE & W. SCHMIEGEL. 1993. Tumor necrosis factor (TNF) up-regulates the expression of p75 but not p55 RNF receptors, and both receptors mediate, independently of each other, up-regulation of transforming growth factor-α and epidermal growth factor receptor mRNA. J. Biol. Chem. **268:** 2762–2766.
67. KALTHOFF, H., C. ROEDER, J. GIESEKING, I. HUMBURG & W. SCHMIEGEL. 1993. Inverse regulation of human ERBB2 and epidermal growth factor receptors by tumor necrosis factor-α. Proc. Natl. Acad. Sci. USA **90:** 8972–8976.
68. DIPPOLD, W.G., R. KLINGEL, M. KERLIN, W. SCHWAEWBLE, M. MEYER & K.-H. MEYER ZUM BÜSCHENFELDE. 1991. Stimulation of pancreas and gastric carcinoma cell growth by interleukin 3 and granulocyte-macrophage colony-stimulating factor. Gastroenterology **100:** 1338–1344.
69. DEDHAR, S., L. GABOURY, P. GALLOWAY & C. EAVES. 1988. Human granulocyte-macrophage colony-stimulating factor is a growth factor active on a variety of cell types of nonhemopoietic origin. Proc. Natl. Acad. Sci. USA **85:** 9253–9257.
70. POBER, J.S., M.A. GIMBRONE, L.A. LAPIERRE et al. 1986. Overlapping patterns of activation of human endothelial cells by interleukin 1, tumor necrosis factor, and immune interferon. J. Immunol. **137:** 1893–1896.
71. BEVILACQUA, M.P., J.S. POBER, D.L. MENDRICK, R.S. COTRAN et al. 1987. Identification of an inducible endothelial-leukocyte adhesion molecule. Proc. Natl. Acad. Sci. USA **84:** 9238–9242.
72. SCHWAEBLE, W., M. KERLIN, M. MEYER ZUM BUSCHENFELDE & W. DIPPOLD. 1993. De novo expression of intercellular adhesion molecule-1 (ICAM-1, CD54) in pancreas cancer. Int. J. Cancer **53:** 328–333.
73. SHIMOYAMA, S., F. GANSAUGE, S. GANSAUGE, U. WIDMAIER, T. OOHARA & H.G. BEGER. 1997. Overexpression of intercellular adhesion molecule-1 (ICAM-1) in pancreatic adenocarcinoma in comparison with normal pancreas. Pancreas **14:** 181–186.
74. IWAI, K., H. ISHIKURA, M. KAJI, H. SUGIURA, A. ISHIZU, C. TAKAHASHI et al. 1993. Importance of E-selection (ELAM-1) and Sialyl Lewis(a) in the adhesion of pancreatic carcinoma cells to activated endothelium. Int. J. Cancer **54:** 972–977.
75. BROWN, T.D., P. GOODMAN, T. FLEMING, J.S. MACDONALD, E.M. HERSH & T.J. BRAUN. 1991. A phase II trial of recombinant tumor necrosis factor in patients with adenocarcinoma of the pancreas: a South-West Oncology Group study. J. Immunother. **10:** 376–378.
76. ABBRUZZESE, J.L., B. LEVIN, J.A. AJANI et al. 1990. A phase II trial of recombinant interferon-gamma and recombinant tumor necrosis factor in patients with advanced gastrointestinal malignancies: results of a trial terminated by excessive toxicity. J. Biol. Response Mod. **9:** 522–527.
77. SCHMIEGEL, W., J. SCHMIELAU, D. HENNE-BRUNS, H. JUHL, C. ROEDER, P. BUGGISCH, A. ONUR, B. KREMER, H. KALTHOFF & E.V. JENSEN. 1997. Cytokine-mediated enhancement of epidermal growth factor receptor expression provides an immunological approach to the therapy of pancreatic cancer. Proc. Natl. Acad. Sci. USA **94:** 12622–12626.

78. YOSHIMURA, T. & E.J. LEONARD. 1990. Secretion by human fibroblasts of monocyte chemoattractant protein-1, the product of gene JE. J. Immunol. **144:** 2377–2383.
79. OKADA, S., T. OKUSAKA, H. ISHII, A. KYOGOKU, M. YOSHIMORI, N. KAJIMURA, K. YAMAGUCHI & T. KAKIZOE. 1998. Elevated serum interleukin-6 levels in patients with pancreatic cancer. Jpn. J. Clin. Oncol. **28:** 12–15.
80. SAITO, K., H. ISHIKURA, T. KISHIMOTO, Y. KAWARADA, T. YANO, T. TAKAHASHI, H. KATO & T. YOSHKI. 1998. Interleukin-6 produced by pancreatic carcinoma cells enhances humoral immune responses against tumor cells: a possible event in tumor regression. Int. J. Cancer **75:** 284–289.

Strategies for the Detection of Disease Genes in Pancreatic Cancer

C. WALLRAPP,[a,d] F. MÜLLER-PILLASCH,[a,d] A. MICHA,[a] C. WENGER,[a] M. GENG,[a] S. SOLINAS-TOLDO,[b] P. LICHTER,[b] M. FROHME,[c] J.D. HOHEISEL,[c] G. ADLER,[a] AND T.M. GRESS[a,e]

[a]*Universität Ulm, Abteilung Innere Medizin I, Robert Koch Str. 8, 89081 Ulm, Germany*
[b]*Deutsches Krebsforschungszentrum, Abteilung Organisation komplexer Genome, Im Neuenheimer Feld 280, 69120 Heidelberg, Germany*
[c]*Deutsches Krebsforschungszentrum, Labor für Funktionelle Genomanalyse, Im Neuenheimer Feld 506, 69120 Heidelberg, Germany*

ABSTRACT: The present review summarizes our strategies aimed at identifying and characterizing genetic alterations occurring at the transcriptional and chromosomal level in pancreatic cancer. To study transcriptional alterations we have used a number of techniques including modified versions of differential hybridizations and cDNA RDA (representational difference analysis). These approaches have led to the identification of more than 500 genes with differential expression in pancreatic cancer. To study chromosomal aberrations occurring in pancreatic cancer tissues we used comparative genomic hybridization (CGH). This allowed the identification of a number of chromosomal regions containing putative tumor suppressor genes or oncogenes. Genes isolated in both approaches represent potential new disease genes for pancreatic cancer and are at present being characterized by individual or serial analysis.

INTRODUCTION

Pancreatic cancer is the fifth cause of cancer-related deaths in industrialized countries, with a dismal prognosis, an increasing incidence and no or only ineffective means of treatment.[31,32] The development of new treatment modalities, diagnostic and preventive approaches requires the understanding of the molecular mechanisms of the complex multistep process of tumorigenesis in the pancreas. At present mutations or alterations of gene expression have been described for a number of individual genes (for reviews, see Refs. 19 and 22). However, a much larger number of genes are warranted to be involved in primary and secondary processes responsible for the development of the phenotype of pancreatic cancer cells. Identification of these genes is essential as a basis for the development of new treatment or diagnostic modalities. The Genome Project provides the methodologies for a large scale analysis of these complex genetic alterations in cancer. In the recent

---

[d]C.W. and F.M.-P have contributed equally to the work presented in this review, and should both be considered first authors.
[e]Corresponding author: PD.Dr.Thomas Gress, Abteilung Innere Medizin I, Universität Ulm, Robert Koch Str. 8, 89081 Ulm, Germany. Phone, +49 731-502-4311/4385; fax, +49 731-502-4302; e-mail, thomas.gress@medizin.uni-ulm.de

years the major focus of our group has been to modify and adapt Genome Project technology for the study of transcriptional and chromosomal alterations in pancreatic cancer. The present review arcticle summarizes our strategies and some of the results obtained in our large-scale approaches during the past few years.

ALTERATIONS OF GENE EXPRESSION

Early studies using mRNA/cDNA saturation-hybridization techniques showed that the complexity of the mRNA of wild-type and transformed cells may differ up to 10% (e.g., Ref. 16). Taking into account newest estimates, the total number of human genes ranges between 80,000–100,000,[7] of which only a fraction (12–20%) is transcribed depending on cell type and differentiation. Any mammalian cell, with the exception of fetal brain cells, should thus have an average expressed gene number of 10,000–20,000. Based on the mRNA/cDNA saturation-hybridization results named above, we may deduce from these figures that the expression of up to 1000–2000 genes may change as the result of primary and secondary processes during cancerogenesis.

Expression Profiling Using Automated cDNA Library Technology and Differential Hybridizations

Gridded arrays of gene libraries, which have been successfully used for the mapping and sequencing of complex genomes (e.g., Refs. 26 and 46) were invaluable to study the complex alterations of gene expression occurring in pancreatic cancer cells. We used gridded cDNA libraries from pancreatic cancer cell lines for differential hybridizations with labeled probes of the complete mRNA of pancreatic cancer and pancreatic control tissues (FIG. 1).[13] These hybridizations allowed the detection of clones containing sequences abundantly expressed in the tissues used to generate

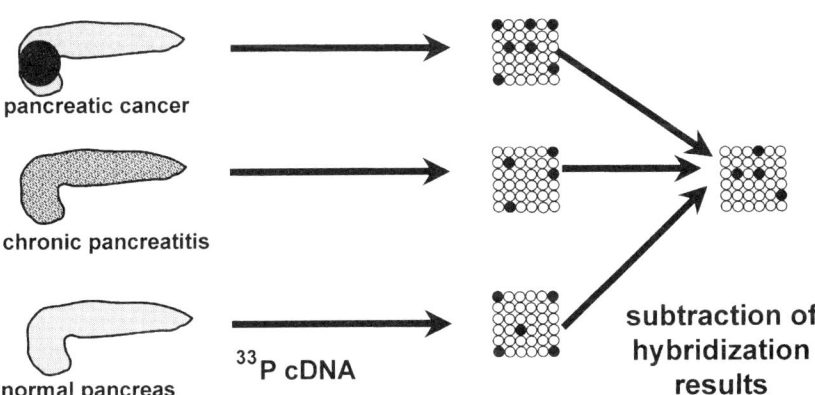

FIGURE 1. Schematic drawing summarizing the principle of differential hybridizations with gridded cDNA library clones for the isolation of genes with differential expression in pancreatic cancer.

TABLE 1. The expression pattern of PATU 8988s cDNA library clones in pancreatic cancer (PACA), chronic pancreatitis (CP) and control pancreatic (CO)

Pancreatic cancer	Chronic pancreatitis	Control pancreas	Hybridizing clones
+	+	+	26%
+	−	−	4%
+	+	−	5.5%
−	−	+	2%
−	+	+	2%
−	+	−	1.5%

Note: Data are based on differential hybridizations with cDNA pool probes synthetized from poly(A) mRNA pools derived from 10 tissue samples each. Clones were classified as + or − upon the strength of the signal obtained in each differential hybridization as determined by image analysis. (Modified from Gress et al.[13])

the probe (FIG. 2). Hybridizing clones were scored by use of an Image Analysis System and stored in our local computer database, allowing an automated data processing. Each hybridization with cDNA pool probes yielded approximately 7000–9000 positive clones on each cDNA library filter. Computerized subtraction analysis revealed that 4% of the total number of clones (approximately 800 in each cDNA library) were selectively overexpressed in pancreatic carcinoma. TABLE 1 summarizes data obtained from the evaluation of hybridizations with cDNA pool probes from 10 tissues in each group and illustrates differential expression patterns.

A total of 410 cDNA clones (369 distinct clones) classified as preferentially expressed in pancreatic cancer were isolated from one cDNA library and characterized

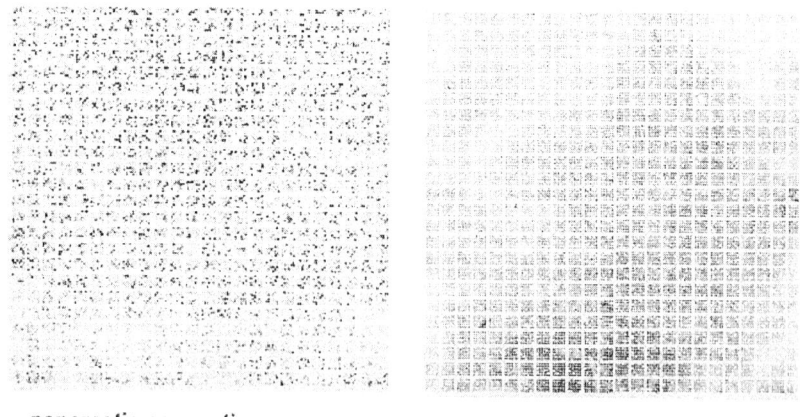

pancreatic cancer tissue
total ^{33}P cDNA

vector

FIGURE 2. Hybridizations of the cDNA library grid of the pancreatic cancer cell line PATU 8988s with vector DNA and a cDNA pool probe synthetized from pooled poly(A) mRNA of 10 pancreatic cancer tissues. (Modified from Gress et al.[13])

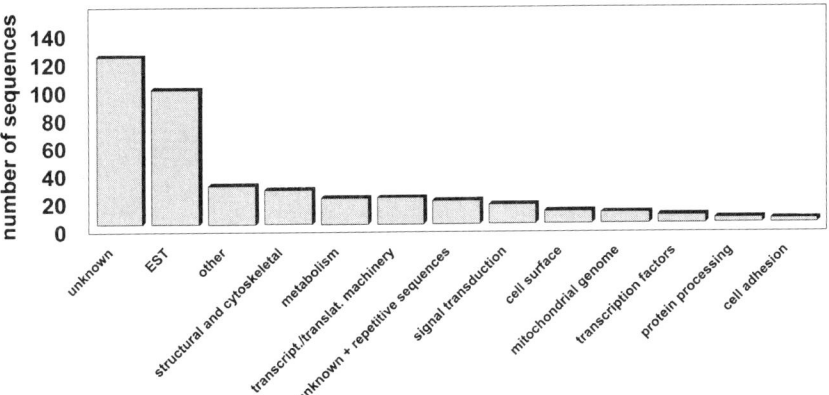

FIGURE 3. Three hundred sixty-nine (369) distinct ESTs classified as preferentially expressed in pancreatic cancer tissues were sorted into functional categories based on data provided by Gen-Bank or found in the literature. The Y-axis shows the number of ESTs in each category (no.). (Modified from Gress et al.[13])

by Northern blot hybridizations, EST-sequencing (generation of short sequence tags of approximately 200–400 bp per clone) and by screening nucleic acid or protein databases for sequence homologies. Northern blot hybridizations of 100 selected clones confirmed the hybridization pattern for approximately 90% of the clones. EST-sequencing of the selected differentially expressed sequences identified novel genes (32.5%) or homologues to EST-sequences with unknown function (26.3%). Homologies to known genes allowed to describe a pancreatic cancer-specific expression profile. The expression profile is summarized in FIGURE 3.

A number of these genes or gene families have already been associated with other malignancies or with pancreatic cancer. Most of the genes summarized in the group metabolism encoded enzymes involved in aerob glycolysis, which is in line with the observation that aerob glycolysis is turned on in tumor cells due to increased energy metabolism (e.g., Refs. 39 and 42). Increased glycolysis and glucose turnover has as well been observed in pancreatic tumors and is being used for diagnostic purposes as, e.g., for positron emission tomography with labeled glucose.[23] This study identified the genes that may be responsible for this phenomenon. A large number of preferentially expressed genes are classified as structural and cytoskeletal or are part of the transcriptional and translational machinery. In the same way as assumed for increased glucose metabolism in cancer cells, these observations are most likely an indication for increased turnover and synthesis in cancer cells and may thus be of secondary nature. However, knowledge of the genes involved in these mechanisms will help to understand the processes leading to increased proliferation and growth of cancer cells and as described for the increased glucose metabolism in cancer cells may represent the basis for the development of treatment or diagnostic modalities. Other individual genes that are known to be associated with the malignant phenotype of pancreatic cancer or other cancer cells are, e.g., annexin II (e.g., Ref. 40), urokinase[34], or amplaxin.[37] Other potential "disease genes for pancreatic cancer" isolated in this approach have been previously discussed in detail.[13]

However, one of our major interests besides the description of an expression profile of known genes was the identification of novel overexpressed genes. In the same way as for the known genes we expected that around 90% of the 217 new genes (120 novel sequences and 97 previously sequenced ESTs) would be overexpressed in pancreatic cancer due to secondary alterations as, e.g., increased metabolism or cell turnover of tumor cells. For this reason we had to develop strategies to select relevant genes for further characterization.

Initially we selected a number of differentially expressed cDNA-sequences showing homologies to interesting genes or to sequence motifs of gene families of potential interest for pancreatic cancerogenesis. A selection of these genes is described below.

One gene highly overexpressed in pancreatic cancer was found to encode a novel protein with four K-homologous (KH) domains and was named *koc* (**KH** domain

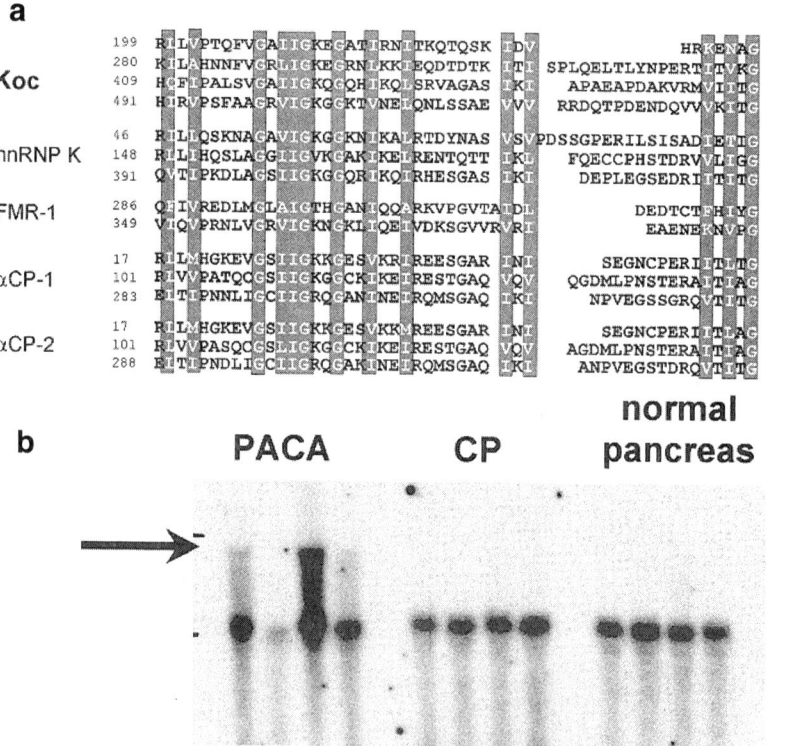

FIGURE 4. The koc-gene. (**a**) Alignment of the four KH domains of koc to the KH domains found in hnRNP K, FMR-1, αCP-1 and αCP-2. The *shaded* amino acids are the most highly conserved KH domain consensus sequences. (**b**) Northern blot of total RNA from human normal pancreas, chronic pancreatitis (CP) and human pancreatic cancer (PACA) tissues. The *arrow* points on the koc transcript. The additional 1.9-kb band, detected at the same level in all examined cancer and control tissues and cell lines, is most likely due to unspecific hybridization in Northern blots with total RNA. This transcript disapears on Northern blots with Poly(A)+ RNA. (Modified from Müller-Pillasch *et al.*[28])

a

```
      L6H        1  MCTGKCARCVGLSLITLCFVCIVANALLLVPNGETSWTNTNHLSLQVWLMGGFIGGGL-MVLCPGIAAVR---
   mouse L6      1  MCYVKCARYIGYSLVWAAVFCIVANALLYFPNGETKYATEDHLSRFVWYFAGIVGGGLLMLL-PAFVFIGMDE
  humanTAL6      1  MCYGKCARCIGHSLVGLALLCIAANILLYFPNGETKYASENHLSRFVWFFSGIVGGGLIMLL-PAFVFIGLEQ
  mesau TAL6     1  MCSSKCTRYIGHSLVVFAVLCIVANILLYFPNGETKYAYEDHLSRFVWFFAGIVGGGLLIL-PAFVFLGLEG
  human ILT4     1  MCTGGCARCLGGTLIPLAFFGFLANILLFFP  GGKVIDDNDHLSQEIWFFGGILGSGVLMIF-PALVFLGLKN

      L6H       70  AGGKGCCGAGCCGNRCRMLRSVFSSAFGVLGAIYCLSVSGAGLRNGPRCLMN-GEWGYHFEDTAGAYLLNRT
   mouse L6     73  EDCCGCCGYENYGKRCSMLSSVLAALIGIVGSAYCVIVASLGLAEGPKCSDAHGVWNYTFASTEGQYLLNSS
  humanTAL6     73  DDCCGCCGHENCGKRCSMLSSVLAALIGTAGSGYCVIVAALIGLAEGPLCLDSLGQWNYTFASTEGQYLLDSS
  mesauTAL6     73  EDCCGCCWSCENYGKRCTMLSSIMAALIGIAGSSGYCVIVAALIGLAEGPKCGDSHGMWNYTFANTDGQYLLDPT
  human ILT4    73  NDCCGCCGNEGCGKRFAMFTSTIFAVVGFLGAGYSFIISAISINKGPKCLMANSTWGYPF--HDGDYLNDEA

      L6H      141  LWDRCEAPPRVVPWNVTLFSLLVAASCLEIVLCGIQLVNATIGVFCGDCRKKQDTPH
   mouse L6    145  MWSKCYEPKHIVEWHVTLFSIILIAFFAAVEFILCLLQVINGMLGGLCGYCCSRQQQYNC
  humanTAL6    145  TWSECTEPKHIVEWNVSLFSIILALGGIEFILCLIQVINGVLGGICGFCCSHQQQYDC
  mesauTAL6    145  TWSKCHEPNNIVEWNVTLFSIILLALGGLEFILCLIQVINGVLEGMCSYCCSHQQQYDC
  human ILT4   143  LWNKCREPLNVVPWNLTLFSILLVVGGIQMVLCAIQVVNGLLGTLGDCQCCGCCGGDGPV
```

FIGURE 5. The TM4SF5 gene. (**a**) The predicted TM4SF5 amino acid sequence is homologous to a number of tetraspan transmembrane proteins. Homology was found to mouse (mouse TAL6), human (human TAL6), and hamster (mesau TAL6) L6 antigen and the interstitial tetraspan membrane protein (human ILT4). Residues shared by at least three members of the family are shown in *shaded boxes*. Homologies are also present in the extracellular domains (30–42 and 132–154). (**b**) Representative Northern blot containing total RNA (30 μg/lane) from human healthy pancreas ($n = 4$), chronic pancreatitis ($n = 4$), and human pancreatic cancer tissues ($n = 4$) hybridized with TM4SF5. (**c**) Northern blot of total RNA (30 μg) from different cancer tissues (1, soft tissue sarcoma; 2, gastric cancer; 3–4, colon carcinoma; 5, carcinoma of the papilla vaterii; 6, gastric cancer) probed with TM4SF5. (**d**) Northern blot containing total RNA from different human intestinal tissues (7, esophagus; 8, stomach; 9, intestine; 10, colon; 11, uterus; 12, placenta; 13, bladder; 14, adipose tissue) hybridized with TM4SF5. (Modified from Müller-Pillasch *et al.*[29])

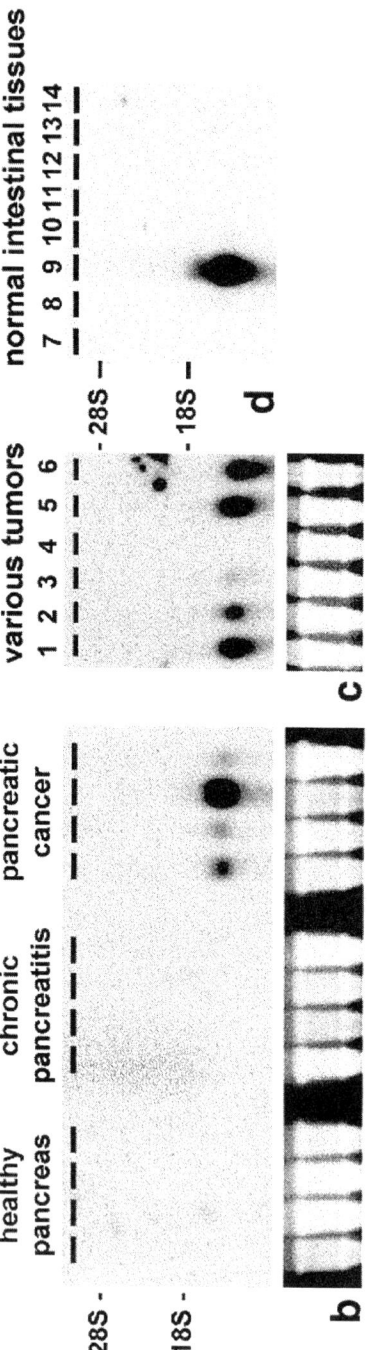

FIGURE 5. *Continued*

containing protein overexpressed in cancer) (Ref. 28, and references therein). KH-domains are found in a subset of RNA-binding proteins, including pre-mRNA-binding (hnRNP) K protein and the fragile X mental retardation gene product (FMR1). The cloned koc cDNA has a 250-bp 5'UTR, a 1740-bp ORF and a 2168-bp 3'UTR. The koc protein with 580 amino acids has a relative molecular mass (M_r) of approximately 65,000 (65K). The Koc transcript was highly overexpressed in pancreatic cancer cell lines and in pancreatic cancer tissue as compared to both normal pancreas and chronic pancreatitis tissue. High levels of expression were found as well in tissue samples of other human tumors (FIG. 4). As the KH domain has been shown to be involved in the regulation of RNA synthesis and metabolism, we speculate that koc may be involved in the regulation of tumor cell proliferation by interfering with transcriptional and/or posttranscriptional processes.[28]

A further overexpressed gene encoded a novel putative tetraspan transmembrane protein highly homologous to the tumor-associated antigen L6 and was named *TM4SF5* (**t**rans**m**embrane **4** **s**uper**f**amily member **5**).[29] The cloned *TM4SF5* cDNA has a 32-bp 5'-untranslated region (UTR), a 591-bp open reading frame (ORF) and a 85-bp 3'UTR. The predicted TM4SF5 protein with 197 amino acids contains three N-terminal hydrophobic transmembrane regions, followed by an extracellular hydrophilic domain containing two potential N-linked glycosylation sites and a C-terminal hydrophobic transmembrane region. These structural features are shared by the L6 antigen and a number of related cell surface proteins associated with cell growth. *TM4SF5* was overexpressed in pancreatic cancer tissues as compared to both normal pancreas and chronic pancreatitis tissues and was detected at high levels in other tumor tissues (FIG. 5). Although the precise function of TM4SF5 remains to be elucidated, it may be useful in a clinical setting for tumor diagnosis and/or therapy (Ref. 29 and references therein).

Another interesting differentially expressed gene encoded a novel putative transmembrane protein with two Kunitz-type serine protease inhibitor domains and was named *kop* (**K**unitz domain containing protein **o**verexpressed in **p**ancreatic cancer). The Kunitz domain is found in a subset of proteins, including the tissue factor pathway inhibitor (TFPI), the amyloid β precursor protein (βAPP) of Alzheimer's disease and the inter-α-trypsin inhibitor (IαTI). The cloned kop cDNA has a 365 5'UTR, a 756-bp ORF and a 444-bp 3'UTR. Besides the two Kunitz domains the KOP protein with 252 amino acids revealed a putative signal sequence with 28 amino acids, two glycosylation sites and a possible transmembrane region. Kop was detected at high levels in pancreatic cancer cell lines and was overexpressed in pancreatic cancer tissue as compared to both normal pancreas and chronic pancreatitis tissue (FIG. 6). Being a member of the Kunitz-type serine protease inhibitor family, this new gene may participate in tumor cell invasion and metastasis and in the development of the marked desmoplastic reaction typical for human pancreatic cancer tissues. In this context the fact that Kop has a putative transmembrane domain may have functional implications of particular interest. Moreover, as it has been shown that the Kunitz domain of βAPP has a transactivating potential, KOP protein may as well be associated with tumor cell proliferation (Ref. 30 and references therein).

As only a small fraction of the 217 new genes contained homologies to protein motifs allowing to draw functional conclusions, we had to devise the methodology

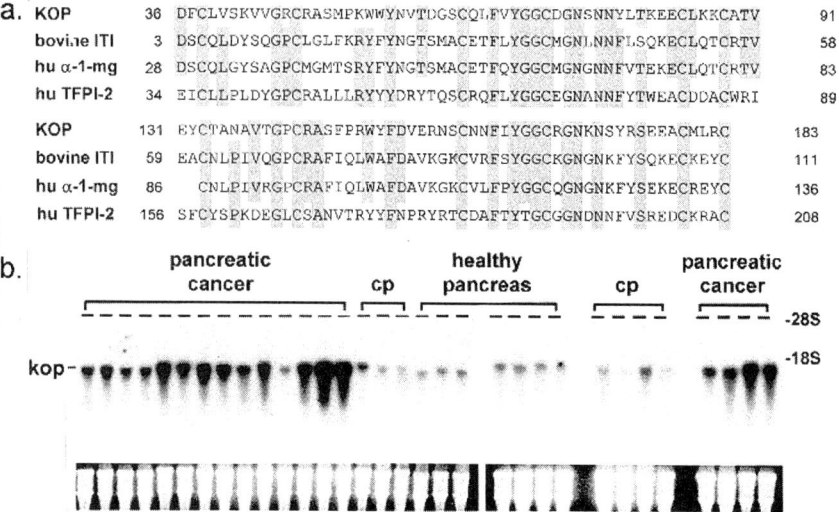

FIGURE 6. The kop gene. (**a**) An alignment of the two Kunitz-type protease inhibitor domains of kop to the Kunitz family signature found in bovine inter-alpha-trypsin inhibitor (ITI), human alpha-1-microglobulin (α-1-mg) and human tissue factor pathway inhibitor-2 (TFPI-2) is shown. The *shaded* amino acids are the most highly conserved Kunitz type protease inhibitor domain consensus sequences. (**b**) Northern blots containing total RNA from human healthy pancreas ($n = 7$), chronic pancreatitis (cp) ($n = 7$) and human pancreatic cancer tissues ($n = 18$) hybridized with kop. (Modified from Müller-Pillasch *et al.*[30])

to identify and characterize the relevant novel disease genes. In this context we developed a serial characterization approach allowing us to identifiy genes associated, e.g., with the invasive/metastatic potential of pancreatic cancer cells, embryonal development or transcriptionally regulated by growth factors as epidermal growth factor (EGF) or transforming growth factor-β (TGF-β).[9] In this serial characterization approach all cDNA clones classified as differentially expressed were spotted in duplicate onto 9×13 cm nylon membranes to facilitate automated analysis. To identifiy, e.g., TGF-β or EGF target genes these small sublibraries are hybridized with cDNA probes from cell lines treated with the respective growth factor or from untreated cells. In this context the use of subtracted and enriched cDNA probes, e.g., generated by use of RDA-technology (see below) has shown to be superior to standard differential hybridizations.[10] The principle of this serial characterization approach is summarized in FIGURE 7.

Analysis of Differential Gene Expression by Use of cDNA Representational Difference Analysis (RDA)

Although the differential screening approach described above was highly efficient and successful, it was laborious and time consuming. In addition, despite the improvement of protocols for probe generation, probe competition and hybridization, as well as the availability of sophisticated image analysis systems, the analysis

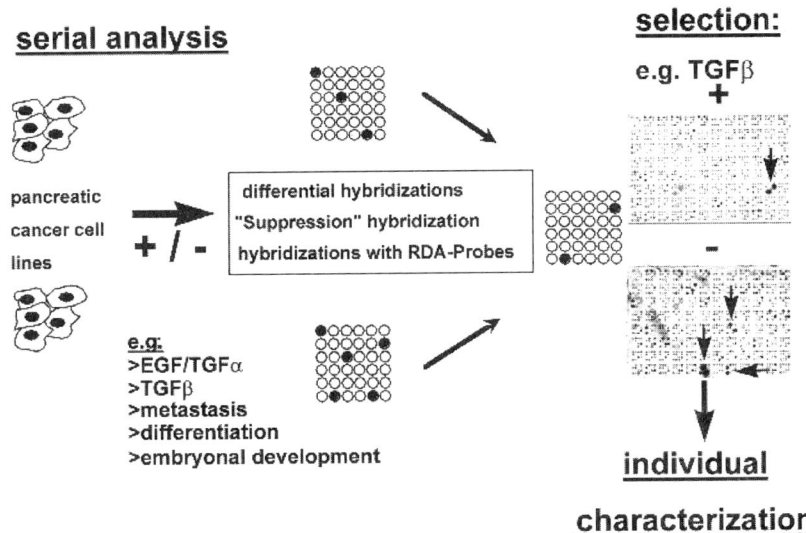

FIGURE 7. Schematic drawing of our strategy employed for the serial characterization of differentially novel expressed genes.

and interpretation of hybridization results remains a challenge. New image analysis systems are costly and their use will be restricted to a small number of specialized laboratories. Furthermore, hybridizations with labeled cDNA probes preferably detect mRNA species expressed at middle to high abundance, thus often missing rare transcripts such as tissue-specific transcription factors and putative tumor suppressor genes. To isolate this sort of genes, representational difference analysis (RDA) appeared to be the ideal technique.

cDNA representational difference analysis (cDNA RDA) represents an iterative process of subtractive hybridization and selective polymerase chain reaction (PCR) amplification allowing to select differentially expressed genes with a highly reproducible specificity. RDA was originally devised to clone differences between complex genomes.[25] An iterative process of subtraction hybridization and selective PCR amplification ensures the isolation of amplifiable restriction fragments present in the tester and absent in the driver. The RDA protocol was later adapted for the use with cDNA to study differential gene expression between two mRNA populations.[20] The standard cDNA RDA protocol is ideally suited to rapidly reduce the number of candidate genes in a highly specific manner, thus allowing to focus on a small number of differential genes. In brief, Poly(A)$^+$-RNA of a tester (e.g., cancer tissues) and a driver (e.g., control tissues) is initially reverse transcribed in cDNA. Each cDNA is then restriction digested with *Dpn*II and ligated to a DNA-adapter cassette. Subsequent to PCR amplification with an adaptor-specific primer, the driver and tester amplicon are again *Dpn*II-digested for the removal of the adapter cassette and the tester is ligated to new adaptor cassette different in sequence. Driver and tester are then mixed at a 100:1 ratio, denatured, reannealed at 67°C for 48 hr and PCR amplified using tester-specific PCR primers to form the first difference product (DP1). DP2

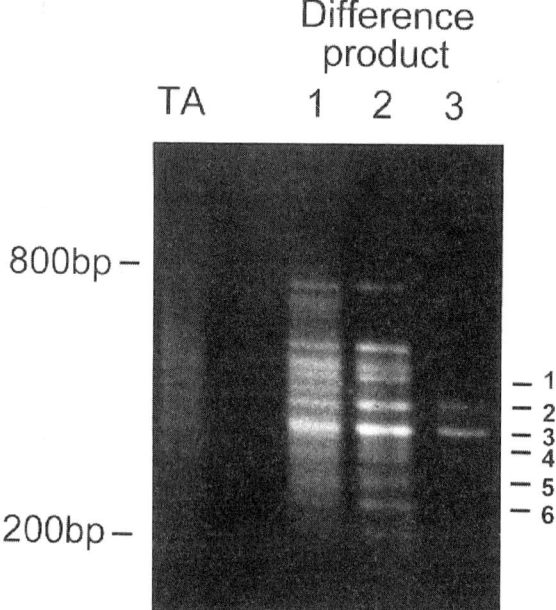

FIGURE 8. cDNA RDA. Agarose gel electrophoresis of the tester amplicon and the difference products obtained after the first (1), second (2) and third (3) cycle of cDNA RDA. Six distinct gene fragments were obtained in the difference product 3 as indicated on the *right margin*. (Modified from Gress *et al.*[14])

(ratio 800:1) and DP3 (400,000:1) are prepared accordingly in iterative rounds of RDA, always using the latest DP product as tester. The DP products are size fractionated on agarose gels, which usually renders more and more distinct band with increasing driver/tester ratios (FIG. 8). These bands can be excised, cloned, sequenced and hybridized onto Northern blots to verify the expression pattern.

We used the standard cDNA RDA protocol as an alternative method to isolate differentially expressed genes in pancreatic cancer.[14] Poly(A) mRNA pooled from pancreatic cancer tissue samples was used as tester. Initially pooled poly(A) mRNA prepared from healthy control tissues was used as driver. This led to the isolation of 24 unique gene fragments. Most of the fragments isolated in this first cDNA RDA were expressed in chronic pancreatitis tissue samples as well (FIG. 9a). Chronic pancreatitis is an inflammatory disease of the pancreas characterized by a strong stromal reaction (fibrosis and interstitial inflammation) similar to the one observed in pancreatic cancer tissues. Sequence analysis revealed that the majority of these fragments were most likely derived from stromal and inflammatory cells. Due to the strong desmoplastic reaction present in most of the pancreatic cancer tissues, this represents a common problem and has hampered most attemps to isolate pancreatic cancer-specific, differentially expressed sequences.

To reduce the influence of stromal tissue components in a second set of experiments, pooled poly(A) mRNA from chronic pancreatitis tissue samples was mixed

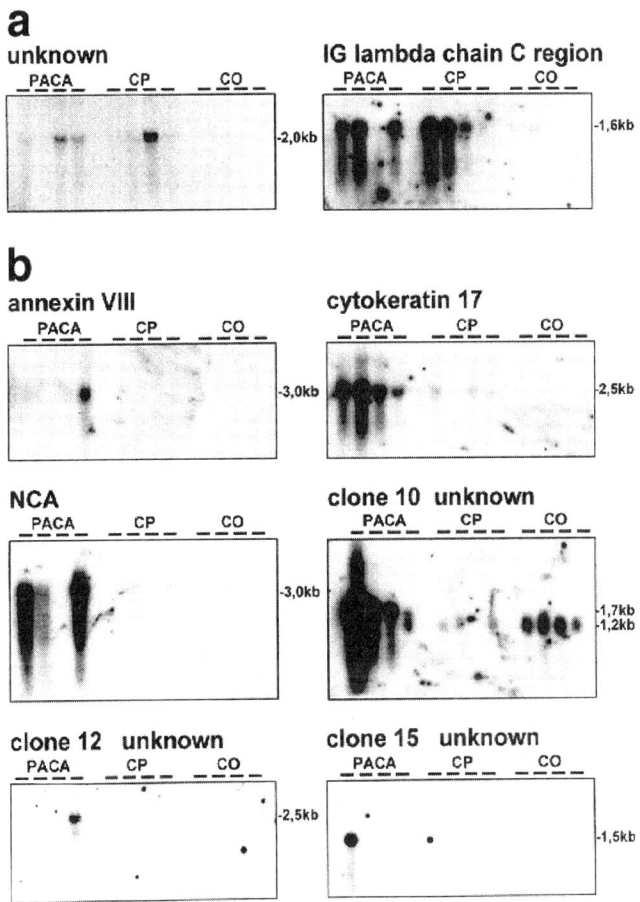

FIGURE 9. Northern blot analysis of differentially expressed sequences isolated by cDNA RDA. (**a**) This panel shows the expression pattern of two DP3 RDA fragments (clone 13/24 = unknown and clone 7/24 = Ig-lambda chain C region) obtained using pooled mRNA from healthy control tissues as driver only. The method clearly identifies gene fragments absent in healthy pancreas (driver). However, due to the strong stromal and inflammatory reaction present in most of the pancreatic cancer tissues, the DP3 gene fragments were also expressed in chronic pancreatitis tissue. They were thus not cancer cell-specific and most likely of stromal origin. For this reason pooled poly(A) mRNA from 10 chronic pancreatitis tissue samples was added to the driver. This led to the identification of 16 gene fragments with cancer tissue-specific expression as verified by Northern blot analysis. (**b**) A selection of the Northern blot hybridizations obtained with the 16 cancer-specific expressed gene fragments. One of these gene fragments was identified by RDA as it showed differential splicing in cancer tissue (no. 10). (Modified from Gress et al.[14])

with the pooled poly(A) mRNA from healthy control pancreatic tissues to form the driver. The use of this mixed driver in the second cDNA RDA led to the identification of 16 distinct gene fragments, of which 13 were overexpressed in pancreatic cancer tissues only (see FIG. 9b). Clone 10 (FIG. 9b) was identified by cDNA RDA as it is differentially spliced and shows a pancreatic cancer-specific splice variant. Nine of 16 gene fragments were expressed at low abundance and required prolonged exposure times. Only two RDA fragments detected no transcript in any of the pancreatic tissues (cancer, chronic pancreatitis or control) on the Northern blot. As both fragments hybridized back only to Southern blots of the initial tester representation and not to the driver representation, it appears likely that these gene fragments were expressed below the level of detection of standard Northern blot analysis with total RNA. This indicates that the sensitivity of cDNA RDA is much higher than standard Northern blot analysis. Sequence analyses revealed homologies to 5 genes that have already been associated with cancerogenesis in the pancreas or in other tissues. The role of the indivdual genes has previously been discussed in detail.[14]

In conclusion, cDNA RDA is a powerful, reproducible and highly efficient method to identify novel cancer-specific expressed genes of potential biomedical importance. The addition of chronic pancreatitis mRNA to the driver ensures the isolation of cancer-specific differentially expressed gene fragments by eliminating mRNA of stromal origin. Thus, cDNA RDA allows to eliminate the influence of stromal tissue components on the isolation of cancer-specific expressed genes, without the necessity to enrich for cancer cells in the tissue sample (e.g., tissue microdissection, nude mice xenografts). In addition cDNA RDA allows the identification of genes differentially expressed at a low expression level, which is difficult to achieve with methods such as, e.g., differential hybridizations. Besides the ability to detect differences in expression levels, cDNA RDA is also suitable to detect cancer-specific splice variants.

Use of cDNA RDA Difference Products as Hybridization Probes on Gridded cDNA Libraries to Study Differential Gene Expression

Standard cDNA RDA allowed to isolate a number of differentially expressed genes in pancreatic cancer with a high specificity. However, the yield was low and the standard protocol does not allow to study complex alterations of gene expression on gridded cDNA library arrays. For this reason we decided to test the use of RDA products as probes on cDNA library arrays.[10] The aim of this approach was to provide a straightforward and reliable protocol, which eliminates the problems usually encountered during standard differential hybridizations with cDNA probes as, e.g., high background, time-consuming image analysis and the need for sophisticated equipment. The difference products (DPs) of representational difference analyses (RDA) were used as hybridization probes on cDNA arrays. The effectiveness of RDA products obtained with increasing driver/tester ratios (DP1 = 100:1, DP2 = 800:1, DP3 = 400,000:1) to isolate differentially expressed genes in pancreatic cancer was compared with the effectiveness of conventional differential hybridizations (FIG. 10). Since RDA allowed to produce a single driver by combining cDNA from chronic pancreatitis and normal pancreas and to subtract tester and driver prior to hybridization, only one autoradiography had to be analyzed in the approach using RDA probes. The vast majority of signals (>80%) obtained—even at low driver/tester ratios—were clearly above background (FIG. 10, D–F), facilitating analysis. With the DP1 probe, 172 clones were classified as differentially expressed. Northern blot analyses demonstrated that a large number of these genes, besides being overexpressed in pancreatic cancer, were also moderately overexpressed in chronic pancreatitis. DP2 and DP3 experiments identified 99 and 27 clones, respectively, all of which from transcripts that were found to be expressed at a higher level in pancreatic cancer than in both controls (FIG. 10, G). Whereas some highly abundant, nondifferential genes as, e.g., housekeeping genes were still detected with the DP1 probe, they were eliminated by iterative rounds of RDA in the DP2/DP3 products (FIG. 10). None of the vector control probes gave a signal with any of the DP products. The fraction of pancreatic cancer-specific expressed genes increased with rising driver/tester ratios, whereas in parallel the total yield of differential clones decreased. In the presented approach the hybridization with the DP2 product obtained after the second round of RDA at a driver/tester ratio of 800:1 represented the best compromise between yield and specificity. The yield was comparable to standard differential hybridizations, whereas the fraction of genes selectively overexpressed in pancreatic cancer tissues was higher (FIG.10, G).

In summary this new technique represents a valuable alternative for the isolation of genes differentially expressed in cancer tissues combining the advantages of gridded library arrays and cDNA representational difference analysis. This technique is superior to conventional differential hybridizations with gridded arrays, as it provides a higher specificity and produces hybridization results allowing a reliable and convenient data analysis with an automated system or even by eye. As compared to conventional cDNA RDA, which is highly specific to isolate a small number of differentially expressed genes, the presented technique allows to study the expression patterns of arrayed cDNA clones or whole libraries. We are convinced that in the future hybridizations with cDNA RDA probes and gridded library arrays will represent a valuable technique to study differential gene expression in a variety of biological systems, without the necessity to purchase expensive equipment.

GENOMIC ALTERATIONS

Multiple cytogenetic aberrations of primary tumors and of cell lines derived from pancreatic carcinoma have been described (e.g., Refs. 2 and 15). According to these studies, chromosomal aberrations of chromosome 1, loss of 6q, gain of chromosomes 7 and 20, and aberrations involving chromosomes 17 and 18 seem to be the most frequent rearrangements present in this tumor. However, it is difficult to obtain sufficient metaphase spreads of good quality from such tumor specimens for cytogenetic analysis. This could also result in the selection of analyzed clones that are not representative of the tumor. Moreover, many aberrant chromosomal regions may not have been identified due to the high complex karyotype of cultured cancer cells carrying both multiple numerical and structural abnormalities. Two major approaches have been used to generate more reliable data concerning chromosomal aberrations in pancreatic cancer. An extremely successful approach to define chromosomal arms that may harbor additional tumor suppressor genes was applied by the group of Scott Kern (The Johns Hopkins University School of Medicine, Baltimore, MD, USA) and

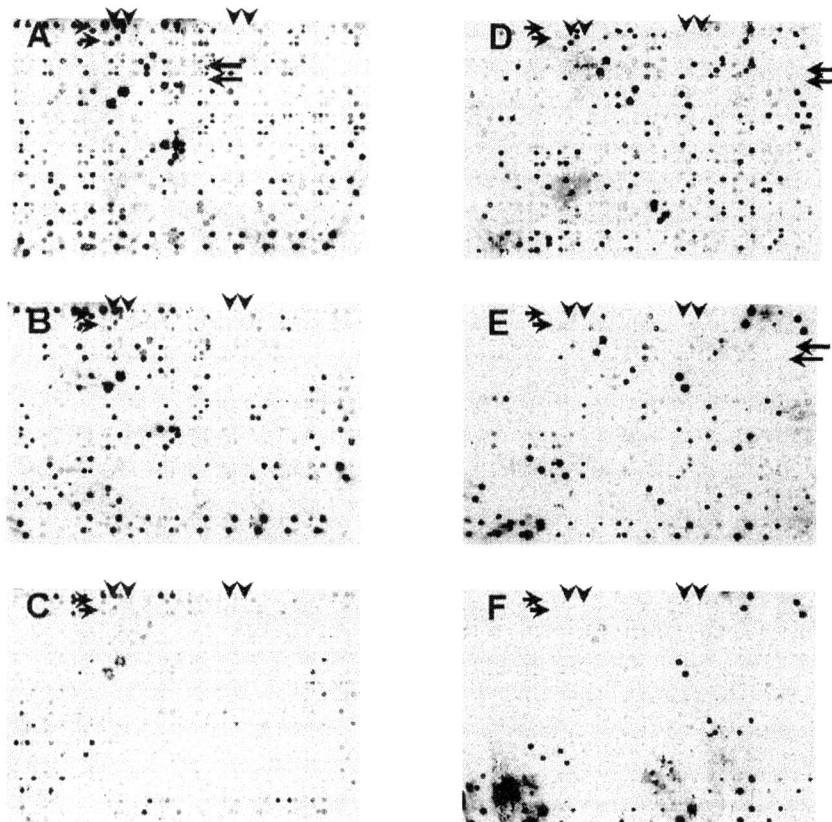

FIGURE 10. Typical hybridization patterns obtained with tissue cDNA probes isolated from (**A**) pancreatic cancer, (**B**) chronic pancreatitis and (**C**) healthy pancreas tissues. Clones were classified as differentially expressed by substracting signal intensities in (B) and (C) from those in (A). Hybridizations of RDA products are shown in (**D**) DP1, (**E**) DP2 and (**F**) DP3. All clones were spotted in duplicate. The positions of a selection of clones spotted as controls are highlighted on all autoradiographies by *arrowheads* (two mitochondrial genes) and *small arrows* (vector only clone). Vector clones were spotted at the same position in each 4 × 4 clone array in the first three rows of each grid to control for unspecific hybridization. Please note that none of the vector clones gave a specific signal in any of the hybridizations. The two housekeeping genes gave strong signals with all tissue cDNA probes (A–C) and with the DP1 product (D), whereas they gave no signal in the hybridizations with the DP2/DP3 products (E/F). (**G**) Graphical representation of the results obtained

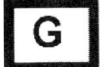

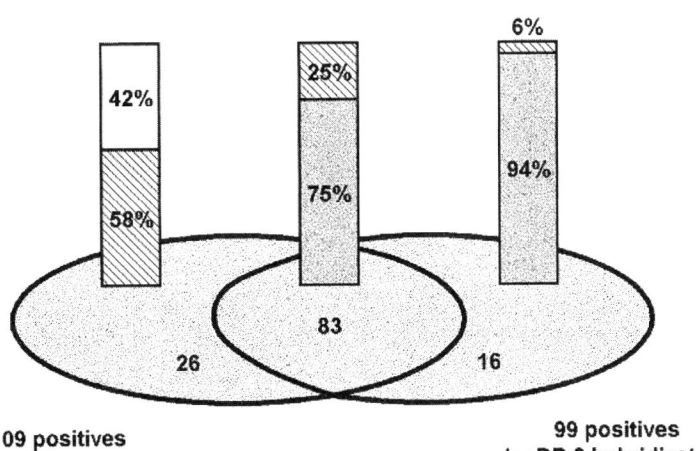

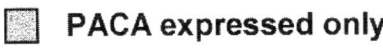

- PACA expressed only
- PACA expression + lower CP expression
- Similar expression levels in CP + PACA

by standard differential hybridizations and by hybridizations with the DP2 RDA probe. One hundred nine (109) cDNA clones were classified as differentially expressed in pancreatic cancer after subtraction of the hybridization results obtained with tissue cDNA probes. Ninety-nine (99) clones hybridized with the DP2 RDA probe. Eighty-three (83) clones were detected with both methods. Sixteen (16) clones were only classified as differential by the DP2 product and were shown to contain genes selectively overexpressed in pancreatic cancer. Twenty-six (26) clones were only detected in the differential hybridization approach. These genes were expressed in both, pancreatic cancer and chronic pancreatitis. The *bars* show the results of Northern blot hybridizations done with selected clones from each group to verify the differential expression pattern. A total of 50 Northern blots were done. PACA: pancreatic cancer; CP: chronic pancreatitis. (Modified from Geng *et al.*[10])

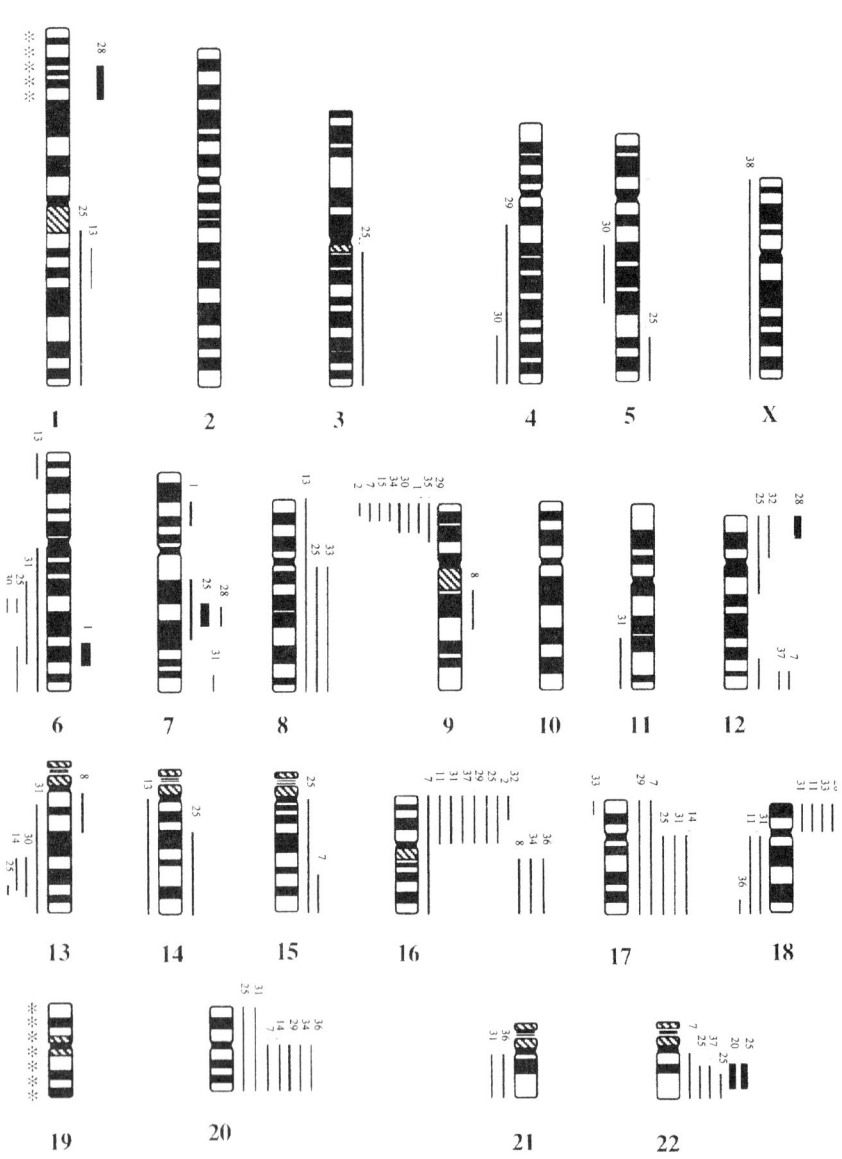

has led to the identification of important tumor suppressor genes in pancreatic cancer as, e.g., *DPC4 (deleted in pancreatic cancer 4*[18]). This approach is based on the generation of an allelotype of pancreatic cancer using a xenograft enrichment technique.[17] Xenografted tumors were allelotyped using polymorphic markers spanning the whole genome to detect allelic loss. This approach detected highly frequent allelic loss (>60%) at chromosomes 1p, 9p, 17p, and 18q and moderately frequent allelic loss (40–60%) at 3p, 6p, 6q, 8p, 10q, 12q, 13q, 18p, 21q, and 22q. Our approach was to use comparative genomic hybridzation (CGH)[36] to detect chromosomal imbalances in pancreatic cancer tissues, with the major advantage of detecting both, loss and gain of chromosomal material. This approach is described below.

Comparative Genomic Hybridization

Twenty-seven cases of pancreatic adenocarcinoma were analyzed by CGH (comparative genomic hybridization).[36] This approach does not require metaphase preparation of the tumor sample and thus circumvents the limitations of karyotypic analysis possibly influenced by short-term culturing of tumor cells. CGH is based on the use of genomic DNA of tumor cells as a probe for fluorescence *in situ* hybridization to normal metaphase chromosomes.[6,21] The probe is cohybridized with genomic DNA, isolated from normal lymphocytes, and visualized with a different fluorochrome. Comparison of the signal intensities from tumor and control DNA probes allows the detection of chromosomal imbalances. Gains or losses of chromosomal material in the tumor are indicated by the increase and decrease of the ration of the fluorescence signal intensities, respectively. Regions showing gains of chromosomal material may harbor putative oncogenes, whereas areas with loss of chromosomal material may contain putative tumor suppressor genes. Of the 27 tumors analyzed in this study, 23 showed chromosomal imbalances (FIG. 11). Gains of chromosomal material were much more frequent than losses. The most common overrepresentations were observed on chromosomes 16p (eight cases), 20q (seven cases), 22q (six cases), and 17q (five cases) and underrepresentations on a subregion of chromosome 9p (eight cases). Distinct high-level amplifications were found on 1p32–p34, 6q24, 7q22, 12p13, and 22q. These data provided evidence for a number of new cytogenetically defined recurrent aberrations that are characteristic of pancreatic carcinoma. The overrepresented or underrepresented chromosomal regions represent candidate regions for potential oncogenes and tumor suppressor genes, respectively, possibly involved in pancreatic tumorigenesis. The most common chromosomal imbalances are being studied in ongoing experiments in our laboratory. The following part of this review summarizes data we have generated for the high-level amplification on 6q23–24 and the area on 9p showing the most frequent loss of chromosomal material.

FIGURE 11. Summary of genetic imbalances detected in 27 pancreatic adenocarcinomas. *Vertical lines on the left*, chromosome ideogramms indicate loss of genetic material; *vertical lines on the right*, gain of genetic material. *Bold lines*, high-level amplifications. *Numbers above each line*, case analyzed. The distal part of chromosome 1p and chromosome 19 are labeled with (*), since in these two regions only high copy number amplifications were scored. (Modified from Solinas-Toldo *et al.*[36])

Characterization of High Copy Number Amplifications

Distinct high-level amplifications are usually confined to DNA segments of <1 MB and provide a good basis for the identification of candidate protooncogenes.

To identify the most likely candidate oncogene involved in the high-level amplification on 6q23-24 amplification, the extension of the amplification in pancreatic cancer tissues and cell lines was determined by Southern blot analysis with probes from genes located in the proximity of 6q24.[41] This initial analysis revealed a clear high copy number amplification including the locus of the *c-myb* oncogene. To isolate the candidate oncogene a contig covering the amplified region was constructed. For this purpose a first YAC clone was isolated with a *c-myb* gene probe and the ends of this YAC clone were used for the identification of overlapping YACs. Southern blot analysis with the ends of all YAC clones allowed to identify the minimal commonly amplified region in pancreatic cancer tissues (FIG. 12). As the complete minimally amplified region was contained in the first isolated YAC, we used this clone to isolate additional candidate genes by exon trapping. This approach led to the identification of several gene fragments from the 6q24 region, however only the protooncogene *c-myb* and *eRF3b* (Wallrapp *et al.* in preparation), a novel putative translation termination factor, were found to be amplified in the cancer tissues containing the minimal commonly amplified region (FIG. 12). Only a part of the restriction fragments detected with the *eRF3b* probe on Southern blots were found to be coamplified with *c-myb*. These data suggest that *eRF3b* is presumably located in the breakpoint of the amplification in the tissue containing the minimally amplified region. Expression studies revealed enhanced transcript levels of *eRF3b* only in the amplified pancreatic carcinoma tissue no. 1 and pancreatic cancer cell line PC2. A clear overexpression could not be found in tissue no. 7, which supports our suggestion that only parts of the gene are positioned inside the amplified region in this tissue (see FIG. 12). This and the finding that *eRF3b* is only overexpressed in tissues harboring a large 6q24 amplification suggest that this gene is not of general importance for pancreatic carcinogenesis, but simply represents a gene coamplified with the relevant oncogene.[41]

The second gene amplified in pancreatic cancer at 6q24 was the protooncogene *c-myb*, which encodes a transcriptional activator protein with repeated helix-turn-helix DNA-binding motifs. In hematopoiesis, *c-myb* appears to control both proliferation and differentiation.[11] *c-myb* is known to be activated as an oncogene through amplification in several tumor cells, for example, in some acute myelogenous leukemic cell lines,[35] primary breast cancer[47] and in a few additional cases in established adenocarcinoma cell lines from colon carcinoma[1] and small cell lung carcinoma.[24] Our data represent the first report describing an amplification of the *c-myb* locus in pancreatic cancer. This amplification appears to occur at a moderate frequency of 10% as compared to the amplification rates observed in primary breast cancer (3%)[47] and in colon cancer (23%).[12]

The selective increase of the copy number of the *c-myb* oncogene should result in increased RNA expression. Therefore, we examined the abundance of *c-myb* transcripts in different pancreatic tissues by reverse transcriptase polymerase chain reaction (RT-PCR) with c-*myb* specific primers. Using these conditions c-*myb* expression was barely detectable in healthy pancreas and chronic pancreatits, a control tissue with a similar degree of fibrosis and interstitial inflammation as cancer tis-

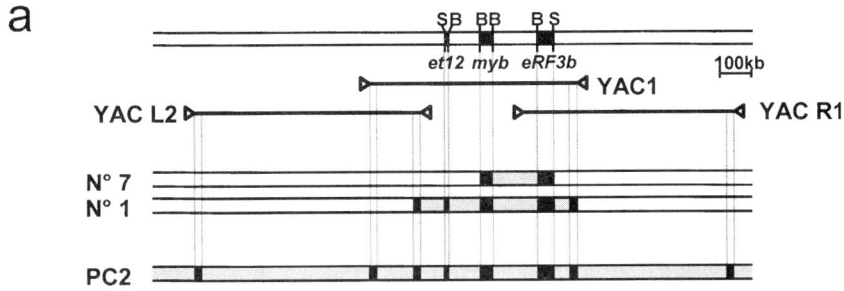

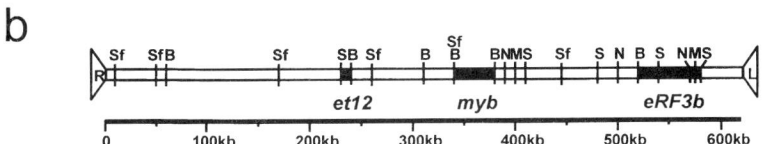

FIGURE 12. (a) Schematic drawing of the 6q24 region. YAC ends from the clones YAC1 (ICRFy900A0311Q), YAC R1 (ICRFy900K107Q9) and YAC L2 (ICRFy900E218Q) and some gene fragments isolated by exon trapping with YAC1-DNA (et12: novel gene, coding for a SH3-domain containing protein, homologue to protooncogene YES, GeneBank/NCBI accession no. U93815; eRF3b: eukaryotic release factor 3b, a novel putative translation termination factor, GeneBank/NCBI accession no. U87791) were hybridized on Southern blots of pancreatic carcinoma tissue and pancreatic cancer cell lines. Probes, which identified a high copy number amplification are marked by *black squares*; presumably coamplified regions are drawn in *gray*. (b) Restriction map of YAC1 (ICRFy900A0311Q) covering the minimally amplified region and localization of some trapped gene fragments. Sf: *Sfi*I; B: *Bss*HII; S: *Sal*I; N: *Nru*I; M: *Mlu*I. (Modified from Wallrapp *et al.*[41])

sue. Significantly enhanced expression was found in the pancreatic cancer tissues and cells showing amplifications at 6q24, thus confirming that DNA amplification is one of the genetic mechanisms leading to an upregulation of *c-myb* gene expression. Interestingly, overexpression was found not only in the tissues and cells showing amplifications but also in 70% of the examined pancreatic cancer tissues and 54% of the examined pancreatic cancer cell lines. Therefore, we suggest that enhanced *c-myb* expression is an important pathogenetic factor for pancreatic carcinogenesis and that other mechanisms besides DNA amplification lead to *c-myb* activation.

Interestingly, in addition to high copy number amplifications other genetic alterations of the *c-myb* locus were detectable. Loss of heterozygosity was found in 14% of the examined pancreatic cancer tissues and 15% of the examined pancreatic cancer cell lines. It has been suggested, that genetic imbalances of the *myb* locus, both amplification and deletion, might occur along with tumor progression or metastasis.[45] In fact, the DNAs showing amplification or loss of heterozygosity (LOH) were obtained from tumors of advanced stage, which had already metastasized to regional lymph nodes or other organs. Therefore, we postulate that genetic alterations of the

TABLE 2. Results of the PCR reactions with primer pairs from 35 microsatellite markers covering the region 9p13 to 9pter done to search for homozygous deletions in pancreatic cancer cell lines

Cytogenetic localization	STS	Capan1	Capan2	HPAF	PATU8902	PANC1	AsPc1	PC44	MIAPACA	PC2	PC3	PaTu2	DanG	SKPC1	MIMPC2	PATU8988t
9p24	D9S1858															
	D9S54															
	D9S178															
	D9S230															
9p23	D9S288															
	D9S281															
	D9S286															
	D9S144															
9p22	D9S256															
	D9S269															
	D9S268															
	D9S267															
	D9S274															
	D9S285															
	D9S156															
	D9S157															
	D9S162															
	D9S1648	■														
	D9S1778															
	IFNB							■					■			
	IFNA PCR															
	IFNA PCR												■			
9p21	D9S1814															
	D9S1870					■										
	D9S1846															
	D9S1751															
	D9S736												■			
	D9S1749															
	D9S1748					■										
	D9S1752					■										
	D9S966					■										
	D9S265	■														
	D9S171	■											■			
	D9S126	■											■			
	D9S259	■											■			
	D9S169	■														
9p13	D9S263	■														
	D9S165															

Note: The *black bars* indicate the deleted areas in the individual cell lines. STS = sequence tagged sites.

c-myb gene locus in pancreatic carcinoma may be associated with tumor progression or may be indicative for highly metastatic or invasive tumors.

Characterization of Deletions

By use of CGH the most frequent loss of chromosomal material was found on 9p in a region ranging from 9p21 to 9pter. This region is known to show both homozygous deletions and LOH in a variety of cancer tissues and cell lines (e.g., Refs. 3 and 8). *Cyclin-dependent kinase inhibitor 2* (*CDKN2*) was identified to be the most likely tumor suppressor gene involved in this deletion, in particular in pancreatic cancer.[3,4,33] However, additional deletions on 9p, not involving *CDKN2*, have been detected in a number of other tumors,[43,38] and it has been suspected that one or more tumor suppressor genes are located in this area. In pancreatic cancer the precise extension of the deletion on 9p21 has not been determined.

Since our CGH-data[36] showed that the deletion on 9p in pancreatic cancer tissues may extend from 9p21 to 9pter we assumed the involvement of additional, more distal gene loci. As these additional deleted loci may harbor new tumor suppressor genes, we decided to generate a fine map of the deletion on 9p in pancreatic cancer cell lines.

PCR reactions with primer pairs from 35 microsatellite markers and 11 known genes covering the region 9p13 to 9pter were done to search for homozygous deletions (cell lines). Six of 15 pancreatic cell lines showed homozygous deletions at 9p with an average length of 2.5 MB (see TABLE 2). The minimal commonly deleted region included markers located close to the *CDKN2* locus on the proximal side and markers located close to the interferon-α (INF–α) locus on the distal side of the deletion. One cell line (PANC1) displayed two separate homozygous deletions on 9p21, one comprising the *CDKN2* locus and a second one located close to the *INF-α* locus. This may serve as an indication that, as described for other tumors, 9p in addition to CDKN2 contains further tumor suppressor genes, which may be of importance for a small fraction of pancreatic tumors. Data in the literature suggest, that *INF-α* may be one of the candidate genes with tumor suppressor activity on 9p21.[27,5]

ACKNOWLEDGMENTS

We thank U. Lacher, S. Hähnel and K. Bartels for invaluable technical assistance. This work was supported by grants from the German Ministry of Science and Education (BMBF, Grant KBF 01 GB 9401), from the Deutsche Forschungsgemeinschaft (GR-1010-3-2) and the European Community (BMH1-CT92-0401). We thank Dr. G. Varga (Institute of Experimental Medicine, Budapest, Hungary), Dr. F. Gansauge and Prof. H.G. Beger (Department of General Surgery, University of Ulm, Germany) and Dr. H. Friess (Inselspital, University of Bern, Switzerland) for providing the pancreatic tissue samples used in this study.

REFERENCES

1. ALITALO, K., R. WINQVIST, C.C. LIN *et al.* 1984. Aberrant expression of amplified *c-myb* oncogene in two cell lines from a colon carcinoma. Proc. Natl. Acad. Sci. USA **81:** 4534–4538.

2. BARDI, G., B. JOHANSSON, N. PANDIS et al. 1993. Karyotypic abnormalities in tumours of the pancreas. Br. J. Cancer **67**: 1106–1112.
3. CAIRNS, P., T.J. POLASCIK et al. 1995. Rates of p16 (MTS1) mutations in primary tumors with 9p loss. Science **265**: 415–416.
4. CALDAS, C., S.A. HAHN, L.T. DA COSTA et al. 1994. Frequent somatic mutations and homozygous deletions of the p16 (MTS1) gene in pancreatic carcinoma. Nat. Genet. **8**: 27–32.
5. DIAZ, M.O., S. ZIEMIN, M.M. LE BEAU et al. 1988. Homozygous deletion of the alpha- and beta 1-interferon genes in human leukemia and derived cell lines. Proc. Natl. Acad. Sci USA **85**: 5259–5263.
6. DU MANOIR, S., M.R. SPEICHER, S. JOOS et al. 1993. Detection of complete and partial chromosome gains and losses by comparative genomic in situ hybridization. Hum. Genet. **90**: 590–610.
7. FIELDS, C., M.D. ADAMS, O. WHITE & C. VENTER. 1994. How many genes in the human genome? Nat. Genet. **7**: 345–346.
8. FOUNTAIN, J.W., M. KARAYIORGOU, M.S. ERNSTOFF et al. 1992. Homozygous deletions within human chromosome band 9p21 in melanoma. Proc. Natl. Acad. Sci. USA **89**: 10557–10561.
9. GENG, M.M., G. ADLER & T.M. GRESS. 1998a. Identification of TGFβ target genes in pancreatic cancer cells by representational difference analysis [abstract]. Gastroenterology **114**(Part 2): A600.
10. GENG, M., C. WALLRAPP, F. MÜLLER-PILLASCH et al. 1998b. Isolation of differentially expressed genes by combining representational difference analysis (RDA) and cDNA library arrays. BioTechniques. In press.
11. GRAF, T. 1992. Myb: a transcriptional activator linking proliferation and differentiation in hematopoietic cells [published erratum appears in Curr. Opin. Genet. Dev. 1992 Jun; 2(3): 504]. Curr. Opin. Genet. Dev. **2**: 249–255.
12. GRECO, C., G.M. GANDOLFO, F. MATTEI et al. 1994. Detection of c-myb genetic alterations and mutant p53 serum protein in patients with benign and malignant colon lesions. Anticancer Res. **14**: 1433–1440.
13. GRESS, T.M., F. MÜLLER-PILLASCH, M. GENG et al. 1996. A pancreatic cancer-specific expression profile. Oncogene **13**: 1819–1830.
14. GRESS, T.M., C. WALLRAPP, M. FROHME et al. 1997. Identification of genes with pancreatic cancer-specific expression by use of cDNA representational difference analysis. Genes Chromosomes Cancer **19**: 97–103.
15. GRIFFIN, C.A., R.H. HRUBAN, P.P. LONG et al. 1994. Chromosome abnormalities in pancreatic adenocarcinoma. Genes Chromosomes Cancer **9**: 93–100.
16. GROUDINE, M. & H. WEINTRAUB. 1980. Activation of cellular genes by avian RNA tumor viruses. Proc. Natl. Acad. Sci. USA **77**: 5351–5354.
17. HAHN, S., A.B. SEYMOUR, A.T.M. HOQUE et al. 1995. Allelotype of pancreatic adenocarcinoma using xenograft enrichment. Cancer Res. **55**: 4670–4675.
18. HAHN, S.A., M. SCHUTTE, A.T.M. HOQUE et al. 1996. DPC4. A candidate tumor suppressor gene at human chromosome 18q21.1. Science **271**: 350–353.
19. HRUBAN, R.H., G.M. PETERSEN, P.K. HA & S.E. KERN. 1998. Genetics of pancreatic cancer. From genes to families. Surg. Oncol. Clin. North Am. **7**: 1–23.
20. HUBANK, M. & D.G. SCHATZ. 1994. Identifying differences in mRNA expression by representational difference analysis of cDNA. Nucleic Acids Res. **22**: 5640–5648.
21. JOOS, S., H. SCHERTHAN, M.R. SPEICHER et al. 1993. Detection of amplified DNA sequences by reverse chromosome painting using genomic DNA as probe. Hum. Genet. **90**: 584–589.
22. KERN, S.E. 1998. Advances from genetic clues in pancreatic cancer. Curr. Opin. Oncol. **10**: 74–80.
23. KLEVER, P., R. BARES, J. FASS, U. BÜLL & V. SCHUMPELICK. 1992. PET with fluorine-18 deoxyglucose for pancreatic disease. Lancet **340**: 1158–1159.
24. KIEFER, P.E., G. BEPLER, M. KUBASCH et al. 1987. Amplification and expression of protooncogenes in human small cell lung cancer cell lines. Cancer Res. **47**: 6236–6242.

25. LISITSYN, N., N. LISITSYN & M. WIGLER. 1993. Cloning the differences between two complex genomes. Science **259**: 946–951.
26. MEIER-EWERT, S., E. MAIER, A. AHMADI *et al.* 1993. An automated approach to generating expressed sequence catalogues. Nature **361**: 375–376
27. MIYAKOSHI, J., K.D. DOBLER, A. TURNER *et al.* 1990. Absence of IFNA and IFNB genes from human malignant glioma cell lines and lack of correlation with cellular sensitivity to interferons. Cancer Res. **50**: 278–283.
28. MUELLER-PILLASCH, F., U. LACHER, C. WALLRAPP *et al.* 1997. Cloning of a gene highly overexpressed in cancer coding for a novel KH-domain containing protein. Oncogene **14**: 2729–2733.
29. MÜLLER-PILLASCH, F., C. WALLRAPP, U. LACHER *et al.* 1998a. Identification of a new tumor associated antigen TM4SF5 and its expression in human cancer. Gene **208**: 25–30.
30. MÜLLER-PILLASCH, F., C. WALLRAPP, K. BARTELS *et al.* 1998b. Cloning of a new Kunitz-type protease inhibitor overexpressed in pancreatic cancer. Biochim. Biophys. Acta **1395**: 88–95.
31. MURR, M.M., M.G. STARR, A.J. OISHI & J.A. VAN HEERDEN. 1994. Pancreatic cancer. CA Cancer J. Clin. **44**: 304–318.
32. MYERS, M.H & L.A. GLOECKLER-RIESS. 1989. Cancer patients survival rates: SEER programmee for 10 years of follow-up. CA Cancer J. Clin. **39**: 21–32.
33. NAUMANN, M., N. SAVITSKAIA, C. EILERT *et al.* 1996. Frequent codeletion of p16/MTS1 and p15/MTS2 and genetic alterations in p16/MTS1 in pancreatic tumors. Gastroenterology **110**: 1215–1224.
34. NEKARDA, H., M. SCHMITT, K. ULM *et al.* 1994. Prognostic impact of urokinase-type plasminogen activator and its inhibitor PAI-1 in completely resected gastric cancer. Cancer Res. **54**: 2900–2907.
35. PELLICI, P.G., L. LANFRANCONE, M.D. BRATHWAITE *et al.* 1984 Amplification of *c-myb* oncogene in a case of human acute myelogenous leukemia. Science **224**: 1117–1121.
36. SOLINAS-TOLDO, S., C. WALLRAPP, F. MÜLLER-PILLASCH *et al.* 1996. Mapping of chromosomal imbalances in pancreatic carcinoma by comparative genomic hybridization. Cancer Res. **56**: 3803–3807.
37. SCHUURING, E., E. VERHOEVEN, W.J. MOOI *et al.* 1993. The product of the EMS-1 gene, amplified and overexpressed in human carcinomas, is homologue to a v-src substrate and is located in cell-substratum contact sites. Mol. Cell. Biol. **13**: 2891–2898.
38. TAKITA, J., Y. HAYASHI, T. KOHNO *et al.* 1997. Deletion map of chromosome 9 and p16 (CDKN2A) gene alterations in neuroblastoma. Cancer Res. **57**: 907–912.
39. VAN ERP, H.E, J.A.M. UNNIK, G. RIJSKEN, J.G. SMITS & G.E. STAAL. 1991. Cellular expression of k-type pyruvate kinase in normal and neoplastic tissues. Cancer **15**: 2595–2601.
40. VISHWANATHA, J.K., Y. CHIANG, K.D. KUMBLE *et al.* 1993. Enhanced expression of annexin II in human pancreatic carcinoma cells and primary pancreatic cancer. Carcinogenesis **14**: 2575–2579.
41. WALLRAPP, C., F. MÜLLER-PILLASCH, S. SOLINAS-TOLDO *et al.* 1997. Characterization of a high copy number amplification at 6q24 in pancreatic cancer identifies myb as candidate oncogene. Cancer Res. **57**: 3135–3139.
42. WEINHOUSE, S. 1983. Isozyme alterations, gene regulation and neoplastic transformation,. Adv. Enzyme Regul. **21**: 369–386.
43. WIEST, J.S, W.A. FRANKLIN, J.T. OTSTOT *et al.* 1997. Identification of a novel region of homozygous deletion on chromosome 9p in squamous cell carcinoma of the lung: the location of a putative tumor suppressor gene. Cancer Res. **57**: 1–6.
44. YAMADA, K., S.K. AKIYAMA, T. HASEGAWA *et al.* 1985. Recent advances in research on fibronectin and other cell attachment proteins. J. Cell. Biochem. **28**: 78–98.
45. YOKOTA, J., Y. TSUNETSUGU YOKOTA, H. BATTIFORA *et al.* 1986. Alterations of *myc*, *myb*, and *rasHa* proto-oncogenes in cancers are frequent and show clinical correlation. Science **231**: 261–265.

46. ZEHETNER, G. & H. LEHRACH. 1994. The Reference Library System-sharing biological material and experimental data. Nature **367:** 489–491.
47. ZHOU, D.J., H. AHUJA & M.J. CLINE. 1989. Proto-oncogene abnormalities in human breast cancer: *c-ERBB-2* amplification does not correlate with recurrence of disease. Oncogene **4:** 105–108.

p22/PRG1: A Novel Early Response Gene in Pancreatic Cancer Cells Regulated by p53 and NFκB

WOLFGANG E. SCHMIDT,[a,b,c] ALEXANDER ARLT,[a] ANIA TRAUZOLD,[a] AND HEINER SCHÄFER[a]

[a]*Laboratory of Molecular Gastroenterology and Hepatology, I. Department of Medicine, Christian-Albrechts-University of Kiel, Kiel, Germany*

[b]*Department of Medicine I, St. Josef-Hospital, Ruhr-University of Bochum Medical School, Bochum, Germany*

INTRODUCTION

Pancreatic cancer belongs to the most malignant gastrointestinal tumors in Western countries and is responsible for several fatal tumor cases, still with increasing incidence. The extremely poor prognosis of pancreatic carcinomas is due to less defined and rather unspecific symptoms leaving progression of the disease undiscovered for a long time. Thus, most pancreatic carcinomas are diagnosed very late, a situation that precludes an adequate and successful therapeutic intervention. In order to improve our management of this devastating disease, it is therefore necessary to augment our understanding of the molecular mechanisms that account for malignant pancreatic cell growth. The discovery of multiple genetic alterations in various forms of cancers has advanced our knowledge of how malignant tumors develop.

In an attempt to identify and characterize genes related to the induction of proliferation and apoptosis, we recently cloned a novel early response gene from proliferating rat pancreatic carcinoma cells, designated p22/PACAP response gene 1 (p22/PRG1).[1] This gene also exists in man, known as IEX-1/DIF2,[2,3] and in mice, known as gly96.[4] Its expression has been shown to be associated with the induction of cell growth as well as with stress response and cellular adaptation.[1–4] In accordance with these multiple conditions of stimulated p22/PRG1 expression, the promoter of this novel gene contains binding sites for various important transcription factors—including AP-1/Ets-1, myc/max, SP-1 and NFkB—that account for the early and transient induction of p22/PRG1.[1,4,5] Another important transcription factor that regulates p22/PRG1 expression in rats is the tumor suppressor p53.[6] Although the exact cellular function of p22/PRG1 is not known, it can be speculated that this novel gene is implicated in growth regulation under various cellular yet undefined conditions.

In this study, we describe cloning of the human p22/PRG1 promoter and characterization of functional p53 and NFκB binding sites. Furthermore, we elucidate the

---

[c]Corresponding author: Wolfgang E. Schmidt, M.D., Ph.D., Professor of Medicine, Department of Medicine I, St. Josef-Hospital, Ruhr-University of Bochum Medical School, Gudrunstrasse 56, D-44791 Bochum, Germany. Phone, +49 234-509-2310/-11; fax, +49 234-509-2309; e-mail, wolfgang.e.schmidt@ruhr-uni-bochum.de

expression of human p22/PRG1 in response to activated p53 as well as NFκB and discuss an involvement in the control of apoptosis.

METHODS

Cloning and Sequencing of the Human p22/PRG1 Promoter

Using the *PromoterFinder* human genomic DNA-walking kit (Clontech), polymerase chain reaction (PCR) fragments of the hp22/PRG1 promoter were generated. As gene-specific primers we first used two reversed primers targeted to the human p22/PRG1 gene:

5'AGGTCAGGTCGAGGCCTCTGGAGT3',
5'GTTCCCCAGTGACTCCAGGGCAGCGCA3'

and in a second run a third p22/PRG1 specific primer:

5'TGAGCCAGCGGAGTGTAAGGCCAAGT3'.

PCR products comprising the entire human p22/PRG1 gene fragment were generated by PCR on 2 µg of human genomic DNA using the following primers:

forward, 5'CCTCACTTATAAGTGGGAACCA3'/
reverse, 5'GGCGATCTCGACAGTCGCTC3'.

PCR conditions were as described.[5] PCR products were checked by nested PCR, cloned into the TA cloning vector (*In vitro* Gene) and submitted to automatic sequencing (LICOR 4000L) using labeled universal sequencing primers or inserting specific primers (MWG-Biotech).

Gel Shift and Supershift Assays

For p53 gel shifts, purified recombinant baculovirus expressed wt-p53 or double mutated p53-C5 (80 ng) were incubated in incubation buffer (Stratagene) together with a γ^{32}P-labeled oligonucleotide (*aggtgccacatgctccgacatgtgcctgca*) containing the p53 binding site from the human p22/PRG1 promotor. For NFκB gel shifts, nuclear extracts from tumor necrosis factor-α (TNF-α)-stimulated Jurkat cells were incubated with a γ^{32}P-labeled oligonucleotide (*aatcgtcggaatttccagcccg*) containing the NFκB binding site from the human p22/PRG1 promoter or a consensus NFκB-binding site. After 30 min incubation at room temperature, samples were submitted to native polyacrylamide gel electrophoresis (PAGE). Gels were dried and exposed to X-ray Hyperfilm (Amersham). For supershift assays, a monoclonal p53 antibody (Ab1, Calbiochem) or anti-p65/p50 NFκB antibodies (Santa Cruz) were added for 1 hr at 4°C.

Reverse Transcriptase Polymerase Chain Reaction

For reverse transcriptase polymerase chain reaction (RT-PCR), 2 µg of total heat-denatured (75°C, 3 min) RNA was submitted to reverse transcription and subsequent PCR using appropriate primers. For the analysis of p22/PRG1 expression the specific targeted primers 5'cggcttaccatgtgtcactctcgca3' (*sense*) and 5'ggtcgaaggtgaagatctcaggacc3' (*antisense*) were used, for the glyceraldehyde-3-phosphate dehydrogenase (GAPDH) or β-actin mRNA control *Amplimer* PCR primers (Clontech). PCR was carried out at 95°C, 60 sec; 58°C, 35 sec; and 72°C, 45 sec for 18–24 cycles (p22/PRG1) or 12–16 cycles (GAPDH) and a 10-min extension at 72°C (Perkin Elmer Thermocycler 9600). PCR products were analyzed by polyacrylamide gel electrophoresis and subsequent staining with ethidium bromide. Bands were quantified by densitometry (BIO-DOC).

Generation of CAT-Reporter Gene Constructs

Using appropriate composite Hind-III/Xba-I and Sal-I/Xba-I PCR primers, PCR fragments of the human p22/PRG1 promoter were generated containing deletions in positions −226/−244 and −106/−111 (Δ^{p53}, $\Delta^{-NF\kappa B}$) or shortened at the 5' end (pos. +1 to −439, −335, −285, −225, −180, and −110). Products were cloned into the CAT-basic vector (Promega) and checked by nucleotide sequencing.

Cell Transfection and CAT-Reporter Gene Assay

HeLa cells were cultured in 6-well plates and transiently transfected (Lipofectamine®; GIBCO-BRL) with pCAT vectors (1.5 µg) containing human p22/PRG1 promoter fragments and 0.5 µg pCMV-lacZ as internal control. For cotransfection, 0.1 µg of cytomegalovirus (CMV) early enhancer promoter-driven expression plasmids for wild-type p53 (pCMV-p53) or mutant p53 (pCMV-c5p53) were added. After 24 hr culture, CAT expression (ng) was determined by enzyme-linked immunosorbent assay (ELISA, Boehringer) and normalized to β-galactosidase expression (β-gal ELISA, Boehringer).

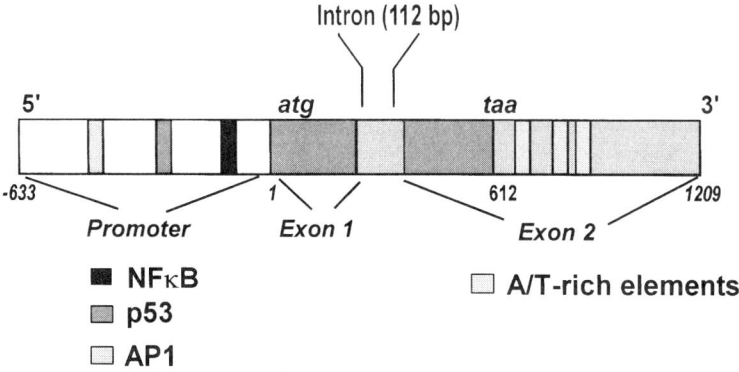

FIGURE 1. Gene structure of human p22/PRG1. Exon/intron organization of the human p22/PRG1 gene and the 5' flanking region harboring the putative promoter. Binding sites for transcription factors are indicated.

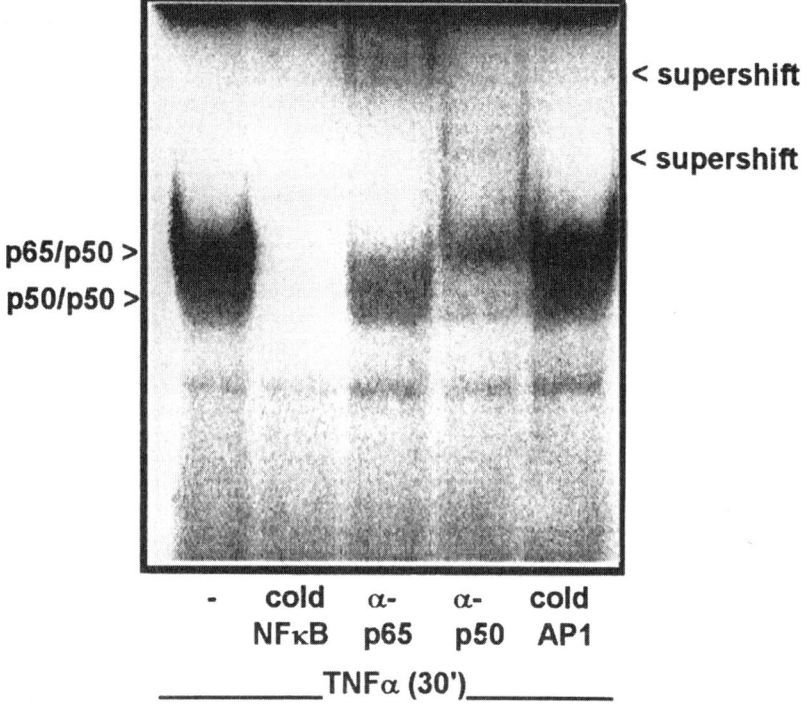

FIGURE 2. Gel shift and supershift assay. (**a**) Using nuclear extracts from TNF-α-stimulated Jurkat cells, we performed gel shift assays with equal amounts of the [γ^{32}P]-labeled oligonucleotide containing the NFκB binding site of the human p22/PRG1 promoter. (**b**) Using baculovirus recombinant wild-type p53 (*lanes 1,3,4*) or recombinant mutant p53-C5 (*lane 2*), we performed gel shift assays with equal amounts of the [γ^{32}P]-labeled oligonucleotide containing p53 binding site of the human p22/PRG1 promoter. Assays were conducted in the absence or presence of a 50-fold molar excess of unlabeled oligo, or in the presence of a monoclonal antiody against p65/p50 (a) or the C-terminal domain of wild-type p53 (b). C1, shifted band; C2, supershifted band.

RESULTS

Structural Organization of the p22/PRG1 Gene

Employing the genome walking strategy a PCR product was generated from human genomic DNA and sequenced. This product contained a 1.842-bp fragment of the human p22/PRG1 gene encompassing two exons, an intron and a putative promoter region consisting of 633 bp (FIG. 1). This promoter contains a TATA-like box (pos. −30) and potential binding sites for several transcription factors, including NFκB (pos. −113), SP1 (pos. −452), AP1 (pos. −382), Ets (pos. −520 and −417), c-

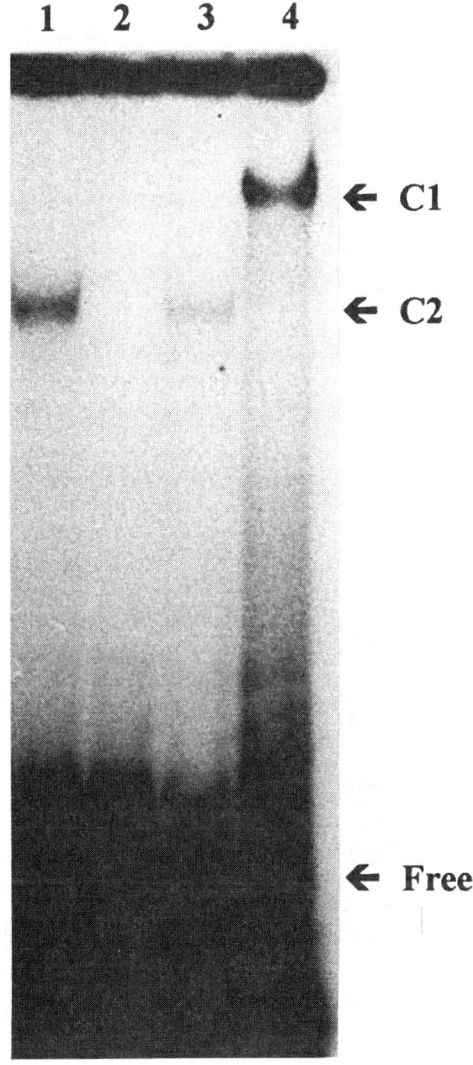

FIGURE 2b

myc (pos. −172) and two sites for the tumor suppressor protein p53 (pos. −245 and −163). Two repetitive polynucleotide regions, A_{15} and A_7TA_5, are located at positions −305 and −470, respectively.

TABLE 1. NFκB-dependent transcriptional activity of the p22/PRG1 promoter in response to TNF-α

	0.2 nM TNF-α	PBS
(−439/−1)-CAT	396 ± 32	100
(−439/$^{\Delta NFκB}$/−1)-CAT	78 ± 12	100
(−145/−1)-CAT	467 ± 53	100
(−110/−1)-CAT	80 ± 8	100

NOTE: HeLa cells were transiently cotransfected with CAT reporter gene vectors containing the indicated fragments of the human p22/PRG1 promoter and pCMVlacZ, as transfection control. Upon subsequent stimulation with 0.2 nM TNF-α for 6–8 hr, CAT expression was quantified by a CAT-ELISA and normalized to β-galactosidase activity. Basal activity was determined in cells treated with phosphate-buffered saline (PBS). Mean ± SD, $n = 4$.

Functional Analysis of Transcription Factor Binding Sites in the p22/PRG1 Promoter

p53 Gel Shift Assays

In order to verify site-specific binding of p53 and NFκB to the human p22/PRG1 promoter, gel shift assays were conducted. As shown in FIGURE 2a, coincubation of an oligonucleotide containing the p53 binding site of the human p22/PRG1 promoter with recombinant wt-p53 produces an intensively labeled protein/DNA complex. Labeling of this complex was diminished in the presence of the unlabeled homologous oligonucleotide at a 50-fold molar excess. No protein/DNA complex was observed when coincubating the p53-oligo with recombinant mutant p53 incapable of site-specifc DNA binding. The specificity of the labeled protein/DNA complex was confirmed by the addition of a p53 specific monoclonal antibody producing a ternary protein/DNA complex visualized as supershifted band.

NFκB Gel Shift Assays

For gel shift assays on NFκB, nuclear extracts from TNF-α-stimulated Jurkat cells were used. As shown in FIGURE 2b, an intensively labeled protein/DNA complex could be detected when coincubating the nuclear extract and the NFκB probe derived from the p22/PRG1 promoter. The addition of an excess of the homologous unlabeled oligo completely reduced labeling of the protein/DNA complex, whereas an unrelated oligo like AP1 did not compete with the probe. The specificity of the identified protein/DNA complex was underlined by the appearance of a supershifted ternary complex with monoclonal antibodies against p65 and p50 (FIG. 2b)

p53 and NFκB CAT Reporter Gene Assays

The capacity of NFκB and p53 binding sites to transcriptionally induce the human p22/PRG1 promoter was checked by CAT reporter gene assays using various modified promoter fragments of human p22/PRG1. As shown in TABLE 1, strong transcriptional induction (>400%) of the CAT gene by TNF-α was observed in HeLa cells transiently transfected with CAT constructs of the human p22/PRG1 promoter containing the NFκB binding site. No such TNF-α-dependent increase of CAT ex-

TABLE 2. p53-dependent transcriptional activity of the p22/PRG1 promoter

	pCMV[p53]	pCMV[C5p53]	pCMV[lacZ]
(−439/−1)-CAT	445 ± 70	89 ± 21	100
(−439/$^{\Delta p53}$/−1)-CAT	135 ± 19	92 ± 7	100
(−335/−1)-CAT	387 ± 51	107 ± 14	100
(−285/−1)-CAT	564 ± 44	95 ± 9	100
(−185/−1)-CAT	119 ± 28	82 ± 11	100

NOTE: HeLa cells were transiently cotransfected with 0.1 µg of pCMV-p53 or pCMV-C5p53 plus 1.5 µg of various CAT reporter gene constructs of the human p22/PRG1 promoter and 0.5 µg pCMV-lacZ as control. Basal activity was determined by cotransfection without p53 expression vectors, CAT expression was quantified by a CAT-ELISA and normalized to β-galactosidase activty. Mean ± SD, $n = 4$.

pression was observed in cells that received CAT reporter gene constructs lacking the NFκB binding site. Instead, in these transfectants CAT expression was slightly decreased (up to 20%) by TNF-α.

A p53 binding site-restricted increase of CAT expression could be demonstrated in HeLa cells transiently cotransfected with CAT-promoter constructs and a CMV promoter-driven expression vector for wild-type p53.[7] As shown in TABLE 2, the level of CAT expression was elevated up to 6-fold in cells receiving promoter constructs containing the p53 binding site, but not in transfectants lacking this site. In contrast, cotransfection with an expression plasmid for mutant p53 (pCMV-c5p53) resulted in no site-restricted increase of CAT expression, like cotransfection with the control vector pCMV(lacZ).

Overexpression of p53 Elevates Expression of Endogenous p22/PRG1

To verify induction of endogenous p22/PRG1 transcription in HeLa cells upon expression of ectopic active p53, mRNA levels of p22/PRG1 were analyzed by RT-PCR in the same panel of transfected cells described above. As shown in FIGURE 3, a 2–3-fold increase of p22/PRG1 mRNA was obeserved in HeLa cells transfected with pCMV(p53) compared to mock- or pCMV(lacZ)-transfected cells. When transfected with pCMV(C5p53), this elevation of the p22/PRG1 mRNA level did not occur. No alteration of the mRNA contents was noted for the housekeeping gene GAPDH in all HeLa-transfectants (FIG. 3).

TNF-α Induces Expression of p22/PRG1 Probably via NFκB

The exposure to TNF-α was followed by a rapid increase of NFκB binding to its binding site in the human p22/PRG promoter (see above). Along with the increase of NFκB activity, p22/PRG1 mRNA levels were strongly elevated, as shown in FIGURE 4. This elevation was maximal after 1 hr and amounted to 8–10-fold, followed by a rapid decline within 2–3 hr. In contrast, mRNA levels of the housekeeping gene β-actin remained unaltered in Jurkat cells under these conditions. Blocking the for-

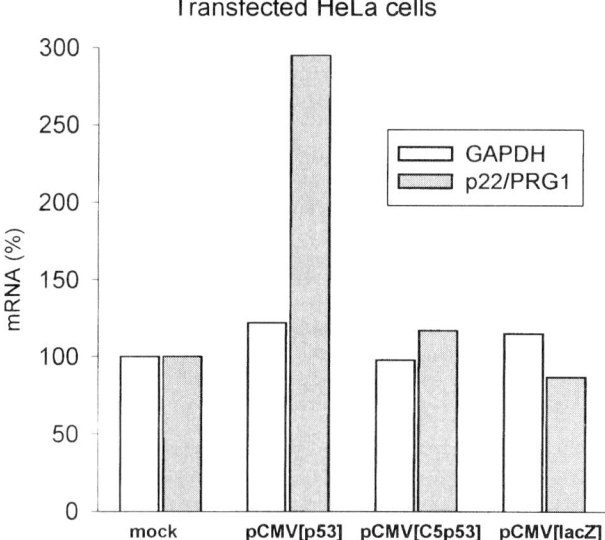

FIGURE 3. Wild-type p53 specifically induces p22/PRG1 expression in transiently transfected HeLa cells. HeLa cells were transiently transfected with an empty vector (mock), pCMV-p53, pCMV-C5p53 or pCMV-lacZ. Upon 24 hr, including a 6-hr period of serum withdrawal, total RNA was submitted to RT-PCR using primers for p22/PRG1 and GAPDH. PCR products were quantified by densitometry of ethidium bromide stained PAA gels.

mation of active nuclear NFκB by addition of gliotoxin abolished the inducing effect of TNF-α, as shown in FIGURE 4.

DISCUSSION

The promoter of human p22/PRG1 contains highly conserved binding sites for NFκB and p53 at almost identical positions compared to its rodent counterparts. This high degree of conservation indicates an essential role of these promoter elements. In accordance with the significant structural identity with the corresponding consensus sequences,[8–10] both binding sites turned out to be functional in terms of NFκB- and p53-dependent transactivation. Since endogenous p22/PRG1 expression was inducible under conditions of NFκB and p53 activation, it can be hypothesized that p22/PRG1 serves as a target gene for these two important transcription factors. In support of our recent finding that p22/PRG1 expression is induced by TNF-α in pancreatic carcinoma cells resistent to TNF-α cytotoxicity,[11] recruitment of p22/PRG1 by TNF-α in HeLa cells seems to be related to NFκB-dependent activation of the human p22/PRG1 promoter. Therefore, it can be assumed that p22/PRG1 is involved in biological actions of TNF-α mediated via NFκB. Similar to stress response (UV light, γ-irradiation)[3] that also involves NFκB activation, recruitment of p22/PRG1 by TNF-α may contribute to a cellular survival and regeneration signal. This signal

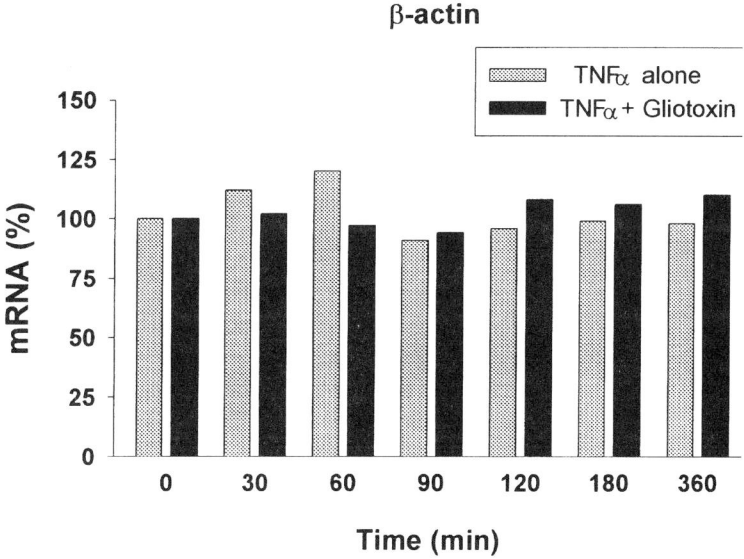

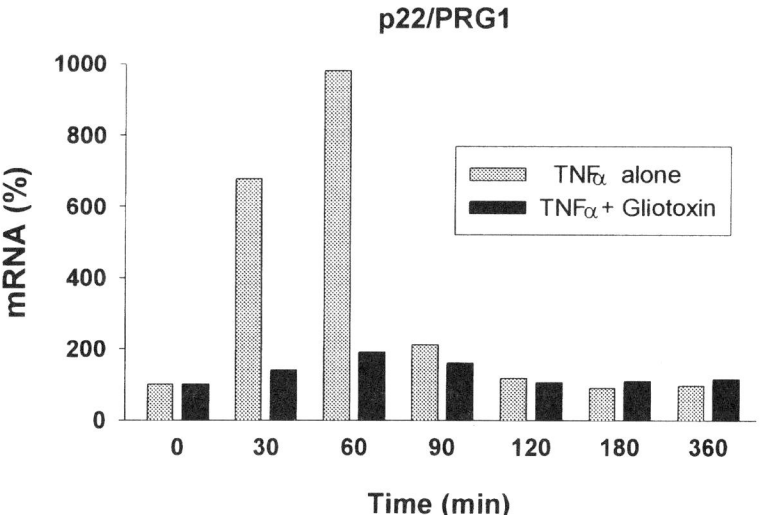

FIGURE 4. TNFα induces NFκB-dependent expression of p22/PRG1. Jurkat cells were treated with 0.3 nM TNFα for various periods in the presence or absence of the NFκB inhibitor gliotoxin (0.5 μg/ml). Then total RNA was prepared and submitted to RT-PCR for the detection of p22/PRG1 mRNA, and β-actin mRNA as control. PCR products were submitted to PAGE followed by EtBr staining and subsequent densitometric evaluation. Data represent the result of a representative experiment ($n = 3$).

initiates at the TNFR-1 receptor and its interaction with TRAF-2,[11] and requires NFκB-dependent gene transcription. Still, these genes need to be defined, and p22/PRG1 can be regarded as a novel candidate. This assumption is supported by the recent demonstration of an antiapoptotic role of a longer splicing variant of p22/PRG1—termed IEX-1L—that protects from TNF-α and Fas-mediated apoptosis in a variety of cells.[12] However, the detailed cellular function of both isoforms of p22/PRG1/IEX-1 in this context is unknown.

The identity of human p22/PRG1 as a target gene for p53 is another interesting issue, yet the role in this context is rather speculative. In its predominant function as transcription factor,[13] p53 recruits genes that are involved in growth arrest and DNA repair as well as in apoptosis,[14] hereby preventing the propagation of potentially mutated cells. The lack of such a p53-dependent growth control is a major cause of cancer. The recruitment of p22/PRG1 by p53 may be related to another mode of p53-dependent growth regulation,[15,16] in that cells recovered from DNA damage are allowed to reenter the cell cycle and thus to survive. Current studies focus on the function and the interrelation of IEX-1L and its shorter isoform p22/PRG1 during NFκB-mediated cellular survival on the one hand, and p53-mediated growth control on the other. As a major goal, these studies may provide a novel mechanism by which tumors become resistant against apoptotic elimination.

REFERENCES

1. SCHÄFER, H., A. TRAUZOLD, E.G. SIEGEL, U.R. FÖLSCH & W.E. SCHMIDT. 1996. Cancer Res. **56:** 2641–2648.
2. KONDRATYEV, A.D., K.N. CHUNG & M.O. JUNG. 1996. Cancer Res. **56:** 1498–1502.
3. PIETZSCH, A., C. BÜCHLER, C. ASLANIDIS & G. SCHMITZ. 1996. Biochem. Biophys. Res. Commun. **235:** 4–9.
4. CHARLES, C.H., J.K. YOON, J.S. SIMSKE & L.L. LAU. 1993. Oncogene **8:** 797–801.
5. PIETZSCH, A., C. BÜCHLER & G. SCHMITZ. 1998. Biochem. Biophys. Res. Commun. **245:** 651–657.
6. SCHÄFER, H., A. TRAUZOLD, T. SEBENS, W. DEPPERT, U.R. FÖLSCH & W.E. SCHMIDT. 1998. Oncogene **16:** 2479–2487.
7. STÜRZBECHER, H.W., P. CHUMAKOV, W.J. WELCH & J.R. JENKINS. 1987. Oncogene **1:** 201–211.
8. EL-DEIRY, W.S., S.E. KERN, J.A. PIETENPOL, K.W. KINZLER & B. VOGELSTEIN. 1992. Nat. Genet. **1:** 45–49.
9. ZAMBETTI, G.P., J. BARGONETTI, K. WALKER, C. PRIVES & A.J. LEVINE. 1992. Genes Dev. **6:** 1143–1152.
10. KUNSCH, C., S.M. RUBEN & C.A. ROSEN. 1992. Mol. Cell. Biol. **12:** 4412–4421.
11. HSU, H., H.B. SHU, M.G. PAN & D.V. GOEDDEL. 1996. Cell **84:** 299–308.
12. WU, M.X., Z. AO, K.V.S. PRASAD, R. WU & S.R. SCHLOSSMAN. 1998. Science **281:** 998–1001.
13. UNGER, T., M.M. NAU, S. SEGAL & J.D. MINNA. 1992. EMBO J. **11:** 1383–1390.
14. KO, L.J. & C. PRIVES. 1996. Genes Dev. **10:** 1054–1072.
15. XIAO, Z.X., J. CHEN, A.J. LEVINE, N. MODJTAHEDI, J. XING, W.R. SELLERS & D.M. LIVINGSTON. 1995. Nature **375:** 694–698.
16. SHIN, T.H., A.J. PATERSON & J.E. KUDLOW. 1995.. Mol. Cell. Biol. **15:** 4694–4701.

Protein Tyrosine Dephosphorylation and the Maintenance of Cell Adhesions in the Pancreas

J. SCHNEKENBURGER, J. MAYERLE, P. SIMON, W. DOMSCHKE, AND M.M. LERCH[a]

Department of Medicine B, Westfälische Wilhelms-Universität, Münster, Germany

ABSTRACT: Cell-cell contacts are important regulatory elements in tissue development, organ morphogenesis and malignant tumor invasion. In recent *in vivo* studies we have identified the members of the cadherin/catenin family of cell adhesion proteins that are differentially expressed in the pancreas and have determined their cell biological dynamics during dissociation and repair of adherens junctions. To further characterize these events, epithelial cell culture systems were used and a number of type II protein tyrosine phosphatases (PTPs) were found to colocalize and interact with the cadherin/catenin complex. These observations suggest that tyrosine dephosphorylation in general and PTPs in particular are involved in cell contact formation. Our most recent experiments indicate 1) that inhibition of PTPs alone dissociates pancreatic adherens junctions, 2) that cytosolic and transmembrane PTPs are differentially expressed in acinar cells, and 3) that a subset of them can associate with proteins of the cadherin/catenin complex at pancreatic cell-cell adhesions.

TRANSMEMBRANE PROTEIN TYROSINE PHOSPHATASES AND CELL CONTACT FORMATION

A key element in the regulation of cell-cell and cell-matrix adhesion is the tyrosine phosphorylation of proteins that are localized at focal adhesions and at intercellular junctions.[1] While much is known about the protein tyrosine kinases involved in the phosphorylation of cell adhesions, very little information exists about the protein tyrosine phosphatases (PTPs), which are thought to be responsible for the dephosphorylation of these structural complexes. Probable candidates are those receptor-like PTPs, which contain a cell adhesion molecule-like extracellular domain and could therefore regulate their intrinsic phosphatase activity in response to cell contact. Recent reports suggest that some PTPs do, in fact, possess properties that resemble those of classical cell adhesion molecules.[2] A direct involvement in cell contact formation has so far been demonstrated for PTPμ[3,4] and PTPκ,[5] where a homophilic interaction between the extracellular domains of these PTPs on neighboring cells was found. Moreover, the localization of PTPμ was found to be restricted to sites of cell-cell contacts,[2,6] and its surface expression is increased in a cell density-dependent manner.[6] Direct association of PTPμ with members of the cadherin/catenin family suggested further that proteins of the cell adhesion complex

---

[a]Address for correspondence: Dr. M.M. Lerch, Department of Medicine B, Westfälische Wilhelms-Universität, Albert-Schweitzer-Strasse 33, 48129 Münster, Germany. Phone, +49 251-834-7559; fax, +49 251-49504; e-mail: markus.lerch@uni-muenster.de

represent physiological substrates for this PTP.[4] For another receptor-like PTPase, PTP LAR, which was found to associate with focal cell-substratum adhesions via the newly identified LAR interacting protein-1, a possible regulatory function in cell-matrix adhesion, has been proposed.[7] PTPμ,[8] PTPκ,[9] LAR,[10] and PTPσ[11] are members of the so called type II receptor-like PTPs. In their extracellular portion, they all present a variable number of immunoglobulin (Ig)-like and fibronectin type III (FN III)-like domains. In addition to their sequence homology, these PTPs share characteristics in their biosynthesis, they all undergo proteolytic processing by a furin-like endoprotease, and they are expressed at the cell surface in two subunits, which are not covalently linked.[6,9,11,12] It was shown for LAR[12] and other PTPs[6,11] that the E-subunit, which contains the cell adhesion molecule-like extracellular domain, is shed from the cell surface when cells are grown to a high density. Although the cell density-dependent expression pattern and the shedding of the E-subunit of class II PTPs would suggest a critical role in cell contact formation, the biological function of the extra- and intracellular domains of these phosphatases during this event is still poorly understood.

EPITHELIAL CELL ADHERENS JUNCTIONS AND TYROSINE DEPHOSPHORYLATION

Most research addressing the signaling mechanisms involved in growth, development and cell contact formation has focused on the identification and characterization of novel receptor tyrosine kinases.[13] During the search for protein tyrosine phosphatase partners that would potentially counteract the biological function of these tyrosine kinases in epithelial cells, the human homologue of PTPκ (hPTPκ) was identified.[14] The expression of this phosphatase depended on the relative density to which epithelial cells in culture were grown and hPTPκ was found to colocalize with two members of the arm family of classical cell-adhesion proteins, β-catenin and γ-catenin/plakoglobin, at adherens junctions. By using *in vitro* and *in vivo* binding assays, a specific complex formation between endogenous PTPκ and β- and γ-catenin could be demonstrated. In addition, evidence was found that β-catenin represents a possible substrate for the catalytic activity of PTPκ. These data indicate that PTPκ might be involved in the regulation of epithelial cell-cell adhesions. When a novel member of the same family of receptor-type PTPs (PCP2) was identified and characterized in the pancreas, this phosphatase was found to colocalize with E-cadherin and β-catenin as well.[15] This observation lends further support to the hypothesis that class II PTPs may have a highly related biological function in the formation and maintenance of adherens junctions between epithelial cells.

Another class II PTP, PTPσ, was found to undergo biosynthesis and proteolytic processing in a manner that highly resembles that of the closely related PTP LAR.[16] Moreover, further proteolytic processing of PTPσ as well as of LAR could be induced by treatment of the cells with tissue plasminogen activator (TPA) or the calcium ionophore A23187. This inducible processing took place in the extracellular segment of the P-subunit in a juxtamembrane position and led to shedding of the E-subunit. Both, LAR and PTPσ were predominantly localized in adherens junctions and desmosomes. The inducible shedding of the E-subunit of LAR and PTPσ was followed by a redistribution of the PTP within the cell membrane or by an internalization of the cleaved P-subunits. It therefore represents a mechanism through which the phosphatase activity of these PTPs can be regulated in response to cell contact. The cell adhesion molecule-like character of LAR and PTPσ was further supported by the fact that the internalization of LAR and PTPσ occurred independently of the proteolytic processing if cells were grown in calcium-depleted growth medium. The parallels in specific localization as well as in intracellular behavior of PTPσ and LAR with classical cell adhesion molecules of the cadherin/catenin family extended the observations made for the other receptor type phosphatases mentioned above. Although these data strongly suggested a direct involvement of class II protein tyrosine phosphatases in the formation and maintenance of intercellular contacts between epithelial cells, it remained unknown whether and how these mechanisms apply to an intact organ system such as the pancreas where cells of different phenotypes form functional units.

CELL-CELL ADHESIONS IN THE EXOCRINE PANCREAS

In the exocrine pancreas a number of different cell types interact, and this interaction determines the organ's physiological function.[17] They are exocrine cells, which produce large amounts of excretable protein and whose intercellular contacts form secretory acini, centroacinar cells that secrete bicarbonate and thus regulate the zymogen granule membrane recycling from the luminal surface of acinar cells,[18] duct cells that line the excretory channels, interstitial cells that synthesize and secrete extracellular matrix proteins, and endothelial cells. A number of pathological conditions can disrupt cellular interactions. Acute pancreatitis, for example, is a disease that can lead to significant loss of cells by either necrosis or apoptosis,[19,20] and regeneration from this loss of tissue requires de novo formation of intercellular contacts between cells of different phenotypes on a very large scale. In a milder variety of pancreatitis that is not associated with significant loss of tissue, the rapid interstitial fluid collections, termed pancreatic edema, require the dissociation of numerous cell-cell contacts either before or during their formation.[21]

Data derived from experiments with dispersed pancreatic acinar cells suggest that several of the initial cell biological disturbances observed during acute pancreatitis could be caused by alterations within the acinar cells' cytoskeleton.[22] Recent experiments have indicated that similar destructive mechanisms may be operative at cell-cell contacts during pancreatitis.[23,24] The vast majority of intercellular contacts between polarized epithelial cells belong to the class of adherens junctions.[25] At these specialized regions of the basolateral plasma membrane, actin filaments insert in a functional complex that is formed by members of the cadherin/catenin family of cell-adhesion molecules.[26] Cadherins, in turn, anchor adjacent cells to each other by means of Ca^{++}-dependent homophilic interaction and are therefore considered master molecules for the maintenance of cellular integrity and polarized function. Because of this localized and tight association between actin filament bundles and membrane-spanning cadherin bridges, the adherens junctions are generally believed to be directly involved in the structural and functional stability of polarized epithelial cells.[27] However, whether and how these mechanisms apply to the exocrine pancreas was, until recently, not known.

In two recent investigations we have attempted to characterize interactions between the pancreatic cytoskeleton and adherens junctions. When we studied microfilaments and microtubules of acinar cells during the initial hours of experimental pancreatitis,[23] we found that as early as 30 minutes after induction of the disease these cytoskeletal elements progressively dissociated. In parallel to this disassembly their structural proteins, actin and β-tubulin, were found to be proteolytically degraded. These observations not only provided an explanation for the prominent disturbance of intracellular vesicle transport and segregation,[28,29] but, since microfilaments insert in the lateral plasma membrane at sites of cell-cell contacts, also suggested a mechanism through which intercellular junctions might be disrupted. When we followed the dynamics of E-cadherin, β-catenin, α-catenin and actin during the first 12 hr of acute experimental pancreatitis,[30] our data suggested that adherens junctions are rapidly disassembled during the early disease phase, thus allowing for extravasated fluid to accumulate in the interstitial space. This disassembly of adherens junctions was paralleled by an upregulation of E-cadherin and α-catenin mRNA and a modest decrease in intracellular E-cadherin. More importantly, E-cadherin, which is predominantly localized at the basolateral cell membrane under physiological conditions, was distributed to the cytosol soon after the start of pancreatitis, but, unlike the cytoskeletal proteins actin and β-tubulin, did not undergo intracellular proteolytic degradation. Instead, adherens junctions were rapidly reassembled while pancreatitis was still in progress, and E-cadherin was relocalized to form intercellular anchors. We concluded that the restitution of focal cell-cell contacts, which allows for the later insertion of force-generating actin filament bundles, represents one of the earliest mechanisms of acinar cell reorganization and recovery from acute pancreatitis.

TYROSINE DEPHOSPHORYLATION AND PANCREATIC ADHERENS JUNCTIONS

Having identified the members of the cadherin/catenin family that are involved in the formation and maintenance of intercellular adhesions in the pancreas and having determined their dynamics in a pathophysiological event that disrupts adherens junctions, we took the next logical step, which was to investigate how these processes, which appear to determine the structural recovery and secretory polarity of the pancreas, are regulated. Studies from our and other laboratories suggest that tyrosin dephosphorylation in general and the action of PTPs in particular may represent the critical regulatory element in acinar cell contact formation and maintenance. In a first set of experiments we tried to determine whether and in what manner tyrosine dephosphorylation would affect the adherens junctions of pancreatic acinar cells. To answer this question, we isolated intact acini from rat pancreas by collagen digestion and incubated them in a medium containing the specific PTP inhibitor orthovanadate (0.5 mM) for 30 min. Acini were then fixed in a mixture of formaldehyde/glutaraldehyde (2%/2%) embedded in Epon, and contrasted thin sections were studied by electronmicroscopy. While maximal or supramaximal stimulation of acini with the

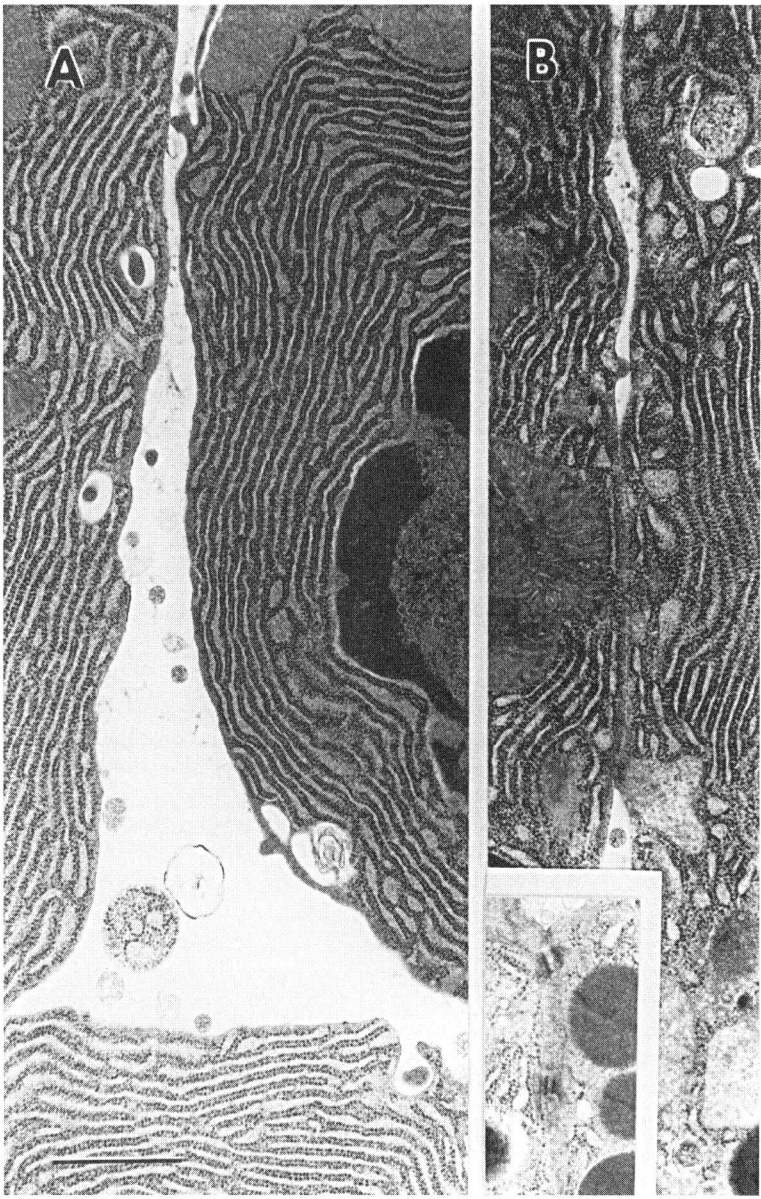

FIGURE 1. Electronmicrograph of an isolated pancreatic acinus after incubation with orthovanadate (0.5 mM, 30 min) in (**A**). Cell-cell contacts along the lateral cell membrane are disrupted as indicated by the widened interstitial space. The acinus in (**B**) was incubated with a supramaximal concentration of caerulein (10^{-7} M) and its adherens as well as tight junctions (*inset*) remained intact. Bar: 10 μm.

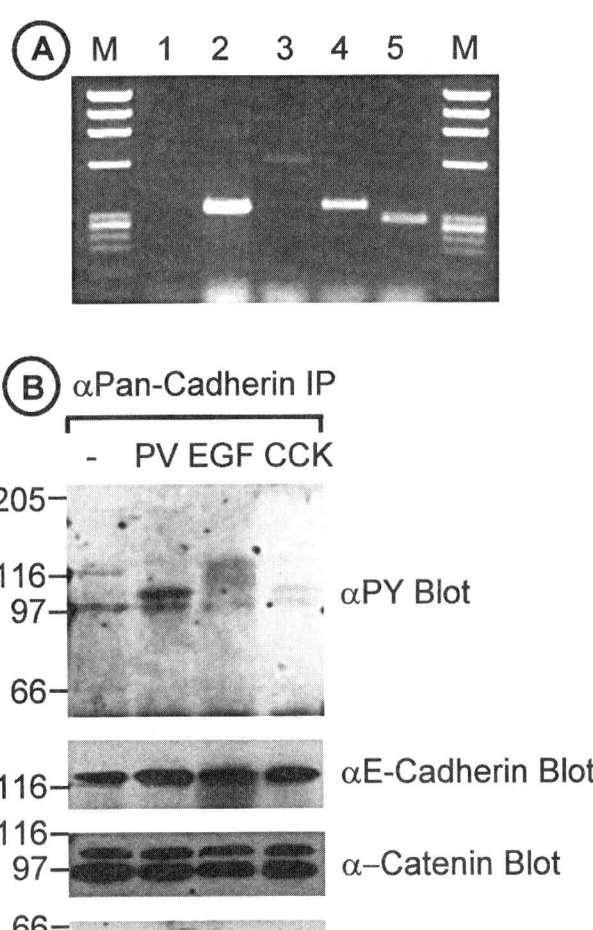

FIGURE 2. Protein tyrosine phosphatases in pancreatic acinar cells. (**A**) RT-PCR detection was performed with total RNA from acinar cells as a template and specific primers for the murine PTP-sequences. Control (*lane 1*), PTP SHP-2 (*lane 2*, bp 39–59 and 363–383), PTP SHP-1 (*lane 3*, bp 106–126 and 375–395), RPTPκ (*lane 4*, bp 1088–1108 and 1421–1440) and RPTPμ (*lane 5*, bp 350–369 and 627–647). (**B**) Association of the protein tyrosine phosphatase SHP-1 with proteins of the cadherin/catenin complex in isolated pancreatic acini after 3 min stimulation with either 0.5 mM pervanadate (PV), 20 ng/ml epidermal growth factor (EGF) or 100 pM cholecystokinin (CCK). Two (2) mg of the lysate were used for immunoprecipitation with monoclonal anti-pan-cadherin antibody. Immunoprecipitates were blotted after polyacrylamide gel electrophoresis (PAGE) separation, labeled with a monoclonal anti-phosphotyrosine antibody, and reblotted with monoclonal antibodies specific for E-cadherin, α-catenin, β-catenin and SHP-1. The pan-cadherin antibody precipitated a constitutive complex composed of E-cadherin, α-catenin and β-catenin (not shown). Pervanadate stimulation lead to tyrosine phosphorylation of α-catenin and β-catenin and an association of the cytosolic protein tyrosine phosphatase SHP-1 with this complex.

secretagogue caerulein did not result in an ultrastructural dissociation of acinar cell adherens junctions, PTP inhibition with orthovanadate did (FIG. 1). The interstitial space between acinar cells was found to be progressively widened along the lateral cell membranes, and multiple adherens junctions were found to be dissociated. The tight junctions that form acinar cell-cell contacts at the apical pole and seal the interstitial space towards the acinar lumen were, by contrast, not found to be affected by orthovanadate treatment. These observations suggest that tyrosine dephosphorylation and the activity of PTPs is required to maintain functional adherens junctions between acinar cells. They indicate further that the inhibition of PTP activity alone is sufficient to dissociate cell-cell contacts at the lateral acinar cell membrane but insufficient to disrupt tight junctions at the apical pole. Because adherens and tight junctions of acinar cells are composed of different subsets of adhesion molecules, it appears likely that pancreatic adherens junction proteins (i.e., the cadherin/catenin complex) depend on a dephosphorylated state to maintain their biological function, whereas tight junction proteins (e.g., ZO-1) do not. This conclusion is in accordance with the observation that tyrosine phosphorylation impairs the Ca^{++}-dependent homophilic interaction of cadherins.[31] To identify PTPs that are potentially involved in the maintenance of acinar cell adherens junctions, we used monospecific antibodies as well as reverse transcriptase polymerase chain reaction (RT-PCR) with specific 300-bp primers under high stringency conditions to identify transmembrane and cytosolic PTPs with sufficient expression levels in the pancreas to be likely candidates in this context. Initial experiments indicated that the class II PTPs, PTPμ and PTPκ, as well as the intracellular PTPs, SHP-1 and SHP-2, are expressed in acinar cells (FIG. 2A). When tyrosine phosphorylation in dispersed acini was stimulated with pervanadate, classical cell adhesion proteins were recovered in an intact cadherin/α-catenin/β-catenin complex on immunoprecipitation studies, and this complex was further found to be tyrosine phosphorylated (FIG. 2B). Reblotting experiments revealed not only that α-catenin and β-catenin were the tyrosine phosporylated components within the complex, but also that SHP-1 associated with cell adhesion proteins following pervanadate stimulation.

These data provide the first direct evidence that endogenous PTPs do, in fact, play a physiological role in the cell-cell contact formation of an intact epithelial organ such as the pancreas. The association of SHP-1 with members of the cadherin/catenin complex can so far only be regarded as a preliminary indication of the involvement of PTPs in this process. The differential subcellular expression and distribution patterns of PTPs as well as the biological function of their various protein domains clearly require further analysis. However, this raises the possibility that dephosphorylation of cell adhesion proteins and the activity of a cell type- and organ-specific subset of PTPs are critical elements in pancreatic development, regeneration from pancreatitis-induced injury, as well as metastatic spread of pancreatic cancer.

ACKNOWLEDGMENTS

This work was supported by Grants Le 625/4-1 and Le 625/5-1 from the Deutsche Forschungsgemeinschaft and Grant 01KS9604-IKF/D9 from the German Federal Ministry for Education and Research.

REFERENCES

1. KEMLER, R. 1993. From cadherins to catenins: cytoplasmic protein interactions and regulation of cell adhesion. Trends Genet. **9:** 317–321.
2. BRADY-KALNAY, S.M., A.J. FLINT & N.K. TONKS. 1993. Homophilic binding of PTPμ, a receptor-type protein tyrosine phosphatase, can mediate cell-cell aggregation. J. Cell. Biol. **122:** 961–972.
3. GEBBINK, M.F.B.G., G.C.M. ZONDAG, R.W. WUBBOLTS et al. 1993. Cell-cell adhesion mediated by a receptor-like protein tyrosine phosphatase. J. Biol. Chem. **268:** 16101–16104.
4. BRADY-KALNAY, S.M., T. MOURTON, J.P. NIXON et al. 1998. Dynamic interaction of PTPμ with multiple cadherins in vivo. J. Cell Biol. **141:** 287–296.
5. SAP, J., Y.P. JIANG, D. FRIEDLANDER et al. 1994. Receptor tyrosine phosphatase R-PTP-κ mediates homophilic binding. Mol. Cell. Biol. **14:** 1–9.
6. GEBBINK, M.F.B.G., G.C.M. ZONDAG, G.M. KONINGSTEIN et al. 1995. Cell surface expression of receptor protein tyrosine phosphatase RPTPμ is regulated by cell-cell contact. J. Cell Biol. **131:** 251–260.
7. SERRA-PAGES, C., N.L. KEDERSHA, L. FAZIKAS et al.. 1995. The LAR transmembrane protein tyrosine phosphatase and a coiled-coil LAR interacting protein co-localize at focal adhesions. EMBO J. **14:** 2827–2838.
8. GEBBINK, M.F.B.G., I. VAN ETTEN, G. HATEBOR et al. 1991. Cloning, expression and chromosomal localization of a new putative receptor-like protein tyrosine phosphatase. FEBS Lett. **290:** 123–130.
9. JIANG, Y.P., H. WANG, P. D'EUSTACHIO et al. 1993. Cloning and characterization of R-PTP-κ, a new member of the receptor protein tyrosine phosphatase family with a proteolytically cleaved cellular adhesion molecule-like extracellular region. Mol. Cell. Biol. **13:** 2942–2951.
10. STREULI, M., N.X. KRUEGER, L.R. HALL et al. 1988. A new member of the immunoglobulin superfamily that has a cytoplasmic region homologous to the leucocyte common antigen. J. Exp. Med. **168:** 1553–1562.
11. PULIDO, R., N.X. KRUEGER, C. SERRA-PAGES et al. 1995. Molecular characterization of the human transmembrane protein-tyrosine phosphatase δ. J. Biol. Chem. **270:** 1–7.
12. STREULI, M., N.X. KRUEGER, P.D. ARINIELLO et al. 1992. Expression of the receptor-linked protein tyrosine phosphatase LAR: proteolytic cleavage and shedding of the CAM-like extracellular region. EMBO J. **11:** 897–907.
13. CIOSSEK, T., M.M. LERCH & A. ULLRICH. 1995. Cloning, characterization and differential expression of MDK2 and MDK5, two novel receptor tyrosine kinases of the eck/eph family, in the mouse. Oncogene **11:** 2085–2095.
14. FUCHS, M., T. MÜLLER, M.M. LERCH et al. 1996. Association of human protein-tyrosine phosphatase K with members of the armadillo family. J. Biol. Chem. **271:** 16712–16719.
15. WANG, H., Z. LIAN, M.M. LERCH et al. 1996. Characterization of PCP-2, a novel receptor protein tyrosine phosphatase of the MAM domain family. Oncogene **12:** 2555–2562.
16. AICHER, B., M.M. LERCH, T MÜLLER et al. 1997. Cellular redistribution of protein tyrosine phosphatases LAR and PTPσ by inducible proteolytic processing. J. Cell Biol. **138:** 681–696.
17. SLACK, J.M. 1995. Developmental biology of the pancreas. Development **121:** 1569–1580.
18. FREEDMAN, S.D. & G.A. SCHEELE. 1994. Acid-base interactions during exocrine pancreatic secretion. Primary role for ductal bicarbonate in acinar lumen function. Ann. N. Y. Acad. Sci. **713:** 199–206.
19. LERCH, M.M., A.K. SALUJA, R. DAWRA et al. 1992. Acute necrotising pancreatitis in the opossum: earliest morphologic changes involve acinar cells. Gastroenterology **103:** 205–213.

20. GUKOVSKAYA, A.S., P. PERKINS, V. ZANINOVIC et al. 1996. Mechanisms of cell death after pancreatic duct obstruction in the opossum and the rat. Gastroenterology **110:** 875–884.
21. LERCH, M.M., H. WEIDENBACH, T.M. GRESS et al. 1995. Effect of kinin inhibition in experimental acute pancreatitis. Am. J. Physiol. **269:** G490–G499.
22. O'KONSKI, M.S. & S.J. PANDOL. 1990. Effects of caerulein on the apical cytoskeleton of the pancreatic acinar cell. J. Clin. Invest. **86:** 1649–1657.
23. JUNGERMANN, J., M.M. LERCH, H. WEIDENBACH et al. 1995. Disassembly of the rat pancreatic acinar cell cytoskeleton during supramaximal secretagogue stimulation. Am. J. Physiol. **268:** G328–G338.
24. FALLON, M.B., F.S. GORELICK, J.M. ANDERSON et al. 1995. Effect of cerulein hyperstimulation on the paracellular barrier of the rat exocrine pancreas. Gastroenterology **108:** 1863–1872.
25. FARQUHAR, M.G. & G.E. PALADE. 1963. Junctional complexes in various epithelia. J. Cell. Biol. **17:** 375–412.
26. NÄTHKE, I.S., L. HINCK, J.R. SWEDLOW et al. 1994. Defining interactions and distributions of cadherin and catenin complexes in polarized epithelial cells. J. Cell. Biol. **125:** 1341–1352.
27. TAKEICHI, M. 1995. Morphogenetic roles of classical cadherins. Curr. Opin. Cell Biol. **7:** 619–627.
28. LERCH, M.M., A.K. SALUJA, R. DAWRA et al. 1993. The effect of chloroquine administration on two experimental models of acute pancreatitis. Gastroenterology **104:** 1768–1779.
29. LERCH, M.M., A.K. SALUJA, M. RÜNZI et al. 1995. Luminal endocytosis and intracellular targeting by acinar cells during early biliary pancreatitis in the opossum. J. Clin. Invest. **95:** 2222–2231.
30. LERCH, M.M., M.P. LUTZ, H. WEIDENBACH et al. 1996. Dissociation and reassembly of adherens junctions during experimental acute pancreatitis. Gastroenterology **113:** 1355–1366.
31. KYPTA, R.M., H. SU & L.F. REICHARDT. 1996. Association between a transmembrane protein tyrosine phosphatase and the cadherin-catenin complex. J. Cell Biol. **134:** 1519–1529.

Differentially Expressed Genes in Normal and Tumor Pancreatic Tissue

C. BACKHAUS,[a] S. SCHNEUER, R. JESNOWSKI, S.LIEBE, AND M. LÖHR

Department of Medicine, Division of Gastroenterology, University of Rostock, Rostock, Germany

INTRODUCTION

Pancreatic cancer is one of the leading causes of cancer death in industrialized Western countries with an overall five-year survival rate that is under 1%. The majority—more than 90%—of cancers of the exocrine pancreas arise from pancreatic ducts.

It is increasingly evident that neoplastic transformation occurs as a result of a multistep process, which may include the overexpression of growth factors and their receptors, activation of protooncogenes, and inactivation of tumor suppressor genes.

For example, it has already been shown that pancreatic tumors overexpress the epidermal growth factor receptor and transforming growth factors alpha and beta.[1,2] Moreover, a large percentage of pancreatic tumors show a mutation in the k-ras oncogene.[3] Ras mutations are detected in the early stages of tumorigenesis as well as in more advanced stages. Taking into consideration the high incidence of ras mutations, we may conclude that mutations in the k-ras gene mark an important event in the development of pancreatic cancer.

Therefore, the identification of alterations in gene expression that occur during tumorigenesis may provide critical information in regard to early diagnosis of pancreatic cancer.

Consequently, the aim of our studies was to identify genes that are over- or underexpressed in pancreatic tumor tissue relative to normal pancreatic tissue.

Furthermore, we wanted to investigate the effect of a defined single gene defect on gene expression in pancreatic duct cells. For this purpose we stably transfected an immortalized bovine epithelial pancreatic duct cell line with a cDNA coding for the mutated ras oncogene. This *in vitro* model may reveal critical information about ras-mediated up- or downregulation of genes, which may contribute to carcinogenesis.

In order to accomplish this aim we employed differential display reverse transcriptase polymerase chain reaction (DDRT-PCR). Differential mRNA display, as first described by Liang and Pardee, is a powerful method for identifying differentially expressed genes.[4,5] It allows the comparison of expressed mRNAs from different populations of cells and tissues.

---

[a]Corresponding author: Christiane Backhaus, M.S., Div. of Gastroenterology, Dept. of Medicine, University of Rostock, Ernst-Heydemann-Str. 6, 18057 Rostock, Germany. Phone, +49 381-494-7497; fax, +49 381-494-7348; e-mail, loehr@med.uni-rostock.de

METHODS

RNA was isolated from normal pancreatic tissue ($n = 7$) and tumor tissue ($n = 9$), pooled and subjected to DDRT-PCR. The most important requirement is the complete absence of DNA, which is achieved by Dnase I treatment. Differential display was performed with 1 µg of RNA according to the manufactorer's instructions (MoBiTec).

The general strategy of the differential display method is to amplify partial cDNA sequences from subsets of mRNAs by reverse transcription using a set of anchored primers and subsequent polymerase chain reaction. Using a radioactive nucleotide, PCR amplification of cDNA species of each fraction is performed with the appropriate anchored primer and a set of arbitrary primers.

Resulting fragments are electrophoretically seperated (FIG. 1). Different cDNA fragments are reamplified and cloned.

Differential expression was verified by reverse Northern blot. The cloned fragments are blotted onto a nylon membrane, which is hybridized with Dig-labeled cDNA from either normal or tumor pancreatic tissue as a probe. S6 was used as a control to equalize differences in efficiency of reverse transcription between the two populations. Further confirmation was independently obtained by quantitative RT-PCR.

Differentially regulated fragments were sequenced to determine whether they correspond to known or unknown genes.

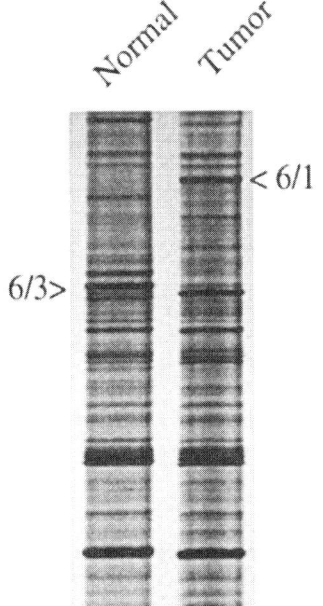

FIGURE 1. DDRT gel from tumor and normal pancreatic tissue. Differentially expressed cDNAs are marked.

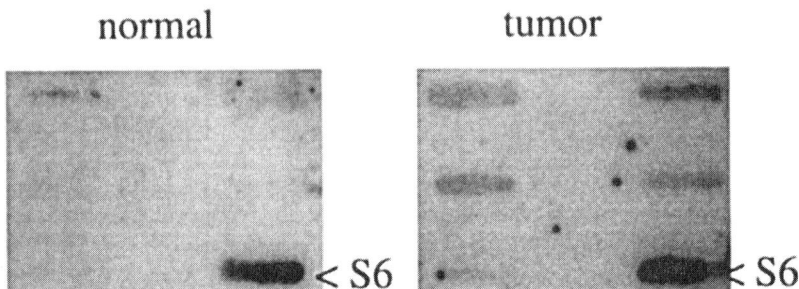
FIGURE 2. Reverse Northern blot of fragment 6/1.

RESULTS

Most electrophoretically separated fragments were common to both cancer tissue and normal tissue samples. Differentially regulated cDNAs were excised from the gel and cloned. To exclude false-positive clones, differential expression was confirmed by another independent method. As an example, FIGURE 2 shows a reverse Northern blot: different clones of the fragment 6/1 were blotted onto a nylon membrane. As a probe, Dig-labeled cDNA from tumor and normal pancreatic tissue was used.

Subsequent sequencing identified fragment 6/1 to be coding for the c-region of immunglobulin kappa light chain, which is clearly upregulated in pancreatic tumor tissue.

TABLE 1 summarizes the genes so far identified. Five of the isolated clones were overexpressed and four were downregulated in tumor tissue. Sequence analysis showed that six clones were unknown genes, as they did not match any sequence in the database. Three other cloned fragments revealed sequence homologies to known genes. Two of them have already been described as tumor specific in regard to other malignant tumors. These are MGC24, a polymorphic epithelial mucin[6] found in gastric carcinoma, and a tumorspecific L-arginine:glycine-amidinotransferase[7] so far exclusively found in a kidney carcinoma cell line.

CONCLUSION

DDRT-PCR is a suitable method for identifying differentially expressed genes. It enables us to investigate genetic alterations in normal and tumor pancreatic tissue, resulting in both activation of oncogenes and inactivation of tumor suppresor genes.

Our studies could identify some unknown cDNA-fragments, potentially playing a critical role in pancreatic cancer.

Three other fragments revealed homology to known genes. These are MGC 24, L-arginine:glycine-amidinotransferase and the c-region from immunglobulin kappa light chain.

TABLE 1. Differentially expressed genes in tumor and normal pancreatic tissue

Clone	Expression		Sequence homology
	Normal	Tumor	
7/4/03	∅	++	none
6/1/01	∅	+++	IG kappa chain C region
7/8/02	∅	++	MGC-24
14/4/01	+++	∅	L-arginine:glycine-amidinotransferase
13/8/02	++	∅	none
6/3/06	+++	+	none
8/2	∅	++	none
13/9	++	∅	none
13/10	+	+++	none

NOTATION: ∅ = no, + = low, ++ = moderate, +++ = high expression.

Isolating complete cDNAs of the unknown genes by rapid amplification of cDNA ends (RACE)-PCR,[8] their sequencing and analysis of their potential function are our aims for the future.

ACKNOWLEDGMENTS

This work was supported by Pinguin-Stiftung, Düsseldorf and BMBF, FKZ 994027.

REFERENCES

1. KORC, M. *et al.* 1986. Enhanced expression of epidermal growth factor receptor correlates with alterations of chromosome 7 in human pancreatic cancer. Proc. Natl. Acad. Sci. USA **83:** 5141–5144.
2. SMITH, J.J. *et al.* 1987. Production of transforming growth factor alpha in human pancreatic cancer cells: evidence for a superagonist autocrine cycle. Proc. Natl. Acad. Sci. USA **84:** 7567–7570.
3. HRUBAN, R.H. *et al.* 1993. K-ras oncogene activation in adenocarcinoma of the human pancreas: a study of 82 carcinomas using a combination of mutant-enriched polymerase chain reaction and allele-specific oligo-nucleotide hybridisation. Am. J. Pathol. **143:** 545–554.
4. LIANG, P. & A.B. PARDEE. 1992. Differential display of eucaryotic messenger RNA by means of the polymerase chain reaction. Science **257:** 967–971.
5. LIANG, P. *et al.* 1992. Differential display and cloning of messenger RNA from human breast cancer versus mammary epithelial cells. Cancer Res. **52:** 6966–6968.
6. MASUZAW, Y. *et al.* 1992. A novel core protein as well as polymorphic epithelial mucin carry peanut agglutinin binding sites in human gastric carcinoma cells: sequence analysis and examination of gene expression. J. Biochem. **112:** 609–615.
7. HUMM, A. *et al.* 1994. The amino acid sequences of human and pig L-arginine:glycine amidinotransferase. FEBS Lett. **339:** 101–107.

8. FROHMAN, M.A. *et al.* 1988 Rapid production of full length cDNAs from rare transcripts: amplification using a single gene-specific oligonucleotide primer. Proc. Natl. Acad. Sci. USA **85:** 8998–9002.

Typing of Leukocytes in Pancreatic Tissue Surrounding Human Pancreatic Carcinoma

JÖRG EMMRICH,[a] GISELA SPARMANN, ULRICH HOPT,[b] MATTHIAS LÖHR, AND STEFAN LIEBE

Division of Gastroenterology, Department of Internal Medicine, [b]Department of Surgery, University of Rostock, Rostock, Germany

INTRODUCTION

There are tumor infiltrating lymphocytes between carcinoma cells and at the border of carcinoma suggesting antitumor immune response.[1] Pancreatic tissue surrounding carcinoma was expected to be nearly free of infiltrating cells. Recently, we compared quantitatively the patterns of infiltrating leukocytes in normal human pancreas, in chronic pancreatitis tissues, and in the vicinity of pancreatic carcinoma.[2] The leukocyte subset pattern was similiar in pancreatic tissue surrounding carcinoma and in chronic pancreatitis. Here, we present results from a larger number of carcinoma patients using an extended panel of monoclonal antibodies specific to the leukocyte subsets to characterize the cell infiltration.

MATERIALS AND METHODS

A total of 15 patients with pancreatic carcinoma was included in the investigation. Pancreatic tissues surrounding pancreatic carcinoma were obtained from surgical resections. Pancreatic carcinoma were classified histologically to differentiate G2 ($n = 11$), and G3 ($n = 4$).

Surgical specimens were immediately snap frozen and stored at −80°C. Serial sections 5 µm thick were cut and air dried at room temperature followed by fixing in acetone for 10 min. The fixed samples were stored at −80°C until immunohistochemical labeling.

The pancreatic specimens were labeled with clones of monoclonal antibodies (MoAb) as listed here: MT 310 (CD4, T helper/inducer), DK 25 (CD8, T suppressor/cytotoxic), UCHL-1 (CD45R0, memory lymphocytes), ACT-1 (CD25, IL-2 receptor), Ber-ACT18 (MLA, mucosa specific lymphocyte antigen), To 15 (CD22, B cells), T 16 (CD38, plasma cells), EBM11 (CD68, monocytes/macrophages), TÜK4 (CD14, monocytes). The clone T 16 was obtained from DIANOVA, Hamburg, FRG. All other antibodies were purchased from DAKO, Glostrup, Denmark.

Antibody binding was shown by using the alkaline phosphatase monoclonal antialkaline phosphatase (APAAP) method.[3] The specimens were incubated sequen-

---

[a]Address for correspondence: Prof. Dr. med. Jörg Emmrich, Div. of Gastroenterology, Dept. of Medicine, University of Rostock, Ernst-Heydemann-Str. 6, D-18057 Rostock, Germany. Phone, +49 381-494-7484; fax, +49 381-494-7482; e-mail: joerg.emmrich@med.uni-rostock.de

tially with unlabeled primary mouse monoclonal antibody, rabbit anti-mouse IgG (DAKO) and monoclonal mouse APAAP complex (DAKO). Alkaline phosphatase activity was visualized by incubating the specimens with substrate solution containing new fuchsin, sodium nitrite, levamisole and naphthol AS-BI (all Sigma, St. Louis, MO, USA). Cell nuclei were counterstained using hematoxylin followed by mounting in glycogel.

An ocular grid consisting of a simple square lattice of 0.625 mm^2 was used to enumerate positively stained cells at ×400 magnification. Results are given in counts per mm^2. Evaluation was done blindly by two investigators. Reproducibility was tested after decoding with SD < 10%.

RESULTS

In pancreatic tissue surrounding pancreatic carcinoma, a high number of infiltrating mononuclear leukocytes could be found (350.4 ± 121.1 cells/mm^2). The predominant cell populations in leukocyte infiltrations were T lymphocytes (53.5%) and macrophages (32.4%). Regarding the T cell subsets, the CD4+/CD8+ ratio was 1.12. Infiltrations with CD4+ and CD8+ lymphocytes are shown in FIGURE 1 and FIGURE 2, respectively. Nearly 80% of T lymphocytes expressed CD45R0 identifying memory cells. Only 4.1% of T cells expressed the interleukin-2 (IL-2) receptor on the cell surface. The **m**ucosa-specific **l**ymphocyte **a**ntigen (MLA) could be shown in 8.7% of lymphocytes.

In pancreatic tissue surrounding carcinoma, 5.7% of lymphocytes were recognized by the B cell-specific MoAB. There was a higher percentage (8.4%) of plasma cells (CD38+) in the infiltrations. Macrophages were characterized by expression of CD68. A mean of 113.6 ± 46.8 cells/mm^2 was found for macrophages representing 32.4% of leukocytes. By using antibodies against CD14, 66.2% of macrophages stained positive.

DISCUSSION

In pancreatic tissues surrounding pancreatic carcinoma there were high numbers of infiltrating mononuclear cells compared to our results in normal pancreatic tissues.[2] Leukocyte infiltrations were also found in cases without a marked obstruction of the pancreatic duct. In normal pancreatic tissue, T lymphocytes (31.3%) and macrophages (56.3%) were the predominant mononuclear cell populations without a special pattern of spatial distribution.[2] The pancreatic tissues obtained from patients with carcinoma were histologically characterized by a higher percentage of T lymphocytes (53.5%). Only a low number of cells expressed the IL-2 receptor as a marker of proliferating cells. Compared to our results in a smaller number of carcinoma patients,[2] the CD4+/CD8+ ratio was elevated (1.12 versus 0.78), indicating the slightly preferential accumulation of CD4+ lymphocytes during the ongoing infiltration. Bedossa *et al.*[4] have found in healthy pancreata equal numbers of CD4+ and CD8+ T cells (CD4+/CD8+ ratio ≅ 1) using a semiquantitative score system. These authors also described a predominance of CD8+ subsets in chronic pancreatitis.

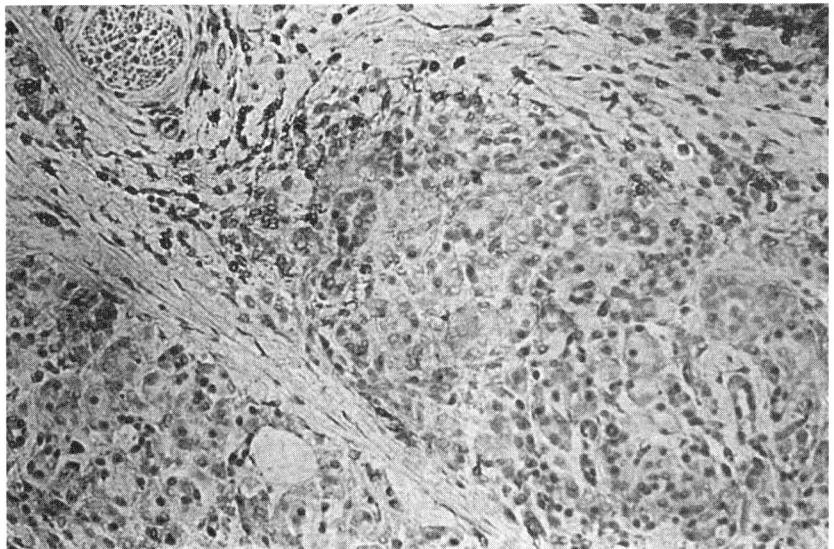

FIGURE 1. Immunohistochemical analysis of CD4+ lymphocytes in pancreatic tissue of pancreatic carcinoma. Tissue specimens were stained by APAAP technique and counterstained with hematoxylin (original magnification, ×400) as described in Materials and Methods.

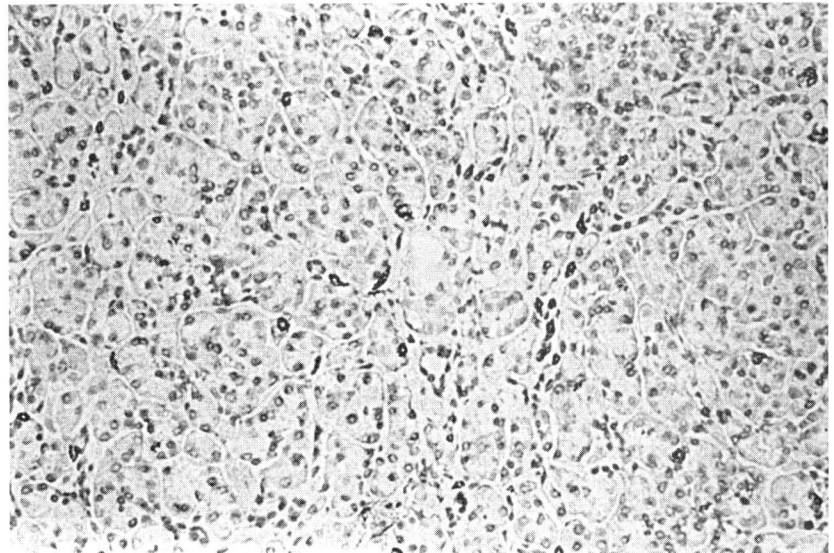

FIGURE 2. Immunohistochemical analysis of CD8+ lymphocytes in pancreatic tissue of pancreatic carcinoma. Tissue specimens were stained by the APAAP technique and counterstained with hematoxylin (original magnification, ×400) as described in Materials and Methods.

CD45R0 is highly expressed on memory T cells primed by contact with a specific antigen.[5] Nearly 80% of T lymphocytes infiltrating pancreatic tissue surrounding carcinoma were characterized by this memory cell marker. Since in the peripheral blood compartments of memory and naive T cells are of similiar size,[6] selective infiltration of memory cells in the pancreas was suggested. Low numbers of B lymphocytes and plasma cells were also shown.

The mucosa-specific lymphocyte antigen (MLA) is a homing receptor of gastrointestinal tract-specific lymphocytes.[7] Only 8.7% of the infiltrating lymphocytes in pancreatic tissue of carcinoma patients expressed this receptor indicating that these lymphocytes do not receive a specification as lymphocytes of the gastrointestinal tract.

By using antibodies against CD14 as a monocyte marker, 66.2% of CD68+ macrophages expressed this receptor as a result of infiltration with monocytes from peripheral blood.

In conclusion, our results suggest that in pancreatic tissue of patients with pancreatic carcinoma, there was a significant increase of mononuclear positive cells compared to the normal pancreas. The predominant cells in these infiltrations are memory T cells indicating specific immune response in the carcinoma surrounding tissues. However, these T cells do not proliferate. It needs further investigation to analyze the specificity and the function of these cells.

REFERENCES

1. GANSS, R. & D. HANAHAN. 1998. Tumor microenvironment can restrict the effectiveness of activated antitumor lymphocytes. Cancer Res. **58:** 4673–4681.
2. EMMRICH, J., *et al.* 1997. Immunohistochemical characterization of the pancreatic cellular infiltrate in normal pancreas, chronic pancreatitis and pancreatic carcinoma. Digestion **59:** 192–198.
3. CORDELL, J.L. *et al.* 1984. Immunoenzymatic labeling of monoclonal antibodies using immune complexes of alkaline phosphatase and monoclonal anti-alkaline phosphatase (APAAP complexes). J. Histochem. Cytochem. **12:** 219–229.
4. BEDOSSA, P. *et al.* 1990. Lymphocyte subsets and HLA-DR expression in normal pancreas and chronic pancreatitis. Pancreas **5:** 415–420.
5. TOUGH, D.H. & J. SPRENT. 1994. Turnover of naive- and memory-phenotype T cells. J. Exp. Med. **179:** 1127–1135.
6. DEPAOLI, P. *et al.* 1988. Age-related changes in human lymphocyte subsets: progressive reduction of the CD4CD45R (suppressor inducer) population. Clin. Immunol. Immunopathol. **48:** 290–296.
7. SCHIEFERDECKER, H.L. *et al.* 1990. The HML-1 antigen of intestinal lymphocytes is an activation antigen. J. Immunol. **144:** 878–884.

Apoptotic Molecules in Pancreatic Carcinoma Cell Lines

B. RINGEL, S.M. IBRAHIM, H. KÖHLER, J. RINGEL,[a] D. KOCZAN, S. LIEBE,[a] M. LÖHR,[a] AND H.-J. THIESEN[b]

Institute of Immunology and [a]Department of Gastroenterology, Rostock University, Schillingallee 70, 18055 Rostock, Germany

INTRODUCTION

Recently, a novel mechanism of immune evasion by tumor cells has been described, namely "the tumor counter-attack model." In this model tumor cells kill activated lymphocytes through functional expression of Fas ligand (FasL).[1–3] FasL and TRAIL are two highly homologous tumor necrosis factor (TNF) family members with the ability to induce apoptosis in susceptible cells through interaction with their membrane receptors Fas and DR4, DR5, respectively.[4,5] To study the role of apoptosis in pancreatic malignancy, we determined the expression pattern of several apoptosis receptors and ligands, FasL/Fas, sFas (an alternatively spliced soluble form of Fas that was shown to protect cells from apoptosis),[6] Trail/DR4 and DR3 in five human adenocarcinoma lines, BxPC3, Panc1, AsPC, PaCa 44, and PancTu using three different methods—reverse transcriptase polymerase chain reaction (RT/PCR), flow cytometry and Western blotting.

RESULTS AND DISCUSSION

All six tumor cell lines expressed the three receptors Fas, DR4, and DR3 as shown by RT/PCR. However, soluble Fas was not detected in any of them (FIG. 1). Expression of Fas was confirmed at the protein level by fluorescence-activated cell sorter (FACS) and Western blotting (FIG. 2). Although all cells expressed the Fas protein, clearly levels of expression were variable. Despite high levels of expression of Fas, pancreatic cell lines tested for susceptibility to Fas-mediated apoptosis were resistant. Additionally, we could also detect high levels of TRAIL expression by RT/PCR in all lines (FIG. 1).

Contrary to what has been shown for other tumors, we could not detect FasL expression by RT/PCR or FACS analysis, using the NOK1 antibody, of intact or permeabilized cells (FIG. 2).[7,8] Only one cell line, AsPC1, showed weak intracellular staining after permeabilization. Strong bands were obtained in Western blotting using two other antibodies, mAb33 and C20. These bands were of different sizes, 36 kD and 65 kD, respectively (the expected size of FasL band is roughly 36 kD),

---

[b]Corresponding author: Dr. H.-J. Thiesen, Institute of Immunology, Rostock University, Schillingallee 70, 18055 Rostock, Germany. Phone, +49 381-494-5870; fax, +49 381-494-5882; e-mail, hans-juergen.thiesen@med.uni-rostock.de

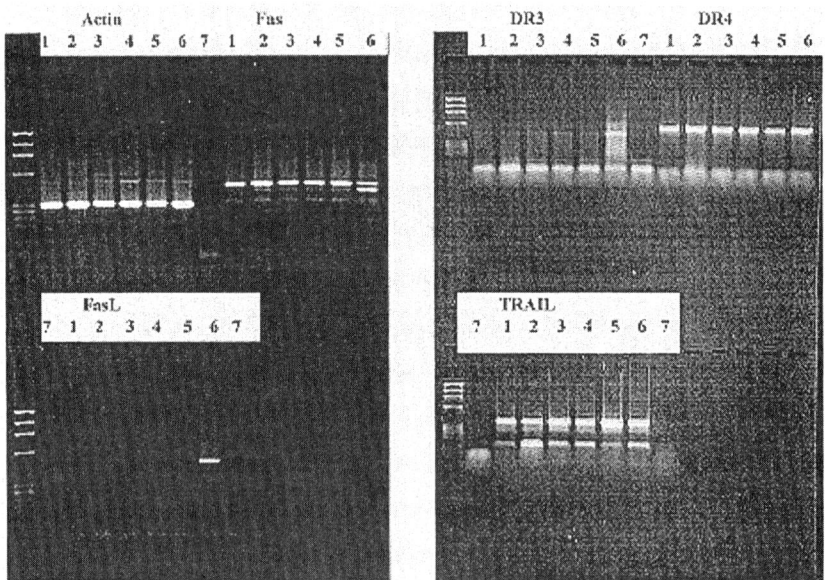

FIGURE 1. RT/PCR of apoptotic receptors and ligands in pancreatic carcinoma cell lines. *Lanes 1–5* represent cell lines: BxPC3, Panc1, AsPC, PaCa 44, and PancTu; *lane 6* represents human peripheral blood lymphocytes (PBLs), and *lane 7* PCR water control. Methods: mRNA was prepared using the Qiagen RNA extraction kit, and cDNA was prepared following standard protocols. PCR was performed using TFL (Thermus flavus) DNA polymerase and a standard buffer supplied by the manufacturer (BioZym, Germany). Conditions were as follows: an initial denaturation step for 2 min at 94°C, then 30 seconds at 94°C, 30 seconds at 60°C, and 50 seconds at 72°C for 30 cycles followed by an elongation step for 7 minutes at 72°C. The following primers were used for PCR:
Actin: 5′ GCCGCCAGCTCACCATGG-3′
and 5′ CTCCTCGGGAGCCACACG-3′;
Fas: 5′ GCAACACCAAGTGCAAAGAGG-3′
and 5′ GTCACTAGTAATGTCCTTGAGG-3′;
Trail: 5′ CAGGATCATGGCTATGATGG-3′
and 5′ GACCTCTTTCTCTCACTAGG-3′;
FasL: 5′ CCAGAGAGAGCTCAGATACGTTGAC-3′
and 5′ ATGTTTCAGCTCTTCCACCTACAGA-3′;
DR4: 5′ ACACAGCAATGGGAACATAGC-3′
and 5′ TTGTGAGCATTGTCCTCAGC-3′;
DR3: 5′ AGATGTTCAGGGTCCAGGTG-3′
and 5′ TCCATCACGTCGTAGAGCTG-3′.

and they could be seen in all cell lines tested. However, the specificities of these antibodies have been called into question in recent reports and as such are not reliable.[9,10] Such a controversy should be solved by microsequencing of the proteins recognized by these antibodies.

We aim to extend our studies to further elucidate the role of TRAIL and FasL in tumor evasion by pancreatic tumor cell lines, identify the mechanisms they employ

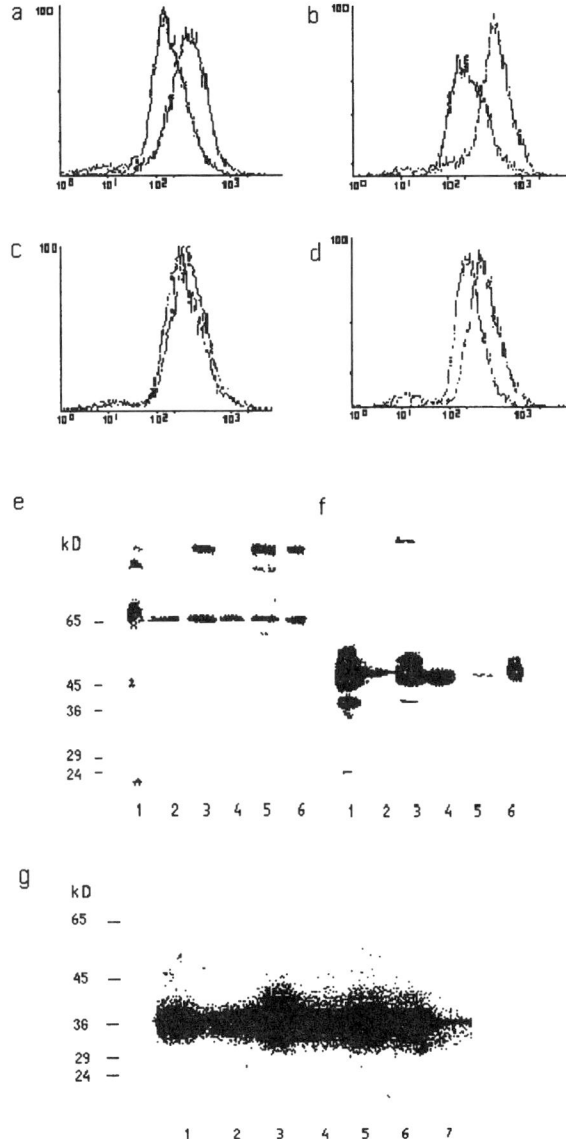

FIGURE 2. Expression of Fas and FasL proteins in pancreatic carcinoma cell lines. FACS analysis of Fas surface expression by AsPC1 (**a**) and PancTu (**b**) was performed using PE-conjugated anti-Fas antibody UB2 (Immunotech, Germany) or by an isotype-matched control mAb. Staining of FasL in nonpermeabilized (**c**) or permeabilized (**d**) AsPC-1 cells was performed using the mAb NOK-1 or an isotype control (Pharmingen, Hamburg, Germany). Western blotting of cell lysates was performed with rabbit anti-FasL (**e**) or anti-Fas (**f**) polyclonal antobodies (C20, Santa Cruz Biotechnology, USA) and with horseradish per-

to resist apoptosis and discover the role these mechanisms play in tumor aggressivity/metastsis.

REFERENCES

1. WALKER, P.R. *et al.* 1997. Role of Fas Ligand (CD95L) in immune escape: the tumor cell strikes back. J. Immunol. **158:** 4521–4524.
2. HAHNE, M. *et al.* 1996. Melanoma cell expression of Fas (Apo-1/CD95) Ligand: implications for tumor immune escape. Science. **274:** 1363–1366.
3. O'CONNEL, J. *et al.* 1996. The Fas counterattack: Fas-mediated T cell killing by colon cancer cells expressing Fas ligand. J. Exp. Med. **184:** 1075–1082.
4. NAGATA, S. 1997. Apoptosis by death factor. Cell. **88:** 355–365.
5. MAIANI, S.M. *et al.* 1998. Differential regulation of Trail and CD95 ligand in transformed cells of the T and B lymphocyte lineage. Eur. J. Immunol. **28:** 973–982.
6. THIESEN, H.-J. *et al.* 1997. The role of apoptosis in autoimmune disease with special reference to juvenile chronic arthritis. Rev. Rheum. **64:** 140–143.
7. UNGEFROREN, H. *et al.* 1998. Human pancreatic adenocarcinomas express Fas and Fas ligand yet are resistant to Fas-mediated apoptosis. Cancer Res. **58:** 1741–1749.
8. RIEGER, J. *et al.* 1998. APO2 ligand: a novel lethal weapon against malignant glioma? FEBS Lett. **427:** 124–128.
9. STOKES, T.A. *et al.* 1998. Constitutive expression of FasL in thyrocytes. Science **279:** 2015a.
10. FIEDLER, P. *et al.* 1998. Constitutive expression of FasL in thyrocytes. Science **279:** 2015a.
11. PAPPOF, G. *et al.* 1998. Constitutive expression of FasL in thyrocytes. Science **279:** 2015a.

---

oxidase (HRP)-conjugated goat anti-rabbit immunoglobulin G (IgG) as a secondary antibody (Boehringer Mannheim, Germany). *Lanes 1–6* represent cell lines PaCa 44, AsPC-1, PancTu, BxPC3, Panc1, and Capan1, respectively. The anti-FasL mAb33 (Transduction Laboratories, USA) followed by AP-conjugated goat anti-mouse IgG antibodies were also used for Western blotting **(g)**. In this case *lanes 1–7* represent cell lines AsPC1, BxPC3, Capan1, Panc1, PancTu, PaCa 44, and a control lysate provided by Transduction Laboratories. Detection was performed by chemiluminescence. Molecular weight markers are indicated.

Genomic Anomalies in Pancreatic Tumors Other Than Common Adenocarcinoma

ALDO SCARPA[a] AND GIUSEPPE ZAMBONI

Istituto di Anatomia Patologica, Università di Verona, Verona, Italy

ABSTRACT: In recent years enormous advances have been made in the understanding of the molecular mechanisms governing pancreatic ductal adenocarcinoma. However, little is known about other pancreatic neoplasms, which include intraductal papillary mucinous (IPMT), serous cystic (SCT), mucinous cystic (MCT), solid pseudopapillary (SPT), acinar and islet cell tumors. In addition, the study of tumors grouped under the unfortunate term of periampullary cancers will help distinguish the pathogenetic features of these neoplasms, often confused with pancreatic head neoplasms. The available data suggest that the less common pancreatic tumor types do not generally follow the same molecular pathway as the more common ductal carcinoma. IPMT seems to contain chromosomal anomalies similar to those found in ductal cancers, whereas papilla of Vater and duodenal cancers show genetic anomalies resembling those of gastrointestinal malignancies. The application of genome-wide screening techniques to these less common pancreatic tumors will undoubtedly play a central role in unraveling the complexity behind their pathology.

INTRODUCTION

Despite the conspicuous advances in our understanding of the molecular basis of pancreatic ductal adenocarcinoma,[1] very little is known about molecular abnormalities in pancreatic neoplasms other than common ductal adenocarcinoma. These are tumor entities with distinct clinicopathologic features and include neoplasms originating from either pancreatic ducts or acinar or islet cell precursors.[2] The tumors considered as originating from ductal cell precursors include the common ductal cancer, intraductal papillary-mucinous tumor (IPMT), serous cystic tumor (SCT), mucinous cystic tumor (MCT) and solid pseudopapillary tumor (SPT).

The pancreatic cancer research group of Verona University is focusing on the study of genetic anomalies of carcinomas arising from the epithelium of pancreatic ducts and their terminal excretory structure (papilla of Vater), as well as of tumors originating from islet cells. The molecular characterization of a representative series of different pancreatic tumor types will lead to an understanding of their specific molecular pathogenesis and clinical behavior. As a result, the identification of novel and useful diagnostic/prognostic markers can be expected, as has been the case for cancers of the papilla of Vater.[3] In addition, IPMT, MCT and papilla of Vater tumors represent useful models to search for transformation-related and progression-related

---

[a]Address for correspondence: Aldo Scarpa, M.D., Istituto di Anatomia Patologica, Università di Verona, Strada Le Grazie, 8, I-37134 Verona, Italy. Phone, +39 45-8098-617; fax, +39 45-8098-136; e-mail, scarpa@anpat.univr.it

TABLE 1. Complete or partial studies on chromosomal anomalies of pancreatic tumors

	Cystic	Ductal	Intraductal	Papilla	Mucinous
Karyotype	Yes	No	No	No	
Allelotype	Yes[c]	No[c]	No[c]	No[c]	
Amplotype (ap-pcr)[a]	Yes[c]	No[c]	Yes[c]	No[c]	
CGH[b]	Yes	No	No	No	

[a]ap-pcr, arbitrarily primed-polymerase chain reaction.
[b]cgh, comparative genomic hybridization.
[c]Ongoing studies at Verona University.

genetic anomalies of pancreatic epithelia. In fact, and at variance with ductal adenocarcinoma, the different stages of progression of malignancy are morphologically recognized in these peculiar tumor types.

This presentation is divided into three parts. The first describes the ongoing genomic screenings at Verona University, the second deals with genetic anomalies in the different pancreatic tumors, and the last treats periampullary malignancies.

GENOME-WIDE SCREENING FOR DETECTION OF NONRANDOM CHROMOSOMAL ANOMALIES

The search for specific genes involved in the pathogenesis and progression of malignancy of cancers may be driven by the discovery of nonrandom genomic anomalies.

The available genome-wide screenings for chromosomal anomalies in pancreatic tumors and those that we are applying with the aim of obtaining genomic characterization of different pancreatic tumor types are summarized in TABLE 1. We are using two complementary genome-screening approaches to obtain a genomic fingerprint and a map of chromosomal losses of the different pancreatic tumors, namely, DNA fingerprinting by *arbitrarily primed polymerase chain reaction* (AP-PCR) and *genome-wide allelotyping.*

AP-PCR amplifies DNA fragments that are chromosome specific,[4-7] and it has been demonstrated that decreased intensity of AP-PCR bands in tumor DNA reflects allelic losses, whereas increased band intensity indicates the presence of extra copies of these sequences.[6-8] Being based on a PCR technique, this approach requires only a limited amount of DNA (20 ng/test). This provides a rapid and sensitive tool for the analysis of genetic material extracted from microdissected cancer samples.

Allelotyping studies are based on the detection of loss of heterozygosity (LOH) at chromosomal-specific polymorphic sites in DNA extracted from tumor, when compared to DNA from matched normal tissues. Such "allelotyping" is feasible by PCR amplification of microsatellite repeats, provided the heterozygosity for the studied loci and a neoplastic cellularity higher than 60% in the cancer sample. We are using a set of oligonucleotide primers to amplify 350 chromosomal locus-specific microsatellite repeats. This approach allows the analysis of all chromosomes at an approximate 10-cM resolution. The set of primers was chosen among those fur-

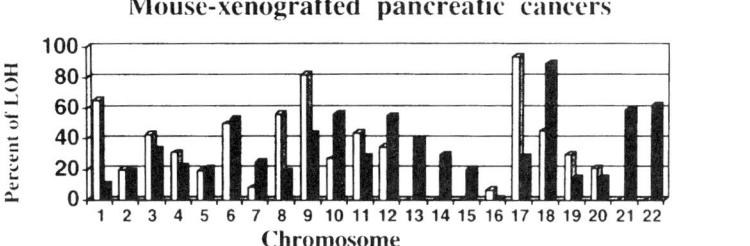

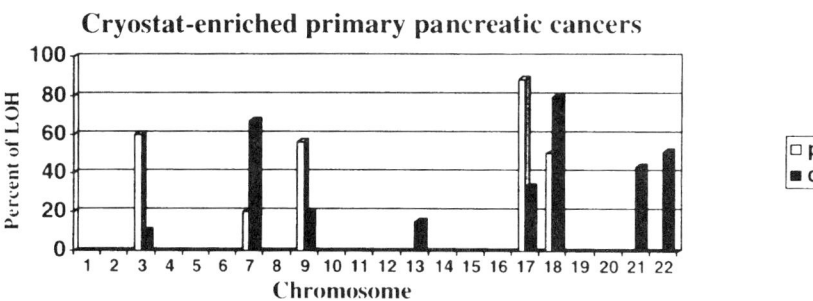

FIGURE 1. Frequency of allelic losses (LOH) on different chromosomal arms in pancreatic cancer cells enriched with different methods. The panel from xenograft-enriched cells is from Hahn *et al.*[10] (publicly available: http://www.path.jhu.edu/pancreas). The panel below is drawn from preliminary data (only for the chromosomes shown) obtained from a panel of cryostat-enriched cancers at Verona University and partially published.[6,43] Note the concordance of the results for chromosomes 17, 18, 21 and 22, whereas chromosomes 3, 7, 9, and 13 show discordant results in the two series.

nished by the "MapPairs collection" (Research Genetics, Huntsville, AL, USA) and from "ABI PRISM Linkage mapping set panels" (Perkin-Elmer). The preliminary data obtained from complete and/or partial allelotyping studies of different pancreatic tumors is summarized in FIGURES 1 and 2.[6, 7, 9–14]

Tumor Cell Enrichment for Genetic Analysis

In the last few years, we have established a frozen tissue bank and a DNA bank from different cryostat-enriched pancreatic tumor types, and we have generated *in vivo* and *in vitro* models of different pancreatic tumors (ductal, papilla of Vater and mucinous cystic tumors), through nude mice-xenografting and *in vitro* culture of primary tumors.

In fact, the main limitation for molecular studies in pancreatic neoplasms is that cancer cellularity is low compared to other tumor types. To overcome this problem, neoplastic cell-enrichment techniques have been developed, such as cryostat dissection of primary cancers[6,15] or xenografting in nude mice.[10,16,17] Each of these methods introduces some bias in the selection of cases. Cryostat enrichment is successful in only about 20% of cases, which represent those with a neoplastic cellularity higher than the average common pancreatic cancer. Xenografting, which allows the neo-

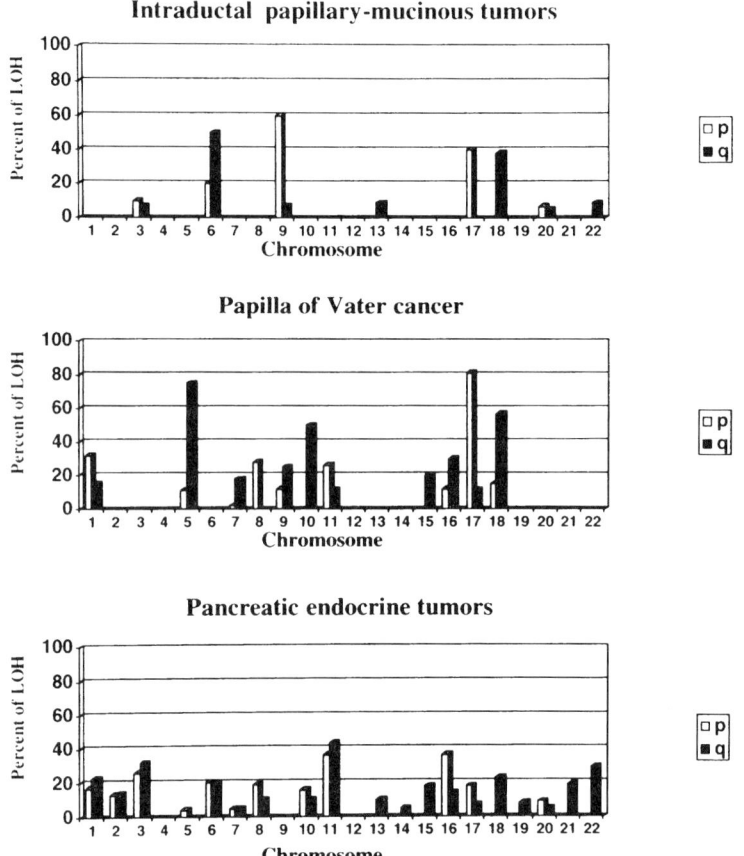

FIGURE 2. Available data on the frequency of chromosome allelic losses (LOH) in different pancreatic tumors. Information is available only for the chromosomal arms shown and is recovered from published data[12,14] and from partially published preliminary results obtained at Verona University.[7,13,54] Note the low frequency of LOH in endocrine tumors with respect to those of exocrine tumors shown in this figure and in FIGURE 2.

plastic enrichment of at least 2–5 times, may also introduce some bias in the panels obtained. For instance, all xenografts show *Ki-ras* mutations and *p53* mutation rates are higher than those found in primary cancer samples,[18] suggesting either a selection for that particular 60% of pancreatic cancers containing a *p53* mutation,[19–21] or perhaps a selection for subclones within a cancer population.[10, 22]

Based on this consideration, the results obtained with either type of material may differ (FIG. 2). In addition, the DNA anomalies found in cryostat-enriched neoplastic tissues represent an average of the anomalies in the different tumor areas, and thus the heterogeneity of the cancer cell population will be hidden. However, consistent anomalies occurring in the large majority of cancer cells are nonetheless observed. The use of microdissection on additional frozen or paraffin-embedded samples then

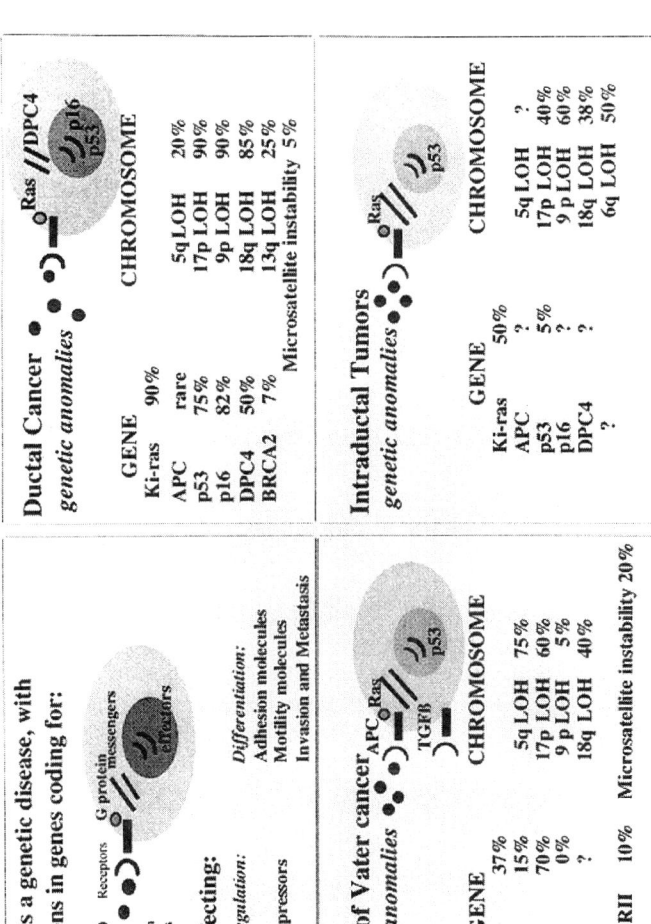

FIGURE 3. Frequency of gene mutations and allelic losses of their corresponding chromosomal site in different tumor types.

allows a precise topographical localization of the anomalies and the study of progression-related events.[7]

GENETIC ANOMALIES

Known Defects

The known genetic anomalies described in ductal, intraductal and papilla of Vater neoplasia, also with the contribution of the group from Verona University, are summarized in FIGURE 3 and discussed below.

In common ductal cancer, these mainly include mutation of the *Ki-ras*, *p53*, *p16^{INK4a}* and *DPC4* genes. Point mutational *Ki-ras* activation is a feature of ductal cancer (reviewed in Refs. 23 and 24) and occurs at precancerous stages, within lesions termed pancreatic intraepithelial neoplasia (PIN).[25, 26] They also seem to be early events in about 35% of papilla of Vater and 50% of IPMT.[27–31] *Ki-ras* mutations have also been found in SCT.[32] *Adenomatous polyposis coli* (*APC*) gene mutations are infrequent events in papilla of Vater cancers in spite of a high frequency of chromosome 5q LOH[7,33] and are exceedingly rare in ductal cancer.[15,34–36]) Biallelic inactivation of the *p53* gene in which one copy of the gene on chromosome 17p is lost and the remaining copy is inactivated by a point mutation is found in about 70% of ductal and papilla of Vater cancers.[3,19–21,27] The occurrence of intragenic 1–2-basepair microdeletions is a peculiarity of ductal cancers in comparison with other tumor types.[19, 21] In papilla of Vater tumors and IPMT, *p53* alterations are believed to accompany the adenoma-carcinoma transition.[27,29] The gene coding for the cyclin-dependent kinase inhibitor *p16^{INK4a}* is frequently inactivated in ductal cancer and in its precursor lesion either by homozygous deletion (48%) or by intragenic mutation (34%).[16,25] It has recently been shown that the gene is transcriptionally silenced by methylation in an additional 16% of ductal cancers.[37] IPMT shows LOH of the *p16^{INK4a}* locus on chromosome 9p21 in 60% of cases,[12] whereas papilla of Vater cancer rarely shows LOH at 9p21 (Scarpa, unpublished data).

The loss of one copy of chromosome 18q occurs at high frequency in ductal cancer.[6,10] The *DPC4* gene is located on this chromosome and is inactivated in about 50% of cases by either intragenic mutation or homozygous deletion.[38] This gene is thought to belong to the transforming growth factor-β (TGF-β) superfamily signaling pathway, and data exist about additional genetic anomalies disrupting the TGF-β pathway.[39] Both IPMT and papilla of Vater tumors show LOH at 18q in 40% of cases, but no data are available for *DPC4* mutations. The *BRCA2* gene was found to be mutated in the germ-line of 7% of pancreatic cancer patients.[40] No data are available for IPMT and papilla of Vater tumors.

Widespread alterations at simple repeat sequences (microsatellite instability) occur in about 20% of papilla of Vater cancers, where it is an early phenomenon and is associated with a good prognosis.[3] The TGF-β signaling pathway is hampered in proportion of this subgroup of papilla of Vater tumors by mutation of the TGF-β–type II receptor (Scarpa, unpublished). At variance, microsatellite instability is a rare event in ductal tumors and seems to be associated with peculiar clinicopathological characteristics.[41]

No or limited data are available on molecular abnormalities of acinar cell,[89] serous cystic,[32,42] mucinous cystic and solid pseudopapillary tumors (SPT).[42] The latter is a low grade malignancy primarily affecting prepuberal and young women, which characteristically show progesterone receptor immunostaining.[96] No genome-wide analysis for chromosomal anomalies in IPMT, papilla of Vater tumors and MCT has been reported to date.

In summary, the limited information about genetic anomalies in tumors other than ductal cancer suggests that IPMT seem to contain chromosomal anomalies similar to those found in ductal cancers, although at a lower frequency,[12] whereas papilla of Vater cancers show genetic anomalies more closely resembling those of gastrointestinal malignancies.[3,7,28]

Chromosomal Losses with No Identified Genes

In ductal cancers there is an additional collection of chromosomal arms for which losses have been seen in at least 50% of cases, including chromosomes 1p, 3p, 6p, 6q, 8p, 10q, 12q, 21q, and 22q.[1] A high frequency of chromosome 7q31–32 LOH has been detected in the highly cellular subgroup of ductal cancers, and 5q LOH has been observed in papilla of Vater cancers (see below).[6,7] Although no target gene has been conclusively identified for the aforementioned chromosomal deletions, the following genes have been excluded: p18 cyclin-dependent kinase inhibitor for chromosome 1p; the retinoblastoma (Rb) for 13q; and neurofibromatosis type 2 Schwannomin (SCH) for chromosome 22q.[10] However, data from our group suggest that the *fragile histidine triad* (*FHIT*) gene at chromosome 3p14.2 might be a target for chromosome 3p deletion.[43]

Our DNA fingerprinting studies of cryostat-enriched pancreatic and papilla of Vater cancers using AP-PCR detected nonrandom anomalies that were further characterized by allelotyping of the chromosome from which the AP-PCR bands were derived. Chromosome 7q LOH is a frequent event (80%) in cryostat-enrichable common pancreatic ductal carcinomas; the smallest common deleted region described by our cases was between 7q31.1 and 7q32 markers.[6] Pax-4 located in this chromosomal region is not the target of this deletion (Scarpa, unpublished). Similarly, 75% of papilla of Vater cancers showed LOH at chromosome 5q, with two smallest common deleted regions at 5q13.3–q14 and at 5q23–q31, which do not include the *APC* gene locus and are similar to those found in gastric cancer.[7]

In the course of allelotyping studies of cryostat-enriched primary pancreatic cancers, we found allelic losses at chromosome 3p14.2 in about 60% of cases and that they occur much more rarely on chromosome 3 outside this region. The *FHIT* gene is located at this site and has been proposed as a candidate tumor suppressor gene, due to its frequent alteration in different cancer types.[44] Further studies have shown that the *FHIT* gene is expressed in the terminal ductules and centrocinar cells of normal pancreas and that 60% of primary pancreatic ductal cancers exhibit various alterations affecting *FHIT* gene expression, often represented by *FHIT* gene intragenic deletions.[43]

PERIAMPULLARY CANCERS

The term "periampullary carcinoma" has been diffusely used to define cancers involving the region of the papilla (ampulla) of Vater. This has rendered it extremely difficult to compare the results of the different clinicopathologic and few molecular studies. In fact, under this definition a heterogeneous group of neoplasms is included, which originate from either the proper ampulla or periampullary anatomical structures, i.e., the pancreatic head, the duodenum and the extraduodenal bile duct. On the other hand, the comparable histopathologic characteristics of the epithelial tumors arising in this region and the advanced stage at which most cases are diagnosed prevent a precise definition of the structure of origin. The exact site of origin can only be determined in small lesions. Only the study of a well-selected series of other types of periampullary tumors may help in understanding the common and/or distinct features in the pathogenesis of this heterogeneous group of neoplasms.

We have studied a series of cancers of unequivocal ampullary origin for genetic alterations including: i) mutations of *Ras*-family, *APC*, *p53* and *p16^{INK4}* genes, ii) AP-PCR and partial or complete allelotyping of different chromosomes (see FIG. 3); iii) presence of a "RER+ phenotype," as defined by the presence of DNA replication errors (RER) at simple repeat sequences (SRS) interspersed throughout the genome.

Ras mutations occur in about 35% of cases and usually affect Ki-ras, but rarely N-ras.[27,28] They are a relatively early phenomena associated with adenomas and a proportion of cancers having an adenomatous phase in their pathogenesis. Ras mutated tumors included three of four cases which mainly involved the intraduodenal bile duct, suggesting that a proportion of Ras-mutated cancers might correspond to those originating from the epithelium of the bile duct component of the ampulla.[28] Interestingly, biliary tract cancers show a relatively high frequency of *Ki-ras* mutations,[45–47] but with peculiar differences according to their location. Motojima *et al.*[45–47] reported a frequency of 9%, 0% and 41% in cancers of proximal, middle and distal bile duct, respectively.

APC gene mutations are not frequent in ampullary cancer pathogenesis.[33] Interestingly, all *APC* mutated cases also contained a Ras gene mutation and were found in tumors with an adenomatous component. This might suggest that *APC* mutations, like Ras gene mutations, are restricted to a proportion of cancers arising on an adenomatous precursor. In contrast with the low frequency of *APC* gene mutations, frequent allelic losses at chromosome 5q (75%) were found, as suggested by AP-PCR fingerprinting.[7] Allelotyping of chromosome 5 located the previously mentioned two smallest common deleted regions at 5q13.3–q14 and at 5q23–q31, which correspond to those found in gastric tumors and do not include the *APC* locus. In addition, the presence of 5q LOH in 6 of 8 adenomas and in 3 of 4 early-stage cancers suggests that such a phenomenon occurs at early stages of neoplastic progression of the ampullary epithelium.

Inactivation of tumor suppressor gene p53 by mutation of one allele and loss of the normal one is a frequent phenomenon and is mainly associated with high-grade advanced-stage disease, irrespective of the presence of adenomatous components and of *Ras*, *APC*, chromosome 5q or RER abnormalities.[3,27] Neither losses nor mutations of the p16 gene were found (Scarpa, unpublished). Finally a RER+ phenotype was detected in 20% of cases and was associated with long survival of patients.[3] A proportion of these tumors also showed mutations in polyadenine tracts of TGF-β-RII, Bax and hMSH3 genes (Scarpa, unpublished).

In conclusion, our data suggest that papilla of Vater tumors arise from two different molecular pathogenetic pathways, characterized by either chromosomal instability (CIN) or microsatellite instability (MIN) with different clinicoprognostic

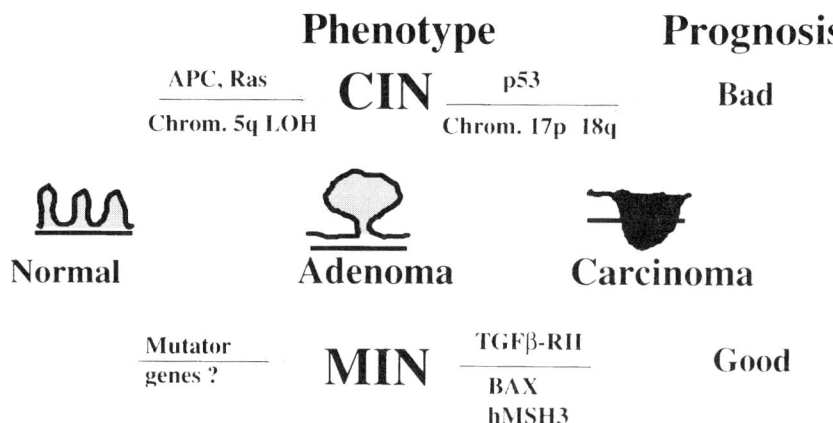

FIGURE 4. Schematic representation of the molecular pathogenesis of papilla of Vater and duodenal cancer. Two molecular pathways lead to papilla of Vater and duodenal cancer, and they may be termed "chromosome instability" (CIN) and "microsatellite instability" (MIN) pathways.[55,56] The more common sporadic cancers (80%) belong to the first and are characterized at the molecular level by allelic losses in an average of at least 25% of randomly chosen DNA sequences. In these cases, the early genetic events include chromosome 5q allelic losses and less frequently APC and Ras gene mutations. p53 gene inactivation by mutation of one allele and loss of the second together with chromosome 18q LOH characterize progression of malignancy. A proportion of about 20% of cancers show a MIN phenotype, characterized by widespread genomic mutations and by rare chromosomal losses. In these cancers, the impaired function of DNA repair genes also causes the mutational activation or inactivation of functional genes,[56] such as the TGF-β–type II receptor (TGF-β-RII), Bax and hMSH3 genes.

features (FIG. 4). We have also demonstrated the existence of these two alternative pathogenetic pathways in duodenal cancer.[48] This scenario parallels that of the common type sporadic colorectal and gastric cancers.[49,50] The decision as to whether papilla of Vater and duodenal adenocarcinoma should be viewed as a gastrointestinal cancer or as a peripancreatic cancer is unclear.[51–53] This is not a trivial question, since it involves the debate about the opportunity and type of a surgical and/or chemotherapic treatment.[51–53] Our findings suggest that both papilla of Vater and duodenal cancers should be considered as gastrointestinal malignancies.

AKNOWLEDGMENTS

Most of the results of our study have been supported by grants from the Associazione Italiana Ricerca Cancro (AIRC), Milan, Italy; Consorzio Studi Universitari and Banca Popolare di Verona, Verona, Italy.

REFERENCES

1. HRUBAN, R., C. YEO & S. KERN. 1998. Pancreatic cancer. *In* The Genetic Basis of Human Cancer. B. Vogelstein & K. Kinzler, Eds.: 603–613. McGraw-Hill. London.

2. KLÖPPEL, G., E. SOLCIA, D. LONGNECKER et al. 1996. Histological typing of tumours of the exocrine pancreas. In International Histological Classification of Tumours. World Health Organization, Ed. Springer-Verlag. Berlin.
3. ACHILLE, A., M. O. BIASI, G. ZAMBONI et al. 1997. Cancers of the papilla of Vater: mutator phenotype is associated with good prognosis. Clin. Cancer Res. **3:** 1841–1847.
4. IONOV, A., M. A. PEINADO, S. MALKHOSYAN et al. 1993. Ubiquitous somatic mutations in simple repeated sequences reveal a new mechanism for colonic carcinogenesis. Nature **363:** 558–561.
5. YASUDA, J., M. NAVARRO, S. MALKHOSYAN et al. 1996. Chromosomal assignment of human DNA fingerprint sequences obtained by arbitrarily primed PCR (AP-PCR). Genomics **34:** 1–5.
6. ACHILLE, A., M. BIASI, G. ZAMBONI et al. 1996. Chromosome 7q allelic losses in pancreatic carcinoma. Cancer Res. **56:** 3808–3813.
7. ACHILLE, A., A. BARON, G. ZAMBONI et al. 1998. Chromosome 5 allelic losses are early events in tumors of the papilla of Vater and occur at sites similar to those of gastric cancer. Brit. J. Cancer **78:** 1653–1660.
8. PEINADO, M. A., S. MALKHOSYAN, A. VELAZQUEZ et al. 1992. Isolation and characterization of allelic losses and gains in colorectal tumors by arbitrary primed polymerase chain reaction. Proc. Natl. Acad. Sci. USA **89:** 10065–10069.
9. GRIFFIN, C., R. HRUBAN, L. MORSBERGER et al. 1995. Consistent chromosome abnormalities in adenocarcinoma of pancreas. Cancer Res. **55:** 2394–2399.
10. HAHN, S. A., A. B. SEYMOUR, A. T. M. SHAMSUL HOQUE et al. 1995. Allelotype of pancreatic adenocarcinoma using xenograft enrichment. Cancer Res. **55:** 4670–4675.
11. SOLINAS-TOLDO, S., C. WALLRAP, F. MÜLLER-PILLASCH et al. 1996. Mapping of chromosomal imbalances in pancreatic carcinoma by comparative genomic hybridization. Cancer Res. **56:** 3803–3807.
12. FUJII, H., M. INAGAKI, S. KASAI et al. 1997. Genetic progression and heterogeneity in intraductal papillary-mucinous neoplasms of the pancreas. Am. J. Pathol. **151:** 1447–1454.
13. BEGHELLI, S., G. PELOSI, G. ZAMBONI et al. 1998. Pancreatic endocrine tumours: evidence for a tumour suppressor pathogenesis and for a tumour suppressor gene on chromosome 17p. J. Pathol. **186:** 41–50.
14. CHUNG, D., S. BROWN, F. GRAEME-COOK et al. 1998. Localization of putative tumor suppressor loci by genome-wide allelotyping in human pancreatic endocrine tumors. Cancer Res. **58:** 3706–3711.
15. SEYMOUR, A. B., R. H. HRUBAN, M. REDSTON et al. 1994. Allelotype of pancreatic adenocarcinoma. Cancer Res. **54:** 2761–2764.
16. CALDAS, C., S. A. HAHN, L. T. DA COSTA et al. 1994. Frequent somatic mutations and homozygous deletions of the p16 (MTS1) gene in pancreatic adenocarcinoma. Nature Genet. **8:** 27–32.
17. REYES, G., A. VILLANUEVA, C. GARCIA et al. 1996. Orthotopic xenografts of human pancreatic carcinomas acquire genetic aberrations during dissemination in nude mice. Cancer Res. **56:** 5713–5719.
18. ROZENBLUM, E., M. SCHUTTE, M. GOGGINS et al. 1997. Tumor-suppressive pathways in pancreatic carcinoma. Cancer Res. **57:** 1731–1734.
19. SCARPA, A., P. CAPELLI, K. MUKAI et al. 1993. Pancreatic adenocarcinomas frequently show p53 gene mutations. Am. J. Pathol. **142:** 1534–1543.
20. PELLEGATA, N. S., F. SESSA, B. RENAULT et al. 1994. K-ras and p53 mutations in pancreatic cancer: ductal and non-ductal tumors progress through different genetic lesions. Cancer Res. **54:** 1556–1560.
21. REDSTON, M. S., C. CALDAS, A. B. SEYMOUR et al. 1994. p53 mutations in pancreatic carcinoma and evidence of common involvement of homocopolymer tracts in DNA microdeletions. Cancer Res. **54:** 3025–3033.
22. GORUNOVA, L., B. JOHANSSON, S. DAWISKIBA et al. 1995. Massive cytogenetic heterogeneity in a pancreatic carcinoma: fifty-four kariotypically unrelated clones. Genes Chromosomes Cancer **14:** 259–266.

23. HRUBAN, R., A. VAN-MANSFELD, G. OFFERHAUS et al. 1993. K-ras oncogene activation in adenocarcinoma of the human pancreas. A study of 82 carcinomas using a combination of mutant-enriched polymerase chain reaction analysis and allele-specific oligonucleotide hybridization. Am. J. Pathol. **143:** 545–554.
24. SCARPA, A., P. CAPELLI, A. VILLANUEVA et al. 1994. Pancreatic cancer in Europe: ki-ras gene mutation pattern shows geographical differences. Int. J. Cancer **57:** 167–171.
25. MOSKALUK, C. A., R. H. HRUBAN & S. E. KERN. 1997. p16 and K-ras gene mutations in the intraductal precursors of human pancreatic adenocarcinoma. Cancer Res. **57:** 2140–2143.
26. BRAT, D., K. LILLEMOE, C. YEO et al. 1998. Progression of pancreatic intraductal neoplasia to infiltrating adenocarcinoma of the pancreas. Am. J. Surg. Pathol. **22:** 163–169.
27. SCARPA, A., P. CAPELLI, G. ZAMBONI et al. 1993. Neoplasia of the ampulla of Vater: Ki-ras and p53 mutations. Am. J. Pathol. **142:** 1163–1172.
28. SCARPA, A., G. ZAMBONI, A. ACHILLE et al. 1994. Ras-family gene mutations in neoplasia of the ampulla of Vater. Int. J. Cancer **59:** 39–42.
29. SESSA, F., E. SOLCIA, C. CAPELLA et al. 1994. Intraductal papillary-mucinous pancreatic tumors are phenotypically, genetically and behaviorally distinct growths. An analysis of tumor cell phenotype, K-ras and p53 genes' mutations. Virchows Arch. **425:** 357–367.
30. HOWE, J., D. KLIMSTRA, C. CORDON-CARDO et al. 1997. K-ras mutation in adenomas and carcinomas of the ampulla of Vater. Clin. Cancer Res. **3:** 129–133.
31. Z'GRAGGEN, K., J. A. RIVERA, C. C. COMPTON et al. 1997. Prevalence of activating K-ras mutations in the evolutionary stages of neoplasia in intraductal papillary mucinous tumors of the pancreas. Ann. Surg. **226:** 491–498; discussion 498–500.
32. BARTSCH, D., D. BASTIAN, P. BARTH et al. 1998. K-ras oncogene mutations indicate malignancy in cystic tumors of the pancreas. Ann. Surg. **228:** 79–86.
33. ACHILLE, A., M. SCUPOLI, A. MAGALINI et al. 1996. APC gene mutations and allelic losses in sporadic ampullary tumours: evidence of genetic difference from tumours associated with familial adenomatous polyposis. Int. J. Cancer **68:** 305–312.
34. HORII, A., S. NAKATSURU, Y. MIYOSHI et al. 1992. Frequent somatic mutations of the APC gene in human pancreatic cancer. Cancer Res. **52:** 6696–6698.
35. MCKIE, A., M. FILIPE & N. LEMOINE. 1993. Abnormalities affecting the APC and MCC tumour suppressor gene loci on chromosome 5q occur frequently in gastric cancer but not in pancreatic cancer. Int. J. Cancer **55:** 598–603.
36. YASHIMA, K., S. NAKAMORI, Y. MURAKAMI et al. 1994. Mutations of the adenomatous polyposis coli gene in the mutation cluster region: comparison of human pancreatic and colorectal cancers. Int. J. Cancer **59:** 43–47.
37. SCHUTTE, M., R. HRUBAN, J. GERADTS et al. 1997. Abrogation of the Rb/p16 tumor-suppressive pathway in virtually all pancreatic carcinomas. Cancer Res. **57:** 3126–3130.
38. HAHN, S. A., M. SCHUTTE, A. T. HOQUE et al. 1996. DPC4, a candidate tumor suppressor gene at human chromosome 18q21.1. Science **271:** 350–353.
39. VILLANUEVA, A., C. GARCÌA, A. PAULES et al. 1998. Disruption of the antiproliferative TGF-beta signaling pathways in human pancreatic cancer cells. Oncogene **17:** 1969–1978.
40. GOGGINS, M., M. SCHUTTE, J. LU et al. 1996. Germline BRCA2 gene mutations in patients with apparently sporadic pancreatic carcinomas. Cancer Res. **56:** 5360–5364.
41. GOGGINS, M., G. J. OFFERHAUS, W. HILGERS et al. 1998. Pancreatic adenocarcinomas with DNA replication errors (RER+) are associated with wild-type K-ras and characteristic histopathology. Poor differentiation, a syncytial growth pattern, and pushing borders suggest RER+. Am. J. Pathol. **152:** 1501–1507.
42. VORTMEYER, A., I. LUBENSKY, F. FOGT et al. 1997. Allelic deletion and mutation of the von Hippel-Lindau (VHL) tumor suppressor gene in pancreatic microcystic adenomas. Am. J. Pathol. **151:** 951–956.

43. SORIO, C., A. BARON, A. ORLANDINI et al. 1999. The *FHIT* gene is expressed in pancreatic ductular cells and is altered in pancreatic cancers. Cancer Res. **59:** 1308–1314.
44. SOZZI, G., K. HUEBNER & C. CROCE. 1998. FHIT in human cancer. Adv. Cancer Res. **74:** 141–166.
45. LEVI, S., A. URBANO-ISPIZUA, R. GILL et al. 1991. Multiple K-ras codon 12 mutations in cholangiocarcinomas demonstrated with a sensitive polymerase chain reaction technique. Cancer Res. **51:** 3497–3502.
46. MOTOJIMA, K., T. TSUNODA, T. KANEMATSU et al. 1991. Distinguishing pancreatic carcinoma from other periampullary carcinomas by analysis of mutations in the Kirsten-ras oncogene. Ann. Surg. **214:** 657–662.
47. IMAI, M., T. HOSHI & K. OGAWA. 1994. K-ras codon 12 mutations in biliary tract tumors detected by polymerase chain reaction denaturing gel electrophoresis. Cancer **73:** 2727–2733.
48. ACHILLE, A., A. BARON, G. ZAMBONI et al. 1998. Molecular pathogenesis of sporadic duodenal cancer. Br. J. Cancer **77:** 760–765.
49. POWELL, S. 1998. Stomach cancer. *In* The Genetic Basis of Human Cancer. B. Vogelstein & K. Kinzler, Eds.: 647–652. McGraw-Hill. London.
50. KINZLER, K. & B. VOGELSTEIN. 1998. Colorectal tumors. *In* The Genetic Basis of Human Cancer. B. Vogelstein & K. Kinzler, Eds.: 565–587. McGraw-Hill. London.
51. BRENNAN, M. F. 1990. Duodenal cancer. Asian J. Surg. **13:** 204–209.
52. ROSE, D. M., S. N. HOCHWALD, D. S. KLIMSTRA et al. 1996. Primary duodenal adenocarcinoma: a ten year experience with 79 patients. J. Am. Coll. Surg. **183:** 89–96.
53. KLEMPNAUER, J., G. J. RIDDER & R. PICHLMAYR. 1995. Prognostic factors after resection of ampullary carcinoma: multivariate survival analysis in comparison with ductal cancer of the pancreatic head. Br. J. Surg. **82:** 1686–1691.
54. SCARPA, A., P. PEDERZOLI & G. ZAMBONI. 1996. Genetics of pancreatic and ampullary tumors. *In* Advances in Pancreatic Disease. C. Dervenis, Ed.: 1–11. Georg Thieme Verlag. Stuttgart.
55. PERUCHO, M. 1996. Microsatellite instability: the mutator that mutates the other mutator. Nat. Med. **2:** 630–631.
56. SHIBATA, D. 1996. Loss of DNA mismatch repair: life in the fast lane? Gastroenterology **111:** 519–521.

Pancreatic Cancer: Development of a Unifying Etiologic Concept

ALBERT B. LOWENFELS[a,c] AND PATRICK MAISONNEUVE[b]

[a]*Department of Surgery and Community and Preventive Medicine, New York Medical College, Valhalla, New York, USA*
[b]*Program of Clinical Epidemiology, European Institute of Oncology, Milan, Italy*

ABSTRACT: Our knowledge of the etiology of all forms of cancer including pancreatic cancer has improved dramatically in the second half of this century. The current model describes a gradual change from a normal pancreatic cell to a fully malignant cell requiring several stages with gradual and progressive alterations appearing at the genetic and the tissue level. Although there are many germ line diseases that are associated with pancreatic cancer it is probable that inherited diseases account for only about 10% of the total burden of pancreatic cancer. Avoidance of smoking and dietary modification are the current best strategies for reducing the risk of this tumor. In addition, newer molecular techniques and imaging procedures should provide clinicians with the ability to detect pancreatic cancer at an early, potentially curable stage.

INTRODUCTION

During the first half of the twentieth century, the aim of cancer research was to identify a single causative agent. Most likely the ability of bacteriologists, such as Koch, to link a single bacteria with a single disease, was responsible for the persistent effort to find a unique cause for cancer. Quite early, certain rodent tumors were found to be associated with viruses, while other tumors could easily be induced by the application of hydrocarbons to the skin. When it became apparent that there might be more than one cause of cancer, researchers became champions of their own favorite theory. A widely quoted statistic in the 1960s and 1970s was that 80–90% of all cancer was environmental. Doll and Peto in their influential monograph, partitioned the cause(s) of cancer into 11 known categories, with tobacco and diet being the leading causes.[1] Much of this compartmentalized thinking was counterproductive.

We now know that it is conceptually imprecise to search for a single cause of cancer and, depending upon one's viewpoint, all tumors might be considered to be genetic, or conversely, to be environmental. For example, consider the rare disease xeroderma pigmentosa, a known genetic disorder with an extremely high risk of early onset skin cancer. Clearly this disease must be considered a splendid example of a gene-related cancer. But an equally strong argument can be put forth that this is an

---

[c]Address for correspondence: Albert B. Lowenfels, M.D., Department of Surgery, New York Medical College, Valhalla, NY 10595. Phone, 914/594-4260; fax, 914/594-4576; e-mail, Lowenfel@nymc.edu

entirely environmental cancer, because in the complete absence of ultraviolet light, tumors do not develop!

In this paper we shall review the development of various models dealing with the problem of cancer causation, using pancreatic cancer as an example.

TOWARDS A UNIFYING THEORY

Early Theories of Cancer Etiology

Medicine in ancient Egypt had deep religious and magical roots. Nevertheless, we do know from sources such as the Smith papyrus that many common diseases including tumors were recognized. Prognosis rather than etiology was the Egyptian physician's major concern. The phrase "This is a disease I will (will not) treat" appears frequently in the Smith papyrus, dating back to about 1600 BC. Undoubtedly a patient suffering from pancreatic cancer with weight loss, jaundice and severe back pain would have been placed in the "do not treat" category.

Hippocratic physicians were greatly interested in cancer and were the first to differentiate between benign and malignant tumors. Their curiosity led them to discard the traditional idea that disease was preordained and to ask, "What is the cause of this person's illness?" The search for the cause of cancer can be traced back to this early era.

Galen, the most prolific and influential physician of ancient times, was strongly influenced by the Hippocratic tradition. Galenic medicine emphasizes the balance of various elements within the body. Disease resulted from an imbalance of an excess or deficiency of a key element. The etiology of cancer would have been attributed to the same causes. Galenic medical views influenced medicine for over 1500 years and even today, the concept of an imbalance or disturbance of body elements or emotions forms the basis of many types of alternative medical paradigms.

Occupation and Cancer Etiology

As we approach the current period, several physicians noted the strong connection between occupation and disease, including cancer. The most well-known example is the excess of scrotal cancer in chimney sweeps. First noticed by the surgeon Percival Pott in the late 1700s, there was a delay of more than a century before coal tar, to which chimney sweeps were exposed, was suspected to be a carcinogen.

Early studies of other occupations have also provided information about cancer etiology. In the 1500s a Swiss physician, Paracelsus noted that miners suffered from many diseases. In the late nineteenth century observations on the Schneeburg miners in Germany noted a high incidence of pulmonary lesions. These mines have since been discovered to contain the element uranium; presumably much of the lung disease noted earlier in Schneeburg miners was unrecognized lung cancer.

Although occupation has proved to be important for tumors such as bladder cancer and certain types of skin cancer, it has never been suspected to be a major determining factor for cancer of the pancreas.

Development of the Concept of Chemical Carcinogenesis

Although Percivall Pott noted in the eighteenth century that continuous exposure to an irritating substance might cause cancer, the full development of this concept did not occur until the middle of the twentieth century. Animal models suggested three stages in the development of cancer: initiation, an irreversible stage; promotion, which is reversible and dependent upon continued application of the promoting agent; and, finally, progression, another irreversible stage with genomic alterations. The chemical carcinogenesis model effectively describes the development of tumors due to specific environmental agents, such as radiation and tobacco degradation products. This model has considerable importance for pancreatic cancer, because smoking is a strong risk factor. Nearly every study has shown an approximately twofold increased risk of pancreatic cancer in smokers compared to nonsmokers. Although the smoking-pancreatic cancer link is not as strong as for lung cancer, it still remains the single commonest reversible risk factor for this lethal tumor.

The concept that cancer arises in various stages grew out of the study of laboratory animals, but was reinforced and strengthened by the evidence provided by looking at the age-incidence curves for various cancers. Epidemiologic data for nearly all tumors show an exponential increase in the incidence of cancer with increasing age. A multistage model requiring approximately four or five intermediate stages before cancer becomes clinically detectable can best explain this relationship. The observed age-specific increase in the incidence of pancreatic cancer fits the multistage model.

CURRENT THEORIES OF CARCINOGENESIS

What is the current most widely accepted model for carcinogenesis, does it relate to any of the earlier models, and is it valid for pancreatic cancer? Unlike the chemical carcinogenesis model, which was developed largely from animal experiments, the current model has been developed in humans, mostly from work done on colon cancer. The current model stresses sequential genomic alterations that develop in cancer cells. Similar to the multistage model, there are many alterations, and the "multihit" concept implies that several mutations must occur before cancer develops. Four main classes of genetic factors have been described: oncogenes, tumor suppressor genes, DNA repair genes, and apoptosis genes.

One of the earliest changes is a mutation in the ras gene, noted in about half of all colon cancers, and in about 80% of all pancreatic cancers.[2-4] In pancreatic cancer, other mutations are frequently observed: p53 is overexpressed in at least 50–70% of pancreatic cancers, the tumor suppressor genes DCC (deleted in colon carcinoma) and MTS1 are observed in more than 50% of all pancreatic cancers.[5,6] DPC4 (deleted in pancreatic cancer) is another tumor suppressor that is altered in about 50% of pancreatic cancers. At the molecular level, there are multiple presumably sequential, time-dependent, somatic changes, which can be detected. For a clinical tumor to develop, a single alteration is probably insufficient. There is great similarity between the present model and earlier multistage models developed prior to the genetic revolution.

At the tissue level we also see evidence of progress from a normal cell to hyperplasia, dysplasia, and finally cancer.[7] These tissue changes increase with age and also with exposure to agents such as alcohol that are known to damage the pancreas.[8]

Knudson's "Two-Hit" Theory

The material presented so far suggests that there are two independent pathways that might lead to the development of cancer. The first is related to external, environmental causes, and the second is internal or genetic. How can the conflict between these two opposing theories be resolved?

In 1971, Knudson, based on observations of a very rare pediatric tumor, retinoblastoma, developed what has been termed the "two-hit" theory for the etiology of cancer.[9,10] Knudson observed that there were two types of retinoblastoma, a dominantly inherited type that is usually bilateral and occurs at an early age, and a sporadic, relatively uncommon uniocular type appearing at a later age.

Knudson reasoned that in the inherited type, one mutation was already present in the retinoblast. Thus, these individuals would develop early tumors, because only a single additional mutation would be required to form a retinoblastoma. In contrast, in sporadic cases two independent, sequential mutations would be required to damage both alleles.

The "two-hit" hypothesis, based on thoughtful reasoning about a unique, rare pediatric cancer, has been widely accepted as a useful model to explain the etiology of common human cancers. A normal cell becomes cancerous only when both alleles are damaged. In the cases of inheritable cancers, one allele is already damaged, so these kindreds are much more likely to develop cancer, since only a single additional mutation is required. Such conditions are rare and probably account for no more than about 10% of all cancers. For persons not carrying a defective gene, cancer rates are lower because a "double hit" is required. The age of onset of cancer is later in sporadic cancers compared to persons carrying a defective gene, such as the RB gene.

Quite recently there has been an intriguing link between the retinoblastoma gene, which is a tumor suppressor gene, and pancreatic cancer. A gene on chromosome 9p, p^{16INK4} has been implicated in susceptibility to malignant melanoma kindreds.[11] In addition to melanoma, these kindreds also have an increased risk of pancreatic cancer. The possible explanation is that p^{16INK4} acts in conjunction with retinoblastoma protein to prevent the growth of human cancer cells.[12]

PANCREATIC CANCER AND INHERITED GENETIC DISORDERS

It is generally believed that only about 10% of pancreatic cancers are directly related to inherited diseases.[13] Probably the most important currently known inherited gene is *BRCA2*, which may account for as many as approximately 5% of all cases of pancreatic cancer.[14] TABLE 1 lists currently known inherited diseases with an increased risk of pancreatic cancer. At this time, the genetic defect is known for all of these diseases with the exception of familial pancreatic cancer.

Generally, pancreatic cancer, when caused by a germ line defect, appears earlier in life than sporadic pancreatic cancer. However, in persons with familial pancreatic cancer, the age of onset is not appreciably different than in nonfamilial pancreatic

TABLE 1. Inherited diseases with an increased risk of pancreatic cancer

Disease	Affected chromosome
Hereditary pancreatitis	7q35
Cystic fibrosis[a]	7q31
Familial pancreatic cancer	??
BRCA2	13
Hereditary non-polyposis colonic cancer (HNPCC)	2 and 3
Familial adenomatous polyposis (FAP)	5q12-21
Li-Fraumeni syndrome	17p13.1
Peutz-Jegher's syndrome	19p
Ataxia-Telangiectasia[a]	11q
Familial atypical malignant melanoma syndrome (FAMM)	9p21

[a]Autosomal recessive genetic disorder. All others are believed to be autosomal dominant.

cancer. The reason is unknown. One possible explanation is that in a large population, sporadic clusters of pancreatic cancer might occur in some families by chance.

CELLULAR DIVISION AND PANCREATIC CANCER

Mutations are the driving force both for natural selection and for neoplasms. It is known that mutations accumulate with each cell division and with age, implying that the number of cell divisions is related to the frequency of mutations. Increased cell turnover as seen in numerous disorders leads to, and, theoretically, should be associated with an increased risk of cancer. There are many examples that reinforce this simplifying concept. It is easy to understand that a damaged organ undergoing repair with increased cell turnover could increase the risk of cancer.

Proliferative changes are common in chronic pancreatitis, and there is a suspected link between cell proliferation, cell division and cancer.[15] If so, we should expect an increased risk of pancreatic cancer in patients with chronic pancreatitis. Our own data support this concept. An international cohort study of 2015 patients with well documented pancreatitis (mostly related to alcohol) followed for an average period of 7.4 years, revealed an approximately 10–20-fold excess risk of pancreatic cancer.[16] The excess risk was found in all types of pancreatitis, in males and females, and in all countries included in the study. The cumulative risk of pancreatic cancer increased over time reaching about 4% in 20 years. Several other more recent studies have found elevated risks of pancreatic cancer in chronic pancreatitis, although the observed increased risk was lower than in our report.

Hereditary pancreatitis and tropical pancreatitis are much less common than alcoholic pancreatitis. Both diseases have an exceptionally high risk of pancreatic cancer.[17,18] In hereditary pancreatitis the relative risk is about 50 times greater than expected in the background population after adjustment for age and sex. The cumulative risk of pancreatic cancer to age 70 is greater than 30%.

The reported increased risk of pancreatic cancer in patients with pancreatitis reinforces the concept that an antecedent benign disease with detectable alteration in ductal structure is a risk factor for pancreatic cancer.

DIET AND PANCREATIC CANCER

What is the role of dietary factors in the etiology of pancreatic cancer? There are several possible links between diet and tumors of the pancreas. These include: the distribution of nutrients (carbohydrates, fats, proteins), the source of ingested food (animal versus plant), the total caloric content, the presence of specific carcinogens, and the presence of antitumor or protective agents in the diet. The risk of pancreatic cancer appears to be somewhat increased in persons consuming high fat, high carbohydrate, or high caloric diets. Conversely, fresh fruits, vegetables, and perhaps fiber appear to be protective.[19–25]

INTERACTION OF INHERITED AND ENVIRONMENTAL FACTORS

Since most persons exposed to environmental factors do not develop cancer, other obligate risk factors (either genetic or environmental) must be required to produce cancer as an endpoint. For example, about 10% of heavy smokers will develop lung cancer; but only about 1–2% will develop pancreatic cancer.

There are several known interactions between various risk factors and the eventual development of tumors in different organs. For example, exposure to either hepatitis B virus or aflatoxins can cause liver cancer. Exposure to both agents results in a markedly increased risk.[26] The high incidence of pancreatic cancer in African-Americans compared to the incidence in whites could be due to an interaction between environmental exposure to tobacco products and a racial difference in the ability to detoxify tobacco-related carcinogens.[27]

DIFFERENCES AND SIMILARITIES BETWEEN PANCREATIC AND NONPANCREATIC TUMORS

A great deal of knowledge about cancer genetics has been obtained from studying colon cancer. Can we assume that the information from the colon cancer model can be applied to pancreatic cancer? On a genetic level there are many similarities.[28,29] On a clinical level there appear to be significant differences. In many ways, clinical and epidemiologic aspects of pancreatic cancer resemble lung cancer more closely than colon cancer. The most striking difference between colon and pancreatic cancer concerns the absence of a premalignant, easily detectable pancreatic lesion similar to the colonic polyp.

AGE AND PANCREATIC CANCER

As with nearly all other forms of cancers, about 75% of pancreatic cancer occurs in persons age 65 or older. Thus age is the strongest risk factor known for this tumor. The reason for the strong association between age and cancer is not entirely clear, but must be related to cellular changes such as decreased efficiency of DNA repair genes and changes in mutation rates.

TABLE 2. Suspected risk factors for pancreatic cancer

Risk Factor	Remarks
Age	Strongest known risk factor. Risk for persons >50 years is approximately 20 times greater than for persons <50 years.
Race	About a 50% excess in African-Americans compared with whites.
Sex	About a 30% excess risk in males compared to females.
Diet	High fat, high caloric diets increase risk. Fresh fruits and vegetables, and fiber lower the risk.
Inherited disorders	About 10% of all pancreatic cancers are related to germ line mutations (ee TABLE 1). BRCA2 may be the most common.
Smoking	Consistently noted to be a strong risk factor. Smokers have at least a two-fold increased risk of pancreatic cancer.
Diabetes	Conflicting evidence; probably not a risk factor.
Coffee	Difficult to separate coffee from smoking. Most recent studies negative. Not considered to be carcinogenic by the International Agency for Research on Cancer.
Pancreatitis	All types of pancreatitis increase the risk of pancreatic cancer. Explains no more than 3-4% of all cases of pancreatic cancer.
Gallstones	Probably not a risk factor.
Miscellaneous Factors	Salmonella carriers have an increased risk of biliary and pancreatic cancer.

We can speculate that patients who develop pancreatic cancer at an early age either have a genetic abnormality or have had an exceptionally strong exposure to a risk factor. It is of interest that patients with any form of pancreatitis (alcoholic, hereditary, or tropical) develop pancreatic cancer several years earlier than patients who do not have pancreatitis. We also know that experimental pancreatic cancer appears sooner in p53-deficient mice than in normal mice.[30,31]

PREVENTION OF PANCREATIC CANCER

Is pancreatic cancer preventable? All-cause mortality doubles every eight years; cancer mortality exhibits a similar exponential increase with age. These age-related changes in cancer frequency are probably related to the accumulation of mutations. But mutations provide the mechanism for evolutionary change, which insures the survival of the species in response to changing external conditions. Cancer may be the price paid by each individual in order to survive as a species.

Life expectancy has increased dramatically in the latter half of the twentieth century. Since cancer and aging are so closely associated, we can predict an increase in the frequency of all cancers, including pancreatic cancer in forthcoming generations. Because age and cancer are so closely related, it will be difficult to eradicate cancer by any easily applicable public health measure.

Rather than the unrealistic goal of eradication of pancreatic cancer, a more realistic target is to reduce the overall burden of this lethal tumor by lowering the incidence and increasing survival. TABLE 2 lists the major risk factors for pancreatic cancer. At present, the strongest risk factor and the one most amenable to reduction is smoking.[32–37] About one third of all pancreatic cancers are directly attributable to this single, avoidable exposure. In the USA and some parts of Europe smoking is becoming less common, but, unfortunately, in Asia and many other parts of the world, smoking is increasing, threatening a global increase in pancreatic and other tobacco-related cancers in the early part of the next millennium.

Although the link between diet and pancreatic cancer is less strong than between smoking and cancer, there is sufficient evidence to recommend widespread adoption of a "prudent" diet—one that has a reduced fat and caloric content, together with an increased amount of fruits, vegetables and fibers. In experimental animals it has long been known that simple caloric deprivation in early life without any dietary modification produces a remarkable reduction in the frequency of cancer.[38]

Reducing exposure to risk factors for pancreatic cancer would most likely increase the age at which pancreatic cancer is diagnosed. Surely contracting pancreatic cancer at age 85 is preferable to developing this tumor at age 65.

Newer diagnostic techniques, in the areas of imaging and molecular diagnosis, will hopefully lead to effective screening protocols for high-risk populations, such as kindreds with familial pancreatic cancer, or patients with pancreatitis. With earlier diagnosis we can hope to detect small (1-cm or less tumors) with a better chance for cure.

ACKNOWLEDGMENTS

This work was supported by grants from the C.D. Smithers Foundation, Solvay Pharmaceuticals, and the Italian Association for Cancer Research.

REFERENCES

1. DOLL, R. *et al.* 1981. The Causes of Cancer. Oxford Medical Publications. New York.
2. BERTHELEMY, P. *et al.* 1995. Identification of K-ras mutations in pancreatic juice in the early diagnosis of pancreatic cancer. Ann. Intern. Med. **123:** 188–191.
3. GANSAUGE, S. *et al.* 1996. Molecular oncology in pancreatic cancer. J. Mol. Med. **74:** 313–320.
4. KALTHOFF, H. *et al.* 1993. p53 and K-RAS alterations in pancreatic epithelial cell lesions. Oncogene **8:** 289–298.
5. ROSEWICZ, S. *et al.* 1997. Pancreatic carcinoma. Lancet **349:** 485–489.
6. HRUBAN, R.H. *et al.* 1998. Genetics of pancreatic cancer. From genes to families. Surg. Oncol. Clin. North Am. **7:** 1–23.
7. KLÖPPEL, G. *et al.* 1980. Intraductal proliferation in the pancreas and its relationship to human and experimental carcinogenesis. Virchows Arch. Pathol. Anat. **387:** 221–233.
8. PITCHUMONI, C.S. *et al.* 1984. Pancreatic fibrosis in chronic alcoholics and nonalcoholics without clinical pancreatitis. Am. J. Gastroenterol. **79:** 382–388.
9. KNUDSON, A.G. 1996. Hereditary cancer: two hits revisited. J. Cancer Res. Clin. Oncol. **122:** 135–140.

10. KNUDSON, A.G. 1971. Mutation and cancer: statistical study of retinoblastoma. Proc. Natl. Acad. Sci. USA **68:** 820–823.
11. GOLDSTEIN, A.M. *et al.* 1995. Increased risk of pancreatic cancer in melanoma-prone kindreds with p16^{INK4} mutations. N. Engl. J. Med. **333:** 970–974.
12. MEDEMA, R.H. *et al.* 1995. Growth suppression by p16^{ink4} requires functional retinoblastoma protein. Proc. Natl. Acad. Sci. USA **92:** 6289–6293.
13. FLANDERS, T.Y. *et al.* 1996. Pancreatic adenocarcinoma: epidemiology and genetics. J. Med. Genet. **33:** 889–898.
14. GOGGINS, M. *et al.* 1996. Germline *BRCA2* gene mutations in patients with apparently sporadic pancreatic carcinomas. Cancer Res. **56:** 5360–5364.
15. PRESTON-MARTIN, S. *et al.* 1990. Increased cell division as a cause of human cancer. Cancer Res. **50:** 7415–7421.
16. LOWENFELS, A.B. *et al.* 1993. Pancreatitis and the risk of pancreatic cancer. International Pancreatitis Study Group. N. Engl. J. Med. **328:** 1433–1437.
17. CHARI, S.T. *et al.* 1994. Risk of pancreatic carcinoma in tropical calcifying pancreatitis: an epidemiologic study. Pancreas **9:** 62–66.
18. LOWENFELS, A.B. *et al.* 1997. Hereditary pancreatitis and the risk of pancreatic cancer. International Hereditary Pancreatitis Study Group. J. Natl. Cancer Inst. **89:** 442–446.
19. BAGHURST, P.A. *et al.* 1991. A case-control study of diet and cancer of the pancreas. Am. J. Epidemiol. **134:** 167–179.
20. BUENO DE MESQUITA, H.B. *et al.* 1991. Intake of foods and nutrients and cancer of the exocrine pancreas: a population-based case-control study in The Netherlands. Int. J. Cancer **48:** 540–549.
21. GHADIRIAN, P. *et al.* 1991. Nutritional factors and pancreatic cancer in the francophone community in Montreal, Canada. Int. J. Cancer **47:** 1–6.
22. GHADIRIAN, P. *et al.* 1991. International comparisons of nutrition and mortality from pancreatic cancer. Cancer Detect. Prev. **15:** 357–362.
23. GOLD, E.B. *et al.* 1985. Diet and other risk factors for cancer of the pancreas. Cancer **55:** 460–467.
24. NEGRI, E. *et al.* 1991. Vegetable and fruit consumption and cancer risk. Int. J. Cancer **48:** 350–354.
25. ZATONSKI, W. *et al.* 1991. Nutritional factors and pancreatic cancer: a case-control study from south-west Poland. Int. J. Cancer **48:** 390–394.
26. ROSS, R.K. *et al.* 1992. Urinary aflatoxin biomarkers and risk of hepatocellular carcinoma. Lancet **339:** 943–946.
27. RICHIE, J.P. *et al.* 1997. Differences in the urinary metabolites of the tobacco-specific lung carcinogen 4-(methynitrosamino)-1-(3-pyridyl)-1-butanone in black and white smokers. Cancer Epidemiol. Biomarkers Prev. **6:** 783–790.
28. ZHANG, L. *et al.* 1997. Gene expression profiles in normal and cancer cells. Science **276:** 1268–1272.
29. HIGASHIKAWA K. *et al.* 1996. Evaluation of CD44 transcription variants in human digestive tract carcinomas and normal tissues. Int. J. Cancer **66:** 11–17.
30. SCHMANDT, R. *et al.* 1993. Genomic components of carcinogenesis. Clin. Chem. **39:** 2375–2385.
31. VOGELSTEIN, B. *et al.* 1992. p53 function and dysfunction. Cell **70:** 523–526.
32. BOYLE, P. *et al.* 1989. Epidemiology of pancreas cancer. Int. J. Pancreatol. **5:** 327–346.
33. DOLL, R. *et al.* 1994. Mortality in relation to smoking: 40 years' observations on male British doctors. Br. Med. J. **309:** 901–911.
34. FALK, R.T. *et al.* 1988. Life-style risk factors for pancreatic cancer in Louisiana: a case-control study. Am. J. Epidemiol. **128:** 324–336.
35. HOWE, G.R. *et al.* 1991. Cigarette smoking and cancer of the pancreas: evidence from a population-based case-control study in Toronto, Canada. Int. J. Cancer **47:** 323–328.
36. MACK, T.M. *et al.* 1986. Pancreas cancer and smoking, beverage consumption, and past medical history. J. Natl. Cancer Inst. **76:** 49–60.

37. ZATONSKI, W.A. *et al.* 1993. Cigarette smoking, alcohol, tea and coffee consumption and pancreas cancer risk: a case-control study from Opole, Poland. Int. J. Cancer **53:** 601–607.
38. AMES, B.N. *et al.* 1997. The causes and prevention of cancer: gaining perspective. Environ. Health Perspect. **105**(Suppl. 4)**:** 865–873.

Hereditary Pancreatitis and Pancreatic Carcinoma

DAVID C. WHITCOMB,[a,b,c,f] SUZANNE APPLEBAUM,[c,d] AND STEPHEN P. MARTIN[e]

[a]*Department of Medicine, Division of Gastroenterology and Hepatology,* [b]*Department of Cell Biology and Physiology,* [c]*Center for Genomic Sciences, and* [d]*Department of Human Genetics, University of Pittsburgh, Pittsburgh, Pennsylvania, USA*
[e]*Department of Medicine, Division of Digestive Diseases, University of Cincinnati, Cincinnati, Ohio, USA*

> ABSTRACT: Few risk factors for pancreatic cancer have emerged except for chronic pancreatitis. Recently, hereditary pancreatitis was estimated to carry a standardized incidence ratio of 53, a risk about 25 times higher than smoking. A review of the ongoing hereditary pancreatitis study of the Midwest Multicenter Pancreatic Study Group suggests that the risk of pancreatic cancer is related to long-standing pancreatitis rather than to the cationic trypsinogen mutations. No recommendations can be made on screening patients with hereditary pancreatitis for pancreatic cancer at this time. However, prospective data, serum, and pancreatic juice should be collected and banked on consenting patients at risk as part of prospective, multicenter trials so that evidence-based recommendations for hereditary pancreatitis and other types of chronic pancreatitis can be made in the future.

INTRODUCTION

Pancreatic cancer remains one of the most deadly and therapeutically resistant cancers faced by mankind. Much of the grim prognosis stems from our relative ignorance of clear risk factors, premalignant states, and tumor biology. Our ignorance, in turn reflects the location of the pancreas, which, until the last decades, has eluded direct or indirect examination except during exploratory surgery, cancer surgery or autopsy. During the past two decades we have witnessed the advent of computed tomography (CT), endoscopic retrograde cholangiopancreatography (ERCP) and other imaging modalities, new molecular biology techniques and more rigorous epidemiological studies. Therefore, new clues are emerging about predisposing risks, possible premalignant lesions, important oncogenes, suppresser genes and other gene, and pancreatic cancer cell biology. Furthermore, new imaging techniques and molecular biological approaches are constantly being developed. But, unfortunately, it is still too early to see the benefit of this new knowledge translated into improved patient survival.

---

[f]Address for correspondence: David C. Whitcomb, MD, PhD, Associate Professor of Medicine, Division of Gastroenterology and Hepatology, 571 Scaife Hall, 3550 Terrace Street, Pittsburgh, PA 15261. Phone, 412/648-7218; fax, 412/383-8913.

Understanding pancreatic cancer biology and cancer prevention strategies have lagged behind other cancer research such as colon cancer because of several major obstacles. In colon cancer, a premalignant lesion, the adenoma, is readily identified on colonoscopy and easily removed by polypectomy. Removing these premalignant lesions results in diminished colon cancer mortality.[1,2] However, in pancreatic cancer the ductal epithelia is remote and generally inaccessible. The only screening technique, ERCP with brushings, introduces several challanges. It is very expensive, relatively invasive, and requires a highly specialized endoscopist, and identifiable abnormalities cannot be removed endoscopically. Furthermore, the clear progression from premalignant lesion to cancer that is recognized in colon cancer has yet to be established for pancreatic cancer. Thus, for example, currently there are no clear prognostic inferences from the finding of k-ras mutations in pancreatic juice. Finally, the current interventions themselves present significant morbidity and mortality, because the dilemma is whether or not to perform a major pancreatic resection rather than the clear decision to perform a polypectomy for preventing colon cancer. On the other hand, late intervention, once pancreatic cancer has become clearly detectable by current imaging techniques, is of little benefit. Because of these obstacles, the early identification of patients at high risk for pancreatic cancer followed by an intervention that clearly saves lives is beyond the current realm medical practice.

RISK FACTORS FOR PANCREATIC CANCER

Many epidemiological studies have been conducted an in attempt to identify dietary and other environmental factors associated with pancreatic cancer.[3] Only minimal risks were identified within the many factors that were examined, and with the exception of cigarette smoking, these trends failed to be confirmed in subsequent studies. The downside of the findings from these efforts was that no consistent predisposing factors could be identified.

CHRONIC PANCREATITIS AND THE RISK OF PANCREATIC CANCER

During the 1980s two small case-control studies noted an increased, albeit non-significant, number of pancreatic cancers among patients with chronic pancreatitis.[4,5] Between 1990 and 1993 three studies noted a small but significantly increased risk of pancreatic cancer in patients with chronic pancreatitis.[6–8]

In 1993 Lowenfels et al.[9] published the results from the International Pancreatitis Study Group's multicenter historical cohort study of 2015 subjects with chronic pancreatitis. These subjects were recruited from clinical centers in six countries. A total of 56 cancers were identified among these patients during a mean follow-up of 7.4 ± 6.2 years. The expected number of cases of pancreatic cancer calculated from country-specific incidence data and adjusted for age and sex was 0.150. For subjects with a minimum of five years of follow-up, the standardized incidence ratio was 14.4. The cumulative risk of pancreatic cancer in subjects with chronic pancreatitis for 10 years was 1.8% and for 20 years 4.0%. Furthermore, the risk of pancreatic cancer was independent of the underlying cause of chronic pancreatitis.

Clearly, the risk of pancreatic cancer in patients with chronic pancreatitis appeared to far exceed any other known risk factor, including cigarette smoking (relative risk from 8 studies varied from 1.2 to 3.1[3]). This finding led to at least 5 additional studies of the risk of pancreatic cancer in patients with chronic pancreatitis.[10–14] Although the estimated risk of pancreatic cancer varied depending on the type of study, all demonstrated a positive association.

HEREDITARY PANCREATITIS AND THE RISK OF PANCREATIC CANCER

The most striking finding has been risk of pancreatic cancer in patients with hereditary pancreatitis. Hereditary pancreatitis was only recognized as a unique disease in 1952.[15] Since then over 100 families have been described world wide.[16,17] Professor DiMagno[18] has pointed out that Comfort and colleagues also described carcinoma of the pancreas associated with chronic elapsing pancreatitis in 1958,[19] and their follow-up of two additional patients included the first documented case of pancreatic cancer in a patient with hereditary pancreatitis. Pancreatic cancer has also been noted in other hereditary pancreatitis kindreds.[20–22] However, the most striking study was that of the International Hereditary Pancreatitis Study Group (IHPSG) headed by Professor Lowenfels.[23] Using surveys sent to the American Pancreatic Association and the International Association of Pancreatology, 37 physicians from 10 countries contributed 245 medical records from patients thought to have hereditary pancreatitis. During the 8531 person-year follow-up, 8 pancreatic adenocarcinomas were identified out of an expected number of 53 yielding a standardized incidence ratio of 0.150. The estimated cumulative risk of pancreatic cancer to age 70 was nearly 40%. Since six of six patients with a known parent-of-origin inherited the disease through the paternal side of the family, the cumulative risk of pancreatic cancer for these patients approximated 75%! Thus, the risk of pancreatic cancer in patients with hereditary pancreatitis appears to be many times higher than the risk of any other factor.

IDENTIFICATION OF THE GENE MUTATION IN HEREDITARY PANCREATITIS

Shortly before completion of the IHPSG study of pancreatic cancer risk in patients with hereditary pancreatitis, we completed a large genetic linkage study[24] and identified the hereditary pancreatitis gene as cationic trypsinogen.[25] The mutation causes an arginine-to-histidine substitution at amino acid residue number 117 (R117H) and results in a mutant trypsin molecule that is resistant to inactivation. We hypothesized that this mutation predisposes affected individuals to episodes of acute pancreatitis during excessive trypsinogen activation within the pancreas at times when activated trypsinogen overwhelms the limited trypsin inhibitory capacity of pancreatic secretory trypsin inhibitor.[25] The active trypsin would then activate all other digestive enzymes, causing acinar cell autodigestion and pancreatitis. Shortly thereafter we identified another mutation in the trypsinogen gene of families without the R117H mutation causing an asparagine-to-isolucine substitution at amino acid residue number 21 (N21I) that resulted in a similar, but slightly less severe phenotype.[26] Thus, most kindreds with hereditary pancreatitis have a mutation in a secreted digestive enzyme expressed in the acinar cell, which is unrelated to the cell type associated with pancreatic cancer. Moreover, mutations in the trypsinogen gene are associated with the highest risk of pancreatic cancer by a log power.

UNANSWERED QUESTIONS

These observations raise a number of important questions. Was the risk of pancreatic cancer in hereditary pancreatitis kindreds overestimated in the IHPSG study because of a selection bias toward the more severely affected patients being seen in a referral center participating in the IHPSG? Are all individuals with trypsinogen R117H mutation at equal risk, or only those who go on to develop chronic pancreatitis? Is the pancreatic cancer typical of sporadic cancers or different in some ways? Does expression of pancreatic cancer require the presence of a germ line oncogene mutation that becomes manifest in the context of hereditary pancreatitis? Should patients with hereditary pancreatitis be screened for pancreatic cancer, and if so, how? Fortunately, several multicenter groups are actively working to answer one or more of these questions.

THE MMPSG HEREDITARY PANCREATITIS STUDY

The Midwest Multicenter Pancreatic Study Group (MMPSG) has continued to expand the number of kindreds initially recruited for mapping and cloning the two known hereditary pancreatitis mutations. As of September 1998 we have tested over 475 individuals and have identified 18 kindreds with cationic trypsinogen R117H mutations, 4 with cationic trypsinogen N21I mutations, and 10 that meet the criteria for hereditary pancreatitis (two or more family members in two or more generations with pancreatitis without identifiable causes) but have neither the cationic trypsinogen R117H or N21I mutations. Additional families meet the criteria for hereditary pancreatitis are undergoing testing and 10 families are incomplete or have a young child with recurrent pancreatitis and uncertain family history (e.g., adopted) and/or very limited family tree. In addition, one child with a suggestive family history who was tested for the cationic trypsinogen R117H mutation because of recurrent pancreatitis was found by her attending physician to have homocystinuria. From these kindreds more than 77 family trees have been constructed. In addition, participating family members were asked through a newsletter whether they, or other family members were diagnosed with pancreatic cancer. To date, 12 pancreatic cancers have been identified in 10 kindreds, and additional cancer cases are being added. Five of the ten families with pancreatic cancer are confirmed hereditary pancreatitis families. In one of the five confirmed families the pancreatic cancer arose from the *unaffected* side of the family.

The current MMPSG Hereditary Pancreatitis Study remains in the recruitment phase. However, because of the importance of the issues being considered at this conference, several preliminary observations have been made. These data are limited in that the hereditary pancreatitis-affected status of many of the individuals within a kindred is based on the data provided by the proband. In other cases, demographic data were unavailable or unattainable. Furthermore, the diagnosis of pancreatic cancer cannot always be made with certainty, because some individuals died years before current diagnostic techniques were available, the diagnosis was ambiguous (e.g., "liver and pancreas cancer"), or the source of cancer or the cause of death is unknown. Therefore, the calculations made below are only rough estimates.

IS THE RISK OF PANCREATIC CANCER IN PATIENTS WITH HEREDITARY PANCREATITIS OVERESTIMATED?

The first question that we asked is whether the risk of pancreatic cancer in patients with hereditary pancreatitis estimated in the IHPSG study[23] was overestimated. In reviewing the cationic trypsinogen R117H mutation-positive kindreds, only 4–6 individuals out of 15 kindreds and more than 200 apparently affected individuals have developed pancreatic cancer. Of these about 100 are over forty years of age. Therefore, as a rough estimate, only about 5% of these individuals at highest risk developed pancreatic cancer. If the risk were associated with having the gene, we would have expected *at least* 12–15 pancreatic cancers in this group. On the other hand, the risk of pancreatic cancer may only be associated with duration of severe chronic pancreatitis. Because of incomplete disease penetrance,[9,24,27] 20% of individuals with the cationic trypsinogen gene R117H mutation are unaffected carriers. Furthermore, only a minority of affected individuals appear to develop significant chronic pancreatitis.[26–28] If one considers that only those with chronic pancreatitis are at risk, then approximately 5 cancers developed in 20–30 individuals at risk. This estimate is well within the confidence intervals calculated in the IHPSG study.[23]

These approximations appear to be internally consistent. Within the cationic trypsinogen R117H mutation kindreds, none of the cancers arose in obligate carriers, and all family members with pancreatic cancer appeared to have prolonged symptoms of hereditary pancreatitis befor pancreatic cancer developed. For example, in the two best characterized cases of pancreatic cancer in families with cationic trypsinogen R117H mutation, the length of time between onset of pancreatitis symptoms and clinical recognition of pancreatic cancer were 33 and 71 years. Likewise, in the IHPSG study, the mean number of years from the onset of symptoms of pancreatitis until diagnosis of pancreatic cancer was 39.6 years.[23] Finally, when we consider the results of the early chronic pancreatitis studies,[6–8] the International Pancreatitis Study Group trial,[9] the IHPSG trial,[23] trials of the risk of pancreatic cancer in tropical pancreatitis,[10] and our own findings, the one consistent risk factor for pancreatic cancer appears to be the duration of chronic pancreatitis. Thus, these preliminary observations suggest that only hereditary pancreatitis family members with *prolonged chronic pancreatitis* are at risk for pancreatic cancer.

IS THE RISK OF PANCREATIC CANCER MUTATION SPECIFIC?

The second observation is that pancreatic cancer occurred in families with cationic trypsinogen R117H, cationic trypsinogen N21I mutations, and in hereditary pancreatitis families that tested negative for both known mutations. Therefore, the occurrence of pancreatic cancer is not mutation specific. This finding also suggests that it is the duration of chronic pancreatitis, rather than the cause that increases the risk of pancreatic cancer.

THE PARENT-OF-ORIGIN EFFECT AND OTHER GERM-LINE MUTATIONS

Third, we are considering the possibility that a second germ line mutation (e.g., an oncogene or tumor suppresser gene) is coinherited in some hereditary pancreatitis kindreds and not others, thereby increasing the risk of pancreatic cancer in selected individuals. This possibility was considered because of the parent-of-origin effect. The parent-of origin effect has been attributed to genetic imprinting. Genetic imprinting is an epigenetic modification of DNA involving the allele-specific methylation of genomic DNA resulting in differential gene expression.[29,30] The earliest methylation-dependent changes in gene expression centered on parent-of-origin diseases such as Prader-Willi syndrome, Angelman syndrome and Beckwith-Wiedemann syndrome.[31] Only a limited number of chromosomal loci are susceptible to this type of imprinting,[29,30] and the trypsinogen gene is not within one of these regions. Since trypsinogen expression is not subject to this type of imprinting, and the trypsinogen gene must be expressed for the disease to be expressed, the paternal parent-of-origin effect cannot be explained by the trypsinogen mutation. Furthermore, if imprinting involves suppression of an oncogene and functional loss of heterozygosity, we might expect to see cancers develop at a young age and for cases of pancreatic cancer to cluster in certain branches of the family tree.

As to the question of cancers clustering within kindreds, to date we have observed 5 cases of pancreatic cancer in the cationic trypsinogen R117H positive kindreds. Of these cancers there was a father-son-affected pair and a father-daughter-affected pair. Thus, the parent-of-origin effect remains unanswered, and pancreatic cancer appears to be related only to the duration of chronic pancreatitis.

SHOULD HEREDITARY PANCREATITIS FAMILY MEMBERS BE SCREENED FOR PANCREATIC CANCER?

The final question is whether the current data should be translated into clinical recommendations and specifically a screening strategy. Certainly, the striking findings of the IHPSG study[23] raised concerns for everyone caring for these families. Should family members be screened for pancreatic cancer? If so, by which technique and how often? What does one do with the results? In the United States and abroad, the high cost of screening must be justified with evidence that clear benefits from screening will be realized. Furthermore, it is recognized that most cancers are inoperable at the time of tumor identification by standard imaging techniques. However, it is the opinion of the authors that no evidence-based recommendations for pancreatic cancer screening can be made at the present time.

THE MMPSG SCREENING STRATEGY

Strategies aimed at the feasibility of screening a high-risk population for the detection of pancreatic cancer at a curable stage were developed by one of the authors (SPM) and were the basis of a consensus position of the MMPSG. Underlying these strategies was the recognition that no accepted screening program exists and that any protocol must be based on a prospective multicenter trial with collection and banking of serum and pancreatic juice for future studies. Potential diagnostic tests (with costs calculated at research rates per test at the University of Cincinnati, July 1998) included: helical CT scan (~$500), ERCP with duct aspirate and/or brushings ($1100), endoscopic ultrasound (EUS) with pancreatic juice from duodenal aspirate ($390) ± fine needle aspiration (FNA) of suspicious lesions, serum tumor markers ($230), pancreatic juice tumor markers ($300), or a combination of these tests. Abdominal ultrasound, magnetic resonance imaging (MRI), and positron emission tomography (PET) were discussed but not given final consideration because of insensitivity, cost and/or general availability.

The cost of screening 72 patients annually for 5 years using, and directly comparing CT, ERCP, EUS, serum and tumor markers is $2520.00 per patient per year for five years costing $907,200.00, with the probability of finding about 4 cancers. Thus, it would cost $226,800 per tumor detected. However, screening with EUS and banking pancreatic juice from duodenal aspirates could be done for ~$400.00 per patient per year for five years costing $144,000. It would therefore cost $36,000 per pancreatic cancer detected. It was reasoned that suspicious lesions would be fully evaluated with health care resources. In addition, experimental imaging techniques (e.g., the combined PET-CT scanner at the University of Pittsburgh) could be used to better define suspicious lesions identified during screening.

The major advantages of EUS considered by the MMPSG include the availability of EUS at each of the MMPSG centers, the ability to obtain pancreatic juice for prospective studies, and the ability to immediately biopsy any suspicious lesions. The major disadvantages include the lower sensitivity in chronic pancreatitis, the unusually operator-dependent nature of the test and potential physician biases toward identification and biopsy of suspicious lesions. Therefore, to minimize variability the data would be collected prospectively according to a standardized protocol and each EUS videotaped for further reference. The pancreatic juice would be banked and retrospectively evaluated in patients who developed pancreatic cancer, using juice from individuals with chronic pancreatitis and two years of pancreatic cancer-free follow-up as disease control and juice from patients without chronic pancreatitis as normal controls. In addition, patients with the most severe and long-standing chronic pancreatitis would be selected to maximize the likelihood of tumor detection during screening. By standardizing this approach and the subsequent results of each patient screened, the MMPSG anticipates that evidence-based recommendations on evaluating and treating patients with long-standing chronic pancreatitis will be forthcoming.

ACKNOWLEDGMENTS

We wish to thank Albert Lowenfels for his assistance on this paper and helpful discussions. This work was supported by Grants Nos. R01DK50236 and R03DK51954 from the National Institutes of Health and by a Veterans Administration Merit Review Award.

REFERENCES

1. MULLER, A.D. & A. SONNENBERG. 1995. Prevention of colorectal cancer by flexible endoscopy and polypectomy: a case-control study of 32,702 veterans. Ann. Intern. Med. **123:** 904–910.
2. SELBY, V.J., G.D. FRIEDMAN, C.P. QUESENBERRY et al. 1992. A case control study of screening sigmoidoscopy and mortality from colorectal cancer. N. Engl. J. Med. **326:** 653–657.
3. GOLD, E.B. 1995. Epidemiology of and risk factors for pancreatic cancer [review]. Surg. Clin. North Am. **75**(5): 819–843.
4. GOLD, E.B., L. GORDIS, M.D. DIENER et al. 1985. Diet and other risk factors for cancer of the pancreas. Cancer **55:** 460–467.
5. MACK, T.M., M.C. YU, R. HANISCH et al. 1986. Pancreas cancer and smoking, beverage consumption and past medical history. J. Natl. Cancer Inst. **76:** 49–60.
6. FARROW, D.C. & S. DAVIS. 1990. Risk of pancreatic cancer in relation to medical history and use of tobacco, alcohol and coffee. Int. J. Cancer **45:** 816–820.
7. JAIN, M., G.R. HOWE, P. ST. LOUIS et al. 1991. Coffee and alcohol as determinants of risk of pancreatic cancer: a case-control study from Toronto. Int. J. Cancer **47:** 384–389.
8. KALAPOTHAKI, V., A. TZONOU, C.C. HSIEH et al. 1993. Tobacco, ethanol, coffee, pancreatitis, diabetes mellitus, and cholelithiasis as risk factors for pancreatic carcinoma. Cancer Causes Control **4:** 1433–1437.
9. LOWENFELS, A.B., P. MAISONNEUVE, G. CAVALLINI et al. 1993. Pancreatitis and the risk of pancreatic cancer. International Pancreatitis Study Group. N. Engl. J. Med. **328**(20): 1433–1437.
10. CHARI, S.T., V. MOHAN, C.S. PITCHUMONI et al. 1994. Risk of pancratic carcinoma in tropical calcifying pancreatitits: an epidemicologic study. Pancreas **9:** 62–66.
11. BANSAL, P. & A. SONNENBERG. 1995. Pancreatitis is a risk factor for pancreatic cancer. Gastroenterology **109:** 247–251.
12. EKBOM, A., J.K. MCLAUGHLIN, B.M. KARLSSON et al. 1994. Pancreatitis and pancreatic cancer: a population-based study. J. Natl. Cancer Inst. **86:** 625–627.
13. FERNANDEZ, E., C. LA VECCHIA, M. PORTA et al. 1995. Pancreatitis and the risk of pancreatic cancer. Pancreas **11:** 185–189.
14. MADEIRA, I., F. PESSIONE, D. MALKA et al. 1998. The risk of pancreatic adenocarcinoma in patients with chronic pancreatitis: myth or reality? Gastroenterology **114:** A481.
15. COMFORT, M. & A. STEINBERG. 1952. Pedigree of a family with hereditary chronic relapsing pancreatitis. Gastroenterology **21:** 54–63.
16. GROSS, J. 1986. Hereditary pancreatitis. *In* The Exocrine Pancreas: Biology, Pathobiology and Diseases. V. Go, Ed.: 829–839. Raven Press. New York.
17. SARLES, H., J. CAMARENA, J.P. BERNARD et al. 1996. Two forms of hereditary chronic pancreatitis. Pancreas **12**(2): 138–141.

18. WHITCOMB, D. 1998. Conference report: the First International Symposium on Hereditry Pancreatitis. Pancreas **18:** 1–12.
19. BARTHOLOMEW, L., J. GROSS & M. COMFORT. 1958. Carcinoma of the pancreas associated with chronic relapsing pancreatitis. Gastroenterology **35:** 473–477.
20. PANDYA, A., S.H. BLANTON, B. LANDA et al. 1996. Linkage studies in a large kindred with hereditary pancreatitis confirms mapping of the gene to a 16-cm region on 7q. Genomics **38**(2): 227–230.
21. MILLER, A.R., D.M. NAGORNEY & M.G. SARR. 1992. The surgical spectrum of hereditary pancreatitis in adults. Ann. Surg. **215**(1): 39–43.
22. KATTWINKEL, J., A. LAPEY, S.A.P. DI et al. 1973. Hereditary pancreatitis: three new kindreds and a critical review of the literature. Pediatrics **51**(1): 55–69.
23. LOWENFELS, A., P. MAISONNEUVE, E. DIMAGNO et al. 1997. Hereditary pancreatitis and the risk of pancreatic cancer. J. Natl. Cancer Inst. **89**(6): 442–446.
24. WHITCOMB, D.C., R.A. PRESTON, C.E. ASTON et al. 1996. A gene for hereditary pancreatitis maps to chromosome 7q35. Gastroenterology **110**(6): 1975–1980.
25. WHITCOMB, D.C., M.C. GORRY, R.A. PRESTON et al. 1996. Hereditary pancreatitis is caused by a mutation in the cationic trypsinogen gene. Nat. Genet. **14**(2): 141–145.
26. GORRY, M., D. GABBAIZADEH, W. FUREY et al. 1997. Multiple mutations in the cationic trypsinogen gene are associated with hereditary pancreatitis. Gastroenterology **113:** 1063–1068.
27. SIBERT, J.R. 1978. Hereditary pancreatitis in England and Wales. J. Med. Genet. **15**(3): 189–201.
28. SOSSENHEIMER, M., C. ASTON, G. EHRLICH et al. 1997. Clinical characteristics of hereditary pancreatitis in a large family based on high-risk haplotype. Am. J. Gastroenterol. **92**(7): 1113–1116.
29. TURKER, M.S. & T.H. BESTOR. 1997. Formation of methylation patterns in the mammalian genome [review]. Mutat. Res. **386**(2): 119–130.
30. YODER, J.A. & T.H. BESTOR. 1996. Genetic analysis of genomic methylation patterns in plants and mammals [review]. J. Biol. Chem. **377**(10): 605–610.
31. LALANDE, M. 1996. Parental imprinting and human disease [review]. Annu. Rev. Genet. **30**(173): 173–195.

Ki-Ras Oncogene Mutations in Chronic Pancreatitis: Which Discriminating Ability for Malignant Potential?

J.L. VAN LAETHEM[a]

Department of Gastroenterology, Erasme University Hospital, Brussels, Belgium

ABSTRACT: Ki-ras mutations are found in the majority of pancreatic adenocarcinomas (85–100%). Ki-ras analysis was increasingly used in ERCP samples in order to differentiate between chronic pancreatitis and pancreatic cancer. However, its sensitivity was recently reported to be low due to a high prevalence of ras mutations in patients with chronic pancreatitis (25–37%). Detection of Ki-ras mutations in microdissected pancreata confirmed their high frequency (55–83%) in pancreatic intraductal lesions (PILs) observed in chronic pancreatitis specimens and in the vicinity of invasive pancreatic carcinoma. There is now molecular evidence that PILs can be precursors of invasive carcinoma, since they can harbor genetic alterations identical to those of the adjacent carcinoma. Similarly, we observed 2 patients with chronic pancreatitis who developed pancreatic cancer 18 and 24 months after the evidence of Ki-ras mutations in pancreatic brushings. However, besides these findings, ras mutations were also identified in nondiseased pancreata coming from autopsy series. The current data on ras analysis in pancreatic juice and brushings or in microdissected pancreata suggest that PILs with Ki-ras mutations do not inevitably lead toward invasive carcinoma. Ki-ras mutations probably have a low discriminating ability for malignant potential and their detection in pancreatic juice is not justified routinely for differentiating between benign and malignant pancreatic diseases. However, prospective follow-up of patients with chronic pancreatitis harboring a mutant ras is probably of major interest by combining the search for other genetic markers that have the ability to characterize patients with the greater risk of malignant transformation.

INTRODUCTION

Ki-ras mutations are found in the vast majority of pancreatic adenocarcinomas, ranging from 85 to 100% of these tumors. These mutations are commonly restricted to the codon 12 and form a "signature" of the disease.[1,2] These results emerged at the end of the nineties and were mainly based on ras analysis on surgically resected specimens of pancreatic adenocarcinomas. In the era of molecular biology, different techniques based on polymerase chain reaction (PCR) analysis were subsequently designed in order to be routinely used for improving the diagnostic approach of ductal adenocarcinoma by detecting codon 12 mutations in pancreatic juice or pancreatic duct brushings collected during endoscopic retrograde cholangio

---

[a]Address for correspondence: J.-L. Van Laethem, MD, PhD, Department of Gastroenterology, Erasme University Hospital, Route de Lennik, 808, B–1070 Brussels, Belgium. Phone, +322-555.37.12; fax, +322-555.46.97; e-mail, jvlaethe@ulb.ac.be

pancreatography (ERCP) or in material obtained by fine needle puncture or in the stool and in the blood.[3–8]

KI-RAS MUTATIONS IN ERCP SAMPLES IN THE DIAGNOSIS OF PANCREATIC DUCTAL ADENOCARCINOMA

In 1995, in a preliminary report, we compared the sensitivity of ras analysis compared to conventional cytological examination. Results based on the study of 40 patients were in favor of the ras analysis, which showed better sensitivity (81 vs 73%), specificity (100 vs 83%) and accuracy (90 vs 58%, $p < 0.01$) as compared to brush cytology.[6] Similar results were reported by other authors who also used ras analysis based on restriction fragment length polymorphism (RFLP).[4,5]

It was therefore tempting to claim that ras analysis in ERCP samples is specific for neoplastic transformation and may help clinicians to differentiate between malignant and benign pancreatic disease.[4–6] In this setting, Ki-ras mutations were basically considered as early markers of malignant changes, as they occur early in the development of neoplastic changes in experimental models of pancreatic ductal carcinogenesis.[9] Nevertheless, this assumption relied only on preliminary results originating from a small number of patients.

We therefore performed a larger study aiming to confirm these promising data.[10] We studied the detection of Ki-ras mtuations in ERCP brushing samples from 125 patients presenting with pancreatic adenocarcinoma ($n = 49$) or chronic pancreatitis ($n = 76$).[10] Ki-ras mutations at codon 12 were found in 78% of our patients with pancreatic cancer, and surprisingly in 25% of our patients with chronic pancreatitis.

By comparison, cytological analysis was positive for malignant cells in 47% of the brushings coming from patients with pancreatic cancer and in 0% of our patients with chronic pancreatitis. Cytology was benign in all brushing samples from our patients with chronic pancreatitis.

The calculated sensitivity of Ki-ras analysis was 81% and therefore better than that of cytological analysis (66%). By contrast, the specificity of Ki-ras analysis was less than that of cytological examination (72 vs 100%). The result was that promising findings regarding ras analysis in differentiating between benign and malignant pancreatic diseases were not confirmed and that conventional cytology remains the gold standard in this type of diagnostic approach.

Therefore, the clinical use of ras analysis from material collected during ERCP is probably not helpful on a routine basis, since the interpretation of the results should be made very cautiously.

KI-RAS MUTATIONS IN CHRONIC PANCREATITIS: WHICH DISCRIMINATING ABILITY FOR MALIGNANT POTENTIAL?

Resulting from the high frequency of Ki-ras mutations found in a population of patients with chronic pancreatitis, the next question will be: is Ki-ras mutation an early marker of malignant transformation or in other terms, should we propose a prompt surgical resection in case we find only a mutant ras in the pancreatic juice without any other evidence of malignancy?

In order to answer this question, an increasing number of studies have focused on the determination of Ki-ras mutations in chronic pancreatitis patients and in pancreatic intraductal lesions (PILs) found in chronic pancreatitis or associated with invasive carcinoma.[11–16]

Chronic pancreatitis may indeed be considered as a premalignant condition on the basis of large epidemiological studies that have shown that these patients have a moderately increased risk of developing pancreatic carcinoma; this risk was evaluated at 2% after 10 years and 4% after 20 years.[17]

Pancreatic intraductal lesions (PILs) have been considered by several authors to be premalignant. They include alterations of cell shape (usually from low cuboidal to tall columnar morphology), differentiation (often from low mucin content to hypermucinous cells) and growth pattern (from a flat single cell layer to a papillary pattern). All these lesions represent deviation from the normal cuboid epithelium and have been categorized as hyperplasia, atypical hyperplasia or dysplasia based on the severity of histological changes.[18–20] Some authors divided these lesions as flat mucous cell hyperplasia, papillary mucous cell hyperplasia and atypical hyperplasia as compared to the normal flat mucosa. For simplification, the noncommittal term PIL (pancreatic intraductal lesion) is currently used to describe any deviation from normal histology of the pancreatic duct epithelium.[21] PILs are frequently seen in pancreatic tissue of patients suffering from chronic pancreatitis, can be encountered in the vicinity of invasive pancreatic adenocarcinoma but can also be observed in nondiseased pancreas. Therefore, it is of major importance to study their molecular profile in order to characterize their malignant potential.

The study of Ki-ras mutations in chronic pancreatitis relies on three different approaches: a) the genetic analysis of pancreatic juice or ductal brushings in patients undergoing ERCP,[3–6,10–12] b) the analysis of surgical specimens without microdissection,[8,13,14] and c) the analysis of pancreatic resection specimen with microdissection in order to focus on intraductal lesions.[8,15,16]

In 1996, our group started a prospective study of patients with chronic pancreatitis without any other evidence of malignancy at the start of the study. Analysis of ras mutations were regularly done in collected ductal brushings during endoscopically therapeutic ERCP performed in these patients for stent exchange or plug extraction. Long-term follow-up is planned in these patients by repeating both ras and cytological analysis every 6–12 months combined with other imaging techniques (e.g., magnetic nuclear resonance and endoultrasonography).

Until now, 76 patients have been enrolled (mean age 48 ± 12 years, range 63 men/ 13 women); the etiology of pancreatitis was alcoholic in 59, idiopathic in 15 and hereditary in 2 of them. Ras mutations were found in 19/76 patients (25%) while cytological examination disclosed benign cells in all patients studied. Ki-ras codon 12 mutations were GAT and GTT in the majority of the cases, quite similar to those found in adenocarcinoma. We did not find any relationship between the presence of mutant ras and the etiology of chronic pancreatitis (alcoholic: 20% of mutant ras, idiopathic: 30%, hereditary: 50%, not significantly different) or the duration of the disease before ras analysis (mean course for mutant ras: 98 ± 79 months; for wild-type ras 73 ± 53 months, not significantly different), the presence of acute attack, the existence of pancreas divisum or the presence of a pancreatic stent.

TABLE 1. Ki-ras mutations in chronic pancreatitis (CP) and pancreatic intraductal lesions (PIL)

Authors ref.	Year	Mutant ras	Specimens
Tada (13)	1991	0/16 (0%)	CP/tissue
Yanagisawa (15)	1993	10/16 (62%)	PIL/micro* CP
Kondo (5)	1994	0/10 (0%)	CP/pancreatic juice
Van Laethem (6)	1995	0/16 (0%)	CP/pancreatic brushing
Iguchi (11)	1996	1/40 (2.5%)	CP/duodenal juice
Tada (22)	1996	12/38 (32%)	PIL/micro^a no pancreatic disease
Moskaluk (21)	1997	18/24 (75%)	PIL/micro^a
Furaya (12)	1997	20/54 (37%)	CP/pancreatic juice
Van Laethem (10)	1998	19/76 (25%)	CP/pancreatic brushing
Gansauge (14)	1998	0/80 (0%)	CP/tisue

^{a}Microdissected specimens.

We have instituted a regular follow-up for 55 of these patients; the mean follow-up was 20 months (range 12–36). They were 12 patients with mutant ras and 43 with wild-type ras. No cancer development was observed within the first period of 6 months. After equivalent periods of follow-up, no pancreatic cancer occurred in the wild-type ras group while in the group harboring mutant ras, and 2 pancreatic cancers were diagnosed after 18 and 24 months of follow-up, emerging from one alcoholic pancreatitis and one idiopathic pancreatitis, respectively (FIG. 1).

Berthelemy *et al.* have observed similar results in their series with two patients developing pancreatic carcinoma 18 and 40 months after the evidence of ras mutations but without any evidence of neoplasia.[4]

By contrast, in a Japanese series of 54 patients, no pancreatic cancer development was observed after a longer mean follow-up of 78 months (range 48–95) in 20/54 patients with chronic pancreatitis harboring a mutant ras.[12]

The report of Ki-ras mutation prevalence in patients with chronic pancreatitis is not definitively achieved, and discordant results have been reported in the literature. TABLE 1 summarizes the different studies reporting the analysis of Ki-ras mutations in chronic pancreatitis and in PIL obtained from ductal samples or resected specimens.

In clinical series assessing the prevalence of Ki-ras mutations in pancreatic juice or brushings, Ki-ras mutations were found in 2.5 to 37% with a percentage of 25 and 37% considering the two larger series.[10,12]

By contrast, results are highly variable with regard to ras analysis in surgical specimens. It clearly appears that the technique of microdissection of pancreatic intraductal lesions is more sensitive than that without microdissection. As an example, Gansauge *et al.* did not find any mutations in ras gene in a series of 80 resected specimens without microdissection, while Ki-ras mutations were consistently found in mucous cell hyperplasia (flat or papillary) with a frequency of 55 to 83% of the mi-

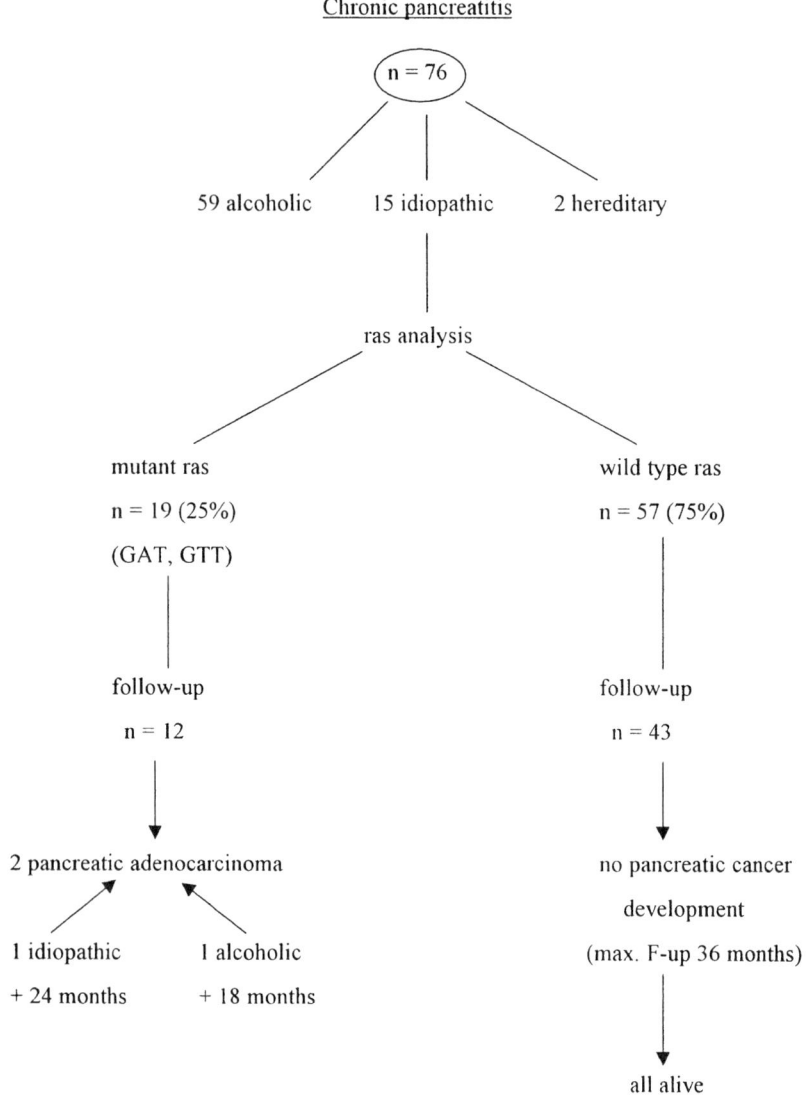

FIGURE 1. Ras analysis in chronic pancreatitis.

crodissected specimens originating from chronic pancreatitis or from the vicinity of infiltrative cancer.[15,16,21] Furthermore, they were highly associated with atypical nuclear features and were more frequent in lesions having a intraductal papillary growth pattern.[21] These conflicting data strongly suggest that the detection of Ki-ras mutations is probably related to the technique used for specimens and DNA collection and furthermore to the technique of ras analysis, which can differ from one study to another.

KI-RAS MUTATIONS IN HYPERPLASTIC DUCT CELLS OF NONDISEASED PANCREAS

Besides the data that support the fact that PILs represent precursor lesions of adenocarcinoma, a provocative study from Tada *et al.* reported the presence of different types of Ki-ras mutations in hyperplastic foci from autopsy samples without pancreatic disease.[22] However, the most frequent mutation types among ductal hyperplasia (i.e., TGT, AGT) were different from those observed in the case of chronic pancreatitis and adenocarcinoma (i.e., GAT, GTT and CGT). Although this report may lead to increase the confusion regarding the role and the relevance of ras mutations in intraductal pancreatic precursor lesions, it clearly questions the ability of ras mutations in discriminating for malignant potential. It also demonstrates that some types of ras mutations are not associated with a malignant potential.

KI-RAS MUTATIONS ASSOCIATED TO p16 GENE ALTERATIONS IN PANCREATIC DISEASES

In search of new genetic markers that might indicate the progression of some pancreatic intraductal lesions toward an invasive phenotype, Moskaluk *et al.* studied mutations at both the Ki-ras and p16 genes within PILs of 10 pancreata resected for adenocarcinoma. Ras mutations were found in all adenocarcinomas studied and in the majority of PILs adjacent to carcinoma. In half the patients, two or more unique Ki-ras mutations were identified among distinct PILs, supporting evidence for the separate clonal evolution of multiple pancreatic neoplasms within individual patients. p16 alterations were found in 4/10 patients; these four pancreata harbored p16 mutations in 3/9 PILs, and two patients had p16 alterations similar to those of the associated carcinomas; p16 mutations were not found in PILs of pancreata with wild-type p16 in the carcinoma, nor were they found in histologically normal ducts.[21]

These findings strongly suggest that PILs can harbor more than one genetic alteration. PILs are precursor lesions to pancreatic adenocarcinoma, but PILs harboring only ras mutations do not inevitably culminate in invasive carcinoma. Ki-ras mutations occur more frequently and earlier than p16 mutations but, as already mentioned, have a low discriminating ability for malignant potential.

CONCLUDING REMARKS AND FUTURE TRENDS

Combining the different approaches of Ki-ras analysis in chronic pancreatitis and PIL, it appears that the interpretation of the results is not easy, either from the clinical or the pathological point of view.

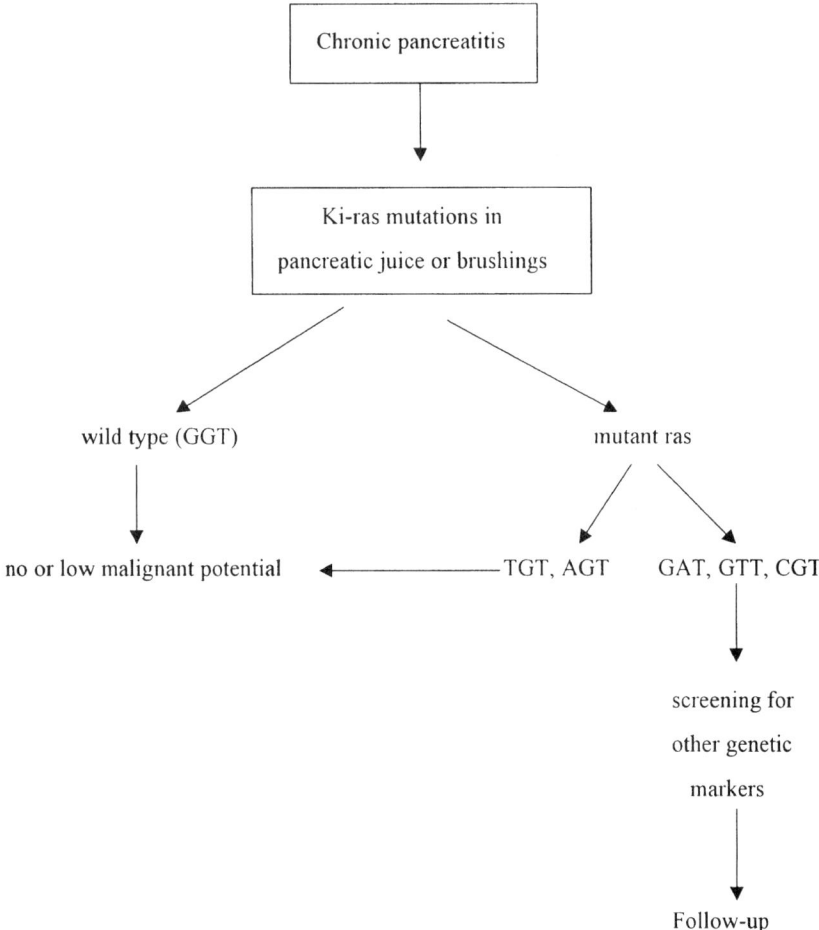

FIGURE 2. Schematic representation of ras analysis in chronic pancreatitis.

Clinically, when chronic pancreatitis is present, finding a mutant ras in pancreatic juice should definitely not be interpreted as the existence of an early cancer, and the relevance of such an analysis in predicting malignant transformation requires further investigation. Patients with mutant ras probably do not require pancreatic resection but need a careful follow-up. In a clinical routine, Ki-ras analysis in pancreatic juice or brushings is probably not justified due to its lack of discriminating potential for differentiating benign and malignant pancreatic disease. Until now, the standard remains conventional cytology, which is less time consuming and more cost effective than ras analysis.

However, ras analysis should be continued in prospective trials aiming to follow large cohorts of patients with chronic pancreatitis. A major question would be to know whether these patients require close follow-up by repeating at regular intervals brush cytology or biopsies using pancreatoscopy. Patients with chronic pancreatitis without mutant ras probably do not carry a risk of malignant transformation. In contrast, chronic pancreatitis with mutant ras might be at higher risk of pancreatic cancer development. Therefore, long-term follow-up studies, such as ours, should be designed to assess the outcome of these patients harboring a mutant ras and the need of repeating investigations. We will be able to determine the incidence of pancreatic cancer development in patients harboring mutant ras within 5 to 10 years and the potential impact, in view of the cost effectiveness of such follow-up, on the survival of these patients.

Ki-ras gene probably does not represent the unique link between chronic pancreatitis and pancreatic cancer. In the future, the study assessment of other genetic markers (e.g., telomerase activity and p16 gene alterations) in pancreatic samples will be able to improve the diagnostic and prognostic approaches of pancreatic neoplasms based on molecular biological methods. Similarly, the detection of ras mutations alone in PILs does not answer the questions about the precursor lesions of pancreatic carcinomas. Molecular analysis is probably better and more sensitive than histology for the identification of the more clinically relevant precursor lesions of pancreatic adenocarcinoma. Therefore, it is of major importance to ascertain other genetic markers that have the ability to characterize PILs harboring the greater risk of malignant transformation. Analogously, identification of these markers in the pancreatic juice of patients with chronic pancreatitis will be of paramount interest, both prospectively and retrospectively in DNA from patients who have developed pancreatic carcinoma (FIG. 2). Combining genetic analysis in microdissected pancreata and pancreatic juice represents the better way to improve our understanding of the sequence of genetic events that occur in pancreatic tumorigenesis and its direct clinical application.

REFERENCES

1. ALMOGUERA, C. et al. 1988. Most human carcinomas of the exocrine pancreas contain c-K ras gene mutations. Cell **53:** 549–554.
2. HRUBAN, R.H. et al. 1993. Ki-ras oncogene activation in adenocarcinoma of the human pancreas: a study of carcinomas using a combination of mutant-enriched polymerase chain reaction analysis and allele-specific oligonucleotide hybridization. Am. J. Pathol. **143:** 545–554.
3. TADA, M. et al. 1993. Detection of ras gene mutations in pancreatic juice and peripheral blood of patients with pancreatic adenocarcinoma. Cancer Res. **53:** 2472–2474.
4. BERTHELEMY, P. et al. 1995. Identification of Ki-ras mutations in pancreatic juice in the early diagnosis of pancreatic cancer. Ann. Intern. Med. **123:** 188–191.
5. KONDO, H. et al. 1994. Detection of point mutations in the Ki-ras oncogene at codon 12 in pure pancreatic juice for diagnosis of pancreatic cancer. Cancer **73:** 1589–1594.
6. VAN LAETHEM, J.L. et al. 1995. Detection of c-Ki-ras gene codon 12 mutations from pancreatic duct brushings in the diagnosis of pancreatic tumours. Gut **36:** 781–787.
7. SHIBATA, D. et al. 1990. Detection of c-Ki-ras mutations in fine needle aspirates from human pancreatic adenocarcinomas. Cancer Res. **50:** 1279–1283.
8. CALDAS, C. et al. 1994. Detection of K-ras mutations in the stool of patients with pancreatic adenocarcinoma and pancreatic ductal hyperplasia. Cancer Res. **54:** 3568–3573.
9. CERNY, W.L. et al. 1992. Ki-ras mutations in an early event in pancreatic duct carcinogenesis in the Syrian golden hamster. Cancer Res. **52:** 4507–4513.

10. VAN LAETHEM, J.L. et al. 1998. Relative contribution of Ki-ras gene analysis and brush cytology during ERCP for the diagnosis of biliary and pancreatic diseases. Gastrointest. Endosc. **47:** 479–485.
11. IGUSHI, H. et al. 1996. Analysis of Ki-ras codon 12 mutations in the duodenal juice of patients with pancreatic cancer. Gastroenterology **110:** 221–226.
12. FURAYA, N. et al. 1997. Long-term follow-up of patients with chronic pancreatitis and Ki-ras gene mutation detected in pancreatic juice. Gastroenterology **113:** 593–598.
13. TADA, M. et al. 1991. Clinical application of ras gene mutation for diagnosis of pancreatic adenocarcinoma. Gastroenterology **100:** 233–238.
14. GANSAUGE, S. et al. 1998. Genetic alterations in chronic pancreatitis: evidence for early occurrence of p53 but not K-ras mutations. Br. J. Surg. **85:** 337–340.
15. YANASIGAWA, A. et al. 1993. Frequent c-Ki-ras oncogene activation in mucous cell hyperplasias of pancreas suffering from chronic pancreatitis. Cancer Res. **53:** 953–956.
16. RIVERA, J. et al. 1997. Analysis of Ki-ras oncogene mutations in chronic pancreatitis with ductal hyperplasia. Surgery **121:** 42–49.
17. LOWENFELS, A.B. et al. 1993. Pancreatitis and the risk of pancreatic cancer. N. Engl. J. Med. **328:** 1433–1437.
18. CUBILLA, A. et al. 1976. Morphological lesions associated with human primary invasive nonendocrine pancreas cancer. Cancer Res. **36:** 2690–2698.
19. KLÖPPEL, G. et al. 1980. Intraductal proliferation in the pancreas and its relationship to human and experimental carcinogenesis. Virchows Arch. A Pathol. Anat. Histol. **387:** 221–233.
20. POUR, P. et al. 1982. Hyperplastic, preoplastic and neoplastic lesions found in 83 human pancreases. Am. J. Clin. Pathol. **77:** 137–152.
21. MOSKALUK, C.A. et al. 1997. p16 and K-ras gene mutations in the intraductal precursors of human pancreatic adenocarcinoma. Cancer Res. **57:** 2140–2143.
22. TADA, M. et al. 1996. Analysis of K-ras gene mutation in hyperplastic duct cells of the pancreas without pancreatic disease. Gastroenterology **110:** 227–231.

Acinar-Ductal-Carcinoma Sequence in Transforming Growth Factor-α Transgenic Mice

ROLAND M. SCHMID,[a,c] GÜNTHER KLÖPPEL,[b] GUIDO ADLER,[a] AND MARTIN WAGNER[a]

[a]*Department of Internal Medicine I, University of Ulm, 89081 Ulm, Germany*
[b]*Department of Pathology, University of Kiel, 24105 Kiel, Germany*

ABSTRACT: Transgenic mice overexpressing transforming growth factor-α (TGF-α) display an expansion of intrapancreatic fibroblasts and a progressive accumulation of extracellular matrix. This massive fibrosis is associated with an increase in pancreatic size and weight. In parallel, tubular complexes appear that are composed of acinar cells with a decreased height. These acinar cells lose zymogen granules and become transitional cells, which subsequently gain duct cell features. In animals older than one year dysplastic lesions develop, which originate from tubular complexes. Occasionally these dysplastic foci transform to papillary and cystic pancreatic carcinoma. These tumors are positive for the duct-specific antigen Duct-1 and carbonic anhydrase activity indicative of ductal differentiation. Tumors overexpress the epidermal growth factor (EGF)-receptor and p53, but lack K-ras mutations. These data suggest an acinar-ductal-carcinoma sequence in TGF-α transgenic mice.

INTRODUCTION

The pancreas consists of acinar, ductal and endocrine cells and is a mitotically quiescent tissue that is highly differentiated. Malignant transformation can occur in all cell types. However, more than 90% of pancreatic carcinomas in humans appear to arise in the exocrine pancreas. It is generally believed that the adenocarcinoma in the human pancreas is of ductal origin and is formed by a muco-protein-secreting cell type.[1–4] Recent advances have been made in defining the molecular basis of pancreatic cancer. Several studies indicate that K-ras gene mutations at codon 12 seem to occur at an early stage of the neoplasm.[5–7] K-ras gene mutations can be detected even in mucinous hyperplasia of the pancreatic duct appearing in association with chronic pancreatitis and in intraductal neoplasia, which are considered as potentially precancerous lesions of ductal carcinoma.[8,9] The second most frequent alterations in pancreatic neoplasms are found in the tumor suppressor gene p16/MTS1.[9–11] An inactivation of one p16 allele can already be detected in noninvasive pancreatic intraductal lesions.[9] The tumor suppressor gene p53 is inactivated with a prevalence between 40 and 60%.[12–15] The inactivation of p53 is associated with a more

---

[c]Address for correspondence: Roland M. Schmid, MD, Department of Internal Medicine I, University of Ulm, Robert-Koch-Str. 8, 89081 Ulm, Germany. Phone, +49 731-50-24305; fax, +49 731-50-24302; e-mail, roland.schmid@medizin.uni-ulm.de

advanced tumor stage and local lymph node involvement, suggesting that p53 mutations are relatively late events in pancreatic carcinogenesis.[15,16] Recently, frequent homozygous deletions and inactivating mutations accompanying loss of heterozygosity (LOH) have been found in the candidate tumor suppressor gene DPC4 (deleted in pancreatic cancer, Smad4).[17] In a limited number of studies DCC (deleted in colon cancer) and APC (adenomatosis polyposis coli) gene mutations have been reported in pancreatic neoplasms.[18,19] These data suggest that these genes may play a potential role in the pathogenesis of pancreatic cancer.

In addition to structural genetic events, the overexpression of growth factors and growth factor receptors is present in a significant number of tumors.[20] The epidermal growth factor (EGF)-receptor, EGF, and transforming growth factor-α (TGF-α) mRNAs and proteins are overexpressed in pancreatic cancer.[21–24] The overexpression of this receptor-ligand system correlates with advanced disease and a worse prognosis, indicating that this signaling cascade plays a significant role in the growth and malignant transformation of pancreatic cells.[24] Furthermore, TGF-α is overexpressed together with the EGF receptor in several human pancreatic ductal carcinoma cell lines, suggesting the existence of an autocrine pathway in the pathogenesis of transformation.[25] TGF-α is more potent than EGF in stimulating anchorage-independent growth of human pancreatic cancer cell lines. An altered acinar cell differentiation has been determined *in vivo* in transgenic mice overexpressing TGF-α. However, the role of TGF-α in the development of pancreatic carcinoma remains unclear.[26,27]

In the present study we present evidence that in TGF-α transgenic mice acinar cells transdifferentiate to duct-like cells within tubular complexes. The latter transform to pancreatic carcinoma significantly more frequently compared to littermate controls. These transformed cells express Duct-1, a duct-specific marker, and are strongly positive for carbonic anhydrase activity. Tumors overexpress the EGF receptor and display strong nuclear staining for p53. However, they lack K-ras mutations. This established for the first time an acinar-ductal-carcinoma sequence in this animal model. Further studies will be needed to define genetic events in tumor progression, since tumor formation is a rather late event and not obligatory in these mice.

MATERIALS AND METHODS

Transgenic Mice

The transgenic mice used in this study have been described previously.[26,28] Mice were maintained as heterozygotes on a BL/6 genetic background. Expression of TGF-α was verified by slot blot analysis.

Gross and Histopathology

Mice were sacrificed at defined ages or when signs of wasting occurred and examined for gross lesions. Pancreata were fixed in 4% paraformaldehyde, embedded in paraffin, sectioned at 4 µM, stained with hematoxylin and eosin, and examined to determine histopathological diagnosis.

Electronmicroscopy

For transmission electron microscopy specimens of the pancreas was fixed by immersion in a mixture of 2% glutaraldehyde and 2% formaldehyde in 0.1 M cacodylate buffer at pH 7.4. After postfixation in 1% osmium tetroxide and standard dehydration, tissue samples were embedded in Epon 812. Thin sections were contrasted with uranyl acetate and lead citrate and examined using a Zeiss EM 10 electron microscope (Zeiss, Oberkochen, Germany).

Immunohistochemistry

Immunohistochemistry was performed as described previously.[28] In brief, frozen sections were airdried and fixed using acetone at −20°C. The antibody Duct-1 (generously provided by R.C. De Listle, Department of Anatomy and Cell Biology, University of Kansas[29]) was used 1:1. Anti-EGF receptor (Santa Cruz Biotechnology, Inc. Santa Cruz, CA) and anti-amylase (Dako, Hamburg, Germany) were used in a 1:250 and 1:100 dilution. Anti-p53 was a gift of W. Deppert, Heinrich-Pette-Institute for Experimental Virology and Immunology, University of Hamburg and used at 1:2000. Signals were visualized with a biotinylated secondary antibody using 3,3'-diaminobenzidine (DAB). Sections were counterstained with hematoxylin.

Carbonic Anhydrase Activity

Carbonic anhydrase activity was detected as described.[30] In brief, frozen sections were repeatedly dipped in a solution of $CoSO_4$ 8.75 mM, KH_2PO_4 5.8 mM, $NaHCO_3$ 157 mM, Triton X-100 0.5% and H_2SO_4 53 mM followed by amonium sulfide solution, washed and counterstained with nuclear fast red. Negative controls were carried out with acetazolamide in the staining solution.

Analysis of K-ras Mutations at Codon 12

The polymerase chain reaction (PCR) assay was performed as earlier described.[28] Tumor DNA was isolated using the QUIamp tissue kit (Quiogen, Hilden, Germany). Mouse K-ras was amplified with primers mK-ras 5': A C T G A G T A T A A A C T T G T G G T G G T T G G A C C T, and mK-ras 3'WT: T A T C T T T T T C A A A G C G G C T G G C T G. After the first round of PCR an aliquot of the amplified product was digested with BstNI (New England Biolabs, Beverly, MA) and subjected to a second round of amplification using primers mK-ras 5' and mK-ras 3'mut: T A T C T T T T T C A A A G C G C C T G G C T G. The amplified products were digested with BstNI, separated on a 4% agarose gel (NuSieve GTG, FCM, Rockland, ME) and stained with ethidium bromide. Wild-type mK-ras is represented as a 114-base pair, while mK-ras mutated in codon 12 results in a 144-base pair fragment. DNA from mouse tails and NIH3T3 cells served as negative, and mutated genomic fragments of mK-ras as positive control.

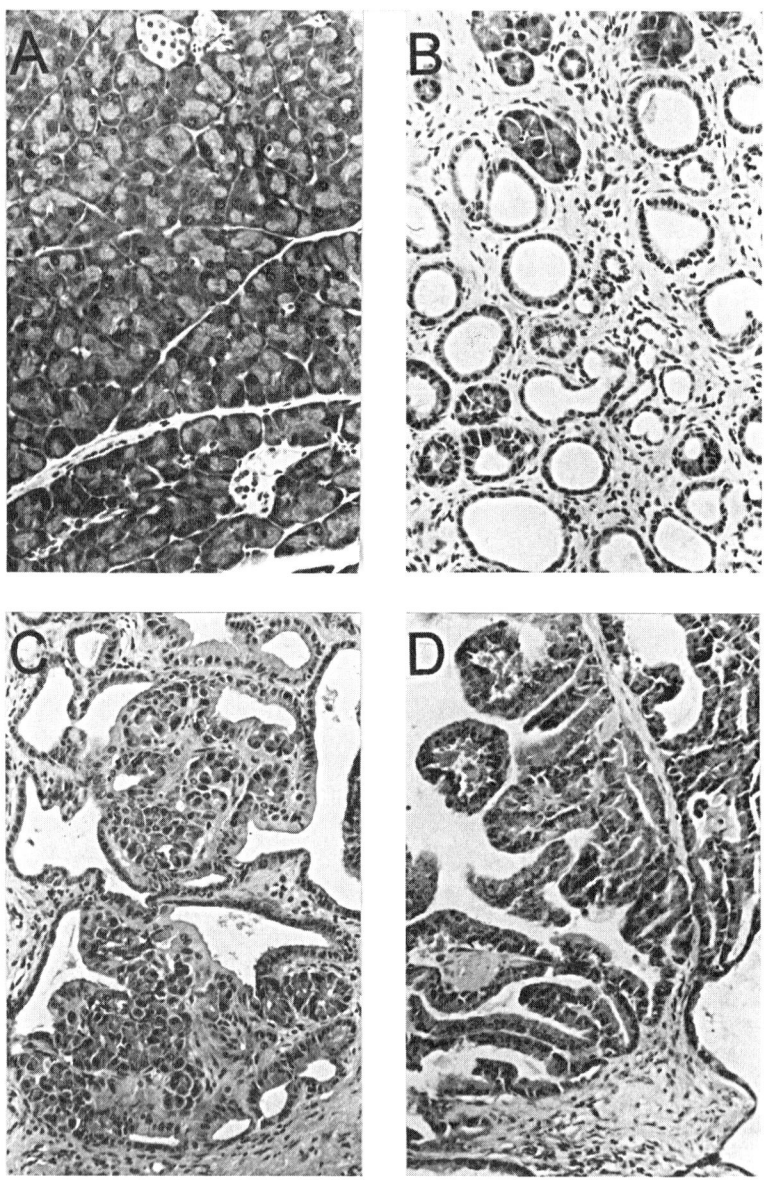

FIGURE 1. Development of fibrosis, tubular complexes, dysplasia and transformation. Wild-type littermate controls show a regular acinar morphology (**A**), whereas TGF-α transgenic mice develop massive pancreatic fibrosis and tubular complexes (**B**). In older animals dysplastic changes occur within tubular complexes (**C**), which occasionally transform to papillary and cystic tumors (**D**). Original magnification 50×.

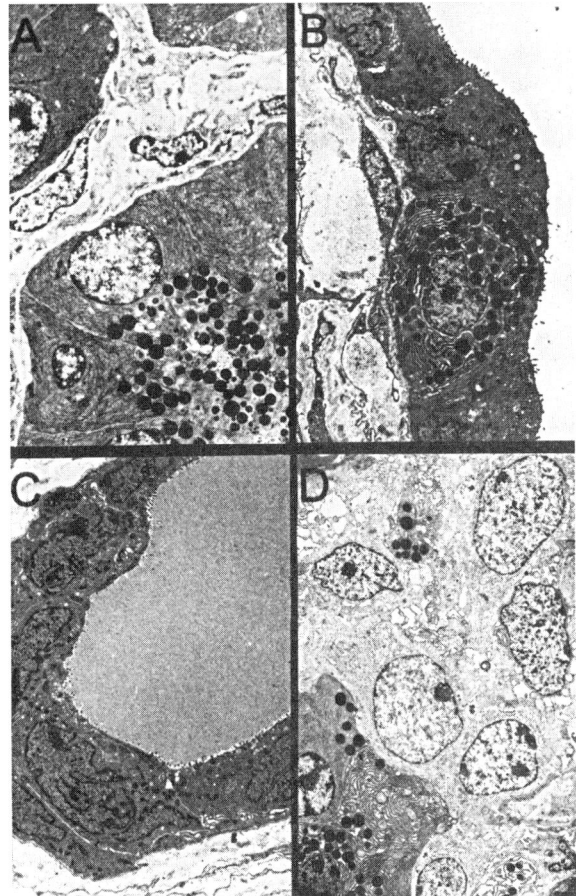

FIGURE 2. Electronmicroscopy of tubular complexes and pancreatic tumors. At day 28 **(A)** decreased acinar cell height with heterogeneous zymogen granules are evident as first changes in acinar morphology in early tubular complexes. At day 180 few cells retained an acinar differentiation, **(B)** while most cells show ductal characteristics like basal tight junctions and mucin granules **(C)**. Tumor cells display altered nuclei as well as vacuolized and dilated endoplasmatic reticulum **(D)**. Original magnification is 2000× (A, B, C) and 1600× (D).

RESULTS

Development of Fibrosis, Tubular Complexes, Dysplasia and Transformation

TGF-α transgenic mice develop a massive enlarged pancreas starting at day 7. Enlargement is due to an excessive fibrosis and matrix accumulation compared to littermate controls (FIG. 1A,B). In addition, an altered acinar differentiation can be observed already at day 14. The first sign of this alteration is a decreased acinar cell height leaving an enlarged acinar lumen. The progression of these changes results in the formation of tubular complexes that are composed of branching and anastomosing tubules with various diameters. The changes are not uniform; areas with these duct-like structures are mixed with areas of unaltered acini (FIG. 1B). In mice older than 270 days we found changes suggestive of dysplasia within tubular complexes (FIG. 1C). The progression of these lesions results in malignant tumors with a papillary cystic phenotype. These tumors occur at multiple foci and show invasive growth characteristics (FIG. 1D).

Electronmicroscopy of Tubular Complexes and Pancreatic Tumors

Electronmicroscopy revealed heterogeneous zymogen granules as well as a total decrease in their number already at day 28 (FIG. 2A). Nuclei were relocated towards the basal membrane. Altered acini gained characteristics of a duct-cell phenotype including basal tight junctions and mucin granules (FIG. 2B). Thus, formation of tubular complexes seems to be a transdifferentiation rather than a dedifferentiation. Tubular complexes in 180-day-old animals appear as structures composed of duct-like cells mixed with cells with acinar characteristics as well as structures composed only of duct-like cells (FIG. 2B,C). Tumor cells display a marked nuclear polymorphism and an increased number of nucleoli. The endoplasmatic reticulum appears dilated and shows vacuolization (FIG. 2D).

Expression of Ductal and Acinar Markers in the Tubular Complexes

Tubular complexes continuously lose expression of acinar markers as shown for amylase (FIG. 3A,B). However, even in 180-day-old animals, cells positive for amylase are present in the tubular complexes (FIG. 3B). This is paralleled by a neoexpression of duct-specific markers as carbonic anhydrase activity (FIG. 3C,D). During the process of transdifferentiation intermediate cells express amylase and display carbonic anhydrase activity.

Expression of Ductal Markers, the EGF Receptor and p53 in Pancreatic Tumors of TGF-α Transgenic Mice

Evidence for a ductal differentiation of tumors is supported by strong carbonic anhydrase activity and the expression of the duct-specific marker Duct-1 (FIG. 4A,B). To investigate whether tumor formation is associated with an autocrine stimulation, we stained tumors with anti-EGF receptor antibodies. Tubular complexes as well as all tumors analyzed are strongly positive for EGF receptor immunoreactivity (FIG. 4C and data not shown). The potential role of p53 in the process of transdifferentiation and transformation is suggested by a strong nuclear immunoreactivity for p53 in tubular complexes as well as in the tumors (FIG. 4D and data not shown).

Tumors Lack K-ras Gene Mutations

Since K-ras gene mutations are frequently detected in human pancreatic cancer, we developed an enriched PCR approach for murine K-ras.[28] Using this assay we are

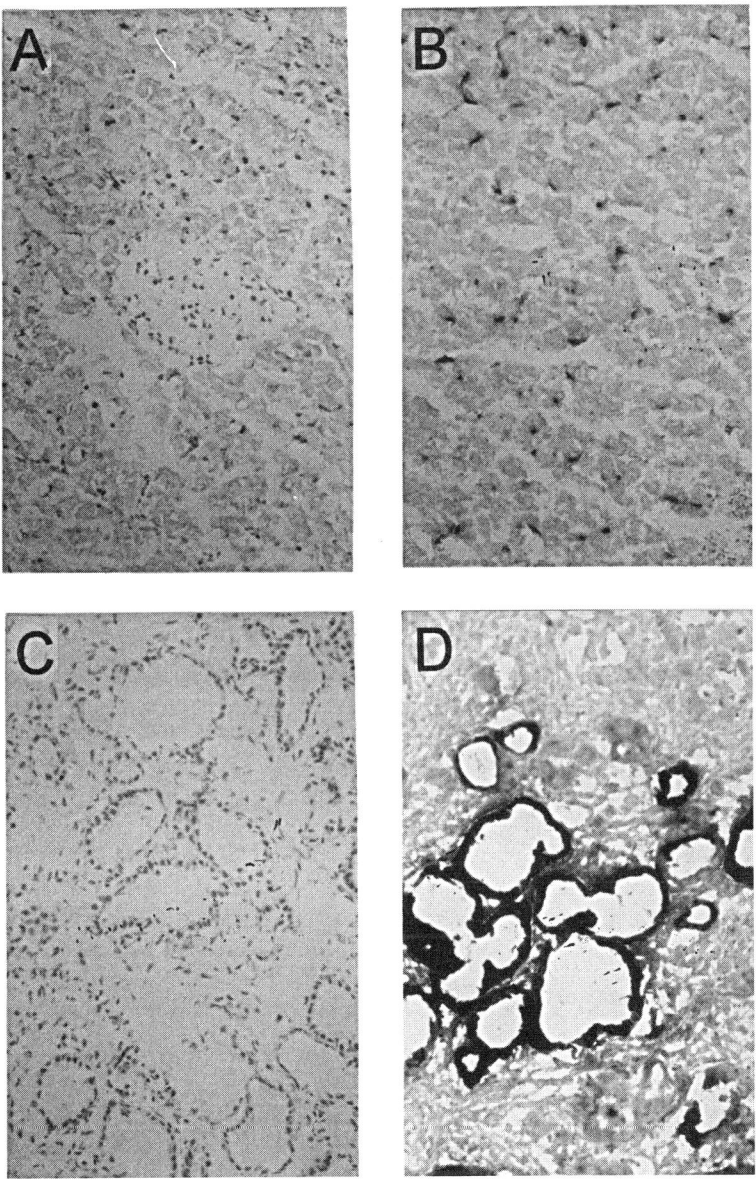

FIGURE 3. Expression of amylase and carbonic anhydrase activity. Wild-type animals show regular immunoreactivity for amylase (**A**), and carbonic anhydrase activity is restricted to the centroacinar region and small ducts (**B**). Tubular complexes lose expression of amylase (**C**) and gain activity of carbonic anhydrase (**D**). Original magnification 50×.

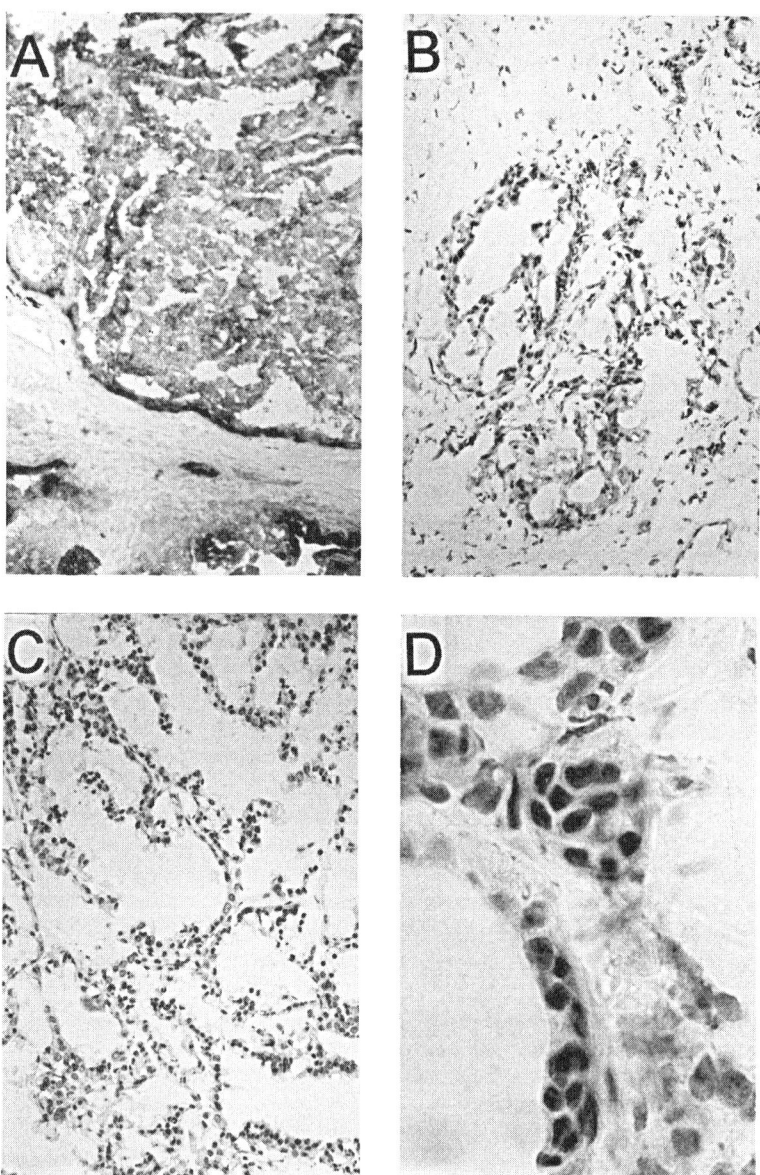

FIGURE 4. Tumors express ductal markers, the EGF receptor and stain for p53. Pancreatic tumors are highly positive for carbonic anhydrase activity (**A**) and show immunoreactivity for Duct-1 (**B**). The EGF receptor is highly expressed in tumor cells (**C**). Multiple foci within tumors show strong nuclear staining for p53 (C). Original magnification 50×.

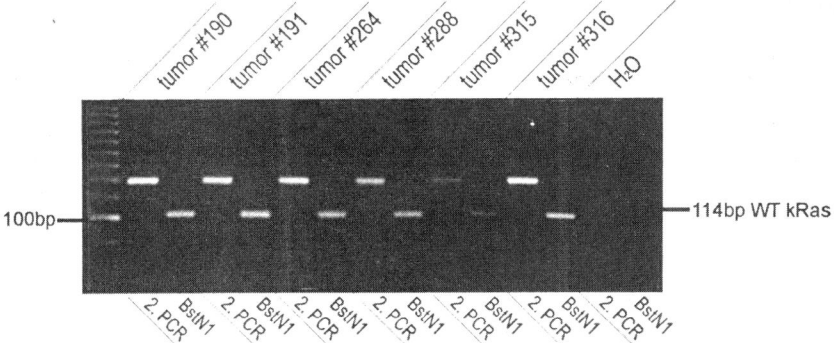

FIGURE 5. K-ras analysis. Genomic DNA was extracted from pancreatic tumors and subjected to two rounds of PCR amplification. The amplified products are loaded before and after BstNI digestion. Only the 114-base pair band indicative of wild-type K-ras can be detected in all samples analyzed.

able to detect one pg in codon 12 mutated K-ras in 50 ng wild-type genomic DNA (data not shown). All tumors analyzed were negative for K-ras mutations in codon 12 (FIG. 5).

DISCUSSION

Mice that overexpress TGF-α in the pancreas show massive fibrosis and a formation of tubular complexes. These tubular structures are composed of flattened acinar cells, which display an intermediate phenotype of acinar and ductal cells. These transitional forms between acinar and ductal cells contain a mixture of granules including dense zymogen granules and lighter granules characteristic of mucin granules. In older animals, almost all cells within tubular complexes lose ultrastructural criteria for acinar cells and gain duct cell features.[31] Occasionally cells within these tubular complexes progress towards a malignant phenotype.[28] Tumors express ductal markers like Duct-1 and are positive for carbonic anhydrase activity suggesting an acinar-ductal-carcinoma sequence in TGF-α transgenic mice.

This raises the question of the very earliest lesions of pancreatic cancer, and in particular, the cell of origin of this neoplasm. There are several different possibilities: Pancreatic cancers arise from (1) duct cells, (2) an undifferentiated stem cell, or (3) centroacinar cells, or (4) there is the possibility that acinar cells retro- or transdifferentiate.

The first possibility is based on the fact that pancreatic carcinomas usually have a ductal phenotype and show no evidence of acinar cell characteristics. Consequently, an origin from normal ductal epithelium has been proposed. In addition, several authors have identified "early lesions" in ducts of the human pancreas.[1–4,32] These ductal lesions include papillary structures lined with cuboidal, mucin-producing cells displaying various dysplastic changes ranging from hyperplasia to carcinoma *in situ*. These duct lesions have been proposed to be the early precursors of pancreatic cancer. The presence of K-ras gene mutations in these lesions supports this hypothesis.[8]

While it is clear that the pancreas originally develops from an undifferentiated duct cell-like progenitor or "stem" cell, the evidence for a stem cell in the adult pancreas is far from being established. The duct cell compartment appears to be the most likely location of the putative stem cells. Only duct cells have been shown to be able to give rise to endocrine cells.[33] Additional evidence supporting the presence of stem cells in the adult pancreas is the capacity of the adult pancreas to regenerate to a modest extent after partial pancreatectomy.[34] This regeneration involves a greater proliferation of insulin cells than of exocrine cells.[35] Since the evidence for the existence of a stem cell in the mature pancreas is only indirect, the hypothesis that pancreatic cancer might originate from such a cell has to remain speculative.

Ultrastructural studies suggest that the earliest lesions in a hamster cancer model involve the centroacinar cells or cells of acinar origin.[36,37] In this model there is evidence that centroacinar cells are the origin for tubular formations. Early neoplastic features are hypertrophy and hyperplasia of centroacinar cells, which form initially tiny and long processes that overlie and underlie the adjacent acinar cells.[37]

In this study we present evidence that acinar cells are the primary site of origin of pancreatic neoplasms in TGF-α transgenic mice. Acinar cells lose zymogen granules and become transitional cells, which subsequently gain duct cell features. In animals older than one year, dysplastic lesions develop, which subsequently transform. In the hamster model a gradual transformation of acinar cells, which lose their apical cytoplasmic portion and zymogen granules is not observed, indicating that the formation of tubular complexes may be different compared to TGF-α overexpressing mice. However, both models provide support for the hypothesis that acinar cells may represent the target population for carcinogenic events in the pancreas. Furthermore, acinar cell hyperplasia has been described in the human pancreas.[38]

In the hamster model mutated K-ras at codon 12 and 13 has been demonstrated and suggested to occur early and may even be the initiating event in this model.[39] Using a PCR-based approach, we were unable to detect K-ras gene mutations in codon 12 in tumors of TGF-α overexpressing mice. We speculate that the overexpression of TGF-α bypasses the need for the activation of K-Ras by mutation and propose that the K-Ras signaling cascade is already maximally activated. Interestingly, the EGF receptor is overexpressed in these tumors, generating an autocrine loop, a feature that is somewhat similar to that reported in humans.[20,22–25]

To screen for alterations that exert a positive selection upon tumor cells, we stained tumor tissue with anti-p53. Tumors in TGF-α transgenic mice show high expression of nuclear p53, which is suggestive of p53 mutations. In normal tissue wild-type p53 protein is difficult to detect, whereas missense mutations of p53 lead to the formation of an abnormal protein product with a prolonged half-life and accumulation of mutant protein in the neoplastic cells.

In summary, the data presented provide strong support for an acinar-ductal-carcinoma sequence in TGF-α transgenic mice, suggesting that the overexpression of TGF-α plays a crucial role in the formation of pancreatic tumors. The precise mechanisms that underlie this transformation process have to be determined.

ACKNOWLEDGMENTS

We are indebted to Elke Wolff-Hieber and Hardi Lührs for technical assistance. We would like to thank Sonja Aigner for assistance with manuscript preparation. This work was in part supported by grant from the Bundesministerium für Bildung und Forschung, IZKF, C4, to Roland M. Schmid and from the Deutsche Forschungsgemeinschaft, Kn 200/4-4, to Guido Adler.

REFERENCES

1. SOMMERS, S.C., S.A. MURPHY, S. WARREN et al. 1954. Pancreatic duct hyperplasia and cancer. Gastroenterology **27:** 629–640.
2. CUBILLA, A.L. & P.J. FITZGERALD. 1975. Morphologial patterns of primary nonendocrine human pancreatic carcinoma. Cancer Res. **35:** 2234–2248.
3. KLÖPPEL, G., G. BOMMER, K. RÜCKERT et al. 1980. Intraductal proliferation in the pancreas and its relationship to human and experimental carcinogenesis. Virchows Arch. A **387:** 221–223.
4. KOZUKA, S., R. SASSA, T. TAKI et al. 1979. Relation of pancreatic duct hyperplasia to carcinoma. Cancer **43:** 1418–1428.
5. ALMOGUERA, C., D. SHIBATA, K. FORRESTER et al. 1988. Most human carcinomas of the exocrine pancreas contain mutant c-K-*ras* genes. Cell **53:** 549–554.
6. SMIT, V.T.H.B.M., A.J.M. BOOT, A.M.M. SMITS et al. 1988. KRAS codon 12 mutations occur very frequently in pancreatic adenocarcinomas. Nucleic Acid Res. **16:** 7773–7782.
7. GRÜNEWALD, K., J. LYONS & A. FRÖHLICH et al. 1989. High frequency of Ki-*ras* codon 12 mutations in pancreatic adenocarcinomas. Int. J. Cancer **43:** 1037–1041.
8. YANAGISAMA, A., K. OHTAKE, K. OHASHI et al. 1993. Frequent c-Ki-ras oncogene activation in mucous cell hyperplasias of pancreas suffering from chronic pancreatitis. Cancer Res. **53:** 953–956.
9. MOSKALUK, C.A., R.H. HRUBAN & S.E. KERN. 1997. p16 and K-ras gene mutations in the intraductal precursors of human pancreatic adenocarcinoma. Cancer Res. **57:** 2140–2143.
10. CALDAS, C., S.A. HAHN, L.T. DA COSTA et al. 1994. Frequent somatic mutations and homozygous deletions of the p16 (MTS1) gene in pancreatic adenocarcinoma. Nat. Genet. **8:** 27–32.
11. NAUMANN, M., N. SAVITSKAIA, C. EILERT et al. 1996. Frequent codeletion of *p16/MTS1* and *p15/MTS2* and genetic alterations in *p16/MTS1* in pancreatic tumors. Gastroenterology **110:** 1215–1224.
12. BARTON, C.M., S.L. STADDON, C.M. HUGHES et al. 1991. Abnormalities of the p53 tumor suppressor gene in human pancreatic cancer. Br. J. Cancer **64:** 1076–1082.
13. RUGGERI, B., S.Y. ZHANG, J. CAAMANO et al. 1992. Human pancreatic carcinomas and cell lines reveal frequent and multiple alterations in the p53 and Rb-1 tumour suppressor genes. Oncogene **7:** 1503–1511.
14. SCARPA, A., P. CAPELLI, K. MUKAI et al. 1993. Pancreatic adenocarcinomas frequently show p53 gene mutations. Am. J. Pathol. **142:** 1534–1543.
15. PELLEGATA, N.S., F. SESSA, B. RENAULT et al. 1994. K-*ras* and p53 gene mutations in pancreatic cancer: ductal and nonductal tumors progress through different genetic lesions. Cancer Res. **54:** 1556–1560.
16. YOKOYAMA, M., Y. YAMANAKA, H. FRIESS et al. 1994. p53 expression in human pancreatic cancer correlates with enhanced biological aggressiveness. Anticancer Res. **14:** 2477–2484.
17. HAHN, S., A. SCHÜTTE, M. HOGQUE et al. 1996. DPC4, a candidate tumor suppressor gene at human chromosome 18q21.1. Science **271:** 350–353.

18. HÖHNE, M.W., M.-E. HALATSCH, G.F. KAHL et al. 1992. Frequent loss of expression of the potential tumor suppressor gene DCC in ductal pancreatic adenocarcinoma. Cancer Res. **52:** 2616–2619.
19. HORII, A., S. NAKATSURU, Y. MIYOSHI et al. 1992. Frequent somatic mutations of the APC gene in human pancreatic cancer. Cancer Res. **52:** 6696–6698.
20. FRIESS, H., P. BERBERAT. M. SCHILLING et al. 1996. Pancreatic cancer: the potential clinical relevance of alterations in growth factors and their receptors. J. Mol. Med. **74:** 35–42.
21. BARTON, C.M., P.A. HALL & C.M. HUGHES. 1991. TGF-α and EGF in human pancreatic cancer. J. Pathol. **163:** 111–116.
22. LEMOINE, N.R., C.M. HUGES & C.M. BARTON. 1992. The epidermal growth factor receptor in human pancreatic cancer. J. Pathol. **166:** 7–12.
23. KORC, M., B. CHANDRASEKAR, Y. YAMANAKA et al. 1992. Overexpression of the epiermal growth factor receptor in human pancreatic cancer is associated with concomitant increase in the levels of epidermal growth factor and transforming growth factor alpha. J. Clin. Invest. **90:** 1352–1360.
24. YAMANAKA, Y., H. FRIESS, M.S. KOBRIN et al. 1993. Coexpression of epidermal growth factor receptor and ligands in human pancreatic cancer is associated with enhanced tumor aggressivenes. Anticancer Res. **13:** 565–570.
25. SMITH, J.J., R. DERYNCK & M. KORC. 1987. Production of transforming growth factor in human pancreatic cancer cells: evidence for a superagonist autocrine cycle. Proc. Natl. Acad. Sci. USA **84:** 7567–7570.
26. SANDGREN, E.P., N.C. LUETTEKE & R.D. PALMITER. 1990. Overexpression of TGF-α in transgenic mice: induction of epithelial hyperplasia, pancreatic metaplasia, and carcinoma on the breast. Cell **61:** 1121–1135.
27. JHAPPAN, C., C. STAHLE, R.N. HARKINS et al. 1990. TGF-α overexpression in transgenic mice induces liver neoplasia and abnormal development of the mammary gland and pancreas. Cell **61:** 1137–1146.
28. WAGNER, M., H. LÜHRS, G. KLÖPPEL et al. 1998. Malignant transformation of ductlike cells originating from acini in mice overexpressing transforming growth factor α in the exocrine pancreas. Gastroenterology **115:** 1254–1262.
29. DE LISTLE, B.C. & C.D. LOGSDON. 1990. Pancreatic acinar cells in culture: expression of acinar and ductal antigens in a growth-related manner. Eur. J. Cell Biol. **51:** 64–75.
30. GITHENS, S., J.J. FINLEY & C.L. PATKE. 1987. Biochemical and histochemical characterization of cultured rat and hamster pancreatic ducts. Pancreas **2:** 427–438.
31. BOCKMAN, D.E. & G. MERLINO. 1992. Cytological changes in the pancreas of transgenic mice overexpressing transforming growth factor α. Gastroenterology **103:** 1883–1892.
32. PARSA, I., D.S. LONGNECKER & D.G. SCARPELLI. 1985. Ductal metaplasia of human exocrine pancreas and its association with carcinoma. Cancer Res. **45:** 1285–1290.
33. DUDEK, R.W., I.E.J. LAWRENCE & R.S. HILL. 1991. Induction of islet cytodifferentiation by fetal mesenchyme in adult pancreas ductal epithelium. Diabetes **40:** 1041–1048.
34. LEHV, M. & P.J. FITZGERALD. 1968. Pancreatic acinar cell regeneration. IV. Regeneration after surgical resection. Am. J. Pathol. **53:** 513–535.
35. BROCKENBROUGH, J.S., G.C. WEIR & S. BONNER-WEIR. 1988. Discordance of exocrine and endocrine growth after 90% pancreatectomy in rats. Diabetes **37:** 232–236.
36. POUR, P.M. 1988. Mechanism of pseudoductular (tubular) formation during pancreatic carcinogenesis in the hamster model. Am. J. Pathol. **130:** 335–344.
37. FLAKS, B. 1984. Histogenesis of pancreatic carcinogenesis in the hamster: ultrastructural evidence. Environ. Health Perspect. **56:** 187–203.
38. LONGNECKER, D.S., H. SHINOZUKA & A. DEKKER. 1980. Focal acinar cell dysplasia in human pancreas. Cancer **45:** 534–540.
39. CERY, W.L., K.A. MANGOLD & D.G. SCARPELLI. 1990. Activation of K-ras in transplantable pancreatic ductal adenocarcinomas of Syrian golden hamsters. Carcinogenesis **11:** 2075–2079.

The Course of Pancreatic Fibrosis Induced by Dibutyltin Dichloride (DBTC)

J. MERKORD,[a,e] H. WEBER,[b] G. SPARMANN,[c] L. JONAS,[d] AND G. HENNIGHAUSEN[a]

[a]*Institute of Experimental and Clinical Pharmacology and Toxicology,*
[b]*Institute of Clinical Chemistry/Pathobiochemistry,* [c]*Department of Medicine,*
and [d]*Institute of Pathology, University of Rostock, Rostock, Germany*

INTRODUCTION

In studies of toxic effects of dibutyltin dichloride (DBTC, 6 mg/kg i.v.) on bile duct and pancreas in rats signs of acute interstitial pancreatitis were observed.[1–3] We characterized the DBTC-induced pancreatitis as a noninvasive experimental model of acute pancreatitis.[3]

The DBTC-induced acute interstitial pancreatitis in rats resembles the human form of this disease concerning activation of enzymes and structural changes of acinar cells in the initial process. Pathogenetically, the DBTC-induced acute pancreatitis is a twofold process, with a biliary and hematogenic component, focusing in an injury of acinar cells and the entire pancreatic gland. The key event for induction of this pancreatitis is the cytotoxic effect of DBTC on the bile duct epithelium caused by the rapid biliary excretion of high concentrations of organotin (10^{-5}–10^{-6} M) in bile. The cytotoxic effects on the biliopancreatic duct epithelium lead to epithelial necrosis with obstruction of the duct, subsequent cholestasis, and interstitial pancreatitis. The hematogenic DBTC effects cause direct injury of pancreatic cells (mitochondrial damage, autophagy, cell necrosis) followed by interstitial edema and inflammation. The development of the DBTC-induced pancreatitis differs from other experimental pancreatitis models with respect to the histomorphological features and course. In addition to the acute pancreatitis DBTC induces pancreatic fibrosis in dependence on the dose and the time after single treatment of the rats.[4–6,9]

Therefore, in the present study the pathohistological changes of rat pancreas and biliopancreatic duct were examined by light microscopy 2–36 weeks after single administration of DBTC (6 and 8 mg/kg body weight (b.w.) intravenously (i.v.)). Furthermore, pathobiochemical parameters of fibrosis (hydroxyproline in urine and hyaluronic acid in serum) and cholestasis (alkaline phosphatase activity and bilirubin concentration in serum) were studied and mRNA expression of collagen type I as well as transforming growth factor-β1 (TGF-β1) were examined by Northern blot analysis.

[e]Address for correspondence: Dr.med. Jutta Merkord, University of Rostock, Institute of Pharmacology and Toxicology, Schillingallee 70, 18057 Rostock, Germany. Phone, +49/3 81/4 94-57 73; fax, +49/3 81/4 94-57 72; e-mail, jutta.merkord@med.uni-rostock.de

MATERIALS AND METHODS

Inbred male rats (LEW-1W, Karlsburg) weighting 150–170 g were used in this study. For single intravenous administration, DBTC (Sigma-Aldrich Chemie GmbH, Steinheim) was first dissolved in 96% ethanol (2 parts) and then mixed with glycerol (3 parts). The DBTC solution was injected into a tail vein with a record syringe at a dose of 6 and 8 mg/kg b.w. The control group received the solvent only.

The animals (7 per group) were sacrificed 2, 4, 8, 15, 21, 24, 32 and 36 weeks after treatment.

Pathohistology

Tissue samples from the pancreatic head region with the adjacent biliopancreatic duct, pancreatic tail region and bile duct were fixed in a stretched manner with calcium formalin and processed for histopathological examination. Paraffin sections were stained with hematoxylin and eosin.

Analytical Methods

Alkaline phosphatase activity (AP) was measured by an optimized method of the German Society of Clinical Chemistry (37°C) with *p*-nitrophenylphosphat as substrate. Bilirubin was determined by the 2.5-dichlorphenyl diazonium (DPD) salt method (37°C). All these parameters were measured on the analyzer Hitachi 717 with test kits from Boehringer-Mannheim (Germany).

Hydroxyproline was assayed by high-performance liquid chromatography (HPLC) with a test kit from BIO-RAD (Munich, Germany).

Hyaluronic acid was assayed by the radioimmunoassay (RIA) technique using a test system purchased from Pharmacia (Freiburg, Germany).

Northern Blot Analysis

Total RNA was prepared from pancreatic tissue according to Sparmann *et al.*[7] Twenty (20) µg of total RNA were electrophoretically separated in a denaturing agarose-formaldehyde gel followed by blotting to nylon membranes. Hybridization was performed with ^{32}P-labeled rat specific cDNA probes.

Statistical Analysis and Evaluation

Means of normally distributed data with similar variances were compared by Student's *t* test. $p < 0.05$ was considered significant.[8]

RESULTS

Morphological Findings

Biliopancreatic Duct Changes

Two weeks after administration of DBTC, the biliopancreatic duct was swollen up to a diameter of 10 mm and filled with a yellow-green secretion. This obstruction

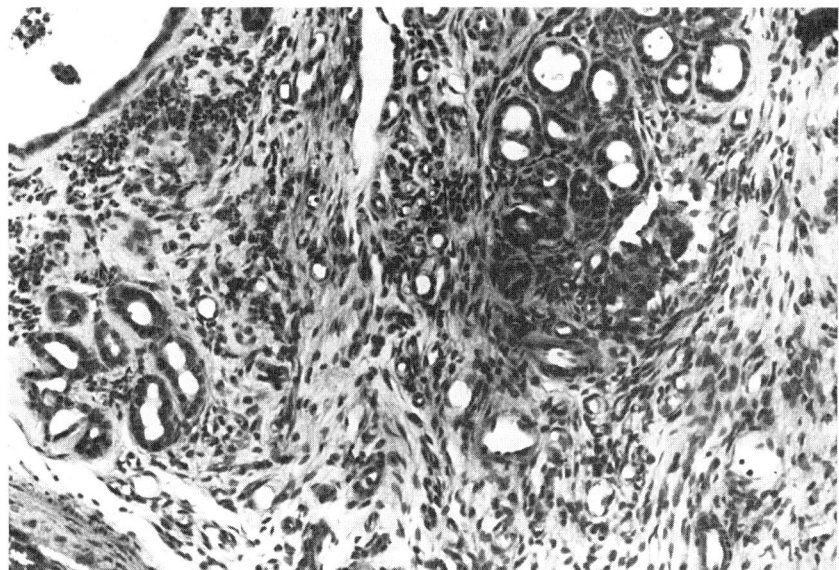

FIGURE 1. Rat pancreas 36 weeks after administration of 6 mg/kg DBTC i.v. Destruction of exocrine parenchyma and fibrosis and beginning changes in endocrine parenchyma were observed. H&E ×40.

persists in 80% of the animals for the entire observation time of 36 weeks. Concretion-like tissue proliferation occurred in the main duct lumen with a consistency of cartilage or connective scar tissue. Total necrosis of the biliopancreatic surface epithelium was found after 2 weeks. Fibrotic areas around the biliopancreatic duct were present. Four to 8 weeks after DBTC administration, the biliopancreatic duct epithelium showed partial regeneration with focal hyperplasia, which sometimes formed papillary connections with the opposite walls of the main duct. Thirty six weeks after DBTC (8 mg/kg i.v.) in some rats the ductal lesions were important (atrophy of epithelium, stenosis, dilatation and hyperplasia). These lesions were often associated with inflammatory infiltration with mononuclear cells and fibrosis (FIG. 1).

Changes in the Pancreas

After 2 weeks, tubular complexes were developed in the damaged exocrine pancreas, and fibrotic areas around the biliopancreatic duct were present. After 4 weeks, one third of the animals (6 mg/kg DBTC i.v.) showed periductal and interstitial fibrosis. The higher DBTC dose (8 mg/kg i.v.) induced periductal and interstitial fibrosis in 50% of the animals after 4 weeks. The interstitial changes in rat pancreas were more prominent than in the acute lesions and consisted of the interacinar septa due to increased numbers of fibroblasts and deposition of collagen fibers. Eight weeks after administration of 8 mg/kg DBTC i.v., we measured an increased mRNA expression of collagen type I as well as TGF-β1 and observed infiltration of lymphocytes and macrophages and an extended pancreatic fibrosis. Pancreatic atrophy and

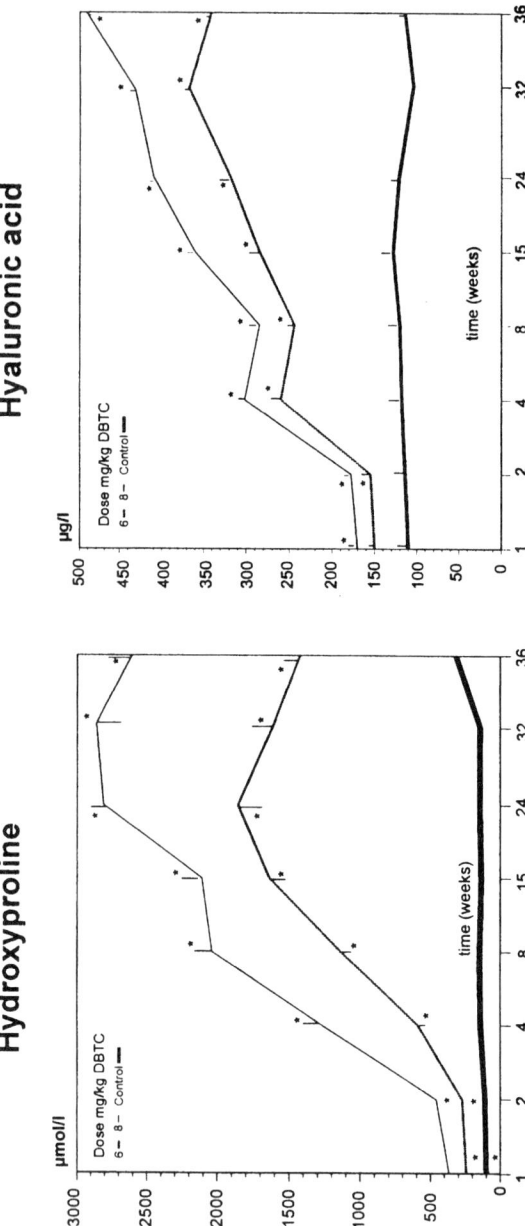

FIGURE 2. Hyaluronic acid in serum and hydroxyproline in urine after single administration of DBTC (6 and 8 mg/kg i.v.). Mean values ± SD, $n = 7$, * $p < 0.05$.

lipomatosis were not observed in these animals. Eight to 15 weeks after DBTC administration, the pancreas was yellow and hard, pancreatic ductules became obstructed by concretions and cellular debris, and acinar and ductular distention occurred. Damaged acini were replaced in time by small cysts, fibrotic tissue, such that only the islets of Langerhans remained. Late in the course of the fibrosis (24–36 weeks), even the islets were affected with diminished insulin production and increased glucose in serum. Thirty-six weeks after administration of DBTC, chronic inflammatory lesions characterized by the destruction of exocrine parenchyma and fibrosis and beginning changes in the endocrine parenchyma were observed (FIG.1).

No changes in pancreas and biliopancreatic duct morphology were noted in samples taken from control animals up to 36 weeks.

Biochemical Changes

The significant increase in hydroxyproline in urine and hyaluronic acid in serum after 2–36 weeks in the DBTC groups with 6 and 8 mg/kg indicates a fibrosis (FIG. 2).

The significant increase in alkaline phosphatase activity and bilirubin concentration in serum 2–36 weeks after treatment with DBTC is a sign of cholestasis.

DISCUSSION

Human chronic pancreatitis is characterized by an irreversible, irregular scarring of exocrine parenchyma with ductal changes subsequent to inflammatory process in the pancreas.[10,11] The mechanisms by which this fibrotic process occurs are not fully understood. In this study, we characterized the DBTC-induced pancreatitis/pancreatic fibrosis during an observation period of 36 months. Two weeks after DBTC administration, increased fibroblast proliferation and fibrosis could be observed. Mononuclear cell infiltration as well as fibrosis and ductal changes persisted until the end of the observation period after 36 months.

Persistently elevated levels of alkaline phosphatase activity and bilirubin concentration indicated obstruction of common biliopancreatic duct during the whole observation period. Duct occlusion may be caused by clotting by necrotic epithelial cells and concretions.[3]

Serum hyaluronic acid has been reported to be a marker of fibrosis in human chronic pancreatitis.[12] In DBTC-induced pancreatic fibrosis, we have found elevated serum hyaluronic acid and hydroxyproline in urine, which indicate a pancreatic fibrosis.

TGF-β1 has been described to play a key role in development of fibrotic diseases, such as liver cirrhosis and pulmonary fibrosis.[13,14] In the DBTC-induced pancreatic fibrosis, we have found a good correlation of the expression of mRNA coding for collagen type I and TGF-β1. On the other hand, high collagen and TGF-β1 transcript levels were paralleled by massive inflammatory cell infiltration in pancreatic tissue.

SUMMARY

In summary, in addition to an acute interstitial pancreatitis the organotin compound DBTC induced a pancreatic fibrosis in rats. The course of the pancreatic fibrosis was studied 2–36 weeks after single i.v. treatment of rats with 6 or 8 mg/kg DBTC.

The pancreatic fibrosis induced by DBTC differs from other experimental models of acute pancreatitis. Extensive infiltration by mononuclear cells is present in fibrotic areas without pancreatic atrophy or lipomatosis. The presence of chronic inflammatory lesions characterized by the destruction of exocrine parenchyma and fibrosis and in the later stages the endocrine parenchyma, indicate a chronic pancreatitis.

In completion of the experimental model of the DBTC-induced acute interstitial pancreatitis in rats, the described late fibrotic effects on rat pancreas may be used as an experimental model of chronic pancreatitis.

REFERENCES

1. MERKORD, J. & G. HENNIGHAUSEN. 1989. Acute pancreatitis and bile duct lesions in rat induced by dibutyltin dichloride. J. Exp. Pathol. **36:** 59–62.
2. MERKORD, J., L. JONAS & G. HENNIGHAUSEN. 1991. Morphological lesions of pancreas and bile ducts in rats induced by dibutyltin dichloride. Arch. Toxicol. Suppl. **14:** 75–79.
3. MERKORD, J., L. JONAS, H. WEBER, G. KRÖNING, H. NIZZE & G. HENNIGHAUSEN. 1997. Acute interstitial pancreatitis in rats induced by dibutyltin dichloride (DBTC): pathogenesis and natural course of lesions. Pancreas **15**(4): 392–401.
4. SPARMANN, G., J. MERKORD, A. JÄSCHKE, H. NIZZE, M. LÖHR, S. LIEBE & J. EMMRICH. 1997. Pancreatic fibrosis in experimental pancreatitis induced by dibutyltin dichloride. Gastroenterology **112:** 1664–1672.
5. MERKORD, J., H. WEBER, L. JONAS, H. NIZZE & G. HENNIGHAUSEN. 1998. The Influence of ethanol on long-term effects of dibutyltin dichloride (DBTC) in pancreas and liver of rats. Hum. Exp. Toxicol. **17:** 144–150.
6. MERKORD, J., H. WEBER, L. JONAS, G. KRÖNING & G. HENNIGHAUSEN. 1998. The DBTC-induced pancreatitis: a new model for acute pancreatitis and pancreatic fibrosis in rats [abstract]. Naunyn-Schmiedeberg's Arch. Pharmacol. **358**(Suppl. 2): 54.22.
7. SPARMANN, G., A. JÄSCHKE, M. LÖHR, S. LIEBE & J. EMMRICH. 1997. Tissue homogenization as a key step in extracting RNA from human and rat pancreatic tisue. Biotechniques **22:** 408–412.
8. SACHS, L. 1992. Angewandte Statistik: Anwendung statistischer Methoden.: 351–360. Springer Verlag. Berlin.
9. MERKORD, J., H. WEBER, G. SPARMANN & G. HENNIGHAUSEN. 1998. Acute pancreatitis and pancreatic fibrosis in rats after single treatment with dibutyltin dichloride (DBTC) in dependence on dose and time [abstract]. Digestion **59**(Suppl. 3): 1325.
10. DI MAGNO, E.P., P. LAYER & J.E. CLAIN. 1993. Chronic pancreatitis. In The Pancreas: Biology, Pathology and Disease. 2nd edit. V.L.W. Go, E.P. Di Magno, J.D. Gardner, E. Lebenthal, H.A. Reber & G.A. Scheele, Eds.: 665–706. Raven Press. New York.
11. KLÖPPEL, G. & B. MAILLET. 1993. Pathology of acute and chronic pancreatitis. Pancreas **8:** 659–670.
12. LÖHR, M., B. SPIES, G. HEPTNER, G. DOMSCHKE & E.G. HAHN. 1991. Parameter des Bindegewebs-stoffwechsels als Marker bei akuter und chronischer Pankreatitis. Z. Gastro-enterol. **29:** 231–236.

13. CASTILLA, A., J. PRITO & N. FAUSTO. 1991. Transforming growth factor $\beta 1$ and α in chronic liver disease: effects of interferon α therapy. N. Engl. J. Med. **324:** 933–940.
14. BROEKELMANN, T.J., A.H. LIMPER, T.V. COLBY & J.A. MCDONALD. 1991. Transforming growth factor-$\beta 1$ is present at sites of extracellular matrix gene expression in human pulmonary fibrosis. Proc. Natl. Acad. Sci. USA **88:** 6642–6646.

CD44, bFGF and Hyaluronan in Human Pancreatic Cancer Cell Lines

JÖRG RINGEL,[a,c] JOACHIM RYCHLY,[a] BARBARA NEBE,[a] CHRISTIAN SCHMIDT,[a] PETRA MÜLLER,[a] JENS RINGEL,[b] JÖRG EMMRICH,[a] STEFAN LIEBE,[a] AND MATTHIAS LÖHR[a]

[a]*Division of Gastroenterology, Department of Internal Medicine, University of Rostock, D-18057 Rostock, Germany*
[b]*Department of Biochemistry, Friedrich Schiller University Jena, D-07749 Jena, Germany*

INTRODUCTION

Altered expression of cell surface molecules and the overexpression of growth factors and their receptors may be involved in malignant progression of human exocrine pancreatic cancer. CD44 is a transmembrane glycoprotein postulated to play a functional role in tumor cell metastasis. A "standard" form of CD44 (CD44st) binds hyaluronan (HA) and is reported to be overexpressed in pancreatic tumors.[2] Alternative splicing gives rise to numerous CD44 isoforms. Variants containing the exon v6 appear to be of major importance for metastatic behavior in a rat pancreas carcinoma model.[1] The published data about the expression of CD44st and CD44 isoforms in pancreatic cancer are contradictive.[2-4] The regulation of CD44 expression is nearly unknown. Recently, a study showed a possible role of basic fibroblast growth factor (bFGF) in endothelial cells. It has been reported that bFGF and its high-affinity receptor (FGF-R) is abundantly present in pancreatic cancer.[5] bFGF is one of the heparin-binding growth factors (FGF, epidermal growth factor (EGF)). The interaction with heparin protects bFGF from proteolytic degradation. Glycosaminoglycan heparin influences the binding of bFGF to the high-affinity receptor, too. Heparin and heparin derivatives can regulate tumor growth and inhibit metastatic behavior. The mechanisms of these regulation processes are poorly understood. Heparin is found exclusively in mast cells. Interestingly, mast cells accumulate by surrounding various neoplastic tissues. We asked whether bFGF alone, bFGF in combination with heparin, heparin alone or the CD44-ligand HA—a member of the glycosaminoglycans—modulates the expression of CD44. Therefore, we used the pancreatic adenocarcinoma cell lines PancTu and Panc-1 (both grade II–III). Furthermore, we investigated the effects of bFGF/heparin on proliferation behavior.

[c]Address for correspondence: Dr. Jörg Ringel, Division of Gastroenterology, Dept. of Internal Medicine, University of Rostock, E. Heydemann Str. 6, D-18057 Rostock, Germany. Phone, +49 (381) 494-7349; fax, +49 (381) 494-7482; e-mail, joerg.ringel@med.uni-rostock.de

MATERIALS AND METHODS

The influence of bFGF/heparin on proliferation was measured using the 3-(4,5-dimethylthiazol-eyl)-2,5-diphenyltetrazolium bromide (MTT) test (Cell Proliferation Kit I, Boehringer). Briefly, both cell lines were cultured in 96-well microtiter plates in medium (without fetal calf serum (FCS)) containing bFGF alone (1, 2, 5, 10, or 100 ng/ml), bFGF and a constant concentration of unfractionated heparin (Sigma, 1 µg/ml) or heparin (0.5; 1, 5, 10, 25; or 100 µg/ml) alone. After 1, 2 or 3 days' incubation, cell proliferation was measured using an enzyme-linked immunosorbent assay (ELISA)-reader. For flow cytometric analysis we used the following monoclonal antibodies (mAbs): SFF-2 (CD44st), anti-CD44v3 (R&D), VFF-8 (CD44v5), VFF-18 (CD44v6), VFF-9 (CD44v7), VFF-17 (CD44v7/8), VFF-14 (CD44v10) (all from Serva), anti-FGF receptor antibody (Chemicon), IgG control antibodies and fluorescein isothiocyanate (FITC)-conjugated anti-mouse IgG (Sigma). For stimulation experiments, 10^6 cells were incubated with bFGF (Boehringer; 1, 5, 10, 100 ng/ml), bFGF and a constant concentration of unfractionated heparin (Sigma) (1 µg/ml) or heparin (0.5; 1, 5, 10, 25; 100µg/ml). After 1, 2 or 3 days the cells were detached. Furthermore, PancTu cells were incubated with hyaluronan (Sigma) (100 µg/ml) for 1 or 2 days. The CD44 expression and CD44st, CD44v3 and v6 expression after stimulation was analysed by fluorescence-activated cell sorter (FACS) flow cytometer.

RESULTS

The FACS analyses revealed the expression of CD44st, v3, v4, v5, v6, v7, v7/8 and v10 on the cell lines Panc-1 and PancTu. Both cell lines also express the flg gene product (FGF high-affinity receptor—FGF-R, data not shown). The incubation with bFGF/heparin for 3 days decreased the expression of CD44st, whereas CD44v6 and CD44v3 were unaffected. In contrast, we found that higher concentrations of unfractionated heparin alone upregulated the CD44st expression. The reasons for this interesting effect are unknown. Furthermore, the incubation with hyaluronan as a CD44-ligand had no influence on CD44st and v6 expression. Various concentrations of bFGF alone and bFGF in combination with 1 µg heparin had no effect on the proliferation of adherent growing Panc-1 and PancTu cells. The MTT proliferation tests also showed that heparin alone had no influence. The blocking of FGF-binding with antibodies reduced the proliferation of PancTu (40%) and Panc1 (30%).

DISCUSSION

We have found that bFGF, heparin and the combination of both have no effect on cell proliferation. However, the blocking of FGF binding with antibodies reduced the proliferation of both pancreatic tumor cell lines. This suggests autocrine loop effects.

We found an expression of CD44st, v3, v4, v5, v6, v7, v7/8 and v10 on the protein level in our human pancreatic cancer cell lines. In correlation with the important cell

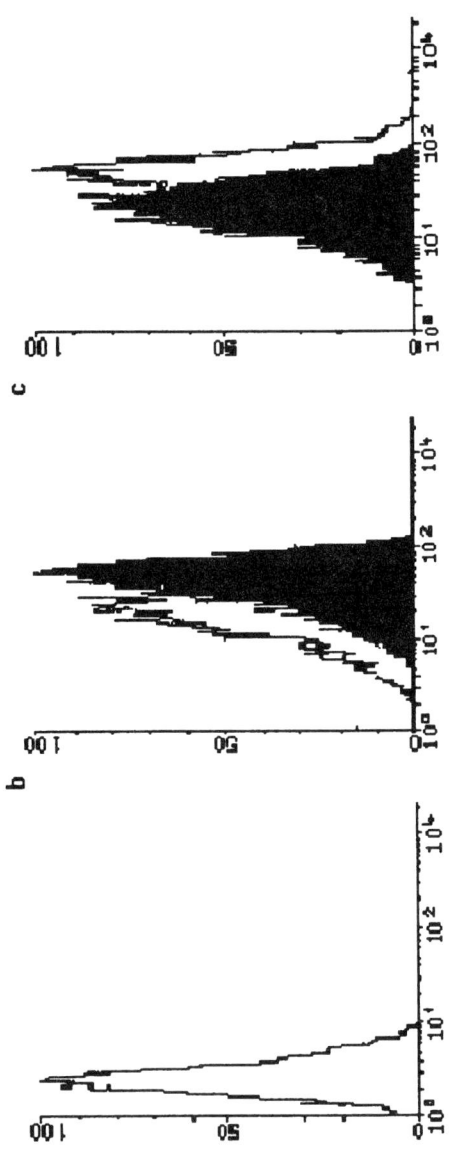

FIGURE 1. FACS analysis of CD44st expression of PancTu cells after stimulation with 5 ng bFGF/ml and **(b)** 1 μg unfractionated heparin ($n = 3$) and **(c)** 25 μg unfractionated heparin alone ($n = 3$) for 72 hours; **(a)** control; *black figure*, CD44st expression of unstimulated cells; *white figure*, stimulated cells.

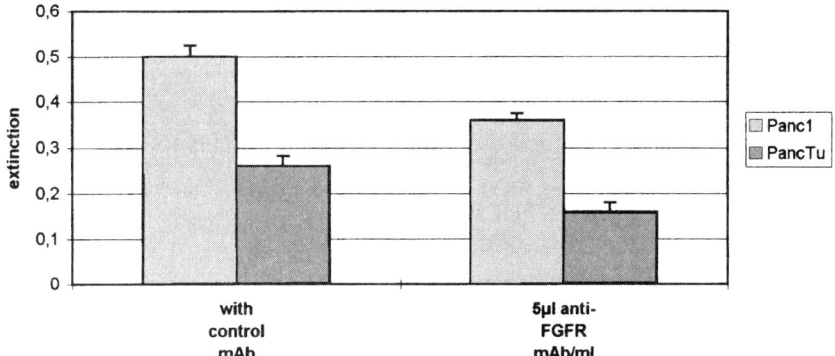

FIGURE 2. MTT test: incubation with mAb (VBS1, Chemicon) blocking the binding of bFGF on FGF receptor or equal amounts of control mAb for 48 hours ($n = 6$).

surface molecule intercellular adhesion molecule-1 (ICAM-1), the expression of CD44st and CD44 variants is weaker on pancreatic cancer cells. But the FACS analysis of CD44 revealed similar results as in other cancer cell lines. The expression of CD44st and CD44v isoforms in abnormal amounts and compositions may play an important role in malignant transformation and cell metastasis. Because CD44 variants expressing v3 have been shown to carry binding sites for heparin binding factors like bFGF, the CD44 expression may play a role in the immobilization and regulation of growth factors in pancreatic cancer. In former studies we could show that interferon-γ (IFN-γ) can modulate the CD44st and CD44v6 expression in pancreatic adenocarcinoma cell lines. In addition, expression of CD44st and variants was unaffected by TGF-β1 using exogenous TGF-β1 incubation and TGF-β1 transfected Panc1 cells. The CD44 ligand hyaluronan does not influence the expression of CD44st and v6. The combination of bFGF and heparin downregulated the CD44st expression. bFGF and heparin had no significant effect on CD44v6 or CD44v3 expression in our cell lines, suggesting an increased gap between CD44st and CD44v6 expression. The reasons for the slightly upregulation of CD44st expression after heparin incubation are unknown. It is possible that added heparin may trigger the biological effects of other heparin-binding factors. Recently, we could show that unfractionated heparin alone can activate mitogen-activated protein (MAP) kinases in a time- and dose-dependent manner in pancreatic adenocarcinoma cell line PaCa44.[6] Whether bFGF/heparin may affect the metastatic behavior of pancreatic carcinomas by the mechanism of up- or downregulation of CD44/CD44 variants has to be investigated further. The mechanism of bFGF/heparin modulation effects has to be proved in further analyses.

REFERENCES

1. GÜNTHERT, U. et al. 1991. A new variant glycoprotein CD44 confers metastatic potential to rat carcinoma cells. Cell **65:** 13–24.

2. TAKADA, M. *et al.* 1994. The significance of CD44 in human pancreatic cancer: I. High expression of CD44 in human pancreatic adenocarcionoma. Pancreas **9:** 748–752.
3. CASTELLÀ, E.M. *et al.* 1996. Differential expression of CD44v6 in adenoarcinoma of the pancreas: an imunohistochemical study. Virchows Arch. **429**(4–5): 191–195.
4. GANSAUGE, F., *et al.* 1995. Differential expression of CD44 splice variants in human pancreatic adenocorcinoma and in normal pancreas. Cancer Res. **55:** 5499–5503.
5. LEUNG, H.Y. *et al.* 1994. Expression and functional activity of fibroblast growth factors and their receptors in human pancreatic cancer. Int. J. Cancer **59:** 667–675.
6. RINGEL, J. *et al.* 1998. The effects of unfractionated heparin on the human pancreatic cancer cell line PaCa44. J. Mol. Med. **76:** A64.

Immunological Escape Mechanisms in Pancreatic Carcinoma

HENDRIK UNGEFROREN, MARTINA VOSS, WOLFRAM V. BERNSTORFF, ANDREAS SCHMID, BERND KREMER, AND HOLGER KALTHOFF[a]

Research Unit for Molecular Oncology, Clinic for General Surgery and Thoracic Surgery, Christian Albrechts University, D-24105 Kiel, Germany

ABSTRACT: Malignancies have developed several strategies to evade immune surveillance. We have investigated pancreatic cancer cell lines and pancreatic cancer surgical specimens to evaluate possibilities of tumor escape in the Fas system, and local immune suppression. Despite Fas expression the majority of cell lines was resistant to Fas-mediated apoptosis. The Fas-associated phosphatase-1 is a strong candidate to confer Fas resistance in pancreatic cancer cells. In addition, all investigated pancreatic cancer cell lines and cancer specimens expressed Fas ligand. Fas ligand was functional in cancer cell lines as shown by coculture assays of pancreatic cancer cell lines with Jurkat cells as targets. Additional local immune suppression was demonstrated by loss of T-cell receptor/CD3-zeta chain of pancreatic cancer infiltrating T-lymphocytes. We conclude that these tumor escape mechanisms may contribute to the poor prognosis of pancreatic cancer but also represent targets for new treatment modalities.

INTRODUCTION

Human pancreatic adenocarcinoma is one of the major causes of cancer death. Less than 20% of patients are alive after two years, and after five years its incidence approximates its death rate.[1] Despite strong infiltration of pancreatic carcinoma tissue with potentially tumor cytotoxic T-lymphocytes (CTLs), the immune system fails to effectively eliminate these malignant cells. Therefore, pancreatic carcinoma cells must have developed strategies to evade CTL-mediated killing. These could result from an impaired interaction between CTLs and tumor cells and may include altered expression of major histocompatibility complex (MHC) class I molecules,[2,3] tumor antigens,[4] and/or costimulatory molecules like B7.[5] In addition, the tumor cells may produce factors that impair CTL function or may even induce cell death in CTLs via secretion of cytotoxic proteins. Fas ligand (FasL) is such a molecule that, when ligated to its receptor Fas (CD95, APO-1), can induce apoptosis in cells expressing functional Fas.[6] Tumor escape mechanisms associated with the Fas system might thus include downregulation or loss of Fas,[7] dysregulation of Fas signal transduction, and/or expression of functional FasL.

---

[a]To whom requests for reprints should be addressed: Research Unit Molecular Oncology, Clinic for General Surgery and Thoracic Surgery, Christian Albrechts University, Arnold-Heller-Strasse 7, D-24105 Kiel, Germany. Phone, +49 431-597-1938; fax, +49 431-597-1939; e-mail, hkalthoff@email.uni-kiel.de

EXPERIMENTAL CONDITIONS

Tissues and Cell Lines

Primary pancreatic cancer specimens including adjacent normal tissue as well as peritumoral lymphnodes were obtained following surgery. Specimens were snap frozen in liquid nitrogen and either stored at −80°C or subjected to cryosectioning. The human pancreatic carcinoma cell lines A818-1, AsPC1, BxPC3, Capan1, Colo357, Panc89, and PancTuI and the human T-cell line Jurkat were kept in RPMI 1640 supplemented with 10% fetal bovine serum, 2 mM glutamine and 1 mM sodium pyruvate.

Immunohistochemistry

Frozen tissue sections from pancreatic tumor tissues were fixed in acetone, followed by successive blocking of unspecific binding sites with normal horse serum, avidin, and biotin (all Vector Laboratories, Burlingame, CA), then incubated with primary antibodies for CD3-zeta chain (clone TCR-zeta, Coulter Immunotech, Krefeld, Germany), CD3-epsilon chain (clone UCHTT-1, Ancell Corporation/Alexis, Grünberg, Germany), CD4 and CD8 receptors (Ancell Corporation/Alexis), or with immunoglobulin G (IgG) matched negative control antibodies (Pharmingen, Hamburg, Germany). Subsequently, sections were immunolabeled by an avidin-biotin complex using an immunoperoxidase technique with the Vectastain ABC kit (Vector Laboratories). Expression of CD3-zeta or -epsilon chains was scored as follows: 2 = moderate to large amounts of tissue infiltrating lymphocytes; 1 = few numbers of infiltrating lymphocytes; 0 = no lymphocytes.

Western Blot Analysis

Cells were lysed in RIPA buffer (0.1% sodium dodecylsulfate (SDS), 1% NP40, 0.5% sodium deoxycholate) and protein extracts subjected to standard 12.5% polyacrylamide gel electrophoresis (PAGE). Fractionated proteins were blotted onto a polyvinylidene difluoride membrane. Following blocking in 5% nonfat milk with 0.1% Tween 20 in Tris-buffered saline (TBS), blots were incubated with primary anti-FasL antibody (clone 33, Transduction Laboratories/Dianova, Hamburg, Germany) for 1 hr at room temperature. Positive signals were developed using a chemoluminescent detection system (ECL kit, Amersham-Buchler, Braunschweig, Germany).

Reverse Transcriptase Polymerase Chain Reaction (RT-PCR)

Total RNA was isolated from cells using RNA Clean (AGS, Heidelberg, Germany). Oligo(dT)$_{16}$-primed total RNA (1–5 µg) was reversely transcribed using Superscript II reverse transcriptase (Life Technologies, Inc.) to yield first-strand DNA. Fas-associated phosphatase-1 (FAP-1)- and glyceraldehyde-3-phosphate dehydrogenase (GAPDH)-specific sequences were amplified in a duplex PCR reaction using:

FAP-1-sense (5′-GAATACGAGTGTCAGACATGG-3′),
FAP-1-antisense (5′-AGGTCTGCAGAGAAGCAAGAATAC-3′),
GAPDH-sense (5′-GGCGTCTTCACCACCATGGAG-3′), and
GAPDH-antisense (5′-AAGTTGTCATGGATGACCTTGGC-3′)

primers. Cycling was performed with a hot-start-touch-down program with an initial annealing temperature of 65°C that was lowered every second cycle by 2°C to reach 55°C at which 30 cycles were performed.

Apoptosis Assays

Apoptosis in response to anti-Fas antibody treatment was evaluated either morphologically at the single cell level by 4,6-diamidino-2-phenylidole (DAPI) staining or by measuring DNA fragmentation with the JAM assay.[8] For the JAM assay tumor cells were labeled for 3 hr with [^{3}H]thymidine, washed, and incubated for 16 hr with anti-Fas antibody (clone CH11, Coulter Immunotech, Heidelberg, Germany).

RESULTS

The Majority of Pancreatic Carcinoma Cell Lines Is Resistant to Fas-Induced Apoptosis

We have investigated a panel of human pancreatic tumor cell lines for expression of Fas and their susceptibility to undergo Fas-induced apoptosis upon incubation with anti-Fas agonistic antibody. Seven out of 7 cell lines were positive for Fas by

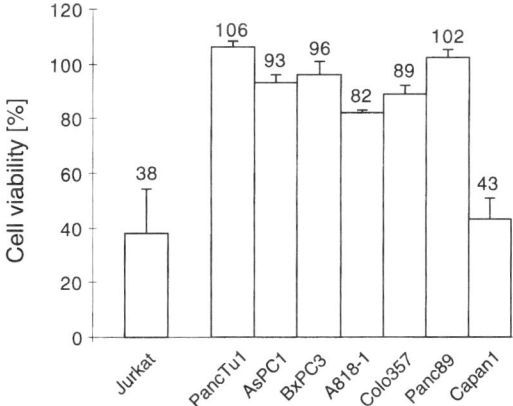

FIGURE 1. Resistance of pancreatic tumor cell lines to Fas-induced apoptosis. The indicated cell lines were labeled with [^{3}H]thymidine and subsequently treated with anti-Fas antibody for 16 hr. The amount of nonfragmented DNA, reflecting viability of cells, was assessed with the JAM assay. Data are given as percentages of untreated controls set arbitrarily at 100 (not depicted). Results from one representative experiment (out of three independent experiments) are shown. The data of each column are the means of 6-fold determinations. Error bars represent standard deviations.

immunoperoxidase staining, and 9/9 exhibited positive membrane staining for Fas in fluorescence-activated cell sorting (FACS) analyses (data not shown). Upon Fas activation, 6/7 pancreatic tumor cell lines (A818-1, AsPC1, BxPC3, Colo357, Panc89, and PancTu1) showed little or no DNA fragmentation in the JAM assay (indicating resistance to Fas-induced killing), while only one (Capan1) displayed an apoptotic rate comparable to that of the Fas-sensitive Jurkat cell line (FIG. 1). It is therefore concluded that the signal transduction cascade that finally leads to the activation of apoptotic effectors is blocked at some point in most pancreatic adenocarcinoma cells.

Resistance of Human Pancreatic Adenocarcinoma Cells to Fas-Mediated Apoptosis Could Result from Overexpression of Fas-Associated Phosphatase-1 (FAP-1)

Recently, the protein tyrosine phosphatase FAP-1 has been identified to inhibit Fas signal transduction.[9] Strikingly, we found high levels of FAP-1 mRNA in 6/6 of the Fas-resistant pancreatic tumor cell lines using RT-PCR. In contrast, the Capan1 cell line as well as two nonpancreatic tumor cells (Jurkat and HL-60), all of which are sensitive to Fas-mediated apoptosis, did not express FAP-1 mRNA (FIG. 2). Prompted by this strong correlation of FAP-1 expression with resistance to Fas-mediated apoptosis, we decided to further investigate the role of FAP-1 as a molecule that can block Fas-triggered apoptosis. The functional role of FAP-1 was evaluated after 1) inhibition of the putative anti-apoptotic function of FAP-1 through disruption of its interaction with Fas in a Fas-resistant, FAP-1 expressing pancreatic carcinoma cell line; and 2) stable transfection of a FAP-1 expression plasmid in a Fas-sensitive FAP-1-negative pancreatic carcinoma cell line.

Based on previous findings that FAP-1 has to interact with the C-terminal end of Fas *in vitro* in order to exert its anti-apoptotic function, we abolished this interaction in a Fas-resistant, FAP-1-expressing pancreatic tumor cell line (Panc89) by microin-

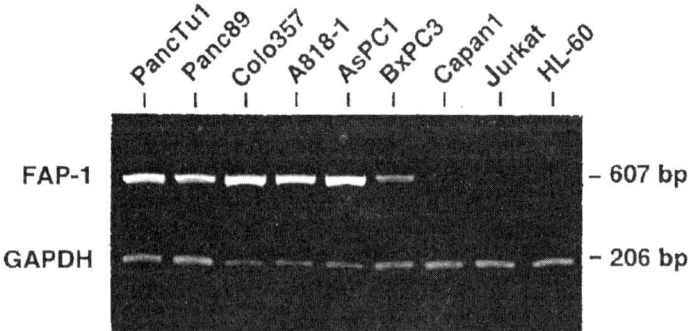

FIGURE 2. Expression of FAP-1 mRNA by pancreatic carcinoma cells. First-strand cDNA from the indicated cell lines was amplified simultaneously with oligonucleotide primers specific for FAP-1 and GAPDH in a PCR reaction. Note strong signals for FAP-1 in the Fas-resistant pancreatic tumor cells and the lack of FAP-1 expression in the Fas-sensitive pancreatic cell line Capan1.

jection of a tripeptide (Ser-Leu-Val) that mimics the most critical amino acids for FAP-1 binding in the C-terminus of Fas. This resulted in a dramatically increased apoptotic rate of microinjected Panc89 cells (after anti-CD95 stimulation) in comparison to cells microinjected with a negative control peptide (Ser-Leu-Tyr) (data not shown). In a parallel approach, the Fas-sensitive, FAP-1-negative cell line Capan1 was genetically engineered to stably express FAP-1 mRNA and protein. Preliminary results indicate that anti-Fas-triggered apoptotic killing was significantly reduced in these FAP-1-expressing cells in comparison to wild-type and vector-transfected control cells. These results point to FAP-1 as a candidate molecule, through which pancreatic tumor cells can protect themselves against Fas-mediated apoptosis.

Pancreatic Tumor Cells Can Kill Activated CTLs by Production of Fas Ligand

Besides the passive escape mechanisms described above, pancreatic tumor cells have also developed active strategies. Recently, several tumor cell types have been reported to produce the cytotoxic molecule FasL, an ability that could enable these tumor cells to kill activated tumor-infiltrating lymphocytes. Therefore, we investigated several primary pancreatic carcinomas as well as several pancreatic carcinoma cell lines for expression of Fas ligand. In contrast to the surrounding stroma, primary carcinoma tissues displayed strong staining for FasL as detected by immunohistochemistry (data not shown). In 6/6 pancreatic carcinoma cell lines FasL mRNA was detected by RT-PCR (data not shown). FasL synthesis by pancreatic tumor cell lines was confirmed by Western blotting (FIG. 3) and other methods (data not shown). The biological activity of the tumor cell-derived FasL was evaluated in coc-

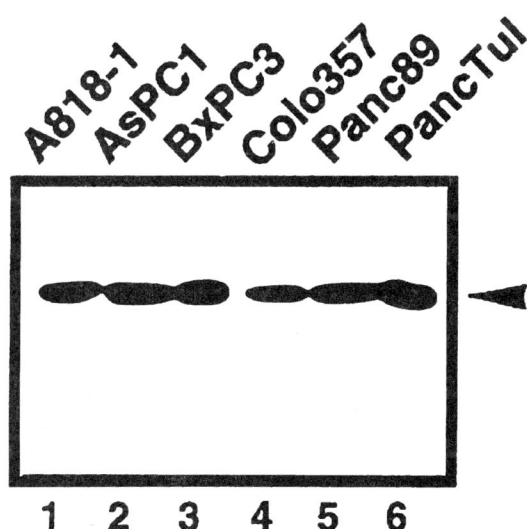

FIGURE 3. FasL protein is present in protein extracts of pancreatic carcinoma cells. The membrane-bound form of FasL (M_r 38,000, *arrowhead*) is shown in a Western blot.

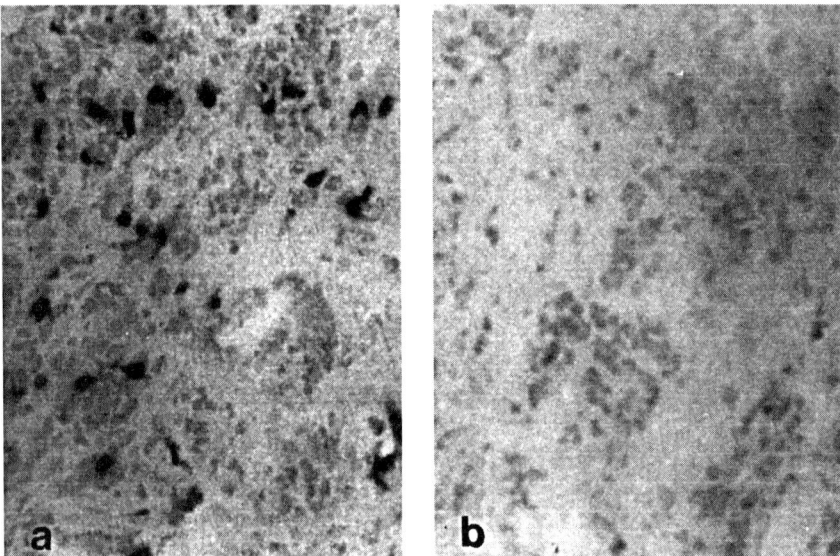

FIGURE 4. Loss of CD3-zeta chain expression of tumor-infiltrating T-lymphocytes in pancreatic adenocarcinoma. Fresh frozen serial sections of pancreatic specimens were stained by immunoperoxidase technique using (**a**) anti-CD3-epsilon (lymphocytes appear as *black spots*) and (**b**) anti-CD3-zeta antibodies. Note that CD3-zeta chains were completely lost in this specimen.

ulture experiments using the pancreatic tumor cell lines AsPc1 and A818-1 and the Fas-sensitive T-cell leukemia cell line Jurkat as target. Coculture of AsPc1 and A818-1 cells with Jurkat cells at an effector-to-target ratio of 2:1 and 10:1, respectively, resulted in a comparable amount of specific DNA fragmentation in Jurkat cells as determined by the JAM assay. This killing was effectively blocked by treatment of the cocultures with a FasL-neutralizing antibody, indicating that Jurkat cell killing was specifically caused by FasL (data not shown).

TCR/CD3-Zeta Chains Are Lost in Tumor-Infiltrating Lymphocytes from Pancreatic Adenocarcinoma

More than 20 specimens of pancreatic ductal adenocarcinomas and in approximately half of these cases corresponding specimens of tumor-free peritumoral lymphnodes were immunohistochemically analyzed for their expression of CD3-epsilon and -zeta chains. A low-grade non-Hodgkin lymphoma was used as an additional control. Significant downregulation or loss of CD3-zeta chains was observed in almost half of the cancer specimens. In 3 specimens no lymphocytes were detected within the limited amount of tissue. In contrast, no loss of CD3-zeta chain expression was observed in any of the lymphnode specimens. Also, no loss of CD3-zeta chain expression was observed in the lymphoma specimen that was heavily infiltrated by lymphocytes.

DISCUSSION

It is becoming increasingly evident that solid tumors in general and pancreatic tumors in particular escape surveillance of the host immune system. A variety of active and passive escape mechanisms have been described.[10,11] These give tumor cells a survival advantage, which finally leads to an increase in tumor size. One mechanism employs the production or secretion of factors with a more general immunosuppressive or anti-inflammatory effect, e.g., transforming growth factor-β (TGF-β)[12] and prostaglandins.[13] Other strategies have been discovered, e.g., those that are aimed at preventing tumor cell-directed activation of CTLs. Here we present evidence for selective loss of T-cell receptor (TCR)/CD3-zeta chains in pancreatic tumor-infiltrating lymphocytes. This is an important finding, since the CD3-zeta chain is an essential component for TCR signal transduction. Although this tumor-suppressive effect has been previously observed in other tumor types,[14,15] the nature of the factor(s) mediating CD3-zeta chain loss remains to be elucidated.

Once the CTL is activated, tumor cells may secrete or produce factors to prevent further interactions of those CTLs with the tumor cells that could otherwise result in tumor cell death. The intriguing finding of production of functional FasL by pancreatic cancer cells[16,17] raises the exciting possibility that tumor cells are capable of killing infiltrating lymphocytes by inducing apoptosis through a distinct pathway originating from the death receptor Fas. The ability to produce FasL was originally thought to be confined to cells of the immune system, being one component of the armament of CTLs. Therefore, the unexpected scenario of tumor cells fighting back the immune system with their own weapons has recently gained much interest and has been termed "the counterattack model."[18] In order to render the counterattack even more effective, it was proposed that tumor cells have, in one way or another, become resistant to the deadly action of the FasL molecule. It was therefore not too surprising that the vast majority of pancreatic tumor cell lines tested so far were resistant to Fas stimulation.[16,17] Generally, resistance can be achieved by several different mechanisms, of which some have indeed been found, e.g., Fas downregulation or loss in hepatocellular carcinomas,[7] mutations in Fas, or expression of a protein(s) that block(s) the intracellular signal transduction downstream of Fas.[9] The latter possibility seems to operate in pancreatic adenocarcinoma cells, since we have tentatively identified the protein tyrosine phosphatase FAP-1 as an anti-apoptotic molecule that can rescue these cells from Fas-mediated apoptosis. Since preliminary experiments indicated that FAP-1 does not completely protect pancreatic carcinoma cells from Fas-mediated apoptosis, it is likely that other inhibitory molecules exist that act in concert with FAP-1 to bring about the resistant phenotype. Interestingly, we found high expression of Bcl-X_L in some pancreatic tumor cell lines (H. Ungefroren, unpublished observation). In conclusion, the concept of active and passive immune escape mechanisms is impressively exemplified in the Fas system. Loss of CD3-zeta chain by tumor infiltrating lymphocytes is an additional example of the local immune suppression by tumors. It can be anticipated that similar types of immune escape strategies will be discovered in the near future and that these represent new targets for promising therapeutical interventions.

ACKNOWLEDGMENTS

This work was supported by a grant from the Bundesminister für Bildung, Wissenschaft, Forschung und Technologie, Bonn (01 GB 9502) and in part from the Medical Faculty, University of Kiel (Grant 443/IZKF), Germany. The excellent technical support of Martina Jansen is gratefully acknowledged.

REFERENCES

1. JANES, R.H., J.E. NIEDERHUBER, J.S. CHMIEL, D.P. WINCHESTER, K.C. OCWIEJA, L.H. KARNELL, R.E. CLIVE & H.R. MENCK. 1996. National patterns of care for pancreatic cancer. Ann. Surg. **223:** 261–272.
2. CORDON-CARDO, C., Z. FUKS, M. DROBNJAK, C. MORENO, L. EISENBACH & M. FELDMAN. 1991. Expression of HLA-A, B, C antigens on primary and metastatic tumor cell populations of human carcinomas. Cancer Res. **51:** 6372–6380.
3. RESTIFO, N.P., F. ESQUIVEL, Y. KAWAKAMI, J.W. YEWDELL, J.J. MULE, S.A. ROSENBERG & J.R. BENNINK. 1993. Identification of human cancers deficient in antigen processing. J. Exp. Med. **177:** 265–272.
4. FLEUREN, J.G., A. GORTER, P.J.K. KUPPEN, S. LITVINOV & S.O. WARNAAR. 1995. Tumor heterogeneity and immunotherapy of cancer. Immunol. Rev. **145:** 91–122.
5. CHEN, L., S. ASHE, W.A. BRADY, I. HELLSTRÖM, K.E. HELLSTRÖM, J.A. LEDBETTER, P. MCGOWAN & P.S. LINSLEY. 1992. Costimulation of antitumor immunity by the B7 counter-receptor for the T lymphocyte molecules CD28 and CTL-4. Cell **71:** 1093–1102.
6. NAGATA, S. & P. GOLSTEIN. 1995. The Fas death factor. Science (Washington DC) **267:** 1449–1456.
7. STRAND, S., W.J. HOFMANN, H. HUG, M. MULLER, G. OTTO, D. STRAND, S.M. MARIANI, W. STREMMEL, P.H. KRAMMER & P.R. GALLE. 1996. Lymphocyte apoptosis induced by CD95 (APO-1/Fas) ligand-expressing tumor cells—a mechanism of immune evasion? Nat. Med. **2:** 1361–1366.
8. MATZINGER, P. 1991. The JAM test: a simple assay for DNA fragmentation and cell death. J. Immunol. Methods **145:** 185–192.
9. SATO, T., S. IRIE, S. KITADA & J. C. REED. 1995. FAP-1: a protein tyrosine phosphatase that associates with Fas. Science (Washington DC) **268:** 411–415.
10. O'CONNELL, J., M.W. BENNETT, G.C. O'SULLIVAN, J.K. COLLINS & F. SHANAHAN. 1997. The Fas counterattack: a molecular mechanism of tumor immune privilege. Mol. Med. **3:** 294–300.
11. CHOUAIB, S., C. ASSELIN-PATUREL, F. MAMI-CHOUAIB, A. CAIGNARD & J.Y. BLAY. 1997. The host-tumor immune conflict: from immunosuppression to resistance and destruction. Immunol. Today **18:** 493–497.
12. SULITZEANU, D. 1993. Immunosuppressive factors in human cancer. Adv. Cancer Res. **60:** 247–271.
13. LEUNG, K.H. 1989. Inhibition of human NK cell and LAK cell cytotoxicity and differentiation by PGE_2. Cell. Immunol. **123:** 384–395.
14. CORREA, M.R., A.C. OCHOA, P. GHOSH, H. MIZOGUCHI, L. HARVEY & D.L. LONGO. 1997. Sequential development of structural and functional alterations in T cells from tumor-bearing mice. J. Immunol. **158:** 5292–5296.
15. NAKAGOMI, H., M. PETERSSON, I. MAGNUSSON, C. JUHLIN, M. MATSUDA, H. MELLSTEDT, J.L. TAUPIN, E. VIVIER, P. ANDERSON & R. KIESSLING. 1993. Decreased

expression of the signal-transducing ζ chains in tumor-infiltrating T-cells and NK cells of patients with colorectal carcinoma. Cancer Res. **53:** 5610–5612.
16. UNGEFROREN, H., M. VOSS, M. JANSEN, C. ROEDER, D. HENNE-BRUNS, B. KREMER & H. KALTHOFF. 1998. Human pancreatic adenocarcinomas express Fas and Fas ligand yet are resistant to Fas-mediated apoptosis. Cancer Res. **58:** 1741–1749.
17. BERNSTORFF, W.V., R.A. SPANJAARD, A.K. CHAN, D.C. LOCKHART, N. SADANAGA, I. WOOD, M. PEIPER, P.S. GOEDEGEBUURE & T.J. EBERLEIN. 1999. Pancreatic cancer cells can evade immune surveillance *via* nonfunctional Fas (APO-1/CD95) receptors and aberrant expression of functional Fas ligand. Surgery **125:** 73–84.
18. O'CONNELL, J., G.C. O'SULLIVAN, J.K. COLLINS & F. SHANAHAN. 1996. The Fas counterattack: Fas-mediated T cell killing by colon cancer cells expressing Fas ligand. J. Exp. Med. **184:** 1075–1082.

The Novel Trk Receptor Tyrosine Kinase Inhibitor CEP-701 (KT-5555) Exhibits Antitumor Efficacy against Human Pancreatic Carcinoma (Panc1) Xenograft Growth and *In Vivo* Invasiveness

SHEILA J. MIKNYOCZKI,[a] CRAIG A. DIONNE,[b] ANDRES J.P. KLEIN-SZANTO,[c] AND BRUCE A. RUGGERI[b,d]

[a]*Department of Pathology and Laboratory Medicine, Allegheny University of the Health Sciences, Philadelphia, Pennsylvania, USA*
[b]*Division of Oncology, Cephalon, Inc., West Chester, Pennsylvania, USA*
[c]*Fox Chase Cancer Center, Philadelphia, Pennsylvania, USA*

ABSTRACT: The survival rate for patients with pancreatic ductal adenocarcinoma (PDAC) is among the poorest for all cancers. The factors that contribute to this poor prognosis are lack of effective early detection, high rate of metastases and a generally refractory response to available treatment modalities.
   The most commonly used treatment methods—chemotherapy and radiation therapy—are mainly used for symptom palliation, with surgery being the only "curative" treatment option. The use of combinations of treatment modalities is the only therapy available to patients with locally advanced disease or that which is surgically unresectable. These options are still not sufficient to increase patient survival time significantly.
   The aggressive behavior and poor prognosis of this cancer is associated with an increased expression of many growth factors and their cognate receptors. We have demonstrated previously the aberrant expression of the Trk receptors (Trks A, B, and C) in PDAC specimens and human PDAC-derived cell lines and a biphasic, dose-dependent response of specific neurotrophic agents on the *in vitro* invasiveness of PDAC cells. Based on these data we have evaluated the therapeutic potential of inhibiting neurotrophin-Trk interactions using a selective Trk tyrosine kinase inhibitor (CEP-701) on subcutaneous (s.c.) and tracheal xenografts derived from the poorly differentiated PDAC cell line, Panc1.
   We demonstrate that CEP-701 administration at 10 mg/kg s.c. BID for 21 days inhibited tumor growth of the Panc1 s.c. xenografts in a statistically-significant manner ($p < 0.01$) compared to vehicle controls, in the absence of morbidity and mortality. A T/C value of 25% was observed for CEP-701-treated s.c. xenografts. In addition, CEP-701 administration inhibited tumor cell invasion in the s.c. tracheal xenograft model of *in vivo* invasiveness. Taken together, these data suggest that further studies are warranted to evaluate CEP-701 as a potential therapeutic agent in the treatment of PDAC.

[d]To whom correspondence and reprint requests should be addressed: Cephalon, Inc. 145 Brandywine Parkway, West Chester, PA 19380. Phone, 610/738-6637; fax, 610/344-0065; e-mail, bruggeri@cephalon.com

INTRODUCTION

Pancreatic ductal adenocarcinoma (PDAC) is the fifth most common cause of cancer deaths in the United States with an estimated 28,100 deaths in 1997.[1] The survival rate for patients with PDAC remains among the poorest for all cancers due to the fact that in the majority of the cases by the time the cancer is diagnosed, the tumor is surgically unresectable, or has metastasized to distant organ sites such as the liver, lung and duodenum.[1,2] The median survival time after diagnosis is approximately four to six months, with a patient five-year survival rate of 1–4%.[1]

Treatment options available for patients with PDAC have proved to be largely ineffective. The most commonly used drugs for chemotherapy—5-fluorouracil and mitomycin—are mainly used for palliative and adjuvant therapy. These drugs, used either alone or in combination, cause tumor regression in only 10–30% of patients. In addition, the drugs have not produced any remissions and do not significantly increase survival time.[1–3] Gemcitabine, the first chemotherapeutic agent to be approved for use in patients with pancreatic cancer in 35 years, has been shown to improve quality of life in phase II trials.[4,5] In clinical trials evaluating the effectiveness of gemcitabine and 5-fluorouracil, objective response rates were determined to be 5.4% and 0, respectively. The median survival time was 5.7 months for gemcitabine and 4.4 months for 5-fluorouracil, with one-year survival rates of 18 and 2%, respectively.[4] Relief from symptoms occurred within 7 weeks of starting therapy with gemcitabine and lasted approximately 18 weeks and was generally better tolerated than 5-fluorouracil.[1,4] Other treatment methods, such as external beam radiation therapy, aid in local control of the cancer, but offer no benefit for increasing patient survival.[2,3,5] In addition, radiation and chemotherapy cause toxic side effects such as nausea, vomiting, mucositis, neutropenia, thrombocytopenia, and anorexia.[2,5] Finally, only 5–15% of patients with PDAC are candidates for surgical resection, with a long-term survival rate of only 10%.[1,3,5] Thus, a treatment that would cause tumor regression or increase patient survival without toxic side effects would be of great benefit in the treatment and management of this disease.

The aggressive behavior and poor survival rate of PDAC has been associated with genetic mutations such as mutations in the *p53* tumor suppressor gene and the *KRAS* oncogene, as well as aberrant overexpression of various growth factors and their corresponding receptors.[6–14] Recently we have demonstrated the expression of the neurotrophin (NT) growth factor family and aberrant expression of their corresponding Trk receptors in human PDAC specimens. Furthermore, we showed that at low nanomolar concentrations there was a significant increase in the *in vitro* invasiveness of human PDAC-derived cell lines through growth factor-reduced Matrigel (submitted). Based on our data demonstrating aberrant Trk expression in PDAC and a biological response of PDAC cells to specific NTs, we have examined the antitumor efficacy of a newly developed Trk tyrosine kinase inhibitor CEP-701 on the development and progression of PDAC.

NT-Trk receptor interactions are known to be inhibited *in vitro* by the indolocarbazole K252a. However, *in vivo* experiments with this compound failed to show any antitumor efficacy.[15–17] CEP-701 (FIG. 1) along with its parent compound CEP-751 are members of a family of recently discovered synthetic derivatives of K252a. This drug is the *O*-desmethyl metabolite of CEP-751, and both are selective inhibitors of

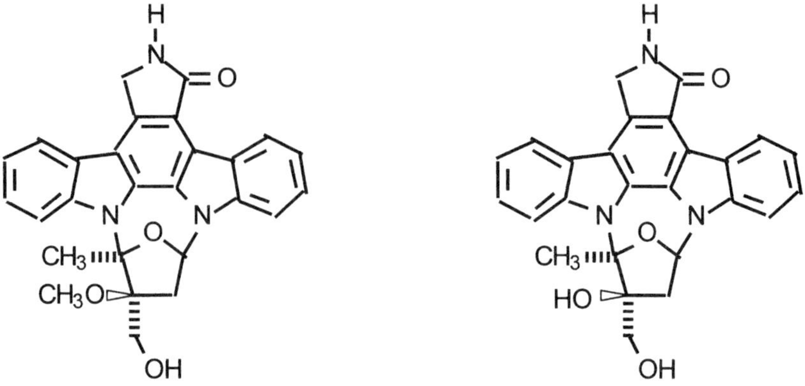

FIGURE 1. The structure of CEP-701 and its parent, CEP-751.

the Trk tyrosine kinase receptor family, protein kinase C, the vascular endothelial growth factor receptor (Flk1/KDR/VEGFR2) and the platelet-derived growth factor receptor β.[15,18,19] CEP-751 has also demonstrated antitumor efficacy in nine different animal models of both human and rat prostate cancer and human models of neuroblastoma and medulloblastoma. The lysinyl-β-alanyl-ester of CEP-751 is now undergoing clinical testing as an anticancer drug in the United States (Refs. 15 and 19 and unpublished data).

In animal models for prostate carcinoma, CEP-701 has been demonstrated to slow the rate of tumor growth or cause a regression in tumor development (unpublished data). At this time, CEP-701 is in phase I clinical trials in normal volunteers. Oral administration of this drug exhibits no adverse side effects and seems to be well tolerated (unpublished data).

We have examined the efficacy of s.c. CEP-701 administration on the *in vivo* growth and invasiveness of Panc1 xenografts in athymic nude mice. Treatment of subcutaneous (s.c.) xenografts with CEP-701 (10 mg/kg s.c. BID for 5 days a week for 21 days) revealed a statistically significant reduction ($p < 0.01$) in tumor growth volume starting at day 7 and continuing throughout the remainder of the experiment. These data were corroborated using the s.c. rat trachea model of *in vivo* invasiveness, which showed that at the identical dose of CEP-701, tumor cell invasiveness through the tracheal wall was inhibited as compared to vehicle-treated controls. These preclinical data suggest that further studies are warranted to evaluate CEP-701 as a potential therapeutic agent in the treatment of PDAC.

MATERIALS AND METHODS

Tissue Culture and Reagents

The poorly differentiated cell line Panc 1 (ATCC, Rockville, MD) was cultured in minimum essential medium (MEM) with 10% fetal bovine serum (FBS), and maintained at 37°C in 5% CO_2. The Trk receptor kinase inhibitor CEP-701 was formulated in a vehicle of 40% polyethylene glycol 1000 (Spectrum, Los Angeles, CA), 10% povidone C30 (ISP, Boudbrook, NJ), and 2% benzyl alcohol (Spectrum, Los Angeles, CA) in distilled water.

Animals

Eight- to ten-week-old female Balb/C, athymic nu/nu mice (Harlan Sprague Dawley, Inc. Indianapolis, IN) were maintained at 5/cage in microisolator units. Animals were given a commercial diet and water ad libitum, housed at 48 ± 2% humidity and 22 ± 2°C, and the light/dark cycle was set at 12-hour intervals. Mice were quarantined for at least one week before experimental manipulation and weighed between 22 and 25 g on the day of tumor or tracheal xenograft implantation.

Preparation of Subcutaneous Xenografts

The Panc1 cell line was grown to subconfluency in MEM (Gibco, Gaithersburg, MD) supplemented with 10% FBS. Upon counting viable cells using trypan blue staining (Fisher Scientific, Malvern, PA), 1×10^6 cells in serum-free media were injected s.c. in the left flank of nude mice. When tumors reached 150–200 mm^3, mice were randomized into two groups of 10 mice each, and administration of CEP 701 (10 mg/kg s.c. BID, 5 days a week) or vehicle (s.c. BID, 5 days a week) was begun. Mice were weighed and tumor volumes (mm^3 = $1 \times w(1 + w/2) \times 0.526$) were calculated using a vernier caliper every 3–4 days.[19] Animals were treated for 21 days and were euthanized by CO_2 asphyxiation. Tumors were removed and either fixed in 10% neutral buffered formalin or frozen. The end points for assessing antitumor activity were tumor volume (calculated as above), tumor growth inhibition (T/C%) and specific growth delay (SGD).

$$T/C\% = \frac{\text{mean}(V_t/V_0)\text{CEP-701 group}}{\text{mean}(V_t/V_0)\text{vehicle group}} \times 100$$

Where V_t refers to tumor volume on a given day, and V_0 is the volume of the same tumor at the start of treatment.

$$SGD = \frac{T_{d(\text{CEP-701})} - T_{d(\text{vehicle})}}{T_{d(\text{vehicle})}}$$

Where T_d refers to the time (days) required for the tumor to double *in vivo*.[15,20]

Preparation of Tracheal Xenografts

Rat tracheas (Zivic Miller, Pittsburgh, PA) were cleaned, mounted on polyethylene tubing and de-epithelialized nonenzymatically by repetitive freezing (−80°C) and thawing as detailed.[21,22] Cultures of Panc1 cells were grown to subconfluency in MEM supplemented with 10% FBS, and 5×10^5 cells in serum-free media were inoculated into each trachea and sealed. Female Balb/C nu/nu mice were lightly anesthetized with Metafane (Halocarbon Laboratories, River Edge, NJ), and tracheas were implanted s.c. (one trachea/mouse). One week after implantation, dosing was started with CEP-701 (10 mg/kg s.c. BID, 5 days a week) or vehicle (100 μl s.c. BID, 5 days a week) and continued for 21 days. Mice were weighed and tumor volumes were calculated as above using a vernier caliper every 3–4 days. At the end of dosing, mice were euthanized by CO_2 asphyxiation; tracheas were removed, fixed in 10% neutral buffered formalin, paraffin embedded, and stained with hematoxylin and eosin. The level of invasiveness through the tracheal wall is based on the following criteria: level 0—there is no invasion of the tracheal wall, and cells are confined to the lumen or are lining the luminal surface; level 1—tumor cells are found in the mucosa and superficial lamina propria; level 2—the lamina propria is completely infiltrated by tumor cells, the pars membranacea and trachealis muscle are invaded, but the adventitia is not invaded; level 3—the malignant cells have reached the adventitia, and the whole tracheal wall is invaded.[22]

Statistical Analysis

The effect of treatment on tumor and trachea volumes was analyzed using one-way analysis of variance (ANOVA) and Student-Newman-Keuls method. All analyses were performed using Sigma Stat for Windows (Jandel Scientific, San Rafael, CA).

RESULTS

The Effects of CEP-701 on Subcutaneous Xenografts in Nude Mice

The antitumor efficacy of CEP-701 was determined using xenografts of the poorly differentiated cell line Panc1. Animals were injected with 1×10^6 cells, and dosing with CEP-701 (10 mg/kg body weight s.c. BID five days a week for 21 days) or vehicle (s.c. BID five days a week for 21 days) began when the tumors reached between

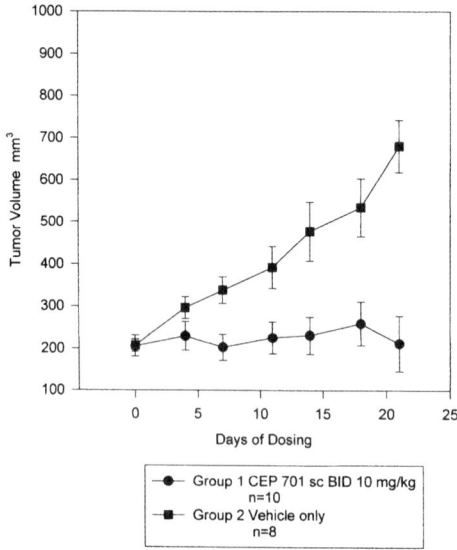

FIGURE 2. Effect of CEP-701 on Panc1 subcutaneous xenografts in athymic nude mice. Athymic nude mice were injected with 1×10^6 cells, and dosing with CEP-701 (10 mg/kg body weight s.c. BID, 5 days a week for 21 days) or vehicle (s.c. BID, 5 days a week for 21 days) began when the tumors reached between 150 and 200 mm^3. Panc1 s.c. xenografts exhibited a marked decrease in tumor volume by day 7 of dosing and significant decreases ($p < 0.01$) in tumor volumes by day 14 and continuing throughout the remainder of the study.

150 and 200 mm^3. In two separate *in vivo* experiments, CEP-701 administration significantly inhibited the growth ($p < 0.05$) of the Panc1 xenografts. The Panc1 xenografts exhibited a marked decrease in tumor volume by day 7 of dosing and significant decreases ($p < 0.01$) in tumor volumes by day 14 and continuing throughout the remainder of the study (FIG. 2). An additional method to determine drug antitumor activity is by calculating T/C values.[23] According to the National Cancer Institute/NIH (NCI), any T/C value ≤42% is considered significant.[20] Based on these criteria, CEP-701 exhibited significant antitumor effects on the Panc1 s.c. xenografts with T/C values of 25% and a specific growth delay (SGD) of 1.1 days. No tumor regressions were observed over the dosing period and regimen used in these studies. All vehicle-treated tumors grew throughout the dosing period (FIG. 2), confirming that inhibitory effects seen were specific to CEP-701 administration.

The Effects of CEP-701 on Tracheal Xenografts in Nude Mice

The rat tracheal xenograft model[21,22] was used to further examine the inhibitory effects of CEP-701 on the growth and invasiveness of human Panc1 tumor cells. Tracheal xenografts require less cells and have a higher take rate and a shorter latency then s.c. xenografts. Further, it is possible to evaluate histologically the *in vivo* invasiveness of the PDAC cells through the tracheal wall (see Materials and Methods).[21,22] Tracheas inoculated with 5×10^5 cells were implanted s.c. in the backs of nude mice. One week after implantation, treatment began using the dosing schedule as above. At the end of dosing, the tracheas were removed, fixed in 10% formalin, stained with hematoxylin and eosin and evaluated histologically for invasiveness through the tracheal wall.[21,22] The growth of Panc1 tracheal xenografts was significantly inhibited ($p < 0.05$) relative to vehicle treated controls by day 14 and throughout the remainder of the study in agreement with our direct s.c. xenograft data (FIG. 3).

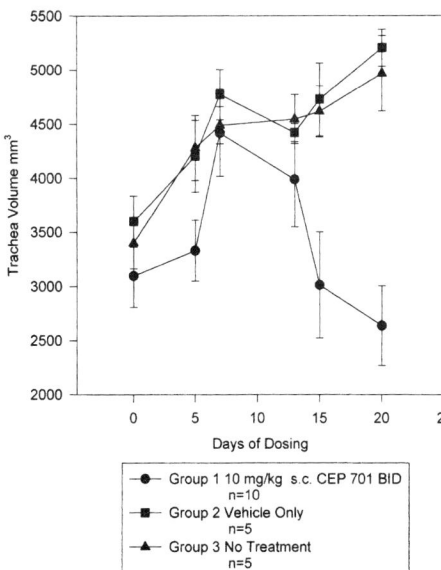

FIGURE 3. Effect of CEP-701 on Panc1 tracheal xenograft growth in athymic nude mice. One week after implantation of tracheal xenografts, dosing began with CEP-701 (10 mg/kg body weight s.c. BID, 5 days a week for 21 days). Panc1 xenografts showed significant decreases in trachea volume throughout the dosing period, achieving statistical significance ($p < 0.05$) by day 14.

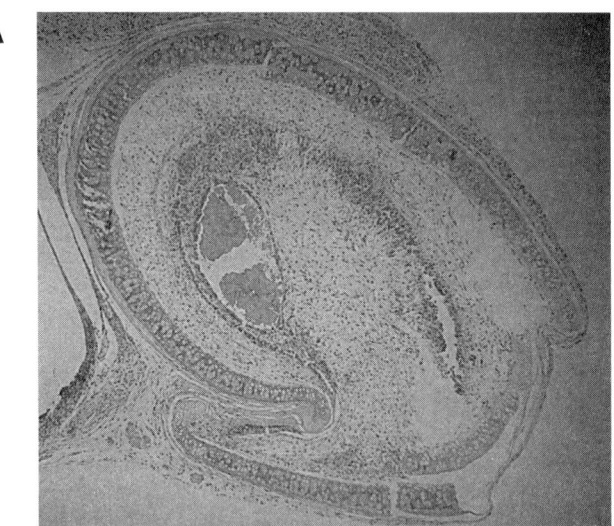

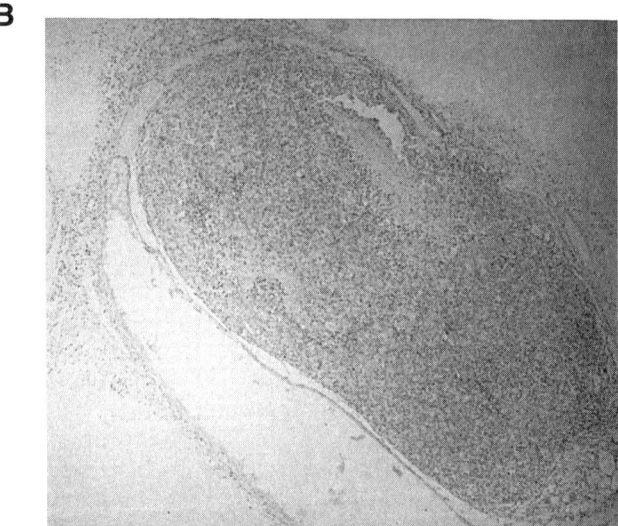

FIGURE 4. Histological sections of CEP-701 and vehicle-treated xenografts in athymic nude mice. One week after implantation of tracheal xenografts, dosing began with CEP-701 (10 mg/kg body weight s.c. BID, 5 days a week for 21 days). (**A**) Panc1 xenografts from CEP-701-treated mice appear to be confined within the mucosal and submucosal tissues (level 1), while (**B**) the corresponding vehicle-treated xenografts totally obscured the lumen and invade the pars membranacea of the trachea and tracheal wall (level 3). Magnification ×200.

Histological evaluation of the levels of invasiveness through the tracheal wall revealed that Panc1 tracheal xenografts had invasive levels for CEP-701 of 1, while vehicle-treated xenografts had an invasive level of 3 (FIG. 4). These data suggest that in this model, CEP-701 treatment inhibits both tumor growth and *in vivo* invasiveness of Panc1 xenografts.

Body weights of CEP-701-treated animals bearing both s.c. and tracheal xenografts were similar to those of the controls throughout the experiment, and no acute signs of drug-associated morbidity (lethargy, abnormal behavior, body weight loss of >10% of initial body weight) or mortality were observed. The absence of gross toxicity in the animals given CEP-701 indicates that the compound is well tolerated at efficacious doses.[15,19]

DISCUSSION

The available treatment options for patients with PDAC have little or no effect on patient survival and are mainly used for symptom palliation.[1,5] In addition, many of the treatments often have adverse side effects, such as nausea, vomiting, and alopecia.[2] To date, surgery remains the only curative treatment; however only 5–15% of PDAC patients are surgical candidates. In addition, postoperative complications such as sepsis and hemorrhaging reduces the surgical survival rate.[24] In the past 35 years only one new drug (gemcitabine) has been approved for use in pancreatic cancer treatment.[4] While this drug shows some promising results, the five-year survival rate still remains low.[1,4]

CEP-701 is a member of a family of synthetic derivatives of the indolocabozole K252a. These drugs target the interactions of the Trk family of tyrosine kinase receptors by competing for the adenosine triphosphate (ATP) binding site.[15,16] Experiments using CEP-751, the parent compound of CEP-701, show that CEP-751 was able to exert antitumor effects against human and rat androgen-dependent and androgen-independent prostate tumors as well as *in vivo* models of human neuroblastoma and medulloblastoma (Refs. 15 and 19 and unpublished data). Here we used CEP-701 to determine its antitumor efficacy against Panc1-derived xenografts in athymic nude mice using two distinct model systems. The rationale for undertaking these studies was based in part on observations that Trk receptor expression is aberrant in a significant percentage of primary PDAC specimens and tumor-derived cell lines as assessed by immunohistochemistry and *in situ* hybridization. Moreover, we have demonstrated significant dose-dependent biphasic effects of the neurotrophins, neurotrophin-3 (NT-3) and brain-derived neurotropic factor (BDNF) on the *in vitro* invasive phenotype of select PDAC-derived tumor cell lines, including Panc1 (Miknyoczki *et al.*, submitted).

Treatment of s.c. xenografts in nude mice with CEP-701 at 10 mg/kg s.c. BID 5 days a week for 21–28 days demonstrated that the Panc1 xenografts exhibited statistically significant reductions in tumor growth as compared to vehicle-treated controls. In addition, no drug-associated effects on morbidity or mortality were noted, indicating that CEP-701 is well tolerated in these animals. A reduction in tumor volume was noted as early as 7 days after dosing commenced, with significant inhibitory effects observed as early as day 14. According to the drug evaluation branch of the division of cancer, National Cancer Institute, a T/C value ≤42% is considered significant antitumor activity. This criterion is mainly used to determine the efficacy of chemotherapeutic agents that are markedly cytotoxic. According to these biological criteria, CEP-701 is an effective antitumor agent against the Panc1 xenografts with a T/C value of 25%. To corroborate the s.c. data, the rat trachea model for tumor growth and invasiveness was used. Histological evaluation revealed that CEP-701 treatment effectively reduced *in vivo* Panc1 tumor cell invasion through the tracheal wall of s.c.-implanted Panc1 xenografts.

In comparison to other drugs tested in the same preclinical models of PDAC, CEP-701 had comparable or more pronounced antitumor efficacy. Previous studies examining the efficacy of adriamycin, cisplatin, and 5-fluorouracil treatment on trocar-implanted MiaPaca2 and Panc1 cell lines in CD1 nu/nu mice demonstrated no effect on tumor growth. Conversely, gemcitabine produced a 69% and 76% inhibition on MiaPaca2 and Panc1 tumor growth, respectively.[25] In another study examining the efficacy of a novel drug delivery system, BXPC3 xenografts showed a 72–79% inhibitory response when treated with 5-fluorouracil, cisplatin, or doxorubicin.[26] Recent studies using trocar-implanted PDAC tumors (HPAC and KCL-MOH1) in severe combined immunodeficient (SCID) mice, evaluated the efficacy of gemcitabine, 5-fluorouracil, taxol, Ara-C, and novel biological agents Bryostatin 1 and Auristatin-PE on PDAC tumor growth. These studies revealed that treatment with gemcitabine was the most effective agent (T/C = 3) followed by Ara-C (T/C = 17), and Bryostatin (T/C = 38); taxol and 5-fluorouracil were ineffective against the tumors, and Auristatin-PE was toxic at the dose used in the study.[20,27] The preclinical data reported in these studies suggest by comparison that CEP-701 may be of clinical value for the treatment of PDAC, used either alone or in conjunction with other available chemotherapeutic agents. We are currently evaluating the antitumor efficacy of CEP-701 alone on additional human PDAC-derived xenografts, and using CEP-701 in combination with gemcitabine in several models of PDAC-derived xenograft models. Currently, CEP-701 is in phase I clinical trials in normal volunteers. Oral administration of this drug exhibits no adverse side effects and seems to be well tolerated (unpublished data).

The mechanism(s) by which CEP-701 and CEP-751 exert their antitumor effects have yet to be determined. CEP-751 has been demonstrated to be selectively cytotoxic to carcinoma cells vs. normal prostate cells *in vivo*, independent of effects on the cell cycle, presumably by inducing apoptosis. Similarly, CEP-701 has been shown to induce apoptosis of neuroblastoma and medulloblastoma cells *in vivo* (Ref 19 and unpublished data). *In vitro* cell viability studies in our laboratories revealed that CEP-701 has moderate dose-dependent cytotoxic effects (IC_{50}s of 270–620 nM) on select PDAC-derived cell lines used here (MiaPaca2, ASPC1, and BXPC3) (data not shown). In addition, it is unclear whether the *in vivo* effects observed in our studies using CEP-701 and in the *in vivo* human prostate models using CEP-701 and CEP-751 are solely due to the inhibition of NT-Trk interactions. This is due to the fact that along with potent inhibition of Trk kinase activity (IC_{50} of <25 nM), CEP-751 and CEP-701 possess inhibitory effects against the vascular endothelial growth factor receptor (Flk1/KDR/VEGFR2) kinase (IC_{50} of 44 ± 10 nM), platelet-derived growth factor-β (PDGF) receptor kinase (IC_{50} 216 ± 34 nM), and protein kinase C (IC_{50} of 226 ± 29 nM).[15,18] Paracrine and/or autocrine influences of aberrantly expressed growth factors, and their receptors play a key role in the development and progression of PDAC.[11,12,14,28,29] Vascular endothelial growth factor (VEGF) expression has been demonstrated to be upregulated in PDAC specimens, and its receptor has been localized to endothelial cells of blood vessels within the tumor stroma.[30] Similarly, the overexpression of the PDGF receptor in PDAC cells concurrent with the expression of PDGF results in an autocrine influence on PDAC development.[12] Therefore, to determine if the antitumor effects demonstrated by CEP-701 are due to disruption of the NT-Trk axis, or are a result of a multimodal mechanism involving the Trks and the VEGF receptors, further studies using Trk-specific and/or VEGF receptor inhibitors are required.

In conclusion, we have demonstrated that CEP-701 administration significantly decreases the *in vivo* growth and invasiveness of poorly differentiated Panc1-derived xenografts in the absence of overt toxicity or morbidity. These results provide preliminary evidence to support further studies investigating the effects of CEP-701 in other preclinical models of human PDAC either alone or in combination with established chemotherapeutic treatment regimes.

REFERENCES

1. NOBLE, S. & K.L. GOA. 1997. Gemcitabine. Drugs **54:** 447–472.
2. LINK, K.H., F. GANSAUGE, J. GORICH *et al.* 1997. Palliative and adjuvant regional chemotherapy in pancreatic cancer. Eur. J. Surg. Oncol. **23:** 409–414.
3. FARRELL, T.J., D.J. BARBOT & F.E. ROSATO. 1997. Pancreatic resection combined with intraoperative radiation therapy for pancreatic cancer. Ann. Surg. **226:** 66–69.
4. REGINE, W.F., W.J. JOHN & M. MOHIUDDIN. 1997. Current and emerging treatments for pancreatic cancer. Drugs Aging **11:** 285–295.
5. CHEN, L.M., D. HARAF, D.G. BRACHMAN *et al.* 1997. Concomitant 5-FU, hydroxurea and cisplatin with external beam radiation therapy for locally advanced pancreatic cancer: a phase II study. Oncol. Rep. **4:** 877–881.
6. LANG, D., S.J. MIKNYOCZKI, L. HUANG *et al.* 1998. Stable reintroduction of wild-type p53 (MTmp53ts) causes the induction of apoptosis and neuroendocrine-like differentiation in human ductal pancreatic carcinoma cells. Oncogene **16:** 1593–1602.
7. RUGGERI, B.A., L. HUANG, D. BERGER *et al.* 1997. Molecular pathology of primary and metastatic ductal pancreatic lesions: analyses of mutations and expression of the p53, mdm-2, and p21/WAF-1 genes in sporadic and familial lesions. Cancer **79:** 700–716.
8. MURR, M.M., M.G. SARR, A.J. OISHI *et al.* 1994. Pancreatic cancer [review]. CA Cancer J. Clin. **44:** 304–318.
9. DAVIS, J.B. & P. STROOBANT. 1990. Platelet-derived growth factors and fibroblast growth factors are mitogens for rat Schwann cells. J. Cell Biol. **110:** 1353–1360.
10. DIRENZO, M.F., R. POULSOM, M. OLIVERO *et al.* 1995. Expression of the met/hepatocyte growth factor receptor in human pancreatic cancer. Cancer Res. **55:** 1129–1138.
11. EBERT, M., M. YOKOYAMA, M.S. KOBRIN *et al.* 1994. Induction and expression of amphiregulin in human pancreatic cancer. Cancer Res. **54:** 3959–3962.
12. EBERT, M., M. YOKOYAMA, H. FRIESS *et al.* 1995. Induction of platelet-derived growth factor A and B chains and over-expression of their receptors in human pancreatic cancer. Int. J. Cancer **62:** 529–535.
13. FRIESS, H., Y. YAMANAKA, M. BUCHLER *et al.* 1993. Enhanced expression of the type II transforming growth factor beta receptor in human pancreatic cancer cells without alteration of type III receptor expression. Cancer Res. **53:** 2704–2707.
14. FRIESS, H., P. BERBERAT, M. SCHILLING *et al.* 1996. Pancreatic cancer: the potential clinical relevance of alterations in growth factors and their receptors. J. Mol. Med. **74:** 35–42.
15. CAMORATTO, A.M., J.P. JANI, T.S. ANGELES *et al.* 1997. CEP-751 inhibits Trk receptor tyrosine kinase activity *in vitro* and exhibits anti-tumor activity. Int. J. Cancer **72:** 673–679.

16. KNUSEL, B. & F. HEFTI. 1992. K-252 compounds: modulators of neurotrophin signal transduction. J. Neurochem. **59:** 1987–1996.
17. TAPLEY, P., F. LAMBALLE & M. BARBACID. 1992. K252a is a selective inhibitor of the tyrosine protein kinase activity of the trk family of oncogenes and neurotrophin receptors. Oncogene **7:** 371–381.
18. ANGELES, T.S., C. STEFFLER, B.A. BARTLETT et al. 1996. Enzyme-linked immunosorbent assay for trkA tyrosine kinase activity. Ann. Biochem. **236:** 49–55.
19. DIONNE, C.A., A.M. CAMORATTO, J.P. JANI et al. 1998. Cell cycle-independent death of prostate adenocarcinoma is induced by the trk tyrosine kinase inhibitor CEP-751(KT6587). Clin. Cancer Res. **4:** 1887–1898.
20. MOHAMMAD, R.M., M.C. DUGAN, A.N. MOHAMED et al. 1998. Establishment of a human pancreatic tumor xenograft model: potential application for preclinical evaluation of novel therapeutic agents. Pancreas **16:** 19–25.
21. BABA, M., A.J. KLEIN-SZANTO, D. TRONO et al. 1987. Preneoplastic and neoplastic growth of xenotransplanted lung-derived human cell lines using deepithelialized rat tracheas. Cancer Res. **47:** 573–578.
22. MOMIKI, S., M. BABA, J. CAAMANO et al. 1991. In vivo and in vitro invasiveness of human lung carcinoma cell lines. Invasion & Metastasis **11:** 66–75.
23. CORBETT, T.H., F.A. VALERIOTE, L. POLIN et al. 1992. Discovery of solid tumor activity agents using a soft-agar-colony-formation-disk-diffusion-assay. In Cytotoxic Anti-Cancer Drugs: Models and Concepts for Drug Discovery and Development. F.A. Valeriote, T.H. Corbett & L.H. Baker, Eds.: 35–89. Kluwer Academic. Boston, MA.
24. STEELE, G.D., JR., R.T. OSTEEN, D.P. WINCHESTER et al. 1994. Clinical highlights from the National Cancer Data Base: 1994. CA Cancer J. Clin. **44:** 71–80.
25. SCHULTZ, R.M., R.L. MERRIMAN, J.E. TOTH et al. 1993. Evaluation of new anticancer agents against the MIA PaCa-2 and Panc1 human pancreatic carcinoma xenografts. Oncol. Res. **5:** 223–228.
26. SMITH, J.P., E. STOCK, E.K. ORENBERG et al. 1995. Intratumoral chemotherapy with a sustained-release drug delivery system inhibits growth of human pancreatic cancer xenografts. Anticancer Drugs **6:** 717–726.
27. MOHAMMAD, R.M., A. AL-KATIB, G.R. PETTIT et al. 1998. An orthotopic model of human pancreatic cancer in severe combined immunodeficient mice: potential application for preclinical studies. Clin. Cancer Res. **4:** 887–894.
28. KORC, M., B. CHANDRASEKAR, Y. YAMANAKA et al. 1992. Overexpression of the epidermal growth factor receptor in human pancreatic cancer is associated with concomitant increases in the levels of epidermal growth factor and transforming growth factor alpha. J. Clin. Invest. **90:** 1352–1360.
29. KOBRIN, M.S., Y. YAMANAKA, H. FRIESS et al. 1993. Aberrant expression of type I fibroblast growth factor receptor in human pancreatic adenocarcinomas. Cancer Res. **53:** 4741–4744.
30. ITAKUREA, J., T. ISHIWATA, H. FRIESS et al. 1997. Enhanced expression of vascular endothelial growth factor in human pancreatic cancer correlates with local disease progression. Clin. Cancer Res. **3:** 1309–1316.

Single-Chain Antibodies in Pancreatic Cancer

DAVID COLCHER,[a,c] GABRIELA PAVLINKOVA,[a] GUY BERESFORD,[a] BARBARA J.M. BOOTH,[a] AND SURINDER K. BATRA[b]

[a]*Department of Pathology and Microbiology and* [b]*Department of Biochemistry and Molecular Biology, University of Nebraska Medical Center, Omaha, Nebraska 68198-3135, USA*

ABSTRACT: Pancreatic cancer is a therapeutic challenge for surgical and medical oncology. Development of specific molecular tracers for the diagnosis and treatment of this lethal cancer has been one of our major goals. Monoclonal antibodies (MAbs) have been successfully used as selective carriers for delivering radionuclides, toxins or cytotoxic drugs to malignant cell populations; therefore, monoclonal antibody technology has led to a significant amount of research into optimizing targeted therapy. This targeted therapy results in the selective concentration of cytotoxic agents or radionuclides in tumors and should lessen the toxicity to normal tissues, which would normally limit the dosage and effectiveness of systemically administered drugs. The MAb CC49 reacts with a unique disaccharide, Sialyl-Tn, present on tumor-associated mucin (TAG-72) expressed by a majority of human adenocarcinomas. The unique Sialyl-Tn epitope has provided a potential target for immunotherapy of cancer. A single chain Fv (scFv) recombinant protein from CC49 MAb was prepared by engineering the DNA fragments for coding heavy-chain and light-chain variable regions with an appropriate oligonucleotide linker. scFv molecules, when compared to intact MAbs and the more conventional enzymatically derived F(ab')$_2$ and Fab' fragments, offer several advantages as carriers for the selective delivery of radionuclides to tumors. The divalent antibody fragments (sc(Fv)$_2$ or (scFv)$_2$) display an affinity constant similar to that of the intact CC49 IgG and are stable with storage, and after radiolabeling. In preclinical studies, both the covalent and the non-covalent dimeric scFvs exhibit excellent tumor targeting properties with characteristics similar to those of the monomer, e.g., the rapid blood clearance, low kidney uptake and small size suitable for rapid penetration through tumor tissue. Increased tumor targeting of the dimers are probably due to their increased functional affinity attributable to valency, coupled with their higher molecular weight and fewer interactions with normal organs. These properties make these constructs superior to monovalent CC49 scFv. The relatively high tumor uptake, the *in vitro* and *in vivo* targeting specificity, and the stability in storage demonstrated by the dimeric CC49 sc(Fv)$_2$ makes it a promising delivery vehicle for therapeutic applications in pancreatic cancer.

INTRODUCTION

Monoclonal antibody (MAb)-based immunodiagnosis and immunotherapy has been pursued for a number of years in experimental murine model systems and more

[c]Corresponding author: Department of Pathology and Microbiology, University of Nebraska Medical Center, 983135 Nebraska Medical Center, Omaha, NE 68198-3135. Phone, 402/559-7935; fax, 402/559-8112; e-mail, dcolcher@unmc.edu

recently in clinical studies. Despite recent advances in understanding the molecular genetics of human cancer, targeted therapeutic approaches still require that a tumor-specific marker, preferably on the cell surface, be defined. Advances in tumor biology have led to the identification of many tumor-associated antigens (TAAs). A number of these antigens, such as carcinoembryonic antigen (CEA),[1,2] CA19-9,[3,4] CA-125,[5] and CA15-3[6] are commonly used as serum markers for disease activity in various malignancies, as well as targeting agents *in vivo*.

Several TAAs have been shown to have many properties consistent with their being a mucin. Tumor-associated epitopes on mucins have been implicated in the pathogenesis of many cancers including pancreatic cancer. Several clinically useful antibodies that recognize epitopes on mucin were originally generated against tumors of secretory epithelial cell origin from the pancreas, breast, colon, and lung, and include (but are not limited to) DUPAN2,[7] HMFG2,[8,9] SM-3,[10] and CA 19-9.[11,12] Some of the antibodies recognize epitopes that are aberrantly expressed on tumor mucin but not on corresponding normal cell populations (SM-3), whereas others recognize epitopes expressed on mucin from both normal and malignant cells from a given organ site (DUPAN2 and CA 19-9). These and other mucin reactive antibodies generally show distinct patterns of tissue reactivity by immunohistochemical analysis.

A unique TAA is TAG-72, a panadeno-carcinoma antigen[13–16] that is expressed by a majority of human adenocarcinomas of the pancreas, colon, ovary, prostate, lung, and esophagus[15–18] and is absent in most normal tissues. TAG-72 has been identified by its immunoreactivity with MAb B72.3, a murine MAb that was developed by the immunization of mice with a membrane-enriched fraction of human metastatic breast carcinoma tissue.[13] The epitope recognized by MAb B72.3 is sialyl-Tn, a unique disaccharide present in multiple copies on the tumor-associated mucin TAG-72. This unique epitope has provided a potential target for active and passive immunotherapy of cancer.

Murine monoclonal antibodies (MAbs) reactive with the sialyl-Tn epitopes B72.3 and CC49 are among the most extensively studied MAbs for cancer therapy. These MAbs after conjugation to potent gamma- and beta-emitting radionuclides have provided selective systemic radiolocalization of disease and have proven therapeutic efficacy in model systems.[19–21] They have also been used clinically to localize primary and metastatic tumor sites.[22,23] However, intact MAbs have practical limitations due to their pharmacology; their relatively long clearance rate results in significant exposure to normal bone marrow and organs,[24,25] limited quantities delivered to tumors,[22,23,25] and relatively poor diffusion of MAb from the vasculature into and through the tumor.[26]

Initial studies attempting to overcome some of these issues were performed using enzymatically derived fragments from antibodies. While the use of $F(ab')_2$ or Fab' fragments helps to improve the relative localization in the tumor as compared to normal tissue in model systems, it is often difficult to generate these immunoglobulin forms in large quantities sufficient for clinical use and in a manner that retains their immunoreactivity. Fab' fragments are normally generated from intact antibodies by enzyme digestion, but the process is tedious and has to be optimized for each antibody.[27] Advances in recombinant DNA technology involving molecular cloning of variable region genes can overcome some of the problems associated in the conventional method for production of Fab'.

Fv fragments of immunoglobulins are one of the smallest size functional modules of antibodies that retain high-affinity binding of an antigen. Their smaller size makes them potentially more useful than a whole antibody for clinical applications. A scFv recombinant protein for a given monoclonal antibody can be prepared by connecting genes encoding for heavy-chain and light-chain variable regions at the DNA level by an appropriate oligonucleotide.[28,29] The resulting translation product forms a single polypeptide chain with a linker bridging the two variable domains.

ScFv molecules, when compared to intact MAbs and more conventional enzymatically derived F(ab')$_2$ and Fab' fragments, offer several advantages as carriers for selective delivery of radionuclides to tumors. First, the rates of clearance of scFv from blood pool and normal tissues have been shown to be much more rapid than that seen with intact immunoglobulin G (IgG), F(ab')$_2$ or Fab' fragments[30,31] offering the possibility of earlier imaging times and, for therapy, a reduction of the radiation-absorbed dose to normal tissues. Secondly, autoradiographic studies have shown that scFv molecules can penetrate into a tumor mass much more rapidly than either intact MAbs or larger enzymatically derived fragments.[32] This may be important for radioimmunotherapeutic applications because of the potential for increasing the homogeneity of radiation dose deposition within tumors. ScFv constructs have been made using a variety of monoclonal antibodies to both complex polypeptide antigens and small molecular weight haptens. In most cases, scFv fragments have been shown to retain antigen-binding affinity of the monovalent Fab' fragment. In general, a decrease in binding affinity of the scFv fragments as compared to intact antibodies[33,31] is noticed. Some antigen-antibody interactions involve both antigen binding sites of an intact antibody, either in binding to multiple epitopes on a single molecule or by bridging two separate cell surface molecules. Thus it is not surprising that a monovalent scFv molecule would have a lower avidity than the divalent IgG molecule.

Multivalency can be an effective means for increasing the functional affinity of an antibody to a surface or a polymeric antigen, and thereby improved performance is achieved for imaging and immunotherapy.[34] Several strategies are being used to produce bivalent scFv fragments. One approach introduced a cysteine at the C-terminus of the scFv, which can be used to covalently link two scFvs *via* a site-specific dimerization. Adams *et al.*[35] prepared divalent-scFvs with the specificity of anti-erbB-2 monoclonal antibody 741F8 using cysteine residues at the carboxyl-terminal. Another approach involves the addition of a short flexible hinge region and an amphiphilic helix at the C-terminus of the scFv fragment.[36,37] Recently, a novel engineered antibody fragment called the minibody was produced by the fusion of T84.66 anti-CEA scFv to the human IgG1 C_H3 domain.[38] Other groups have fused scFvs to protein domains capable of multimerization, e.g., leucine zipper proteins,[39] transcriptional factor p53,[40] streptavidin,[41] or the M-constant region[42] to promote dimer formation. The simplest approach to production of multimeric scFv is based on spontaneous formation of noncovalent dimers such as diabodies[43] or trimers.[44,45] Multiple scFvs with two or more binding sites can also be connected by peptide linker. They show a more favorable *in vivo* clearance rate than monovalent scFv. The multimeric scFv should therefore have a higher percentage of the injected dose per gram localized in the tumor, which would improve the diagnostic and therapeutic potential of these Ig forms. The multivalent scFv molecules should also penetrate better throughout a tumor mass, with less dose heterogeneity, than that obtained with intact IgG.

TABLE 1. Immunohistochemical analysis of pancreatic tumors[a]

	B72.3	DU-PAN-2	CA19-9
% Reactive	86	94	84
>70%[a]	21	16	66
30–70%[a]	45	50	9
1–30%[a]	21	28	9
Negative	14	6	16
Number tested	30	32	32

[a]Percent cell positive; expressed as % of cases in each category. Adapted from M. Tempero et al.[18]

In this paper, we review the unique expression of tumor-associated antigen TAG-72 in pancreatic adenocarcinomas. We have generated and characterized monovalent and divalent forms of single-chain antibody constructs of MAb CC49 that were reactive with TAG-72 antigen. Radiolabeled recombinant CC49 constructs were evaluated for tumor targeting in athymic mice bearing xenograft of adenocarcinoma cell line expressing high levels of TAG-72. The divalent CC49 constructs have shown rapid, high tumor uptake and rapid blood clearance, leading to high tumor:normal tissue ratios as compared to the monomeric scFv form of CC49. Because MAbs B72.3 and CC49 have selective reactivity for primary and metastatic pancreatic tumors, it is possible that the TAG-72 antigen can be a valuable target for radioimmunotherapy of the pancreas.

EXPRESSION OF TAG-72 IN PANCREATIC ADENOCARCINOMAS

Tumor-associated glycoprotein (TAG-72) has been identified by its immunoreactivity with MAb B72.3, a murine monoclonal antibody, developed at the National Cancer Institute following immunization of mice with a membrane-enriched fraction of human metastatic mammary carcinoma tissue.[13] TAG-72 has been partially purified and has characteristics of a mucin. While its function is unknown,[14] immunohistochemical and immunocytochemical analyses have demonstrated preferential localization of this antigen in malignant tissues with uncommon expression in normal tissue; the one significant exception being secretory endometrium.[15]

Lyubsky et al. (1988)[17] performed a retrospective analysis of 25 primary adenocarcinomas of the pancreas, 16 metastatic pancreatic tumors, 8 cases of chronic pancreatitis, and 3 adult normal pancreas for the expression of TAG-72 antigen using MAb B72.3. Twenty-one of 25 (83%) of malignant primary tumors were reactive, and all 16 metastatic sites expressed the B72.3 antigen. In contrast, all cases of pancreatitis and normal pancreas were either weakly reactive or nonreactive. Interestingly, 10 malignant and 2 benign pancreatic fine-needle aspirates showed results similar to those seen with fixed tissues. Tempero et al.[18] examined the incidence and expression of TAG-72 along with other tumor-associated antigens CA19.9, DU-PAN2 and CA125 in serum and tissues of patients with pancreatic cancer. TABLE 1 shows that 83% of tumor tissues demonstrated the expression of 3 or more antigens. The least commonly detected antigen was CA125. Expression of TAG-72 was rare in normal pancreas but was commonly expressed in ductal cells of chronic pancreatitis. Serologic coexpression of elevated antigen levels was less common because 30% of the patients showed increased levels of 3 or more antigens (TABLE 1).

SECOND GENERATION MONOCLONAL ANTIBODIES TO TAG-72

In an effort to produce an improved antibody for therapeutic use in adenocarcinomas Colcher et al.[46] and Muraro et al.[47] have developed and described a series of second generation murine monoclonal antibodies that are reactive with the TAG-72 antigen. To generate these antibodies, purified TAG-72 was used as the immunogen, and 28 second generation IgG monoclonal antibodies were generated. MAb CC49 is one member of this group of antibodies; this antibody is particularly notable for having an 8-fold greater affinity for antigen in comparison to MAb B72.3 and has a more rapid plasma clearance in model systems. MAb CC49 recognizes a slightly different epitope on the TAG-72 antigen from MAb B72.3[48] and exhibits higher reactivity to gastric, pancreatic, and colon adenocarcinomas.[49] Furthermore, radiolocalization studies using a dual labeling technique in athymic mice bearing human tumor xenografts showed a 2-fold improvement in targeting of the radionuclide using MAb CC49 compared to MAb B72.3.[46] Finally, preclinical therapeutic studies using MAb

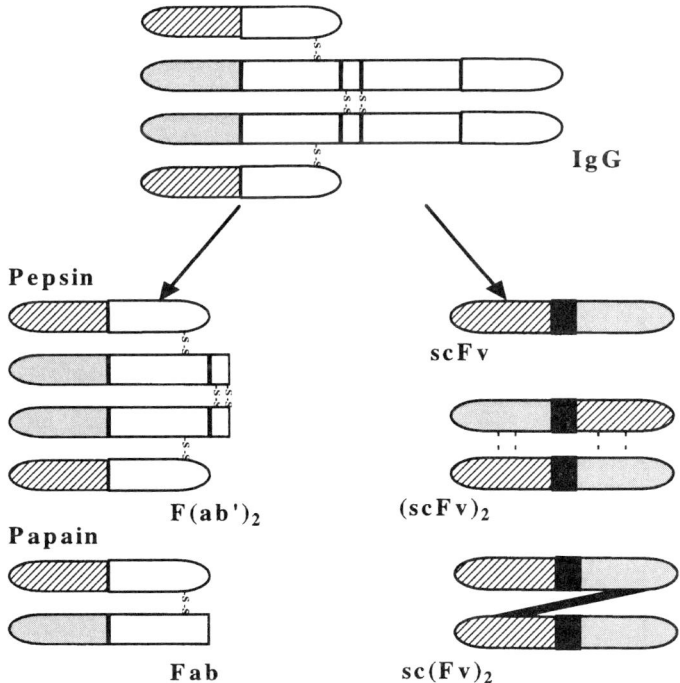

FIGURE 1. A schematic structure of mouse CC49 IgG, F(ab′)$_2$, Fab, scFv, (scFv)$_2$ and sc(Fv)$_2$.

CC49 conjugated to ^{131}I, ^{90}Y, and ^{177}Lu have shown a 3- to 5-fold improvement in therapeutic efficacy, producing cures in these preclinical models.[30,50]

Using DNA recombinant techniques, we have produced a range of smaller fragments called single-chain Fv (scFv) for murine MAb CC49. The valency is one of the hallmarks by which significant improvement in functional affinity and avidity of scFv can be achieved. We have generated and characterized the monovalent and multivalent scFvs for MAb CC49.

GENERATION AND EXPRESSION OF RECOMBINANT scFv CONSTRUCTS

A schematic structure for various enzymatically derived and recombinant forms of CC49 scFvs is shown in FIGURE 1. The monovalent CC49 scFv cDNA (V_L-Linker-V_H) was constructed using the polymerase chain reaction method[51] by combining the V_L region sequence and the V_H region sequence *via* a linker sequence designated a 205C linker. The divalent CC49 sc(Fv)$_2$ (V_L-Linker-V_H-Linker-V_L-Linker-V_H) construct was assembled using the similar polymerase chain reaction in which the linker 205C sequence is also placed between two complete scFv molecules. The

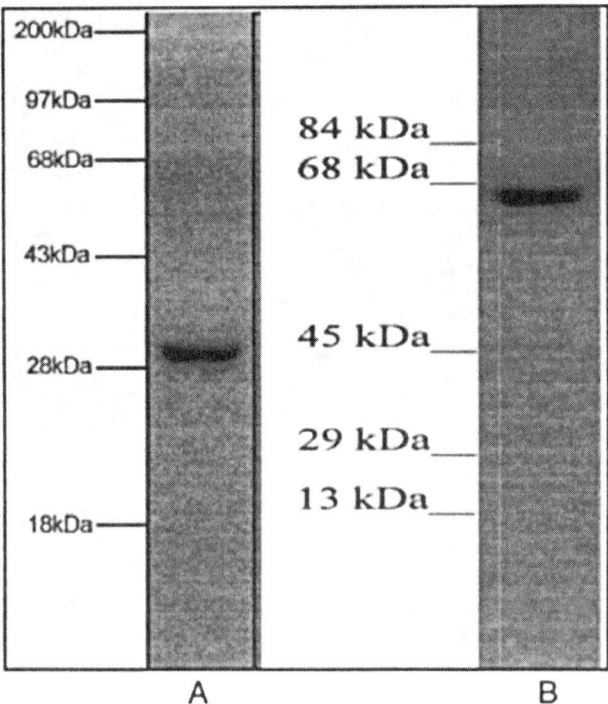

FIGURE 2. SDS-PAGE analysis of purified CC49 scFv under reducing conditions. *Lane A*, purified scFv; *lane B*, sc(Fv)$_2$. Positions and relative molecular weight of marker proteins are indicated.

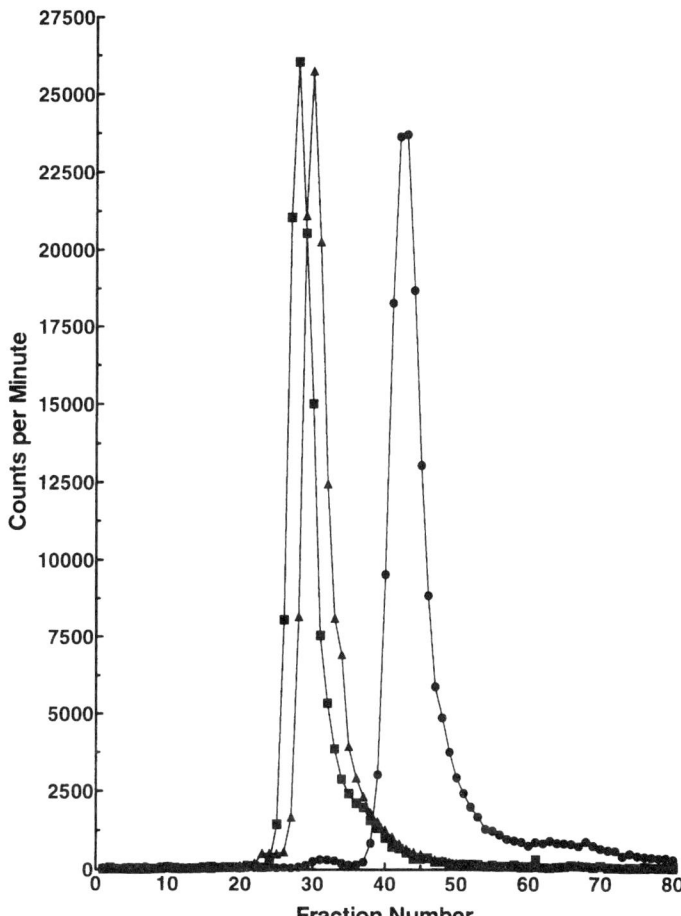

FIGURE 3. HPLC size-exclusion profiles of the radiolabeled CC49 sc(Fv)$_2$, (scFv)$_2$ and scFv. After radiolabeling the iodinated constructs were analyzed using TSK G3000SW and TSK G2000SW size exclusion columns connected in series. The sc(Fv)$_2$ (■), (scFv)$_2$ (▲) and scFv (●) were eluted as single peaks with no evidence of aggregates or breakdown products.

205C linker contained a helical structure,[52] with the first and last amino acids modified resulting in the sequence: LSADDAKKDAAKKDDAKKDDAKKDL. The sequence of the CC49 scFv was confirmed by nucleotide sequence analysis. The scFv fragments were cloned into the pRW83 vector that contained a chloramphenicol resistance gene for recombinant selection, *penP* gene with a penP promoter and terminator, and a pelB signal peptide that directed the recombinant protein to the periplasmic space, where refolding and denaturation of protein occurred resulting in a soluble, biologically active protein. This recombinant protein was purified by ion exchange and gel filtration chromatography.

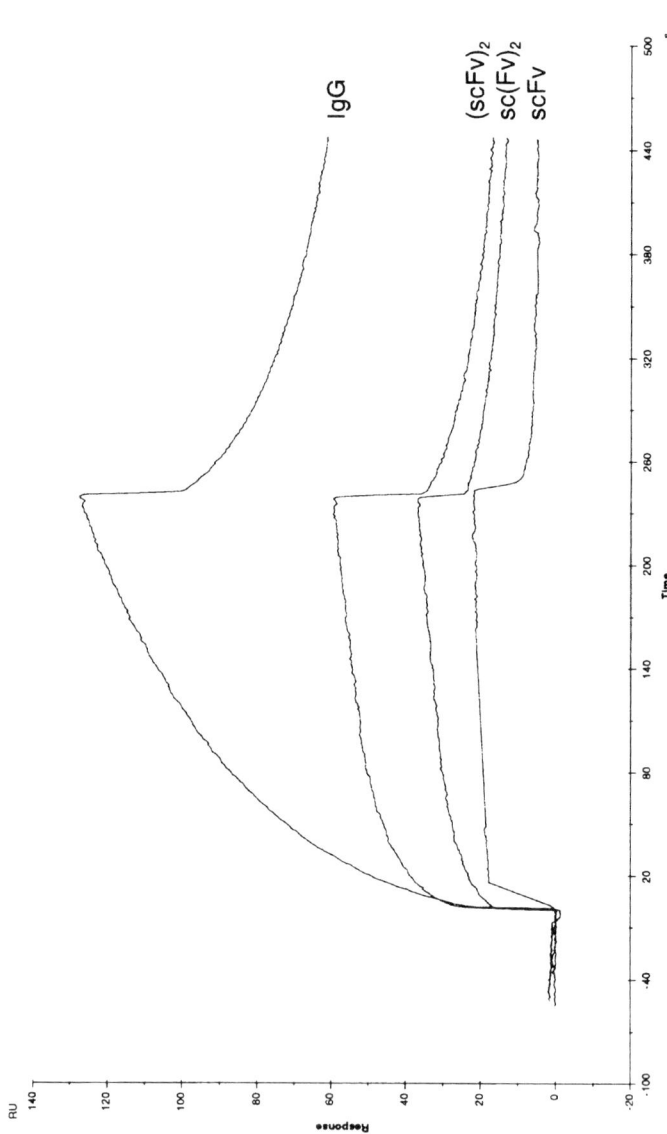

FIGURE 4. BIAcore analysis of CC49 antibody constructs. Sensogram demonstrating the binding and dissociation of MAb CC49 IgG, scFv, (scFv)$_2$ and sc(Fv)$_2$ to BSM on the biosensor chip.

BIOCHEMICAL AND IMMUNOLOGICAL CHARACTERIZATION OF PROTEINS

The purified scFv proteins were analyzed by sodium dodecylsulfate polyacrylamide gel electrophoresis (SDS-PAGE, FIG. 2). The scFv proteins were 90–95% pure and migrated according to its theoretical molecular weights, 28 kDa for scFv and 59 kDa for sc(Fv)$_2$, respectively. The high-performance liquid chromatography (HPLC) analysis evaluating the purity of the radiolabeled CC49 monovalent scFv showed two peaks corresponding to the expected M_r 28 kDa monomeric form (scFv) and a peak (56 kDa) consistent with the dimeric form of the CC49 scFv (scFv)$_2$. The CC49 (scFv)$_2$ was then separated from scFv by using gel filtration chromatography. Additional HPLC analysis of these purified constructs as well as the covalently linked dimeric sc(Fv)$_2$ (≈59 kDa) showed that they eluted as single peaks of the appropriate molecular weights (FIG. 3).

The immunoreactivity of the radiolabeled scFvs was determined by solid phase radioimmunoassay (RIA) using proteins attached to Reacti-Gel beads. Bovine submaxillary mucin (BSM), which contains the epitope recognized by MAb CC49 on the human tumor-associated antigen (TAG-72), was used as a positive control and bovine serum albumin as a negative control. The covalent dimer, sc(Fv)$_2$, showed 94% binding to BSM as compared to 70–83% for the monomeric scFv and 88–94% for the noncovalent dimer (scFv)$_2$. The intact IgG and F(ab′)$_2$ exhibited 87–90% and 81% binding, respectively. All species competed with biotinylated CC49 IgG for the binding to BSM.

To determine the binding kinetics of CC49 IgG, F(ab′)$_2$, Fab′, scFv monomer and dimers, the BIAcore biosensor (Pharmacia Biosensor, Uppsala, Sweden) system was used. This system uses surface plasmon resonance detection and permits real-time kinetic analysis of two interacting species.[53] BSM antigen was immobilized on a CM5 dextran sensor chip. The kinetic constants for association (K_A) and dissociation (K_D) were evaluated using the BIAevaluation 3.0 software supplied by the manufacturer where the experimental design correlated with the Langmuir 1:1 interaction model.[53] The binding affinity constant (K_A) for the intact CC49 IgG, covalent sc(Fv)$_2$, dimeric single-chain Fv (scFv)$_2$ and monomeric single-chain Fv (scFv) were 1.14×10^8 M^{-1}, 3.34×10^7 M^{-1}, 4.46×10^7 M^{-1}, and 1.5×10^7 M^{-1}, respectively.

PHARMACOKINETICS

Pharmacokinetic studies were conducted to determine the blood clearance rates of radiolabeled CC49 scFv forms and to compare them with the blood clearance of the enzymatically derived fragments [Fab′ and F(ab′)$_2$]. As seen in FIGURE 5A, the scFv showed a rapid blood clearance with more than 50% cleared from the blood pool in less than 10 min. The CC49 Fab′ (≈50 kDa) clearance was faster than the clearance of sc(Fv)$_2$ and (scFv)$_2$ with serum half-lives of approximately 30 min, 40 min and 50 min, respectively.

Whole body clearance analyses also displayed a rapid scFv clearance, suggesting that scFvs were not being retained in the extravascular space or in any specific organ,

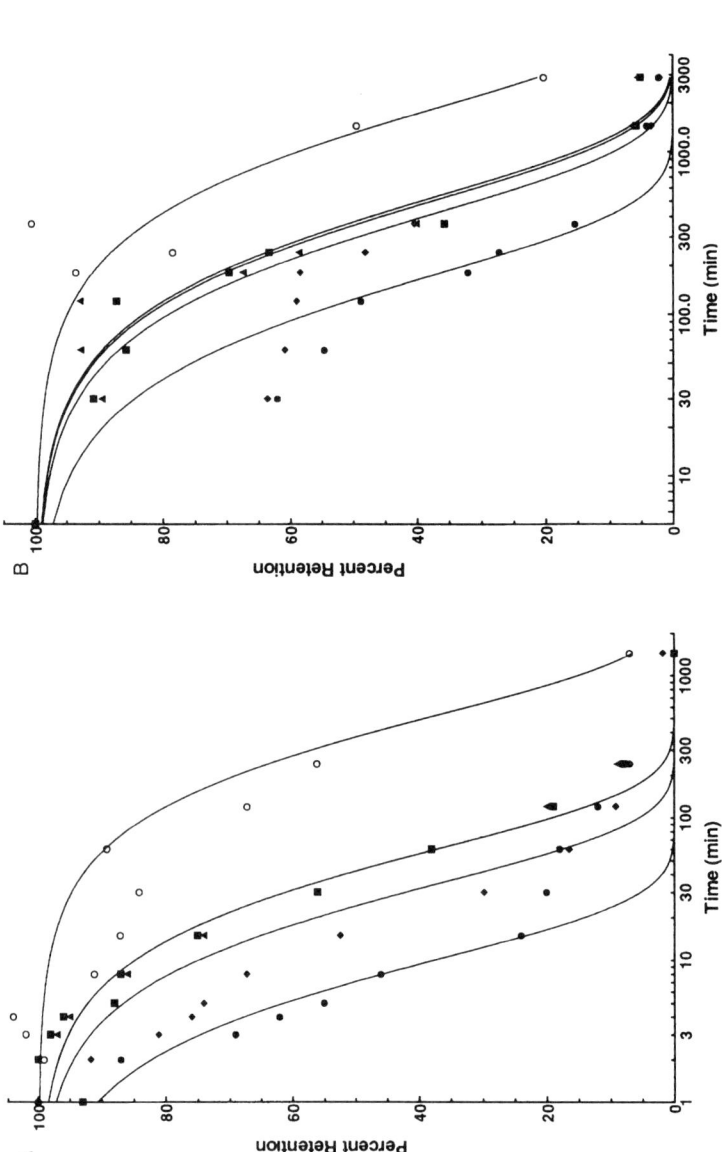

FIGURE 5. Blood and whole body clearance of CC49 constructs. Athymic mice bearing LS-174T colon cancer xenografts were injected with radiolabeled CC49 constructs and (**A**) blood samples (6 per group) were obtained at various times, or (**B**) whole body counts (3 per group) were obtained at various times using a custom-built NaI gamma counter. scFv (●), sc(Fv)$_2$ (■), (scFv)$_2$ (▲), Fab' (◆), F(ab')$_2$ (○).

TABLE 2. Comparative biodistribution studies with CC49 scFv, (scFv)$_2$, sc(Fv)$_2$, Fab', F(ab')$_2$, and IgG (percent injected dose per gram)[a]

Tissue		Time (hours)						
		0.5	1	4	6	24	48	72
scFv:	Tumor	4.74	4.81	2.93	2.01	1.06	0.72	0.27
	Blood	4.66	3.78	1.32	0.77	0.06	0.04	0.05
	Liver	1.79	1.41	0.59	0.37	0.07	0.05	0.05
	Spleen	2.73	2.17	0.84	0.45	0.06	0.04	0.03
	Kidneys	41.24	15.82	2.65	1.48	0.15	0.07	0.06
(scFv)$_2$:	Tumor	5.94	6.37	6.91	6.45	4.29	2.56	1.92
	Blood	19.27	11.89	2.56	1.56	0.10	0.07	0.07
	Liver	6.89	5.72	2.81	2.25	0.30	0.12	0.11
	Spleen	10.82	9.35	3.05	2.28	0.45	0.15	0.07
	Kidneys	32.83	21.50	2.93	1.73	0.42	0.13	0.08
sc(Fv)$_2$:	Tumor	6.12	6.63	6.78	6.27	4.29	2.62	1.94
	Blood	18.30	10.73	2.17	1.35	0.07	0.06	0.07
	Liver	5.65	4.59	2.06	1.63	0.20	0.10	0.09
	Spleen	10.01	8.21	2.04	1.53	0.18	0.08	0.05
	Kidneys	27.85	18.20	2.32	1.34	0.36	0.12	0.07
Fab':	Tumor	4.87	6.29	5.91	3.94	2.96	2.15	nd
	Blood	9.63	5.17	2.38	1.68	0.1	0.06	nd
	Liver	2.59	2.06	1.29	0.93	0.14	0.12	nd
	Spleen	3.44	2.72	1.78	1.16	0.11	0.07	nd
	Kidneys	138.34	132.35	21.50	9.58	0.37	0.16	nd
F(ab')$_2$:	Tumor	14.63	12.48	25.82	35.74	28.06	19.42	13.11
	Blood	30.15	27.88	16.32	10.09	1.68	0.36	0.16
	Liver	7.47	6.79	7.84	6.03	2.24	1.21	1.21
	Spleen	7.13	5.56	7.09	5.64	1.37	0.42	0.48
	Kidneys	11.48	11.31	9.78	7.44	2.10	0.52	0.25
IgG:	Tumor	8.95	nd	30.66	23.12	37.83	42.42	nd
	Blood	28.32	nd	24.20	17.99	11.01	5.34	nd
	Liver	9.65	nd	8.80	7.46	6.19	5.84	nd
	Spleen	8.35	nd	7.90	5.96	4.17	3.34	nd
	Kidneys	7.00	nd	5.29	5.36	2.19	1.18	nd

[a] Iodinated CC49 scFv, (scFv)$_2$, sc(Fv)$_2$, Fab', F(ab')$_2$, and IgG were injected into athymic mice (6/group) bearing LS-174T tumors. The mice were sacrificed at the indicated times and %ID/g for each organ was determined. The values presented are the average of multiple studies. The SEM for the samples were less than 20 %ID/g of the corresponding tissue. nd, not determined.

but they were eliminated from the body apparently through the urine. As seen in FIGURE 5B, the whole body clearance of the scFv dimers was slower than that of the Fab' fragment. The relative rates of clearance observed in the whole body experiments were similar to those observed with the blood clearance.

BIODISTRIBUTION AND TUMOR TARGETING

Dual label biodistribution studies allowed the direct comparison of the antigen-binding ability of the scFvs *in vivo* and their efficiency to target human colon carcinoma (LS-174T) xenografts.[54] These studies were performed with pairs of the CC49 enzyme digested fragments and scFv forms being coinjected in four sets of experiments: ^{125}I-scFv *versus* ^{131}I-Fab′, ^{125}I-(scFv)$_2$ *versus* ^{131}I-F(ab′)$_2$, ^{125}I-scFv *versus* ^{131}I-(scFv)$_2$ and ^{125}I-sc(Fv)$_2$ *versus* ^{131}I-(scFv)$_2$. In a separate dual label study, the intact ^{125}I-IgG and ^{131}I-F(ab′)$_2$ were also compared. At various times after injection, blood, tumor and normal organs were analyzed to determine the amount of each radionuclide retained per gram of tissue. As seen in TABLE 2, the CC49 F(ab′)$_2$ showed %ID/g values similar to those of intact IgG with the exception of a higher uptake in the kidneys at the early time points (<6 hr) and a faster blood clearance that can be easily seen at later points. This faster clearance resulted in somewhat lower %ID/g in the tumor for the F(ab′)$_2$ fragment as compared to the IgG at all time points evaluated after 48 hr. The Fab′, sc(Fv)$_2$, (scFv)$_2$ and scFv %ID/g levels in tissues are generally lower due to a more rapid blood and whole body clearance. As expected, Fab′ and scFv forms showed higher levels in the kidneys at the earliest times evaluated. The Fab′ uptake by kidneys was much higher than that observed for CC49 dimeric and monomeric scFvs (6- to 8-fold higher at 1 hr). The level of uptake of the scFv dimers were elevated in kidneys at the early time points. However, the observed uptake is notably lower, 4-fold (at 30 min) and 6-fold (at 1 hr), than that seen with the Fab′ fragment. The %ID/g in the kidneys observed with the scFv constructs was close to that found in the other major organs by 4 hr post administration. The uptake level at 24 hr of the (scFv)$_2$ in the spleen and liver was 1.5- to 2-fold higher than that seen with the sc(Fv)$_2$ construct. The lower normal tissue levels seen with the covalent dimeric scFv as compared with the noncovalent dimer indicate that the sc(Fv)$_2$ construct may be better for *in vivo* use.

The differential tumor binding of CC49 IgG, F(ab′)$_2$, Fab′, scFv, (scFv)$_2$ and sc(Fv)$_2$ was revealed in the analysis of the *in vivo* tumor targeting. The CC49 IgG and F(ab′)$_2$ %ID/g was as high as 37.8% and 28.1% (TABLE 2), respectively at 24 hr post administration. A higher level of tumor uptake was observed with dimeric scFvs as compared to monomeric scFv and Fab′ fragments, where 4.3 %ID/g was seen for targeting to the LS-174T xenograft as compared to 1.1 %ID/g for monomeric scFv and 3.0 %ID/g for Fab′ at 24 hr post administration. The CC49 F(ab′)$_2$ also showed elevated uptake in the liver, spleen and kidneys compared to (scFv)$_2$ or sc(Fv)$_2$. Dimeric scFvs appear to remain intact *in vivo* as evidenced by the higher tumor uptake than that seen with the monovalent forms of CC49, scFv and Fab′.

An equally important parameter is the radiolocalization index (RI, ratio of the %ID/g in tumor to the %ID/g in normal tissue). The scFv forms exhibited much higher RI values at 24 hr than intact IgG (TABLE 3). Extremely high RIs for well vascularized organs such as liver were obtained with the scFv dimers with tumor:blood and tumor:liver ratios of 42.9 and 14.3, respectively for (scFv)$_2$ and 61.3 and 21.5 for sc(Fv)$_2$, as compared to with 3.4 and 6.1, respectively for IgG and 16.7 and 12.5 for F(ab′)$_2$.

Whole body clearance data showed that 90% of the scFvs had cleared from the body by 24 hr. To investigate whether there is any specific or nonspecific accumula-

TABLE 3. Comparative biodistribution studies of CC49 IgG, F(ab')$_2$, Fab', scFv, sc(Fv)$_2$, and (scFv)$_2$ (Radiolocalization Index) at 24 hours after administration[a]

Tissue	scFv	(scFv)$_2$	sc(Fv)$_2$	Fab'	F(ab')$_2$	IgG
Blood	23.2	42.9	61.3	34.0	16.7	3.4
Liver	16.6	14.3	21.5	16.3	12.5	6.1
Spleen	19.3	9.5	23.8	24.9	20.5	9.1
Kidneys	7.3	10.2	11.9	9.1	13.4	17.3
Lungs	16.6	47.7	61.3	31.2	29.5	7.2

[a]Iodinated CC49 scFv, sc(Fv)$_2$, (scFv)$_2$, Fab', F(ab')$_2$, and IgG were injected into athymic mice (6/group) bearing LS-174T tumors. The mice were sacrificed at the indicated times and radiolocalization index (%ID/g of tumor divided by %ID/g of normal tissue) for each organ was determined.

tion of scFv forms in tissues, the tissue:blood ratios were calculated (FIG. 6). Specific accumulation in the tumor of the CC49 forms is clearly shown by tumor:blood ratios increasing over time. The concentration of Fab' fragments in the kidneys is high at early time points (e.g., 6 hr post injection) and lower at the later time points (e.g., 24 hr). The scFv forms were relatively low in normal tissues at both 6 hr and 24 hr post injection. Differences in the clearance from the normal tissues were observed between the the sc(Fv)$_2$ and the (scFv)$_2$ constructs. The spleen:blood ratio was higher for the (scFv)$_2$ than for the sc(Fv)$_2$ with values of 4.4:1 and 2.6:1, respectively at 24 hr post injection.

CONCLUSIONS

Monoclonal antibodies against tumor-associated antigens are being developed for many clinical applications in pancreatic cancer. Some antigens initially defined only by their reactivity with MAbs are now being used to detect or monitor the progression of the disease (CEA, CA19.9, DU-PAN2). Unfortunately, many of these antigens are commonly expressed in normal tissue, and elevated serum levels occur in many benign gastrointestinal diseases.[55,56] Another antigen highly expressed in gastrointestinal adenocarcinomas is the TAG-72 antigen. The TAG-72 antigen is expressed selectively in a majority of the primary and metastatic pancreatic adenocarcinomas but not significantly in normal pancreas. The restricted expression tumor-associated TAG-72 can be used as a valuable tumor target for active and passive immunotherapy of pancreatic cancer. The preclinical therapeutic studies using radiolabeled MAb CC49 showed a 3- to 5-fold improvement in therapeutic efficacy over the first generation MAb B72.3, producing cures in these preclinical models. In order to further improve the therapeutic efficacy of CC49 IgG, a range of single-chain antibody fragments were engineered.

The divalent antibody fragments (sc(Fv)$_2$ or (scFv)$_2$) displayed an affinity constant similar to that of the IgG CC49 and were stable with storage and after radiolabeling. In biodistribution studies, both the covalent and the noncovalent dimeric scFvs exhibited excellent tumor targeting properties with some characteristics similar to those of the monomer, e.g., the rapid blood clearance, low kidney uptake and small size suitable for rapid penetration through tumor tissue. Increased tumor tar-

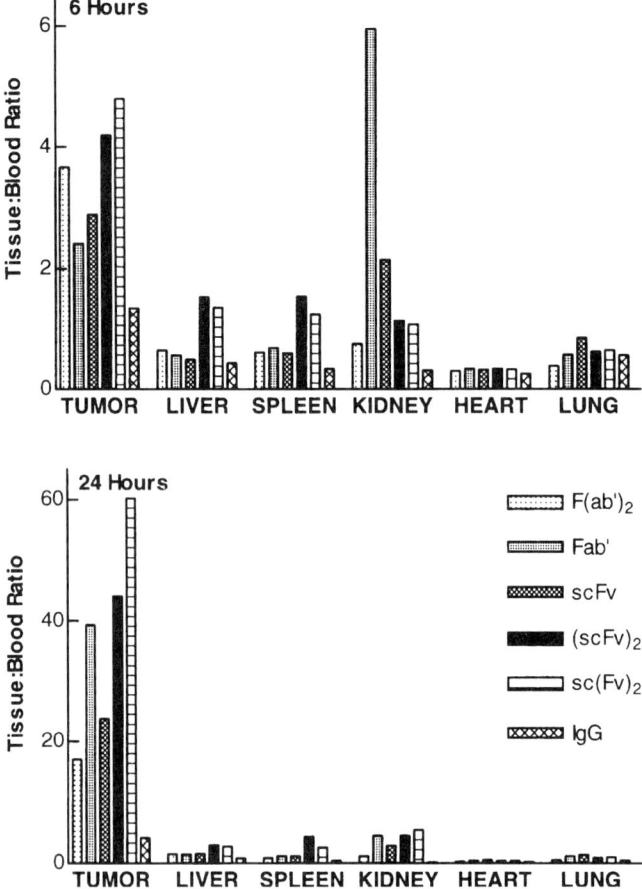

FIGURE 6. Biodistribution studies (tissue:blood ratio) with CC49 scFv, (scFv)$_2$, sc(Fv)$_2$, Fab', F(ab')$_2$, and IgG. Iodinated CC49 Ig forms were injected into athymic mice (6/group) bearing LS-174T tumors. The mice were sacrificed at the indicated times and ratio of %ID/g of tissue to %ID/g of blood was calculated.

geting of the dimers, probably due to its increased functional affinity attributable to valency, coupled with their higher molecular weight and fewer interactions with normal organs, makes these constructs superior to monovalent CC49 scFv. The noncovalent dimeric (scFv)$_2$ showed higher liver and spleen uptake than the covalent sc(Fv)$_2$ construct. High tumor:blood ratios at early times and their rapid clearance makes the scFv constructs excellent candidates for imaging applications. The relatively high tumor uptake, the *in vitro* and *in vivo* targeting specificity, and the stability in storage demonstrated by CC49 sc(Fv)$_2$ makes it a promising delivery vehicle for therapeutic applications.

ACKNOWLEDGMENTS

This study was supported in part by a grant from the United States Department of Energy (DE-FG02-95ER62024) and was conducted in the J. Bruce Henrikson Cancer Research Laboratories. We would like to thank Kathy Niedermyer for help in preparing the manuscript, the Monoclonal Antibody Core Facility for the purification of scFv proteins, the Molecular Interactions Laboratory for the BIAcore analysis, and the Molecular Core Laboratory for sequence analysis. The CC49 scFv construct was a generous gift from the National Cancer Institute Laboratory of Tumor Immunology and Biology and the Dow Chemical Company.

REFERENCES

1. WANEBO, H.J., B. RAO, C.M. PINSKY et al. 1978. Preoperative carcinoembryonic antigen level as a prognostic indicator in colorectal cancer. N. Engl. J. Med. **299:** 448–451.
2. MINTON, J.P., J.L. HOEHN, D.M. GERBER et al. 1985. Results of a 400-patient carcinoembryonic antigen second-look colorectal cancer study. Cancer **55:** 1284–1290.
3. RITTS, R.E., JR., B.C. DEL VILLANO, V.L. GO et al. 1984. Initial clinical evaluation of an immunoradiometric assay for CA 19-9 using the NCI serum bank. Int. J. Cancer **33:** 339–345.
4. SATAKE, K., G. KANAZAWA, I. KHO et al. 1985. A clinical evaluation of carbohydrate antigen 19-9 and carcinoembryonic antigen in patients with pancreatic carcinoma. J. Surg. Oncol. **29:** 15–21.
5. BAST, R.C., JR., T.L. KLUG, E. ST JOHN et al. 1983. A radioimmunoassay using a monoclonal antibody to monitor the course of epithelial ovarian cancer. N. Engl. J. Med. **309:** 883–887.
6. SAFI, F., I. KOHLER, E. ROTTINGER et al. 1991. The value of the tumor marker CA 15-3 in diagnosing and monitoring breast cancer. A comparative study with carcinoembryonic antigen. Cancer **68:** 574–582.
7. METZGAR, R.S., M.T. GAILLARD, S.J. LEVINE et al. 1982. Antigens of human pancreatic adenocarcinoma cells defined by murine monoclonal antibodies. Cancer Res. **42:** 601–608.
8. TAYLOR, P.J., J.A. PETERSON, J. ARKLIE et al. 1981. Monoclonal antibodies to epithelium-specific components of the human milk fat globule membrane: production and reaction with cells in culture. Int. J. Cancer **28:** 17–21.
9. BURCHELL, J., H. DURBIN & P.J. TAYLOR. 1983. Complexity of expression of antigenic determinants, recognized by monoclonal antibodies HMFG-1 and HMFG-2, in normal and malignant human mammary epithelial cells. J. Immunol. **131:** 508–513.
10. BURCHELL, J., S. GENDLER, P.J. TAYLOR et al. 1987. Development and characterization of breast cancer reactive monoclonal antibodies directed to the core protein of the human milk mucin. Cancer Res **47:** 5476–5482.
11. HERLYN, M., Z. STEPLEWSKI, D. HERLYN et al. 1979. Colorectal carcinoma-specific antigen: detection by means of monoclonal antibodies. Proc. Natl. Acad. Sci. USA **76:** 1438–1452.
12. KOPROWSKI, H., Z. STEPLEWSKI, K. MITCHELL et al. 1979. Colorectal carcinoma antigens detected by hybridoma antibodies. Somatic Cell Genet. **5:** 957–971.
13. COLCHER, D., P.H. HAND, M. NUTI et al. 1981. A spectrum of monoclonal antibodies reactive with human mammary tumor cells. Proc. Natl. Acad. Sci. USA **78:** 3199–3203.
14. JOHNSON, V.G., J. SCHLOM, A.J. PATERSON et al. 1986. Analysis of a human tumor-associated glycoprotein (TAG-72) identified by monoclonal antibody B72.3. Cancer Res. **46:** 850–857.

15. THOR, A., N. OHUCHI, C.A. SZPAK et al. 1986. The distribution of oncofetal antigen tumor-associated glycoprotein-72 defined by monoclonal antibody B72.3. Cancer Res. **46:** 3118–3124.
16. OHUCHI, N., A. THOR, M. NOSE et al. 1986. Tumor-associated glycoprotein (TAG-72) detected in adenocarcinomas and benign lesions of the stomach. Int. J. Cancer **38:** 643–650.
17. LYUBSKY, S., J. MADARIAGA, M. LOZOWSKI et al. 1988. A tumor-associated antigen in carcinoma of the pancreas defined by monoclonal antibody B72.3. Am. J. Clin. Pathol. **89:** 160–167.
18. TEMPERO, M., H. TAKASAKI, E. UCHIDA et al. 1989. Co-expression of CA 19-9, DU-PAN-2, CA 125, and TAG-72 in pancreatic adenocarcinoma. Am. J. Surg. Pathol. **13**(Suppl. 1): 89–95.
19. SCHLOM, J., K. SILER, D.E. MILENIC et al. 1991. Monoclonal antibody-based therapy of a human tumor xenograft with a 177lutetium-labeled immunoconjugate. Cancer Res. **51:** 2889–2896.
20. SCHLOM, J., D. EGGENSPERGER, D. COLCHER et al. 1992. Therapeutic advantage of high-affinity anticarcinoma radioimmunoconjugates. Cancer Res. **52:** 1067–1072.
21. SCHLOM, J., A. MOLINOLO, J.F. SIMPSON et al. 1990. Advantage of dose fractionation in monoclonal antibody-targeted radioimmunotherapy. J. Natl. Cancer Inst. **82:** 763–771.
22. CARRASQUILLO, J.A., P. SUGARBAKER, D. COLCHER et al. 1988. Radioimmunoscintigraphy of colon cancer with iodine-131-labeled B72.3 monoclonal antibody. J. Nucl. Med. **29:** 1022–1030.
23. CARRASQUILLO, J.A., P. SUGARBAKER, D. COLCHER et al. 1988. Peritoneal carcinomatosis: imaging with intraperitoneal injection of I-131-labeled B72.3 monoclonal antibody. Radiology **167:** 35–40.
24. FOON, K.A. 1989. Biological response modifiers: the new immunotherapy [published erratum appears in Cancer Res. 1990 Jan 1; **50**(1)**:** 212]. Cancer Res. **49:** 1621–1639.
25. LEICHNER, P.K., G. AKABANI, D. COLCHER et al. 1997. Patient-specific dosimetry of indium-111- and yttrium-90-labeled monoclonal antibody CC49. J. Nucl. Med. **38:** 512–516.
26. JAIN, R.K. 1987. Transport of molecules in the tumor interstitium: a review. Cancer Res. **47:** 3039–3051.
27. MILENIC, D.E., J.M. ESTEBAN & D. COLCHER. 1989. Comparison of methods for the generation of immunoreactive fragments of a monoclonal antibody (B72.3) reactive with human carcinomas. J. Immunol. Methods **120:** 71–83.
28. BIRD, R.E., K.D. HARDMAN, J.W. JACOBSON et al. 1988. Single-chain antigen-binding proteins [published erratum appears in Science 1989 Apr 28; **244**(4903)**:** 409]. Science **242:** 423–426.
29. HUSTON, J.S., D. LEVINSON, M. MUDGETT HUNTER et al. 1988. Protein engineering of antibody binding sites: recovery of specific activity in an anti-digoxin single-chain Fv analogue produced in *Escherichia coli*. Proc. Natl. Acad. Sci. USA **85:** 5879–5883.
30. COLCHER, D., R. BIRD, M. ROSELLI et al. 1990. In vivo tumor targeting of a recombinant single-chain antigen-binding protein. J Natl. Cancer Inst. **82:** 1191–1197.
31. MILENIC, D.E., T. YOKOTA, D.R. FILPULA et al. 1991. Construction, binding properties, metabolism, and tumor targeting of a single-chain Fv derived from the pancarcinoma monoclonal antibody CC49. Cancer Res **51:** 6363–6371.
32. YOKOTA, T., D.E. MILENIC, M. WHITLOW et al. 1992. Rapid tumor penetration of a single-chain Fv and comparison with other immunoglobulin forms. Cancer Res. **52:** 3402–3408.
33. CONDRA, J.H., V.V. SARDANA, J.E. TOMASSINI et al. 1990. Bacterial expression of antibody fragments that block human rhinovirus infection of cultured cells. J. Biol. Chem. **265:** 2292–2295.
34. PLUCKTHUN, A. & P. PACK. 1997. New protein engineering approaches to multivalent and bispecific antibody fragments. Immunotechnology **3:** 83–105.

35. ADAMS, G.P., J.E. MCCARTNEY, M.S. TAI et al. 1993. Highly specific in vivo tumor targeting by monovalent and divalent forms of 741F8 anti-c-erbB-2 single-chain Fv. Cancer Res. **53:** 4026–4034.
36. PACK, P., M. KUJAU, V. M., SCHROECKH et al. 1993. Improved bivalent miniantibodies, with identical avidity as whole antibodies, produced by high cell density fermentation of Escherichia coli. Biotechnology N Y **11:** 1271–1277.
37. PACK, P. & A. PLUCKTHUN. 1992. Miniantibodies: use of amphipathic helices to produce functional, flexibly linked dimeric FV fragments with high avidity in Escherichia coli. Biochem. **31:** 1579–1584.
38. HU, S., L. SHIVELY, A. RAUBITSCHEK et al. 1996. Minibody: a novel engineered anticarcinoembryonic antigen antibody fragment (single-chain Fv-CH3) which exhibits rapid, high-level targeting of xenografts. Cancer Res. **56:** 3055–3061.
39. KOSTELNY, S.A., M.S. COLE & J.Y. TSO. 1992. Formation of a bispecific antibody by the use of leucine zippers. J. Immunol. **148:** 1547–1553.
40. RHEINNECKER, M., C. HARDT, L.L. ILAG et al. 1996. Multivalent antibody fragments with high functional affinity for a tumor-associated carbohydrate antigen. J. Immunol. **157:** 2989–2997.
41. DUBEL, S., F. BREITLING, R. KONTERMANN et al. 1995. Bifunctional and multimeric complexes of streptavidin fused to single chain antibodies (scFv). J. Immunol. Methods **178:** 201–209.
42. MCGREGOR, D.P., P.E. MOLLOY, C. CUNNINGHAM et al. 1994. Spontaneous assembly of bivalent single chain antibody fragments in Escherichia coli. Mol. Immunol. **31:** 219–226.
43. HOLLIGER, P., T. PROSPERO & G. WINTER. 1993. "Diabodies": small bivalent and bispecific antibody fragments. Proc. Natl. Acad. Sci. USA **90:** 6444–6448.
44. ILIADES, P., A.A. KORTT & P.J. HUDSON. 1997. Triabodies: single chain Fv fragments without a linker form trivalent trimers. FEBS Lett. **409:** 437–441.
45. KORTT, A.A., M. LAH, G.W. ODDIE et al. 1997. Single-chain Fv fragments of anti-neuraminidase antibody NC10 containing five- and ten-residue linkers form dimers and with zero-residue linker a trimer. Protein Eng. **10:** 423–433.
46. COLCHER, D., M.F. MINELLI, M. ROSELLI et al. 1988. Radioimmunolocalization of human carcinoma xenografts with B72.3 second generation monoclonal antibodies. Cancer Res. **48:** 4597–4603.
47. MURARO, R., M. KUROKI, D. WUNDERLICH et al. 1988. Generation and characterization of B72.3 second generation monoclonal antibodies reactive with the tumor-associated glycoprotein 72 antigen. Cancer Res. **48:** 4588–4596.
48. KUROKI, M., P.D. FERNSTEN, D. WUNDERLICH et al. 1990. Serological mapping of the TAG-72 tumor-associated antigen using 19 distinct monoclonal antibodies. Cancer Res. **50:** 4872–4879.
49. MOLINOLO, A., J.F. SIMPSON, A. THOR et al. 1990. Enhanced tumor binding using immunohistochemical analyses by second generation anti-tumor-associated glycoprotein 72 monoclonal antibodies versus monoclonal antibody B72.3 in human tissue. Cancer Res. **50:** 1291–1298.
50. SCHLOM, J., D.E. MILENIC, M. ROSELLI et al. 1991. New concepts in monoclonal antibody based radioimmunodiagnosis and radioimmunotherapy of carcinoma. Int. J. Radiat. Appl. Instrum. Part B **18:** 425–435.
51. MULLIS, K.B. & F.A. FALOONA. 1987. Specific synthesis of DNA in vitro via a polymerase-catalyzed chain reaction. Methods Enzymol. **155:** 335–350.
52. PANTOLIANO, M.W., R.E. BIRD, S. JOHNSON et al. 1991. Conformational stability, folding, and ligand-binding affinity of single-chain Fv immunoglobulin fragments expressed in Escherichia coli. Biochemistry **30:** 10117–10125.
53. KARLSSON, R. & A. FALT. 1997. Experimental design for kinetic analysis of protein-protein interactions with surface plasmon resonance biosensors. J. Immunol. Methods **200:** 121–133.
54. TOM, B. H., L.P. RUTZKY, M.M. JAKSTYS, R. OYASU, C.I. KAYE & B.D. KANAN. 1976. Radioimmunoscintigraphy of human colon cancer xenografts in mice with radioiodinated monoclonal antibody B72.3. In Vitro (Rockville) **12:** 180–191.

55. HANSEN, H.J., J.J. SNYDER, E. MILLER *et al.* 1974. Carcinoembryonic antigen (CEA) assay. A laboratory adjunct in the diagnosis and management of cancer. Hum. Pathol. **5:** 139–147.
56. SAKAMOTO, K., Y. HAGA, R. YOSHIMURA *et al.* 1987. Comparative effectiveness of the tumour diagnostics, CA 19-9, CA 125 and carcinoembryonic antigen in patients with diseases of the digestive system. Gut **28:** 323–329.

p53 in Relation to Therapeutic Outcome of Locoregional Chemotherapy in Pancreatic Cancer

FRANK GANSAUGE,[a] SUSANNE GANSAUGE, KARL H. LINK, AND HANS G. BEGER

Department of General Surgery, University of Ulm, 89075 Ulm, Germany

ABSTRACT: Since celiac artery infusion (CAI) led to an increase in survival in palliative chemotherapy in pancreatic cancer, we treated 26 patients with adjuvant CAI following resection for advanced pancreatic cancer. Catheters were placed angiographically into the celiac artery and remained there for five consecutive days. One cycle of chemotherapy consisted of mitoxantrone, 5-fluorouracil (5-FU), folinic acid, and *cis*-platinum. This treatment was repeated five times in monthly intervals. Median survival times in patients who received CAI are 21 months for all patients, whereas in patients who did not receive adjuvant treatment median survival is 10.5 months. In all patients p53 expression of the carcinomas was determined by immunhistochemistry. In 11/26 patients a p53 overexpression was observed. Although p53 overexpression turned out to be associated with poor prognosis in the patients who underwent adjuvant regional cancer treatment, p53 is not a sufficient prognostic parameter in pancreatic carcinoma, since p53 overexpression was more frequent in undifferentiated tumors and in palliative resected tumors.

INTRODUCTION

Cancer of the pancreas still has a devasting prognosis. The overall 5-year survival rate is extremely low ranging between 1% and 2%. To date resection of the tumor at an early stage still offers the only chance for cure. However, even in patients who have undergone resection of the primary tumor, median survival times are seldom higher than 12–18 months, depending on the selection criteria for the patients investigated.[1–3] The overall 5-year survival rates following R0 resection range between 11 and 28%,[3–5] and in UICC stage I carcinomas with a tumor size less than 2 cm the 5-year survival rate was 38%.[6]

Since celiac artery infusion (CAI) based on mitoxantrone, 5-fluorouracil (5-FU), folinic acid, and *cis*-platinum had beneficial effects in regard to increased median survival and pain reduction in patients with unresectable pancreatic cancers,[7] we conducted a study based on that treatment regimen in patients who underwent pancreaticoduodenectomy for pancreatic cancer.

During the past decade numerous studies have investigated molecular alterations in pancreatic cancer.[8] Many among the factors and molecules investigated have been

---

[a]Corresponding author: Frank Gansauge, MD, Department of General Surgery, University of Ulm, Steinhövelstr. 9, 89075 Ulm, Germany. Phone, +49 731-502-7236; fax, +49 731-502-7214.

supposed to have prognostic potential like epidermal growth factor (EGF), transforming growth factor, angiogenin or Cyclin D1.[8] However, in recent study we investigated the prognostic potential of many molecules like EGF, EGF-R, cERB-B2, p53, Cyclin D1, p21WAF, BCL-2, CD95 and KI67 in a large number of pancreatic cancer tissue specimens and found none of these factors to be independent prognostic factors.[9] Since p53 is supposed to be involved in the regulation of enzyme systems that are thought to affect tumor response to chemotherapeutic agents like thymidylatsynthase (TS) or multidrug resistance enzyme 1, we analyzed in the pancreatic cancer tissue of the patients the expression of p53 in order to evaluate the prognostic potential of p53 for response prediction in pancreatic cancer patients undergoing regional chemotherapy.

PATIENTS AND METHODS

Patients

From 12/1992 until 7/1997 we treated a total of 26 patients with CAI following resection for pancreatic cancer. The mean age was 59.3 years ranging from 39 to 75 years. Two of these patients had a pancreatic carcinoma of the tail and underwent left resection. The other 24 patients, 12 female and 12 male, had a pancreatic head carcinoma, and in all cases diagnosis was confirmed by histological examination. One patient had an UICC stage I pancreatic carcinoma, three patients had a locally advanced pancreatic head carcinoma with infiltration of the surrounding tissue (UICC stage II), and 22 patients had pancreatic carcinomas that had already spread into the regional lymph nodes (UICC stage III). In 4 patients a partial duodenopancreatectomy, in one patient a pancreatectomy, in two patients a left resection, and in 19 patients a pylorus-preserving partial duodenopancreatectomy was performed. In 7 patients palliative resections only were performed due to local infiltration of arterial vessels (RII). The mean number of cycles performed per patient was 5.8 (range 2–15).

The control group (resection without adjuvant chemotherapy) consisted of 27 patients who underwent surgery for pancreatic head carcinoma between 01/1993 and 05/1996. The mean age in this group was 60.8 years ranging from 42 to 78 years. The stage distribution was as follows: 1 patient UICC stage I, 3 patients UICC stage II, and 23 patients UICC stage III. In 17 patients a pylorus-preserving duodenopancreatectomy was performed, 8 patients underwent a Whipples's procedure, and in 2 patients a left resection of the pancreas was performed. Out of these 27 patients, 23 were resected without macroscopically visible tumor residues (R0/RI), and in 4 patients tumor residues remained (RII).

Adjuvant CAI

For CAI, catheters were placed in Seldinger's technique with the tip into the celiac axis via the femoral artery and left in place for five consecutive days. The exact position was controlled on the second and fifth day. Heparin (20,000 IU/d) was continously given via the catheter, except during infusion of the drugs. One cycle consisted of mitoxantrone (novantron, Wyeth-Lederle), 10 mg/m^2 (day 1), folinic acid (leucovorin, Wyeth-Lederle), 170 mg/m^2 for 10 minutes, followed by 5-FU (Wyeth-Lederle) 600 mg/m^2 for 120 minutes (days 2–4), and *cis*-platinum (Bristol), 60 mg/m^2 at day 5.

Toxicity was evaluated and graded each cycle according to World Health Organization (WHO) criteria. After the third and sixth cycles an upper abdomen CT-scan and a chest X-ray were performed to evaluate the remission status.

Immunhistochemistry

Tissues were collected immediately after surgical removal, fixed in 4% formalin for 1 day at room temperature, processed, and embedded in formalin. Five-μm-thick sections were placed on 1% silane-coated slide glasses and were boiled up in 0.2% citrate buffer for 20 min. The monoclonal antibody DO1 (Oncogene Science, MA, USA), which recognizes human p53 protein, was used for immunohistochemical staining in a dilution of 1:500. The primary antibody was detected with a biotinylated anti-mouse immunoglobulin G (IgG) secondary antibody and streptavidin-peroxidase complex (Dako, Denmark), followed by incubation with diaminobenzidine tetrahydrochloride as the substrate. The slides were counterstained with Mayer's hemalum.

RESULTS

Toxicity

No severe local side effects at the catheter insertion site occurred. During the treatment cycles no severe systemic or abdominal complications were observed. Systemic side effects WHO I were seen in 31% of the cycles, WHO II in 18%, and WHO III in 8% (mainly gastrointestinal ulcerations), whereas no WHO IV toxic events were observed.

Relapse-Free Survival and Relaspse Pattern

After the sixth cycle the restaging examinations revealed that 17/26 patients were disease free. Three patients had died before the sixth cycle due to local relapses in 2 cases and liver metastases in one case, and 4 patients had local relapses. Two patients finished treatment prior to the sixth cycle.

At present 3/26 patients are without tumor recurrence. Twenty-two of 26 patients died mainly due to local relapses. One patient has had a local recurrence for 15 months.

Survival

In a Kaplan-Meier regression analysis of the 26 patients who received CAI following pancreatic head resection, the median survival is 21 months. In comparison to the control group of patients who only underwent resection, patients who received postoperative regional chemotherapy lived significantly longer (CAI 21 months, no CAI 10.5 months; p <0.005, Fig. 1).

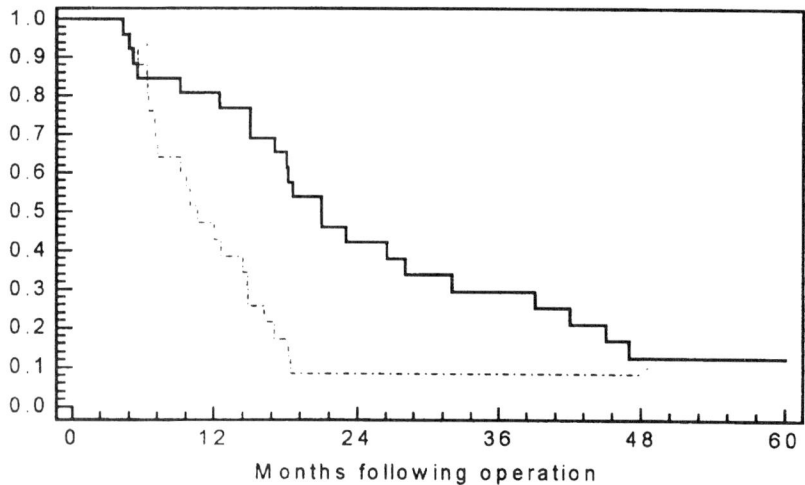

FIGURE 1. Kaplan-Meier regression analysis of all resected pancreatic cancer patients who received CAI (*thick line*, $n = 26$) in comparison to patients who underwent resection only (*thin line*, $n = 27$). Patients with adjuvant CAI lived significantly longer than patients without ($p < 0.005$).

Expression of p53

Overexpression of p53 was observed in 11/26 patients (42%). This p53 overexpression rate is consistant with our previous studies in larger series of pancreatic cancer.[10] In Kaplan-Meier regression analysis, patients whose tissues showed an overexpression of p53 lived a significantly shorter time than those whose tissues stained negatively for p53 (FIG. 2A, $p < 0.01$). However, as reported earlier, p53 overexpression was more frequently found in undifferentiated tumors. Five of 7 (71%) undifferentiated tumors were p53 positive, whereas 13/19 (68%) well or moderately differentiated tumors stained negatively for p53 ($p = 0.08$, Fisher's exact test). Furthermore, in locally advanced tumors that were only resectable under palliative aspects (RII resections), p53 overexpression was also found in 5/7 tumors (71%). In the 26 patients with pancreatic carcinoma who underwent regional chemotherapy, differentiation and resection margins were associated with poor prognosis (FIG. 2B,C). In univariate analysis, p53 turned out to be a dependent parameter with regard

FIGURE 2. Kaplan-Meier regression analysis of patients who underwent regional chemotherapy (**A**) dependent on the p53 status: patients whose tumors stained negatively for p53 (*thick line*, $n = 15$) lived significantly longer than those whose tumors showed an overexpression of p53 (*thin line*, $n = 11$, $p < 0.02$); (**B**) dependent on the tumor grading: *thick line*, well and moderately differentiated tumors ($n = 19$); *thin line*, undifferentiated tumors ($n = 7$, $p < 0.02$); (**C**) dependent on the extent of tumor resection: *thick line*, curative resection ($n = 19$); *thin line*, palliative resection with macroscopic residues of tumor ($n = 7$, $p < 0.0001$).

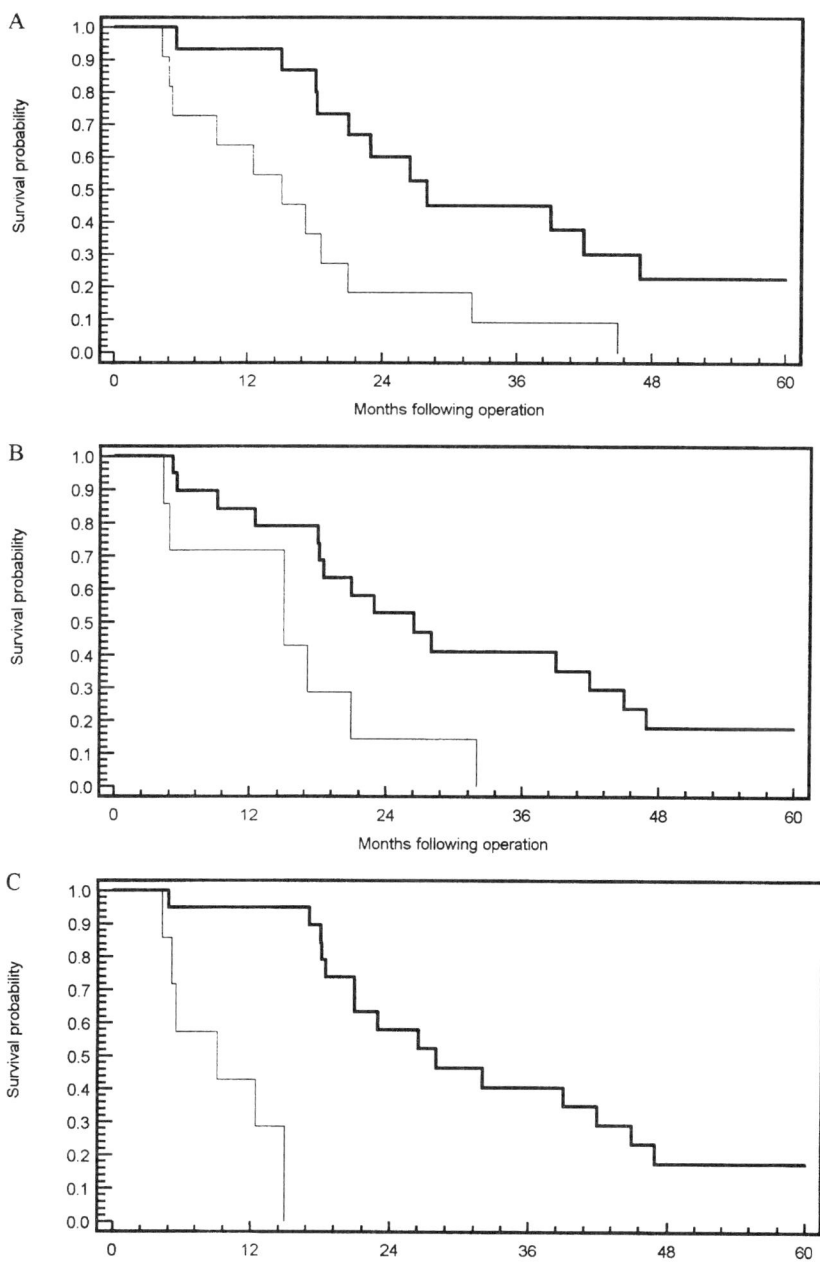

to the resection margins status and the tumor grading, not offering additional information about the outcome of the patients undergoing regional chemotherapy.

DISCUSSION

Systemic chemotherapy has not been accepted as a standard adjuvant procedure in patients who had pancreatic resection for surgical treatment of pancreatic cancer. Postoperative radiochemotherapy based on a 5-FU chemotherapy was firstly introduced by the Gastrointestinal Tumor Study Group (GITSG), and recent studies have confirmed the beneficial effects of this treatment.[5] However, confirmation of this treatment protocol by phase III studies is needed before radiochemotherapy can be recommended as standard adjuvant therapy. These studies (by the European Study Group for Pancreatic Cancer (ESPAC) and in a Dutch multicenter trial) are currently under investigation.

Since our treatment protocol by CAI in the palliative situation in patients with unresectable pancreatic cancer leads to an increase in median survival times,[7] we also used this treatment protocol in the adjuvant situation. Although this treatment is inconvenient for the patient, being immobilized during the treatment for five consecutive days, the compliance was extremely high, which was probably due to the very low toxicity rates and the pain reduction as shown by reduced consumption of analgetics.[11] In all patients treated with CAI in the adjuvant situation following pancreatic head resection for pancreatic cancer, the median survival time according to Kaplan-Meier regression analysis is 21 months, which is twice that observed in a group of patients with pancreatic cancer who did not receive an adjuvant treatment. This increased survival was even higher when only patients who underwent curative resections were included into the analysis. Similar to our results, Ishikawa and co-workers also observed an increase in patients' survival when they treated patients with postoperative hepatic artery and portal vein infusion.[12] Interestingly, p53 overexpression was associated with a worse outcome of the patients undergoing regional chemotherapy. However, detailed analysis of this promising result revealed that p53 overexpression was more frequently found in undifferentiated tumors, which are known to be associated with a worse prognosis, than in well or moderately differentiated tumors. In our series of patients, p53 overexpression was even more frequent in those with macroscopic residues of the tumor, which is also associated with a worse prognosis. In univariate analysis, p53 was dependent on these two parameters, not offering additional information with regard to the prognosis of the patients.

In conclusion, although p53 overexpression is associated with poor prognosis in pancreatic carcinoma patients undergoing adjuvant regional chemotherapy, determination of p53 by using immunhistochemistry does not offer more information with regard to prognosis than tumor grading and resection margins of the pancreatic tumor.

REFERENCES

1. GUDJONSSON, B. 1987. Cancer of the pancreas: 50 years of surgery. Cancer **60:** 2284–2303.

2. NITECKI, S.S., M.G. SARR, T.V. COLBY & J.A. VAN HEERDEN. 1995. Long-term survival after resection for ductal adenocarcinoma of the pancreas. Ann. Surg. **221:** 59–66.
3. BEGER, H.G. & R. BITTNER. 1985. Surgical treatment in carcinoma of the head of the pancreas. Z. Gastroenterol. **23:** 240–247.
4. TREDE, M. 1987. The surgical treatment of pancreatic carcinoma. Surgery **97:** 28–34.
5. YEO, C.J., R.A. ABRAMS, L.B. GROCHOW, T.A. SOHN, S.E. ORD, R.H. HRUBAN, M.L. ZAHURAK, W.C. DOOLEY, J. COLEMAN, P.K. SAUTER, H.A. PITT, K.D. LILLEMOE & J.L. CAMERON. 1997. Pancreaticoduodenectomy for pancreatic adenocarcinoma: postoperative adjuvant chemoradiation improves survival. A prospective, single-institution experience. Ann. Surg. **225:** 621–627.
6. TSUCHIYA, R., T. TOMIOKA, K. IZAWA, T. NODA, K. YAMAMOTO, T. TSUNODA, N. HARADA, T. YAMAGUCHI, R. YOSHINO & T. MIYAMOTO. 1986. Collective review of small carcinomas of the pancreas. Ann. Surg. **203:** 77–81.
7. GANSAUGE, F., K.H. LINK, N. RILINGER, R. KUNZ & H.G. BEGER. 1995. Regional chemotherapy in advanced pancreatic carcinoma. Med. Klin. **90:** 501–505.
8. GANSAUGE, S., F. GANSAUGE & H.G. BEGER. 1996. Molecular oncology in pancreatic cancer. J. Mol. Med. **74:** 313–320.
9. GANSAUGE, F., S. GANSAUGE, J. MULLER, E. SCHMIDT & H.G. BEGER. 1998. Prognostic significance of molecular alterations in pancreatic carcinoma: an immunhistological study. Langenbecks Arch. Chir. **383:** 152–155.
10. HARADA, N., S. GANSAUGE, F. GANSAUGE, H. GAUSE, S. SHIMOYAMA, T. IMAIZUMI, T. MATTFELDT, M.H. SCHOENBERG & H.G. BEGER. 1997. Nuclear accumulation of p53 correlates significantly with clinical features and inversely with the expression of the cyclin dependent kinase inhibitor p21WAF1 in pancreatic cancer. Br. J. Cancer **76:** 299–305.
11. GANSAUGE, F., K.H. LINK, N. RILINGER, R. KUNZ & H.G. BEGER. 1996. Adjuvant regional chemotherapy in locally advanced pancreatic cancer. Chirurg **67:** 362–365.
12. ISHIKAWA, O., H. OHIGASHI & Y. SASAKI. 1994. Liver perfusion chemotherapy via both the hepatic artery and portal vein to prevent hepatic metastasis after extended pancreatectomy for adenocarcinoma of the pancreas. Am. J. Surg. **168:** 361–364.

The Matrix Metalloproteinases and Their Inhibitors in the Treatment of Pancreatic Cancer

LUCIE JONES, PAULA GHANEH, MICHELLE HUMPHREYS, AND JOHN P. NEOPTOLEMOS[a]

Department of Surgery, Royal Liverpool University Hospital, Liverpool L69 3GA, UK

ABSTRACT: Matrix metalloproteinases (MMPs) are a family of zinc-containing proteolytic enzymes that break down extracellular matrix proteins (ECM) in physiological and pathological conditions. Disruption in the tight control of MMP metabolism occurs in cancer, resulting in excessive destruction of the ECM, neovascularization, tumor spread and metastases. Recent studies have shown that overexpression of MMPs is associated with poor prognosis. Several MMP inhibitors have been developed and preclinical trials have confirmed a reduction in tumor spread and metastases. Marimastat is a broad spectrum inhibitor, and recent published results shows the drug is well tolerated in patients with advanced cancer. Phase II studies which have used marimistat alone or in combination with other cytotoxic agents, have produced encouraging results with improved survival. Phase III trials are now underway for the use of marimastat in advanced pancreatic cancer and as an adjuvant therapy in patients following resection of pancreatic cancer.

INTRODUCTION

Pancreatic cancer is characterized by early local invasion of adjacent structures and because of its anatomical position diagnosis is usually late and prognosis poor.[1] Early invasion of local structures includes the surrounding peripancreatic tissue with most patients having lymph node metastasis associated with neural and vascular invasion at presentation.[2–5] During the first steps of cancer cell invasion, the basement membrane surrounding the cancer cell is degraded.[6] Although this membrane is composed of many types of extracellular matrices, the type IV collagen predominates.[7] Two kinds of type IV collagenases have been recognized, gelatinase A (MMP2) and gelatinase B (MMP9).[8] Malignant epithelial cells and induced fibroblasts increase production of these gelatinases along with other matrix metalloproteinases which then degrade the basement membrane and adjacent extracellular matrix (ECM).[9] This results in an intense desmoplastic stromal reaction by the tumor[9] and cancer cell invasion into the surrounding stroma.[6] The loss of type IV collagen and proteoglycans in the basement membrane are a common feature in pan-

---

[a]Address for correspondence: Professor J.P. Neoptolemos, Department of Surgery, 5th Floor UCD Building, Daulby Street, Liverpool L69 3GA, UK. Phone, +44 151-706-4175; fax, +44 151-706-5798; e-mail, j.p.neoptolemos@liverpool.ac.uk

creatic cancer.[11,12] These findings suggest that matrix metalloproteinases may play an important role in the local invasion of pancreatic cancer.

The matrix metalloproteinase (MMP) family are able to degrade all the major structural components of connective tissue.[13] The matrix degrading properties of the metalloproteinases suggest they may play a role in normal ECM remodeling such as in embryonic development and morphogensis. Implantation of an embryo into the uterine wall increases the level of 72-kDa collagenase,[14] whereas MMP activation is known to be important in wound healing and bone resorption.[15,16] There is now increasing evidence that aberrant MMP expression can contribute to the pathogenesis of several diseases including rheumatoid arthritis, atherosclerosis and multiple sclerosis.[17–20] An increase in MMP expression occurs in the synovial fluid of patients with rheumatoid arthritis,[17] and may be related to the extent of cartilage destruction.[18] Dysregulation of MMP control in arterial vessels results in destabilization and disruption of atherosclerotic plaques,[19] and an increased gelatinase activity is present in cerebrospinal fluid of patients with multiple sclerosis.[20] Finally, of great importance is the involvement of MMPs in cancer, tumor invasion and the formation of metastases.[21,22]

STRUCTURE OF MMPs

The MMPs are a family of structurally related proteolytic enzymes and have the following characteristics: (1) they are proteinases which degrade components of the ECM;[22] (2) they all contain a zinc ion in the catalytic domain, which is inhibited by chelating agents;[23] (3) they are secreted as proenzymes and require activation;[24] and (4) they are inhibited by specific natural tissue inhibitors called TIMPs (tissue inhibitors of metalloproteinases).[25,26] Analysis of the primary structure reveals that the MMPs contain several domains each with its own specific function. The predomain is the leader sequence and is required to target the MMP molecule for secretion. This is subsequently removed and is not present in the latent enzyme. The prodomain contains the highly conserved sequence PRCGVPDV; the cysteine residue interacts with the active site zinc ion, sterically blocking the active site. On activation the prodomain is cleaved from the proteinase, freeing the zinc ion to participate in proteolytic cleavage. The catalytic domain contains three conserved histidine residues which are thought to be the zinc binding region. The structure of the active site cleft confers the substrate specificity of each of the MMPs.[23] The final domain, referred to as the hemopexin domain, has a sequence similar to the heme-binding protein and is found in all MMPs except matrilysin (MMP7). The function of this domain is unknown, but may act as a substrate receptor or be involved in the interaction of the plasminogen/urokinase system.[23] Additional domains occur in some of the MMP subgroups. The type IV collagenases and gelatinases (MMPs 2, 3, 9 and 10) contain an additional domain with a sequence homology similar to fibronectin. This fibronectin domain is believed to be involved in substrate binding properties.[27] The membrane-type (MT) MMPs share a transmembrane domain.[25] MMP19 is a recently discovered novel MMP. It exhibits similarities to most MMPs, but lacks a series of structurally distinctive features.[28] These include the amino acid residues Asp, Tyr and Gly near the zinc binding site of the collagenases, the fibronectin-like domain

TABLE 1. MMPs: nomenclature, substrate specificity, activation and inhibition

Group	MMP	Alternative name	Substrate	Activation	Inhibition
Collagenases	MMP1	Type I collagenase/interstitial collagenase	Collagen I, II, III VII, X	Plasmin	Active MMP1
	MMP8	Neutrophil collagenase	Collagen I, II, III		
	MMP13	Collagenase 3	Collagen I	Il-1 TGFβ	
Gelatinases	MMP2	Type IV collagenase(72 kDa)/gelatinase A	Collagen IV, V, VII, X	Plasmin MT-MMP1,2	TIMP1/2
			Fibronectin, gelatins, elastin	MT-MMP3,4	
	MMP9	Type IV collagenase(92 kDa)/gelatinase B	Collagen I, III, IV, V Gelatins	Serine proteases	TIMP1/2
Stromelysins	MMP3	Stomelysin 1 or Transin	Collagen III, IV, V, gelatins proteoglycans, laminin	Plasmin, MMP2 MT-MMP1	
	MMP10	Stromelsin 2 or Transin 2	Collagen III, IV, V, Fibronectin, gelatins		
	MMP11	Stromelysin 3	Serine protease inhibitors		
	MMP19	? Stromelysin 4	Not defined		
Ungrouped	MMP7	Putative MMP (PUMP) or matrilysin	Gelatin, fibronectin, elastin,		
	MMP12	Metalloelastase (MME)	Elastin		
	MMP18	? new subgroup	Not defined		TIMP2
Membrane-bound	MMP14	MT-MMP1	Pro-MMP2		
	MMP15	MT-MMP2	MMP2		
	MMP16	MT-MMP3	MMP2		
	MMP17	MT-MMP4	MMP2		

of the gelatinases and the transmembrane domain of the membrane-type MMPs. MMP19 has similarities to the stromelysin class and has recently been named stromelysin 4 (verbal communication, Graham Wells, British Biotech).

CLASSIFICATION OF MMPs

MMPs are broadly classified according to their substrate specificity. There are four main subgroups: the collagenases (MMP1, 8 and 13), the gelatinases (MMPs 2 and 9), stromelysins (MMPs 3, 10, 11 and 19) and membrane-bound MMPs (MT-MMP 1–4)[29] (TABLE 1). The collagenases all have the unique ability to cleave the chains of type I, II and III collagens. The cleavage "unwinds" the helical collagen fibers and produces a denatured gelatin form that is susceptible to cleavage by the other proteases and MMPs.[30] This loss of collagen leads to irreversible breakdown of the matrix. Collagenases, therefore, play a key role in disruption of the ECM.

The gelatinases/type IV collagenases (MMPs 2 and 9) were originally named for their ability to degrade the triple helix type IV collagen of basal laminae found in the basement membrane.[31] In addition they were also found to possess a potent gelatinolytic activity that degrades collagen types V, VII, IX and X, fibronectin and elastin.[32] Although similar in their structure and function, the two gelatinase enzymes arise from separate mRNA transcripts on separate genes.

The stromelysins consist at present of four members: stromelysins 1, 2, 3 and 4 (MMPs 3, 10, 11 and 19). Stromelysin 1 and 2 (MMPs 3 and 10) are closely related functionally and degrade proteoglycans, laminin, fibronectin, gelatin and the nonhelical portion of the basement membrane collagen.[33] Stromelysin 3 (MMP11) and stromelysin 4 (MMP19) are newly identified, and their specific substrates are not fully established. Stromelysin 3 is effective in degrading serpin α-1 antitrypsin, and it has been found to have a potentiating effect on the serine proteases such as urokinase.[34] Stromelysin 3 (MMP11) has been shown to be expressed in cancerous tissues including breast, bowel and lung, but not in lymphoid neoplasia. Expression of stromelysin 3 appears to be characteristic of tumors of epithelial origin.[35] Stromelysin 4 (MMP19) is a novel MMP, and its substrate specificity has yet to be clarified.[28]

Three enzymes have been identified which on the basis of sequence homology do not belong to the previous groups described. Matrilysin (MMP7, PUMP) is similar to the stromelysins in its substrate specificity, and to interstitial collagenase (MMP1) in the crystal structure of its catalytic domain, but the enzyme is unique in that it lacks the carboxy-terminal segment present in other MMPs.[36] Matrilysin has been shown to cleave extracellular matrix and basement membrane proteins such as fibronectin, collagen type IV, laminin and particularly elastin and proteoglycans. It can also mediate the proteolytic processing of other molecules such as tumor necrosis factor alpha precursor (TNF-α) and urokinase plasminogen activator (uPA).[36] Matrilysin is localized to secretory and ductal epithelium, and is found in a wide variety of tumors such as breast, prostate and stomach.[36]

Metalloelastase (MMP12) degrades elastin.[37] MMP18 is expressed in a wide variety of normal tissues, including mammary gland, placenta, lung and pancreas, and has closest identity to MMPs 1, 3, 10 and 11.[38]

A new subgroup, containing four members, has been identified: MT-MMPs 1–4 (MMPs 14–17). Unlike other MMPs which are secreted, these proteinases have a C-terminal transmembrane domain that anchors them to the cell membrane.[39–41] The substrate specificity of these MT-MMPs is not yet established, but both MT-MMPs 1 and 2 can activate pro-MMP2.[41,42] MT-MMP 1 has also been shown to degrade interstitial collagens and other components of the ECM, giving it a dual role in cleavage of substrates and activation of pro-MMP2.[43]

TIMPs

Like the MMPs, the natural inhibitors of these enzymes also appear to be a multigene family. Four members of the tissue inhibitors of matrix metalloproteinases (TIMPs) family have been characterized so far and called TIMPs 1, 2, 3 and 4.[44–47] The relative molecular mass ranges from 22 to 30 kDa with a 40–50% sequence identity. All TIMPs inhibit active MMPs with relatively low selectivity forming tight noncovalent 1:1 complexes.[46]

It has been suggested that an imbalance between MMPs and TIMPs may be a factor in tumor progression to a more malignant phenotype.[48,49] TIMP1 has been shown to inhibit *in vitro* invasion and metastases in animal models.[50] Furthermore, downregulation of TIMP1 expression by antisense RNA in mouse 3T3 cells, increased their metastatic ability in athymic mice.[51] TIMP2 shows homology to TIMP1, yet the two proteins are immunologically distinct and are encoded by genes on separate chromosomes.[52] TIMP2 also suppresses tumor formation.[53] Injection of recombinant TIMP2 protein has been shown to be an important inhibitor of tumor invasion.[54] The overexpression of TIMP2 in invasive and metastatic *ras*-transformed rat embryo fibroblasts suppressed the formation of lung metastases following intravenous injection in nude mice.[55]

TIMP3 is the only member in the family which is found exclusively in the extracellular matrix.[56] Overexpression of TIMP3 in human colon carcinoma cells induces growth arrest in low serum conditions and inhibits *in vivo* tumor growth.[57] Cells expressing TIMP3 have more TNF-α binding sites; this suggests that TIMP3 may act by protecting receptors from attack by MMPs.[57] TIMP4 is the most recently identified TIMP. This inhibits tumor growth and metastases in human breast cancer cells transfected with TIMP4.[58]

MMP REGULATION

The activity of these degradative enzymes is highly regulated. At the transcriptional level, MMP expression is thought to be controlled by various factors including cytokines, growth factors and oncogenes. Posttranscriptionally, MMP activity is regulated by proteolytic activation of the latent proenzymes and by specific TIMPs.

TRANSCRIPTIONAL ACTIVATION OF MMPs

The MMP genes are not constitutively expressed, but their mRNAs can be induced in physiological and pathological states. The regulation of metalloproteinase transcription has been studied closely and has resulted in a better understanding of how cytokines and oncogenes may control gene expression. The promotor region contains various cis-acting elements such as N-kappa B site, activator protein-1 site (AP-1), PEA3 and Sp-1 site. The AP-1 site plays a predominant role in the transcriptional activation of MMPs. Recent data have shown that transcriptional activation by cytokines and growth factors requires specific interaction of the AP-1 site with other cis-acting elements, particularly the PEA3 site.[59]

Many growth factors stimulate the expression of the protooncogene products c-*fos* and c-*jun*. These proteins form a heterodimeric complex which binds to the AP-1 site, thereby acting as a transcriptional activator for expression of MMPs. Antisense c-*fos* RNA has been shown to block subsequent expression of collagenase and/or stromelysin gene expression.[60] The cytokines, TNF-α and interferon beta (INF-β), prolong activation of c-*jun* and c-*fos*, and therefore the expression of both collagenase and stromelysin genes.[61,62]

In pancreatic cancer there is almost a ubiquitous overexpression of epidermal growth factor receptor (EGFR) and its associated ligand (EGF). This overexpression has been linked with advanced tumor stage in pancreatic cancer.[63–65] The epidermal growth factor binds to its own cell surface receptor and through multiple regulatory pathways induces the nuclear oncogenes encoding for the transcriptional regulatory proteins c-*fos* and c-*jun*. This then selectively increases the production of pro-MMP9 in esophageal cell lines in a dose-dependent manner.[66] Interleukin-1 (IL-1) induces the expression of c-*fos*, c-*jun* and c-*myc* resulting in the transcription of and augmented production of pro-MMP1, pro-MMP3 and TIMP1, but not pro-MMP2 in both human lung cells and cervical fibroblasts.[67,68] This effect was inhibited by protein kinase C (PKC) inhibitors, which suggests that PKC mediates IL-1 production of MMPs and TIMPs.

Protooncogene induction by growth factors appears to be important in the regulation of MMP gene expression. The *ras* family of oncogenes Harvey (H), Kirsten (K) and N-*ras* are the most frequently activated group of transforming genes in human cancer.[69] The *ras* protooncogene may play a role in gene expression of MMPs in pancreatic cancer. Mutations in the K-*ras* gene at codon 12 occur in 75–100% of patients suffering from pancreatic cancer.[70] Collier *et al.* (1988) showed an increased production of MMP2 in bronchial epithelial cell transfected with the *ras* oncogene,[71] whereas Thorgeirsson *et al.* reported that *ras* oncogene transfection of NIH/3T3 fibroblasts induced an increase in MMP9 production *in vitro*.[72]

ACTIVATION OF MMP ENZYMES

With the exception of MT-MMPs which are membrane bound, all MMPs are secreted in an inactive form as proenzymes and require activation to degrade the ECM. Activation of the MMPs is produced by the cleavage of the prosegment from the proteinase. This allows the catalytic zinc ion to participate in proteolytic cleavage. This activation can be induced *in vitro* by organomercurial compounds and *in vivo* by several mechanisms including endogenous activators (e.g., plasmin, serine proteases, cathespins), active MMPs (by positive feedback) and the membrane-bound MMPs

(MT-MMPs).[73] This conversion step from pro- to active enzyme is the next regulatory step after gene transcription at which MMP activity is regulated.

MMP activation can occur at the cell surface through the urokinase plasminogen activator (uPA)/uPAR/plasminogen cascade to produce plasmin which then activates the MMP. Plasmin has been shown to activate procollagenase (MMP1) and prostromelysin (MMP3).[74–76] This process is tightly regulated by plasminogen activator (PA) and plasmin inhibitors as well as TIMPs.

The activation of pro-MMP2 is more complex.[77] In malignant tumor tissue, particularly lung and stomach carcinoma, overexpression of pro-MMP2 correlated with an overexpression of MT-MMP1.[78] MT-MMP1 has subsequently been shown to activate pro-MMP2.[79] This activation requires TIMP2, which inhibits the active form of MT-MMP1, and then acts as an adaptor molecule to mediate pro-MMP2 binding to MT-MMP. This complex then acts as a substrate for other neighboring active MT-MMPs.[77,80] Activation of pro-MMP2 therefore requires at least two MT-MMP molecules on the cell surface.[81] This process localizes active MMP2 onto the cell surface and may trigger invasion and metastases by tumor cells.

The activated MMPs themselves can also act on each other causing a cascade of activity. Knauper *et al.* demonstrated a new activation cascade, possibly significant in breast cancer pathology, where the activation of procollagenase-3 (MMP13) by MT1-MMP was enhanced in the presence of pro-MMP2.[82]

Stromelysin-3 can be processed to the active form by the golgi-associated proteinase, furin. Between the pro- and catalytic domains, there is a peptide sequence or motif which is recognized by this enzyme. Stromelysin-3 can therefore be activated by an obligate cellular proteolytic event.[83]

INHIBITION OF MMP ACTIVITY BY TIMPs

TIMPs bind to MMPs noncovalently to neutralize enzymatic activity. It has been postulated that any small changes in the levels of either leads to a significant alteration in overall enzyme activity.[84]

The N-terminal domains of TIMP1 and 2 are efficient inhibitors of the MMP through their interaction with the active sites.[85] The C-terminal domains of the native inhibitors have at least two other binding sites for gelatinase A (MMP2) and stromelysin 1 (MMP3). It has been proposed that binding of the MMP to the C-terminal domain aligns the N-terminal domain of the TIMP into the active site of the MMP.[85] TIMPs 1 and 2 have been shown to form complexes with both pro-MMP2 and pro-MMP9, although TIMP1 binds preferentially with pro-MMP9 and TIMP2 prefers pro-MMP2. TIMP2 has been shown also to form a complex with active MMP2.[52,53,86] TIMP1, on the other hand, has been shown to bind with MMP9, although it preferentially recognizes the latent form of MMP9.[52,53,86] The TIMPs have not been shown to bind to any other of the latent MMPs, but do form complexes with other active enzymes. TIMP1 binds to active interstitial collagenase (MMP1), active stromelysin 1 (MMP3) and MT-MMP1 (MMP14).[24,26] TIMP2 is thought to bind with the newly discovered MMP19 and MT-MMP1.[28,47,77] TIMP4 has recently been shown to bind in a similar way to TIMP2.[87]

MATRIX METALLOPROTEINASES AND CANCER

Studies looking at the expression of MMPs and TIMPs in human cancer have provided valuable evidence to support the role of these enzymes in tumor growth and metastatic disease. It is hoped that these studies will in the future identify the important individual or subgroups of MMPs in the progression of a particular cancer. This will then provide a foundation for the design of new specific MMP inhibitors which act against a particular subgroup of MMPs, making them more effective in the treatment of cancer. The study of MMP expression in human cancer is difficult; there are a number of different techniques for detecting MMPs, each with its own advantages and disadvantages. Messenger RNA expression of MMPs and TIMPs can be quantified in both normal and cancerous tissue by Northern blot analysis. *In situ* hybridization is required to determine the cellular location of these transcripts. The protein can then be detected by specific antibodies. Enzymatic activity can be measured by substrate gel electrophoresis (zymography).[88]

The overexpression of MMPs and TIMPs has been demonstrated in several cancer studies and correlated with tumor stage and grade. The levels of gelatinase A (MMP2) and gelatinase B (MMP9) were found to be elevated in gastric cancer[89] along with matrilysin (MMP7)[90] and MT1-MMP (MMP14).[91] The prognostic relevance of MMP2 expression in gastric cancer has been studied retrospectively. This immunohistochemical study included 203 patients with gastric cancer and revealed that MMP2 expression was related to a poorer prognosis, although there was no significant difference in survival between high and low levels of MMP2 expressed.[92] Similarly, Sier *et al.* also concluded that activated gelatinase A and progelatinase B in gastric cancer are significant prognostic markers independent of pathological classification.[93] *In situ* hybridization studies on colorectal cancer specimens have indicated increased gelatinase expression,[94] whilst zymographic studies have demonstrated that the active forms of MMP2 and MMP9 are prevalent in cancer specimens and that the active form of MMP2 is absent from normal colonic mucosa.[95,96] Murray *et al.* showed that MMP1 expression was associated with a poor prognosis in colorectal cancer.[97] A series of 64 patients with colorectal tumors showed that interstitial collagenase (MMP1) stained positive in five out of thirty-eight Dukes B tumors and five out of twenty-five Dukes C tumors. The prognosis of patients with collagenase-positive tumors was significantly poorer than that of patients with no collagenase staining. This was independent of tumor stage and patient age. Zeng *et al.* confirmed these findings; gelatinase B mRNA expression correlated inversely to disease-free survival.[94] The MMPs are highly expressed in breast cancer tissue, with all known MMPs and TIMPs expressed except stromyelsin 2 (MMP10) and neutrophil collagenase (MMP8).[98] The levels of MMP2, MMP3 and MMP9 in breast cancer were shown to correlate inversely with the number of nodal metastases, but increased MMP expression did not appear to be related to patient survival.[99]

TIMP1 and 2 levels have also been shown to be elevated in cancer. High expression levels of TIMP1 have been linked to aggressiveness of tumors in gastric cancer.[100] TIMP1 and 2 are both elevated in primary breast carcinoma, and are associated with development of distant metastases.[101] High levels of TIMP2 are related to poor outcome in bladder cancer.[102]

TABLE 2. Studies looking at the expression of MMPs and TIMPs in pancreatic cancer specimens

Author	Number of cases	Method	MMP/TIMPs expressed	Comment
Satoh[105] 1994	30	Immunohistochemistry	MMP 2	Intensity related to invasiveness of tumor
Gress[103] 1995	8	Northern blot analysis	MMP 2,9 TIMP 1,2	MMP1,3 not detected
Bramhall [106] 1996	27	Immunohistochemistry	MMP 2,3 TIMP 1	
Bramhall [84] 1997	17	Northern blot analysis In situ hybridization	MMP 2,7,11 TIMP 1,2 MMP 2,7 MT-MMP1 TIMP 1,2	MMP 1,10 not detected
Koshiba [104] 1998	10	Zymography	Latent MMP 2,9 Active MMP2	Active present only in cancer tissue
Imamura [107] 1998	24	In situ hybridization Immunohistochemistry	MT-MMP1	Intensity related to invasiveness of tumor

PANCREATIC CANCER

Overexpression of several MMPs has been demonstrated in a number of studies in pancreatic cancer (TABLE 2). *In situ* hybridization studies detected high levels of expression of MMP2 and 9 and TIMP1 and 2 in the majority of patients with cancer compared to control pancreatic tissue. MMP1 and 3 were not detected.[103] Transcripts of MMP2 and 9 and TIMP1 and 2 were predominantly detected in tumor epithelium. MMP2 was predominant in the tumor stroma, TIMP1 and 2 distributed evenly between stroma and tumor, while MMP9 was present mostly in the tumor.

Gelatin zymography was used to detect the latent and active forms of MMP2 and 9 in pancreatic cancer specimens in comparison to normal pancreas and chronic pancreatitis tissue.[104] Results confirmed that latent forms of MMP2 and 9 were detected in all samples, but the active form of MMP2 was only detected in cancer specimens. The MMP2 level of activation also corresponded to tumor grade, regional lymph node metastases and distant metastases. An immunhistochemistry study by Satoh *et al.* compared the amount of MMP2 expression in cases of intraductal neoplasia and invasive ductal adenocarcinoma. MMP2 expression was higher in the invasive group, and the intensity of the expression was related to basement membrane disruption.[105] MMP2, MMP3 and TIMP1 protein were detected by immunohistochemistry; they were overexpressed in pancreatic and ampullary cancer. MMP2 immunoreactivity was shown to be related to tumor dedifferentiation and invasive potential.[106] A recent *in situ* hybridization and immunohistochemistry study looked at the expression of MT-MMP1 in 24 pancreatic cancer specimens. Expression was detected in 18 out of 24 cases of pancreatic cancer and in 9 out of 9 cases of secondary liver tumors derived from pancreatic adenocarcinoma.[107] MT-MMP1 expression in tumor stroma cells of common adenocarcinoma may be involved in the processes leading to desmoplastic reaction.

THERAPEUTIC USE OF MMP INHIBITORS

As our knowledge of MMPs in tumor invasion and metastasis increases, the use of an inhibitor as treatment has developed with the possibility of suppressing both primary and secondary tumor growth. There is now the possibility of designing TIMP variants and synthetic inhibitors with potential therapeutic applications. The early synthetic inhibitors were developed from the peptide sequence at the cleavage site in the collagen molecule that is recognized by interstitial collagenase. Recent peptide inhibitors have been designed with the use of X-ray crystallography and computer modeling techniques. Most compounds are nonspecific for the different MMP family subgroups but generally show little or no activity against proteinases outside this group.

The first MMP inhibitors were not orally available, and preclinical trials have involved the administration of the drug by intraperitoneal and intrapleural injection. MMP inhibitors are cytostatic, and therefore may need to be administered for long periods. Orally bioavailable drugs were then subsequently developed for clinical trials.[108,109]

PRECLINICAL TRIALS

One of the first synthetic inhibitor compounds to enter trials in cancer models was a broad spectrum MMP inhibitor called batimastat (British Biotech, BB-94). Batimastat was shown to reduce the tumor burden in nude mice given human ovarian carcinoma xenografts and increased their survival by up to sixfold compared to controls.[110] Autopsy of the mice showed the tumor to be encapsulated in dense tissue stroma with necrosis of some of the tumor cells. This necrosis was thought to be due to inhibition of tumor angiogenesis, another action by which MMP inhibitors control tumor spread. In another xenograft model, fragments of human colorectal tumors were implanted into the intestine wall of nude mice; they were then treated with batimastat.[111] The results showed both a reduction in tumor growth and locoregional invasion. There was also a modest improvement in survival. Batimastat has also been shown to have a significant affect on the growth of primary tumors and the size of spontaneous metastases to the lungs in mice, which were subcutaneously injected with the highly invasive B16-BL6 murine melanoma cells.[112]

An inhibitor developed by Agouron Pharmaceutical, AG 3340, has completed preclinical trials and was shown to be efficacious against the Lewis lung carcinoma model.[109] It resulted in the complete cessation of primary tumor growth in four out of six mice treated with daily intrapleural injections. The treatment also inhibited the formation of lung metastases greater than 5 mm in diameter by 90%. The first MMP inhibitors were not orally available, and preclinical trials have involved the administration of the drug by intraperitoneal and intrapleural injection.

TABLE 3. MMP inhibitors in development[a]

Compound	Company	Indication	Status
AG3340	Agouron	Cancer	Phase II/III
BAY 12-9566	Bayer	Cancer	Phase II/III
Marimastat	British Biotech	Cancer	Phase II/III
CGS 27023A	Novatis	Cancer	Phase II
D2 163	Chiroscience	Cancer	Phase I
Metastat	CollaGenex	Cancer	Preclinical
D5410	Chiroscience	IBD	Phase II
BB-344	British Biotech	Multiple sclerosis	Phase I
Ro 32-3555	Roche	Rheum. Arthritis	Phase II
RS 130830	Roch Biosc.	Osteoarthritis	Phase I

[a]Produced courtesy of P. Brown, British Biotech.

CLINICAL TRIALS

Currently at least ten MMP inhibitors are in clinical trials, six for the treatment of cancer, two for arthritis and one for multiple sclerosis (TABLE 3). Some inhibitors have now finished phase I and II trials, and phase II/III or phase III trials are now underway in patients with cancer. The first MMP inhibitor to be tested in clinical trials was the early nonorally bioavailable batimastat which was administered by intraperitoneal and intrapleural injections to patients with malignant ascites and malignant pleural effusions. The results showed efficacy, but due to the chronicity of the underlying conditions, long-term use was impractical.[113–115] Second generation inhibitors with improved oral bioavailability are now undergoing clinical trials. Marimastat (British Biotech, BB-2516) is a low molecular weight peptide which is a highly potent but reversible inhibitor of MMPs, with only weak activity against unrelated metalloproteinases. Phase I studies of marimastat showed that single and repeated oral doses in healthy male subjects were well tolerated. The drug was rapidly absorbed with high peak levels achieved after oral administration at about three hours after ingestion. The only biochemical changes observed were small, reversible increases in liver transaminases.[116] The inhibitor was well tolerated over a two- to four-week period, but prolonged treatment with marimastat gave rise to reversible musculoskeletal symptoms in a few individuals.[116] All the musculoskeletal symptoms appeared to be dose and duration dependent. Patients taking 100 mg marimastat twice daily developed side effects within 2–3 months of commencing the treatment. Around three-quarters of individuals receiving a lower dose of 25 mg twice daily developed side effects after 4 months of treatment, but at a dose of only 25 mg once daily the incidence of musculoskeletal symptoms was only one in a hundred. All the musculoskeletal symptoms were reversible and stopped after a drug-free period.

The results of a phase I/II trial have been reported where marimastat was given to patients with inoperable or recurrent gastric cancer.[117] The tumor was examined endoscopically and rescoped after 28 days of marimastat treatment. Thirty-five patients were recruited for the study, 30 of these able to complete both 0 and day 28 endoscopy assessment. Six patients had stage II/III disease and 24 patients stage IV disease, and 5 patients were unstaged. The results of repeat endoscopy and repeat biopsy showed that ten patients (of 30) had evidence of increased fibrosis, eight patients had evidence of decreased hemorrhage in the tumor, and three patients had a small decrease in tumor size.[117] To assess the efficacy of marimastat versus placebo in 300 patients from different European centers, a randomized, double-blind, placebo-controlled study for inoperable gastric cancer is now underway. The end point of the study will be survival.

The results of six further trials have just been published. These trials involved patients with advanced colorectal cancer (two studies), ovarian cancer (two studies), pancreatic cancer and prostatic cancer. As marimastat is tumorostatic, serum cancer antigens such as CEA, CA 125, CA 19-9 and PSA were used to indicate biological activity of the tumor, and the changes in the rate of rise were used as a means to detect tumor response to marimastat, in phase I trails. The use of the patients with histologically proven (except pancreatic) cancer were selected for the studies on the basis of the tumor markers being above prespecified levels and values rising by 25% or more over a four-week period.[118] Patients with advanced colorectal cancer showed a dose response with a net fall in CEA serum concentration during treatment at higher marimastat dose levels, whereas patients with ovarian cancer also showed a response, with ten (45%) of 22 patients showing disease stabilization as assessed by serum CA 125 levels.[118–120]

RO-32-3555 (Roche Ltd) is a selective MMP inhibitor. It has been shown to be active against interstitial collagenase (MMP1) with weak activity against gelatinase A (MMP2) and stromelysin 1 (MMP3). Due to its strong interstitial collagenase activity the inhibitor has been developed for the treatment of rheumatoid arthritis and is now in phase II clinical trials. Further MMP inhibitors with a more selective inhibition have been developed and their inhibitory profiles are demonstrated in TABLE 4.

Phase II trial results of marimastat for the treatment of advanced pancreatic cancer have been published.[121–123] The study involved over 100 patients with inoperable pancreatic cancer, most of whom received 25 mg of marimastat once daily for 28 days with the option to continue treatment if disease stabilization was evident. Disease stabilization was diagnosed by CT scan; if it showed there was no increase in the size of the tumor or serologically, the CA 19-9 level remained constant (or declined). Patients with unresectable stage II or III disease had a median survival time

TABLE 4. Inhibitory profiles of MMP inhibitors[a]

Compound	IC_{50}/k_i	MMP1	MMP2	MMP3	MMP7	MMP9
Marimastat	IC_{50}	5	6	230*	16	3
CGS 27023A	k_i	33	20	43	—	8
BAY 12-9556	k_i	>5000*	11	134	—	301
AG3340	k_i	8	0.08	0.27	54*	—
Ro 32-3555	k_i	3	154*	527*	—	59

[a]Produced courtesy of P. Brown, British Biotech.
* > 50-fold weaker inhibition than most potent.

of seven months compared to less than three months in those with stage IV disease. The patients with disease stabilization on CT scan had a median survival of over seven months.[121–123]

A phase IIb study in advanced pancreatic cancer has recently completed recruitment, in which four cohorts of 100 patients each were randomized to gemcitibine or one of three doses of marimastat (5, 10 or 25 mg twice daily). A phase III study in advanced pancreatic cancer, comparing gemcitibine with or without marimastat has also completed recruitment recently. The results of the trials have not yet been published. The phase III study combines two drugs with different modes of action. Gemcitibine is cytotoxic whilst marimastat is a cytostatic agent. In an experimental animal model using the MMP inhibitor CT 1746 (Celltech Ltd) in combination with a cytotoxic agent, the results showed tumor growth and metastasis inhibition occurred synergistically, compared to either alone.[124] The use of marimastat in the adjuvant setting has aroused some interest and British Biotech have recently opened a phase III double-blind randomized study comparing adjuvant chemoradiotherapy with or without marimastat in patients with resectable pancreatic cancer. British Biotech aims to recruit 200 patients with centers primarily based in the USA and Canada.

Phase Ib studies have shown that marimastat given in combination with either 5-fluorouracil folinic acid or gemcitibine does not result in added toxicity.[125] The results of a phase Ib study using a combination of gemcitibine and marimastat in 31 patients with nonresectable cancer revealed a median survival of 290 days (9.7 months).[126] This compared favorably with the phase III study of gemcitibine as first line use in advanced pancreatic cancer which produced a median survival of 5.7 months.[127] The phase Ib gemcitibine/marimastat study also confirmed that the combination treatment was well tolerated and that marimastat did not appear to increase the incidence or severity of chemotherapy-related adverse effects. The data also demonstrated an objective response in 3 of the 31 patients enrolled, based on radiological assessment, and 10 reports of stable disease. Sustained falls in CA 19-9 were also recorded in 14 patients.[125] As a result of this study, a phase III double-blind, placebo-controlled study is underway to assess efficacy of this combination in 200 patients with nonresectable pancreatic carcinoma.

The results of these large random controlled trials will provide important information for the future effective treatment of pancreatic cancer.

REFERENCES

1. NAGAKAWA, T., I. KONISHI, Y. HIGASHINO, K. UENO, T. OHTA, M. KAYAHARA, N. UEDA, K. MACDA & I. MIYAZAKI. 1989. The spread and prognosis of carcinoma in the region of the pancreatic head. Jpn. J. Surg. **19:** 510–518.
2. NAKAO, A., A. HARADA, T. NONAMI, T. KANEKO, H. MURAKAMI, S. INOUE, Y. TAKEUCHI & H. TAKAGI. 1995. Lymph node metastases in carcinoma of the head of the pancreas region. Br. J. Surg. **82:** 399–402.
3. KAYAHARA, M., T. NAGAKAWA, I. KONISHI, K. UENO, T. OHTA & I. MIYAZAKI. 1991. Clinicopathological study of pancreatic carcinoma with particular reference to the invasion of the extrapancreatic neural plexus. Int. J. Pancreatol. **10:** 105–111.
4. CUSACK, J.C., G.M. FUHRMAN, J.E. LEE & D.B. EVANS. 1994. Managing unsuspected tumor invasion of the superior mesenteric-portal venous confluence during pancreatoduodenectomy. Am. J. Surg. **168:** 352–354.

5. NAGAKAWA, T., M. KAYAHARA, K. UENO, T. OHTA, I. KONISHI, N. UEDA & I. MIYAZAKI. 1992. A clinicopathologic study on neural invasion in cancer of the pancreatic head. Cancer **69:** 930–935.
6. LIOTTA, L.A., P.S. STEEG & W.G. STETLER-STEVENSON. 1991. Cancer metastasis and angiogenesis: an imbalance of positive and negative regulation. Cell **64:** 327–336.
7. LEBLOND, C.P. & S. INOUE. 1989. Structure, composition and assembly of basement membrane. Am. J. Anat. **185:** 367–390.
8. STETLER-STEVENSON, W.G., L.A. LIOTTA & D.E. KLEINER. 1993. Extracellular matrix 6-role of matrix metalloproteinase in tumor invasion and metastasis. FASEB J. **7:** 1434–1441.
9. LIOTTA, L.A., K. TRYGGVASON, S. GARBISA, I. HART, C.M. FOLTZ & S. SHAFDIE. 1980. Metastatic potential correlates with enzymatic degradation of basement membrane collagen. Nature **284:** 67–68.
10. MOLLENHAUER, J., I. ROETHER & H.F. KERN. 1987. Distribution of extracellular matrix proteins in pancreatic ductal adenocarcinoma and its influence on tumor cell proliferation *in vitro*. Pancreas **2:** 14–24.
11. LEE, C.S., J. MONTEBELLO, T. GEORGIOU & J. RODE. 1994. Distribution of type IV collagen in pancreatic adenocarcinoma and chronic pancreatitis. Int. J. Exp. Pathol. **75:** 79–83.
12. WANG, Z.-H., T. MANABE, G. OHSHIO, I. IMAMURA, T. YOSHIMURA, H. SUWA, S. ISHIGAMI & T. KYOGOKU. 1994. Immunohistochemical study of heparin sulphate proteoglycan in pancreatic adenocarcinoma and chronic pancreatitis. Pancreas **9:** 758–763.
13. MURPHY, G. & J.J. REYNOLDS. 1993. Extracellular matrix degredation. *In* Connective Tissue and Its Inheritable Disorders. P.M. Royse & B. Steinmann, Eds.: 287–316. Wiley-Liss & Sons, Inc. New York.
14. BRENNER, C.A., R.R. ADLER, D.A. RAPPOLEE, R.A. PEDERSEN & Z. WERB. 1989. Genes for extracellular matrix degrading MMP and their inhibitor TIMP are expressed during early mammalian development. Genes Dev. **3:** 848–859.
15. WOLF, C., M.P. CHENARD, P.D. DE GROSSOUVRE, J.P. BELLOCQ, P. CHAMBON & P. BASSET. 1992. Breast-cancer associated stromelysin-3 gene is expressed in basal cell carcinoma and during cutaneous wound healing. J. Invest. Dermatol. **99:** 870–872.
16. DELAISSE, J.M. & G. VAES. 1992. Mechanism of mineral solublization and matrix degradation in osteoclastic bone resorption. *In* Biology and Physiology of the Osteoclast. B.R. Rifkin & C.V. Gay, Eds.: 290–314. CRC Press. Boca Raton, FL.
17. CAWSTON, T.E. & C. BILLINGTON. 1996. Metalloproteinases in the rheumatic diseases. J. Pathol. **180:** 115–117.
18. CLARK, I.M., L.K. POWELL, S. RAMSEY, B.L. HAZLEMAN & T.E. CAWSTON. 1993. The measurement of collagenases, TIMP and collagenase-TIMP complex in synovial fluids from patients with osteoarthritis and rhematoid arthritis. Arthritis Rheum. **36:** 372–379.
19. GALIS, Z., G. SUKHORA, M. LARK & P. LIBBY. 1994. Increased expression of matrix metalloproteinases and matrix degrading activity in vulnerable regions of human atherioscerotic plaques. J. Clin. Invest. **94:** 2493–2503.
20. CHANDLER, S., K.M. MILLER, J.M. CLEMENTS, J. LURY, D. CORKILL, D.C.C. ANTHONY, S.E. ADAMS & A.J.H. GEARING. 1997. Matrix metalloproteinases, tumor necrosis factor and multiple sclerosis. An overview. J. Neuroimmunol. **72:** 155–161.
21. CHEN, W.T. 1992. Membrane proteases: role in tissue remodeling and tumor invasion. Curr. Opin. Cell Biol. **4:** 802–809.
22. COTTAM, D.W. & R.C. REES. 1993. Regulation of matrix metalloproteinases—their role in tumor invasion and metastasis. Int. J. Oncol. **2:** 861–872.
23. SANCHEZ-LOPEZ, R., C.M. ALEXANDER, O. BEHRENDTSEN, R. BREATHNACH & Z. WERB. 1993. Role of zinc-binding encoded and hemopexin-domain-encoded sequences in the substrate specificity of collagenase and stromelysin-2 as revealed by chimeric proteins. J. Biol. Chem. **268:** 7238–7247.

24. MATRISIAN, L.M. 1990. Metalloproteinases and their inhibitors in matrix remodeling. Trends Genet. **6:** 121–125.
25. MATRISIAN, L.M. 1994. Matrix metalloproteinase gene expression. Ann. N.Y. Acad. Sci. **732:** 42–50.
26. KLEINER, D.E. & S. STEVENSON. 1993. Structural biochemistry and activation of matrix metalloproteinases. Curr. Opin. Cell Biol. **5:** 891–897.
27. STETLER-STEVENSON, W.G. 1990. Type IV collagenase in tumor invasion and metastasis. Cancer Metastasis Rev. **9:** 289–303.
28. PENDAS, A.M., V. KNAUPER, X.S. PUENTE, E. LLANO, M.G. MATTEI, S. APTE, G. MURPHY & C. LOPEZ-OTIN. 1997. Identification and characterization of a novel human matrix metalloproteinase with unique structural characteristics, chromosomal location and tissue distribution. J. Biol. Chem. **272:** 4281–4286.
29. MURPHY, G.J.P., G. MURPHY & J.J. REYNOLDS. 1991. The origin of matrix metalloproteinases and their familial relationships. FEBS Lett. **289:** 4–7.
30. MCCROSKERY, P.A., J.F. RICHARDS & E.D. HARRIS. 1975. Purification and characterization of a collagenase extracted from rabbit tumors. Biochem. J. **152:** 131–142.
31. NETHERY, A. & R.L. O'GRADY. 1989. Identification of a metalloproteinase co-purifying with rat tumor collagenase and the characteristics of fragments of both enzymes. Biochim. Biophys. Acta **994:** 149–160.
32. SENIOR, R.M., G.L. GRIFFIN, C.J. FLISZAR, S.D. SHAPIRO, G.I. GOLDBERG & H.G. WELGUS. 1991. Human 92- and 72-kilodalton type IV collagenases are elastases. J. Biol. Chem. **266:** 7870–7875.
33. WILHELM, S.M., I.E. COLLIER, A. KRONBERGER, A.Z. EISEN, B.L. MARMER, C.A. GRANT, E.A. BAUER & G.I. GOLDBERG. 1987. Human skin fibroblast stromelysin: structure, glycosylation, substrate specificity and differential expression in normal and tumorigenic cells. Proc. Natl. Acad. Sci. USA **84:** 6725–6729.
34. PEI, D., G. MAJMUDAR & S.J. WEISS. 1994. Hydrolytic inactivation of a breast carcinoma cell-derived serpin by human stromelysin-3. J. Biol. Chem. **269:** 25849–25855.
35. KOSSAKOWSKA, A.E., S.A. HUSCHCROFT, S. URBANSKI & D.R. EDWARDS. 1996. Comparative analysis of the expression patterns of MMPs and their inhibitors in breast neoplasia, sporadic colorectal neoplasia, pulmonary cancer and malignant non-Hodgkins lymphoma in humans. Br. J. Cancer **73:** 1401–1408.
36. WILSON, C.L. & L.M. MATRISIAN. 1996. Matrilysin: an epithelial matrix MMP with potentially novel functions. Int. J. Biochem. Cell Biol. **28:** 123–136.
37. SHAPIRO, S.D., D.K. KOBAYASHI & T.J. LEY. 1993. Cloning and characterization of a unique elastolytic metalloproteinase produced by human alveolar macrophages. J. Biol. Chem. **268:** 23824–23829.
38. COSSINS, J., T.J. DUDGEON, G. CATLIN, A.J.H. GEARING & J.M. CLEMENTS. 1996. Identification of MMP-18, a putative novel human MMP. Biochem. Biophys. Res. Commun. **228:** 494–498.
39. SATO, H., T. TAKINO, Y. OKADA, J. CAO, A. SHINAGAWA, E. YAMAMOTO & M. SEIKI. 1994. A matrix metalloproteinase expressed on the surface of invasive tumor-cells. Nature **370:** 61–65.
40. WILL, H. & B. HINZMAN. 1995. cDNA sequence and mRNA tissue distribution of a novel human matrix metalloproteinase with a potential transmembrane segment. Eur. J. Biochem. **231:** 602–608.
41. TAKINO, T., H. SATO, A. SHINAGAWA & M. SEIKI. 1995. Identification of the second membrane-type matrix metalloproteinase (MT-MMP-2) gene from a human placenta cDNA library-MT-MMP forms a unique membrane-type subclass in the MMP family. J. Biol. Chem. **270:** 23013–23020.
42. NAWROCKI, B., M. POLETTE, V. MARCHARD, E. MAQUOI, A. BEORCHIA, J.M. TOURNIER, J.M. FOIDART & P. BIREMBAUT. 1996. Membrane-type MMP-1 expression at the site of human placentation. Placenta **17:** 565–572.
43. D'ORTHO, M.P., H. WILL, S. ATKINSON, G. BUTLER, A. MESSENT, J. GAVRILOVIC, B. SMITH, R. TIMPL, I. ZARDI & G. MURPHY. 1997. MT-MMP 1 and 2 exhibit broad spectrum proteolytic capacities comparable to many MMP. Eur. J. Biochem. **250:** 751–757.

44. SELLERS, A., G. MURPHY, M.C. MEICKLE & J.J. REYNOLDS. 1979. Rabbit bone collagenase inhibitor blocks the activity of other neutral metalloproteinases. Biochem. Biophys. Res. Commun. **87:** 581–587.
45. GREENE, J., M.S. WANG, Y.L.E. LIU, L.A. RAYMOND, C. ROSEN & Y.E. SHI. 1996. Molecular cloning and characterization of human tissue inhibitor of metalloproteinase 4. J. Biol. Chem. **271:** 30375–30380.
46. URIA, J.A., A.A. FERRANDO, G. VELASCO, J.M.P. FREIJE & C. LOPEZ-OTIN. 1994. Structure and expression in breast tumors of human TIMP 3, a new member of the metalloproteinase inhibitor family. Cancer Res. **54:** 2091–2094.
47. GOMEZ, D.E., D.F. ALONSO, H. YOSHIJI & U.P. THORGEIRSSON. 1997. Tissue inhibitors of MMPs: structure, regulation and biological functions. Eur. J. Cell Biol. **74:** 111–112.
48. PONTON, A., B. COULOMBE & D. SKUP. 1991. Decreased expression of tissue inhibitor of the metalloproteinases in metastatic tumor cells leading to increased levels of collagenase activity. Cancer Res. **51:** 2138–2143.
49. MIGNATTI, P., R. TSUBOI, E. ROBBINS & D. RIFKIN. 1989. In vitro angiogenesis on the human amniotic membrane-requirement for basic fibroblast growth-factor induced proteinases. J. Cell Biol. **108:** 671–682.
50. THORGEIRSSON, U.P., L.A. LIOTTA, T. KALEBIC, I.M. MARGULIES, K. THOMAS, M. RIOSCANDELORE & R.G. RUSSO. 1982. Effect of the natural protease inhibitors and a chemoattractant on tumor-cell invasion in vitro. J. Natl. Cancer Inst. **69:** 1049–1054.
51. KHOKHA, R., P. WATERHOUSE, S. YAGEL, P.K. LALA, C.M. OVERALL, G. NORTON & D.T. DENHARDT. 1989. Antisense RNA-induced reduction in murine TIMP levels confers oncogenicity. Science **243:** 947–950.
52. DECLERCK, Y.A., T.D. YEAN, B.J. RATZKIN, H.S. LU & K.E. LANGLEY. 1989. Purification and characterization of two related but distinct metalloproteinase inhibitors secreted by bovine aortic endothelial cells. J. Biol. Chem. **264:** 17445–17453.
53. GOLDBERG, G.I., B.L. MARMER, G.A. GRANT, A.Z. EISEN, S. WILHELM & C.S. HE. 1989. Human 72 kDa type IV collagenase forms a complex with a tissue inhibitor of MMP designated TIMP-2. Proc. Natl. Acad. Sci. USA **86:** 8207–8211.
54. DECLERCK, Y.A., T.D. YEAN, D. CHAN, H. SHIMADA & K.E. LANGLEY. 1991. Inhibition of tumor invasion of smooth muscle cell layers by recombinant human TIMP. Cancer Res. **51:** 2151–2157.
55. DECLERCK, Y., N. PEREZ, H. SHIMADA, T.C. BOONE, K.E. LANGLEY & S.M. TAYLOR. 1992. Inhibition of invasion and metastasis in cells transfected with an inhibitor of metalloproteinases. Cancer Res. **52:** 701–708.
56. BIAN, J.H., Y.L. WANG, M.R. SMITH, H. KIM, C. JACOBS, J. JACKMAN, H.F. KUNG, N.H. COLBURN & Y. SUN. 1996. Suppression of in vivo tumor growth and induction of suspension cell death by tissue inhibitor of metalloprteinase (TIMP-3). Carcinogenesis **17:** 1805–1811.
57. SMITH, M.R., H.F. KUNG, S.K. DURUM, N.H. COLBURN & Y. SUN. 1997. TIMP-3 induces cell death by stabilizing TNF-α receptors on the surface of human colon carcinoma cells. Cytokine **9:** 770–780.
58. WANG, M.S., Y.L.E. LIU, J. GREENE, S.J. SHENG, A. FUCHS, E.M. ROSEN & Y.E. SHI. 1997. Inhibition of tumor growth and metastases of human breast cancer cells transfected with tissue inhibitor of MMP 4. Oncogene **14:** 2767–2774.
59. BENBOW, U. & C.E. BRINCKERHOFF. 1997. The AP-1 binding site and matrix metalloprteinase gene regulation: What is all the fuss about? Matrix Biol. **15:** 519–526.
60. KERR, L.D., D.B. MILLER & L.M. MATRISAN. 1990. TGF-β1 inhibition of transin/stromelysin gene expression is mediated through a fos binding sequence. Cell **61:** 267–278.
61. BRENNER, D.A., M. OHARA, P. ANGEL, M. CHOJKIER & M. KARIN. 1989. Prolonged activation of jun and collagenase genes by tumor necrosis factor alpha. Nature **337:** 661–663.
62. SCIAVOLINO, P.J., T.H. LEE & J. VILCEK. 1994. Interferon-β induces metalloproteinase mRNA expression in human fibroblasts. Role of activator protein-1. J. Biol. Chem. **264:** 21627–21634.

63. CHEN, Y.F., G.Z. PAN, X. HOU, T.H. LIU, J. CHEN, C. YANAIHARA & N. YANAIHARA. 1990. Epidermal growth factor and its receptors in human pancreatic carcinoma. Pancreas **5:** 278–283.
64. LEMOINE, N.R., C.M. HUGHES, C.M. BARTON, R. POULSOM, R.E. JEFFERY, G. KLÖPPEL, P.A. HALL & W.J. GULLICK. 1992. The EGF receptor in human pancreatic cancer. J. Pathol. **166:** 7–12.
65. YAMANAKA, Y., H. FREISS, M.S. KOBRIN, M. BUCHLER, H. BERGER & M. KORC. 1993. Co-expression of EGF receptors and ligands in human pancreatic cancer is associated with enhanced tumor aggressiveness. Anticancer Res. **13:** 565–569.
66. SHIMA, I., Y. SASAGURI, J. KUSUKAWA, R. NAKANO, H. YAMANA, H. FUJITA, T. KAKEGAWA & M. MORIMATSU. 1993. Production of matrix metalloproteinase 9 (92-kDa gelatinase) by human oesophageal squamous cell carcinoma in response to epidermal growth factor. Br. J. Cancer **67:** 721–727.
67. TAKAHASHI, S., T. SATO, A. ITO, Y. OJIMA, T. HOSONO, H. NAGASE & Y. MORI. 1993. Involvement of protein-kinase-C in the interleukin-1 alpha induced gene expression of MMPs and TIMP1 in human uterine cervical fibroblasts. Biochem. Biophys. Acta **1220:** 57–65.
68. MACKAY, A.R., M. BALLIN, M.D. PELINA, A.R. FARINA, A.M. NASON, J.L. HARTZLER & U.P. THORGEIRSSON. 1992. Effect of phorbol ester and cytokines on MMP and TIMP expression in tumor and normal cell lines. Invasion Metastasis **12:**168–184.
69. LEMOINE, N.R. & P.A. HALL. 1990. Growth factors and oncogenes in pancreatic cancer. Clin. Gastroenterol. **4:** 815–832.
70. HRUBAN, R.H., A.D.M. VAN MANSFIELD, G.J.A. OFFERHAUS, D.H.J. VAN WEERING, D.C. ALLISON, S.N. GOODMAN, T.W. KENSLER, K.K. BOSE, J.L. CAMERON & J.L. BOS. 1993. K-*ras* oncogene activation in adenocarcinomas of the human pancreas. A study of 82 carcinomas using a combination of mutant enriched PCR and allele specific oligonucleotide hybridization. Am. J. Pathol. **143:** 545–554.
71. COLLIER, I.E., J. SMITH, A. KRONBERGER, E.A. BAUER, S.M. WILHELM, A.Z. EISEN & G.I. GOLDBERG. 1998. The structure of the human-skin fibroblast collagenase gene. J. Biol. Chem. **264:** 10711–10713.
72. THORGEIRSSON, U.P., T. TURPEENNIEMI-HUJANEN, J.E. WILLIAMS, E.H. WESTIN, C.A. HEILMAN, J.E. TALMADGE & L.A. LIOTTA. 1985. NIH/3T3 cells transfected with human tumor DNA containing activated ras oncogenes in express the metastatic phenotype in nude mice. Mol. Cell. Biol. **5:** 259–262.
73. STETLER-STEVENSON, W.G., H.C. KRUTZSCH, M.P. WACHER, I.M.K. MARGULIES & L.A. LIOTTA. 1989. The activation of human type IV collagenase pro-enzyme. Sequence identification of the major conversion product following organomercurial activation. J. Biol. Chem. **264:** 1353–1356.
74. HE, C.S., S.M. WILHELM, A.P. PENTLAND, B.L. MARMER, G.A. GRANT, A.Z. EISEN & G.I. GOLDBERG. 1989. Tissue cooperation in a proteolytic cascade activating human interstitial collagenase. Proc. Natl. Acad. Sci. USA **86:** 2632–2636.
75. LIM, Y.T., Y. SUGIURA, W.E. LAUG, B. SUN, A. GARCIA & Y.A. DECLERK. 1996. Independent regulation of matrix metalloproteinase and plasminogen activators in human fibrosarcoma cells. J. Cell. Physiol. **167:** 333–340.
76. BARAMOVA, E.N., K. BAJOU, A. REMACLE, C. L'HOIR, H.W. KRELL, U.H. WEIDLE, A. NOEL & J.M. FOIDART. 1997. Involvement of PA/plasmin system in the processing of pro-MMP9 and in the second step of pro-MMP2 activation. FEBS Lett. **405:** 157–162.
77. STRONGIN, A.Y., I. COLLIER, G. BANNIKOV, B.L. MARMER, G.A. GRANT & G.I. GOLDBERG. 1995. Mechanism of cell surface activation of 72 kDa type IV collagenase: isolation of the activated form of membrane matrix metalloproteinase. J. Biol. Chem. **270:** 5331–5338.
78. TOKURAKA, M., H. SATO, S. MURAKAMI, Y. OKADO, Y. WATANABE & M. SEIKI. 1995. Activation of the precursor of gelatinase A/MMP2 in lung carcinomas correlates with the expression of membrane-type matrix metalloproteinase (MT-MMP) and with lymph-node metastasis. Int. J. Cancer **64:** 355–359.
79. WILL, H., S.J. ATKINSON, G.S. BUTLER, B. SMITH & G. MURPHY. 1996. The soluble catalytic domain of membrane type 1 MMP cleaves the propeptide of progelatinase

A and initiates autoproteolytic activation-regulation by TIMP-2 and TIMP-3. J. Biol. Chem. **271:** 17119–17123.
80. ZUCKER, S., M. DREWS, C. CONNOR, H.D. FODA, Y.A. DECLERCK, K.E. LANGLEY, W.F. BAHOU, A.J.P. DOCHERTY & J. CAO. 1998. TIMP-2 binds to the catalytic domain of cell surface receptor, MT-MMP1. J. Biol. Chem. **273:** 1216–1222.
81. KINOSHITA, T., H. SATO, A. OKADA, E. OHUCHI, K. IMAI, Y. OKADA & M. SEIKI. 1998. TIMP-2 promotes activation of progelatinase A by MT-MMP 1 immobilized on agarose beads. J. Biol. Chem. **273:** 16098–16103.
82. KNAUPER, V., H. WILL, C. LOPEZ-OTIN, B. SMITH, S.J. ATKINSON, H. STANTON, R.M. HEMBRY & G. MURPHY. 1996. Cellular mechanisms for human procollagenase-3 (MMP13) activation. Evidence that MT1-MMP (MMP14) and gelatinase A (MMP2) are able to generate active enzyme. J. Biol. Chem. **271:** 17124–17131.
83. PEI, D.Q. & S.J. WEISS. 1995. Furin dependent intracellular activation of human stromelysin-3 zymogen. Nature **375:** 244–247.
84. BRAMHALL, S.R., J.P. NEOPTOLEMOS, G.W.H. STAMP & N.R. LEMOINE. 1997. Imbalance of expression of matrix metalloproteinases and tissue inhibitors of the matrix metalloproteinases in human pancreatic cancer. J. Pathol. **182:** 347–355.
85. WILLENBROCK, F. & G. MURPHY. 1994. Structure and functional relationships of the TIMPs. Am. J. Respir. Crit. Care Med. **150:** S165–S170.
86. MURPHY, G., T.E. CAWSTON & J.J. REYNOLDS. 1981. An inhibitor of collagenase from amniotic-fluid, purification, characterization and action on MMPs. Biochem. J. **195:** 167–173.
87. BIGG, H.F., Y.E. SHI, Y.L.E. LIU, B. STEFFENSEN & C.M. OVERALL. 1997. Specific high affinity binding of TIMP-4 to the C-terminal hemopexin like domain of human gelatinase A-TIMP-4 binds progelatinase A and the C-terminal domain in a similar manner to TIMP-2. J. Biol. Chem. **272:** 15496–15500.
88. KLEINER, D.E. & W.G. STETLER-STEVENSON. 1994. Quantitative zymography: detection of picogram quantities of gelatinases. Ann. Biochem. **218:** 325–329.
89. DAVID, L., J. NESLAND, R. HOLM & M. SOBRINHOSIMOES. 1994. Expression of laminin, collagen IV, fibronectin and type IV collagenase in gastric carcinoma: an immunohistochemistry study of 87 patients. Cancer **73:** 518–527.
90. HONDA, M., M. MORI, H. UEO, K. SUGIMACHI & T. AKIYOSHI. 1996. Matrix metalloproteinase-7 expression in gastric carcinoma. Gut **39:** 444–448.
91. NOMURA, H., H. SATO, M. SEIKI, M. MAI & Y. OKADA. 1995. Expression of membrane-type matrix metalloproteinase in human gastric carcinomas. Cancer Res. **55:** 3263–3266.
92. ALLGAYER, H., R. BABIC, B.C.M. BEYER, K.V. GRUZNER, A. TARABICHI, F.W. SCHILDBERG & M.M. HEISS. 1998. Prognostic relevance of MMP2 (72 kDA collagenase IV) in gastric cancer. Oncology **55:** 152–160.
93. SIER, C.F.M., F.J.G.M. KUBBEN, S. GANESH, M.M. HEERDING, G. GRIFFIOEN, R. HANEMAAIJER, J.H.J.M. VAN KRIEVEN, C.B.H.W. LAMERS & H.W. VERSPAGET. 1996. Tissue levels of matrix metalloproteinases MMP2 and MMP9 are related to the overall survival of patients with gastric carcinoma. Br. J. Cancer **74:** 413–417.
94. ZENG, Z.S. & J.G. GUILLEM. 1995. Distinct pattern of matrix metalloproteinase 9 and tissue inhibitor of metalloproteinase 1 mRNA expression in human colorectal cancer and liver metastases. Br. J. Cancer **72:** 575–582.
95. PARSONS, S.L., S.A. WATSON, H.M. COLLINS, P.A. CLARKE & R.J.C. STEELE. 1996. Colorectal cancer overexpresses gelatinases (matrix metalloproteinases-2 and-9) [abstract]. Gastroenterology **110:** A574.
96. HEWITT, R.E., I.H. LEACH, D.G. POWE, I.M. CLARK, T.E. CAWSTON & D.R. TURNER. 1991. Distribution of collagenase and tissue inhibitor of metalloproteinases TIMPs in colorectal tumors. Int. J. Cancer **49:** 666–672.
97. MURRAY, G.I., M.E. DUNCAN, P. O'NEIL, W.T. MELVIN & J. FOTHERGILL. 1996. Matrix metalloprtoteinase-1 is associated with poor prognosis in colorectal cancer. Nat. Med. **2:** 461–462.
98. HEPPNER, K.J., L.M. MATRISAN, R.A. JENSEN & W.H. RODGERS. 1996. Expression of most matrix metalloproteinase family members in breast cancer represents a tumor-induced host response. Am. J. Pathol. **149:** 273–282.

99. REMACLE, A.G., A. NOEL, C. DUGGAN, E.O. MCDERMOTT, N. O'HIGGINS, J.M. FOIDART & M.J. DUFFY. 1998. Assay of matrix metalloproteinases types 1, 2, 3 and 9 in breast cancer. Br. J. Cancer **77:** 926–931.
100. MIMORI, K., M. MORI, T. SHIRAISHI, T. FUJIE, K. BABA, M. HARAGUCHI, R. ABE, H. UEO & T. AKIYOSHI. 1997. Clinical significance of TIMP expression in gastric carcinoma. Br. J. Cancer **76:** 531–536.
101. HANSEN, R.A., V.A. FLORENES, J.P. BERG, G.M. MAELANDSMO, J.M. NESLAND & O. FODSTAD. 1997. High level of mRNA for TIMP1 and TIMP-2 in primary breast carcinomas are associated with development of distant metastases. Clin. Cancer Res. **3:** 1623–1628.
102. GRIGNON, D.J., W. SAKR, M. TOTH, V. RAVERY, J. ANGULO, F. SHAMSA, J.E. PONTES, J.C. CRISSMAN & R. FRIDMAN. 1996. High levels of TIMP-2 expression are associated with poor outcome in invasive bladder cancer. Cancer Res. **56:** 1654–1659.
103. GRESS, T.M., F. MÜLLER-PILLASCH, M.M. LERCH, H. FREISS, M. BUCHLER & G. ADLER. 1995. Expression and *in situ* localization of genes coding for extracellular matrix degrading proteases in pancreatic cancer. Int. J. Cancer **62:** 407–413.
104. KOSHIBA, T., R. HOSOTANI, M. WADA, Y. MIYAMOTO, K. FUJIMOTO, J.U. LEE, R. DOI, S. ARII & M. IMAMURA. 1998. Involvement of MMP2 activity in invasion and metastases of pancreatic cancer. Cancer **82:** 642–650.
105. SATOH, K., H. OHTANI, T. SHIMOSEGAWA, M. KOIZUMI, T. SAWAI & T. TOYOTA. 1994. Infrequent stromal expression of gelatinase A and intact basement membrane in intraductal neoplasms of the pancreas. Gastroenterology **107:** 1488–1495.
106. BRAMHALL, S.R., G.W.H. STAMP, J. DUNN, N.R. LEMOINE & J.P. NEOPTOLEMOS. 1996. Expression on collagenase (MMP2), stromelysin (MMP3) and tissue inhibitor of the metalloproteinases (TIMP1) in pancreatic and ampullary disease. Br. J. Cancer **73:** 972–978.
107. IMAMURA, T., G. OHSHIO, M. MISE, T. HARADA, H. SUWA, N. OKADA, Z.H. WANG, S. YOSHITOMI, T. TANAKA, H. SATO, S. ARII, M. SEIKI & M. IMAMURA. 1998. Expression of membrane-type matrix metalloproteinase-1 in human pancreatic adenocarcinomas. J. Cancer Res. Clin. Oncol. **124:** 65–72.
108. BECKETT, R.P. 1996. Recent advances in the field of matrix metalloproteinase inhibitors. Exp. Opin. Ther. Pathol. **6:** 1305–1315.
109. SANTOS, O., C.D. MCDERMOTT, R.G. DANIELS & K. APPELT. 1997. Rodent pharmacokinetics and anti-tumor efficiency studies with a series of synthetic inhibitors of matrix metalloproteinases. Clin. Exp. Metastasis **15:** 499–508.
110. DAVIES, B., P.D. BROWN, N. EAST, M.J. CRIMMIN & F.R. BALKWILL. 1993. A synthetic matrix metalloproteinase inhibitor decreases tumor burden and prolongs survival of mice bearing human ovarian carcinoma xenografts. Cancer Res. **53:** 2087–2091.
111. WANG, X., X. FU, P.D. BROWN, M.J. CRIMMIN & R.M. HOFFMAN. 1994. Matrix metalloproteinase inhibitor BB-94 batimastat inhibits colon tumor growth and spread in a patient-like orthotopic model in nude mice. Cancer Res. **54:** 4726–4728.
112. CHIRIVI, C.G., A. GARAFALO, M.J. CRIMMIN, L.J. BAWDEN, A. STOPPACCIARA, P.D. BROWN & R. GIAVAZZI. 1994. Inhibition of the metastatic spread and growth of B16-BL6 murine melanoma by a synthetic matrix metalloproteinase inhibitor. Int. J. Cancer **58:** 460–464.
113. DRUMMOND, A., P. BECKETT & E. BORE. 1995. BB-2516: an orally available matrix metalloproteinase inhibitor with efficiency in animal cancer models [abstract]. Proc. Am. Assoc. Cancer Res. **36:** 100.
114. MACAULAY, V.M., K.J. O'BYRNE, M.P. SAUNDERS, A. SALISBURY, L. LONG, F. GLEESON, T.S. GANESAN, A.L. HARRIS & D.C. TALBOT. 1995. Phase I study of the matrix metalloprotienase inhibitor (BB-94) in patients with pleural effusions [abstract]. Br. J. Cancer **71:** 11.
115. PARSONS, S.L., S.A. WATSON, S.S. AMAR & R.J.C. STEELE. 1996. Phase I/II trial of matrix metalloproteinase inhibitor in patients with malignant ascites [abstract]. Gastroenterology **110:** A575.

116. MILLAR, A., P.D. BROWN, J. MORE, W.A. GALLOWAY, A. CORNISH, T. LENEHAN & K. LYNCH. 1998. Results of single and repeat dose studies of the oral matrix metalloproteinase inhibitor marimastat in healthy male volunteers. Br. J. Pharmacol. **45:** 21–26.
117. PARSONS, S.L., S.A. WATSON, N.R. GRIFFIN & R.J.C. STEELE. 1996. An open phase I/II study of the oral matrix metalloproteinase inhibitor marimastat in patients with inoperable gastric cancer [abstract]. Ann. Oncol. **7:** 47.
118. NEMUNAITIS, J., C. POOLE, J. PRIMROSE, A. ROSEMURGY, J. MALFETANO, P. BROWN, A. BERRINGTON, A. CORNISH, K. LYNCH, H. RASMUSSEN, D. KERR, D. COX & A. MILLAR. 1998. Combined analysis of studies of the effects of the matrix metalloproteinase inhibitor marimastat on serum tumor markers in advanced cancers: selection of a biologically active and tolerable dose for longer term studies. Clin. Cancer Res. **4:** 1101–1109.
119. PRIMROSE, J., H. BLEIBERG, F. DANIEL, P. JOHNSON, J. MANSI, J. NEOPTOLEMOS, M. SEYMOUR & S. VAN BELLE. 1996. A dose-finding study of marimastat, an oral matrix metalloproteinase inhibitor, in patients with advanced colorectal cancer [abstract]. Ann. Oncol. **7:** 35.
120. POOLE, C., M. ADAMS, V. BARLEY, J. GRAHAM, D. KERR, I. LOUVIAUX, T. PERREN, M. PICCART & H. THOMAS. 1996. A dose-finding study of marimastat, an oral matrix metalloproteinase inhibitor, in patients with advanced ovarian cancer [abstract]. Ann. Oncol. **7:** 68.
121. EVANS, J.D., P. GHANEH, A. KAWESHA & J.P. NEOPTOLEMOS. 1997. Role of matrix metalloproteinases and their inhibitors in pancreatic cancer. Digestion **58:** 520–528.
122. EVANS, J.D., S.R. BRAMHALL, A. STARK, H. HINLEY, C. PORTER, L. OSBORNE, F. DANIEL, J. CARMICHAEL, C. IMRIE, C.D. JOHNSON & J.P. NEOPTOLEMOS. 1996. A phase II trial of marimastat (BB-2516) in advanced pancreatic cancer [abstract]. Int. J. Pancreatol. **19:** 218.
123. EVANS, J.D., S.R. BRAMHALL, J. CARMICHAEL, F. DANIEL, C. IMRIE, C.D. JOHNSON, J.P. NEOPTOLEMOS & A. STARK. 1996. A phase II trial of marimastat (BB-2516) in advanced pancreatic cancer [abstract]. Ann. Oncol. **7:** 51.
124. ANDERSON, I.C., M.A. SHIPP, A.J.P. DOCHERTY & B.A. TEICHER. 1996. Combination therapy including a gelatinase inhibitor and cytotoxic agent reduces local invasion and metastasis of murine Lewis lung carcinoma. Cancer Res. **56:** 715–718.
125. CARMICHAEL, J., J.A. LEDERMAN, P.J. WOLL, T. GULLIFORD & R.C.G. RUSSEL. 1998. A phase Ib study of concurrent administration of marimastat and gemcitibine in non-resectable pancreatic cancer [abstract}. ASCO Proc. **17:** 232a.
126. O'REILLY, S.M., S. MARIN, M.J. RATAIN, K.E. BROWN, S. JOHNSON, N.J. VOGELZANG, M.J. KENNEDY, R.C. DONEHOWER & T. RUGG. 1998. Schedules of 5-FU and the matrix metalloproteinase inhibitor marimastat: a phase I study [abstract]. ASCO Proc. **17:** 217c.
127. BURRIS, H.A., M.J. MOORE, J. ANDERSEN, M.R. GREEN, M.L. ROTHENBERG, M.R. MADIANO, M.C. CRIPPS, R.K. PORTENOY, A.M. STORNIOLO, P. TARASSOFF, R. NELSON, F.A. DORR, C.D. STEPHENS & D.D. VAN HOFF. 1997. Improvements in survival and clinical benefit with gemcitibine as first-line therapy for patients with advanced pancreas cancer: a randomized trial. J. Clin. Oncol. **15:** 2403–2413.

Exocrine Pancreatic Function following Pancreatectomy

PAULA GHANEH AND JOHN P. NEOPTOLEMOS[a]

Department of Surgery, Royal Liverpool University Hospital, Liverpool L69 3GA, UK

ABSTRACT: Pancreatic exocrine insufficiency can follow major pancreatic resection and result in the malabsorption of fat, causing symptoms of steatorrhea, abdominal pain and weight loss. The extent of malabsorption will depend on the original disease process and the type and extent of surgical resection. The steatorrhea can be severe and difficult to control, and patients may require high doses of pancreatic enzyme supplements. There have been few studies that have looked at the treatment of steatorrhea postpancreatectomy, and very few randomized studies. Results of the latter have demonstrated that after treatment with oral pancreatic supplements over a third of postpancreatectomy patients still have significant levels of steatorrhea. These results show that even using the best available agents the complete elimination of steatorrhea following major pancreatic resection is not possible at the present time. This indicates a need for further effective therapies.

INTRODUCTION

The extent of pancreatic exocrine insufficiency following pancreatic resection relies on many factors that regulate the mechanisms of nutrient digestion and absorption. The exocrine output of the pancreas in healthy individuals is normally far in excess of that needed for adequate absorption of nutrients. To maintain a standard level of digestion and prevent malabsorption, studies in patients with varying degrees of pancreatic insufficiency have shown that 5–10% of normal pancreatic enzyme output is enough for adequate absorption to occur.[1] The rate of degradation of enzymes in the intestinal lumen is a major factor in the control of nutrient absorption. The half lives and survival activity of the pancreatic enzymes vary considerably: 60% of trypsin and chymotrypsin activity reaches the mid-jejunum and 20% reaches the ileum, whilst amylase is even more stable and most of its activity reaches the terminal ileum. In contrast lipase activity decreases rapidly; most is lost between the duodenum and the ileum and only minimal (<1%) active quantities reach the ileum.[2,3] The main mechanism for loss of enzyme activity is proteolytic degradation: chymotrypsin is the principal factor destroying lipase activity.[4] Lipase is also particularly sensitive to acid destruction.[5] The relatively short half-life of lipase compared with the other enzymes[6] contributes to the early development of fat malabsorption in patients with pancreatic insufficiency (FIG. 1). Efficient fat digestion in the small intestine is exclusively dependent on pancreatic lipase and its cofactors, bile acids

---

[a]Address for correspondence: Professor J.P. Neoptolemos, Department of Surgery, 5th Floor UCD Building, Daulby Street, Liverpool L69 3GA, UK. Phone, +44 151-706-4175; fax, +44 151-706-5798; e-mail, j.p.neoptolemos@liverpool.ac.uk

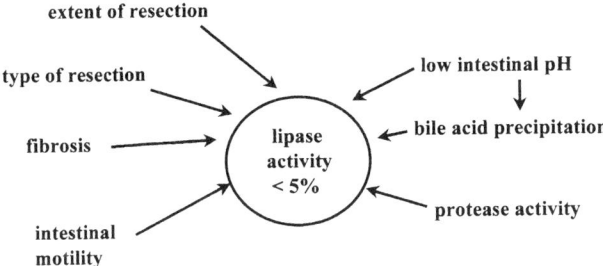

FIGURE 1. Factors affecting lipase activity following pancreatic resection.

and colipase. Therefore, the digestion of fat is intimately related to bile acid secretion, gastric emptying and intestinal motor activity and intestinal pH. A low intraduodenal pH will cause precipitation of bile acids and further compromise lipase activity. The decreased bicarbonate output seen in pancreatic exocrine insufficiency will also contribute to the low intraluminal pH.[5] The amount of nutrient present in the lumen can also affect the activity of the enzymes, and the absorption of nutrients directly correlates with the rate of gastric emptying. In pancreatic insufficiency alterations in gastrointestinal motility contribute to the overall compromise of absorption. There is accelerated gastric emptying and decreased intestinal transit time, which may be due to increased ileal nutrient load of malabsorbed chyme.[7] Attempts to prolong the intestinal transit time have been shown to improve the absorption rate of nutrients with the exception of fat.[8] Extrapancreatic sources of enzymes can compensate for malabsorption of protein and starch, which include salivary amylases, brush border oligosaccharidases, peptidases and gastric proteases. These can prevent malabsorption when trypsin output is less than 10% of normal.[1] A degree of fat absorption can occur due to the action of nonpancreatic lipases; up to 50 g of fat a day can be absorbed in patients without measurable sources of pancreatic enzymes[9] This is due to the actions of gastric lipase, lingual lipase and bacterial lipase present in the gastrointestinal tract. In healthy subjects there is minimal contribution of these lipases to the overall enzyme activity. There is some evidence, however, that the level of extrapancreatic lipase activity increases in patients with established pancreatic exocrine insufficiency.[10]

The aim of treatment of pancreatic exocrine insufficiency is to correct the malabsorption of fat, protein and starch. Fat malabsorption results in steatorrhea and symptoms of abdominal pain and weight loss; it is the earliest manifestation of pancreatic insufficiency and the most difficult to control.

PANCREATIC RESECTION FOR MALIGNANT DISEASE

Major upper gastrointestinal surgery such as gastrectomy and pancreatectomy can result in pancreatic exocrine insufficiency with variable levels of steatorrhea. The principle of curative surgery for pancreatic tumors involves resection of the tumor with a margin of normal pancreas. The majority of patients will undergo Whipple's procedure depending on the origin of the lesion. The extent of resection of

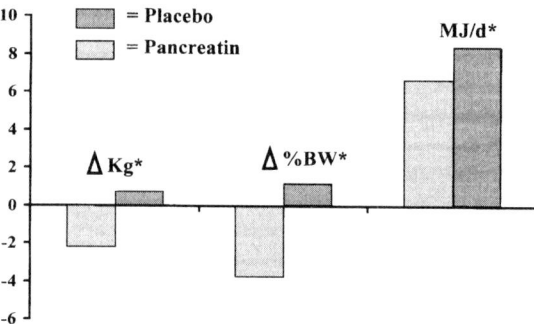

FIGURE 2. Effects of pancreatic enzyme therapy in patients with unresectable cancer of the pancreatic head. ΔKg = change in body weight; Δ%BW = % change in body weight; MJ/d = daily total caloric intake; *$p < 0.05$.

pancreatic parenchyma will contribute to the degree of pancreatic insufficiency. Further contributions to decreased enzyme output can be due to operative occlusion of the pancreatic duct, or a tumor occluding the duct, resulting in fibrosis and atrophy of the distal remnant of the gland. In patients with inoperable tumors of the pancreatic head, causing occlusion of the duct, the use of oral enzyme supplements has had a positive effect on criteria such as the rate of weight loss, which was decreased in the early phases of the treatment (FIG. 2).[11] Coexisting chronic pancreatitis can produce a background of fibrosis which will decrease the enzyme production. In an attempt to preserve pancreatic function in a small series of patients[12] with cystic and islet cell tumors of the neck and body of the pancreas, middle segment pancreatectomy was carried out. After 18 months follow-up no patients required oral pancreatic supplements.[12] The extent of resection has been shown to adversely affect the enzyme output of the pancreas. One study compared pancreatic exocrine function following standard and radical extended pancreatectomy.[13] The latter group demonstrated significantly less pancreatic function compared to the standard resection group (TABLE 1).

TABLE 1. Pancreatic exocrine insufficiency after major pancreatic resection measured by PABA recovery rate[13]

Surgical procedure	Number	Diagnosis	PABA recovery rate (%)
Control	53	control	79 ± 12
Conventional pancreaticodoudenectomy	22	pancreaticoduodenal malignancy	50 ± 17
Extended radical pancreaticoduodenectomy	10	pancreaticoduodenal malignancy	31 ± 14*
Distal pancreatecomy	8	pancreatic cancer or chronic pancreatitis	66 ± 13
Total pancreatecomy	5	pancreatic cancer	20 ± 12*
Side-to-side pancreaticojejunostomy	12	chronic pancreatitis	54 ± 9

NOTATION: PABA = p-aminobenzoic acid; values are mean ± SD; *$p < 0.05$ vs control.

PANCREATIC RESECTION FOR NONMALIGNANT DISEASE

The majority of patients in this group will undergo resection for chronic pancreatitis. The major indication for surgery in these patients is unremitting pain. At the time of surgery most patients will already demonstrate symptoms of pancreatic insufficiency. The standards of pancreatic surgery have improved over recent years with mortality rates as low as 5% in specialist centers with improved supportive care.[14] Thus operations can be tailored to the individual with the hope of improving the long-term outcome. The type of procedure can depend in part on the location of the disease process. The Whipple's procedure is commonly used for right-sided disease. In several studies 50% of patients had pancreatic exocrine insufficiency following Whipple's resection.[15,16] This involves reconstruction of the digestive pathway using pancreatojejunostomy, hepatojejunostomy and gastroenterostomy procedures. The normal physiology of gastric emptying with mixing of food particles, enzymes and bile acids is lost with the resection of the pylorus and duodenum. Increasingly, efforts have been directed at ways to conserve the normal anatomical and physiological mechanisms involved in digestion. The pylorus-preserving pancreatectomy (PPPD) keeps the stomach and proximal 2 cm of duodenum intact to preserve normal gastric emptying. Beger's procedure, which leaves the stomach and duodenum intact, would seem to have the least effect on the physiology of gastric emptying.[17] Several studies have confirmed that there is minimal exocrine insufficiency following this procedure and the nutritional status of the patients improved considerably.[18] Left-sided resection for left-sided disease can reduce pancreatic function depending on the amount of normal tissue removed. Left-sided resections, however, have been associated with more severe levels of exocrine insufficiency when compared to the Whipple's procedure.[19] Left-sided resections are also associated with an increased incidence of diabetes mellitus.[20] If the disease is widespread and multicentric, total or subtotal pancreatectomy may be indicated. This always results in a total loss of exocrine and endocrine pancreatic function with the development of diabetes mellitus. Occasionally this can be compensated for in some patients by extrapancreatic sources of lipase. Drainage procedures such as pancreatojejunostomy may be indicated for dilatation of the pancreatic duct. This results in delivery of enzymes downstream of the duodenum instead of mixing with the chyme, and so there is the potential for insufficiency. The severity of pancreatic insufficiency can also depend on the extent of the fibrosis of the remnant of the gland.[15] Persistent steatorrhea has been described following a variety of procedures for chronic pancreatitis.[21] Necrotizing pancreatitis can result in extensive loss of pancreatic tissue with or without necrosectomy. This can cause profound exocrine insufficiency.[22,23]

DIAGNOSIS OF PANCREATIC EXOCRINE INSUFFICIENCY

Clinical hallmarks of pancreatic exocrine insufficiency include symptoms of fat malabsorption such as steatorrhea (stool fat >7 g/day), weight loss and abdominal pain. Continued malabsorption will result in deficiencies in fat-soluble vitamins such as A, D, E and K. Requirements for oral pancreatic enzyme supplementation will depend on the severity of the patient's symptoms of diarrhea and weight loss despite adequate food intake. Confirmation of the diagnosis can be achieved using direct and indirect measurements of pancreatic function. These will also provide a guide to severity of insufficiency and a baseline to gauge treatment efficacy. The type of test used will depend on the type of surgery undergone by the patient. In addition the local facilities and level of expertise will determine the choice of investigation. Tests such as the secretin-cholecystokinin test are the gold standard but are too time consuming and unfeasible following certain surgical procedures. Direct tests such fecal fat measurement are accurate but are complicated and unpleasant to carry out. Newer procedures such near-infrared spectophotometry are proving to be more simple and rapid.[24] A number of indirect tests of pancreatic function which are noninvasive and easy to perform have been developed. Serum measurements of pancreatic isoamylase, immunoreactive trypsin are widely used but lack sensitivity in mild to moderate chronic pancreatitis. Other tests such as the pancreolauryl test (PLT), which has been optimized to detect moderate cases of chronic pancreatitis,[25] measurement of fecal chymotrypsin and enzyme-linked immunosorbent assay (ELISA) for fecal elastase 1 are in current use. A recent study found that fecal elastase 1 measurement was excellent for the diagnosis of severe chronic pancreatitis but has limited value in mild to moderate chronic pancreatitis.[26] ^{14}C breath tests and the cholesteryl octanoate test are useful, but interference with results can be due to certain metabolic and pulmonary disorders.[27] Newer procedures such as magnetic resonance cholangiopancreatography (MRCP) to image pancreatic intensity following secretin administration are currently being evaluated.[28]

MANAGEMENT OF PANCREATIC EXOCRINE INSUFFICIENCY FOLLOWING PANCREATECTOMY

Once the diagnosis has been confirmed, the aims of treatment are to correct malabsorption of fat, protein and carbohydrate. This will consist of correction of diabetes mellitus if present and oral pancreatic enzyme supplements (pancreatin). Reduction of dietary fat intake is not necessary in the vast majority (if any!) of cases. The preparation of enzymes must contain adequate concentrations of lipase, protease and amylase. Delivery of 20,000–30,000 U lipase into the duodenum may be required to alleviate steatorrhea, and in some cases this dose may need to be doubled to achieve adequate control. Even so, simply replacing lipase does not always abolish steatorrhea, and increasing the dose does not produce the expected increase in control of symptoms.[29] In cases of chronic pancreatitis there may be gastric hypersecretion. Lipase is extremely sensitive to acid destruction; therefore, oral preparations are rapidly destroyed in the stomach.[30] Enteric-coated preparations which are acid resistant and release enzyme only when intraluminal pH is more than 6 have been developed to overcome this obstacle. Reduction of gastric acid output using H_2 antagonists and proton pump inhibitors will protect and enhance the activity of oral lipase.

Ideally the enzymes should be delivered simultaneously with the food bolus into the duodenum. In the normal state, food particles are allowed into the duodenum once they are less than 2 mm in size.[31] This has prompted the development of enteric-coated microspheres (ECPM) which are 1–1.5 mm in diameter. Studies which

TABLE 2. Effects of pancreatic enzyme replacement therapy in patients with pancreatic exocrine insufficiency following pylorus preserving and conventional pancreaticoduodenectomy[39]

Procedure	Healthy control ($n = 9$)	Pylorus-preserving pancreaticoduodenectomy ($n = 5$)	Whipple's resection ($n = 7$)
Diagnosis	control	Pancreatic cancer	Pancreatic cancer
Age (yrs)	21–30	58 ± 10	66 ± 5
Post-op diabetes mellitus (n)	—	2	1
Gastric transit time of test meal vs ECPM (min)	—	50 ± 20 vs 119 ± 43*	53 ± 31 vs 79 ± 59
Mean PABA:PAS ratio before treatment	0.91	0.5*	0.52*
Mean PABA:PAS ratio after treatment	0.91	0.62*	0.98

*$p < 0.05$ versus control; ECPM = enteric-coated pancreatin microsphere; n = number; PABA = para aminobenzoic acid; PAS = para aminosalicylic acid.

have measured the rate of entry of these preparations into the duodenum have shown synchronous entry with a test meal as opposed to delayed entry with larger >2-mm microspheres. One recent study, however, indicated that 2-mm microspheres may pass into the duodenum faster than a solid meal.[32] The rate of gastric emptying can vary greatly from individual to individual thus complicating comparative studies. Microsphere preparations have shown superior efficacy over other pancreatic preparations, and the use of smaller microspheres has been shown to increase the intraluminal digestion of lipids.[33,34] Acid stable lipases which, in contrast to human lipase, are active at a low pH and are relatively stable to proteolytic degradation, represent a possible alternative to conventional enzyme preparations. Preparations which are fungal or bacterial in origin have been used to successfully treat steatorrhea. Although fungal preparations have not been shown to be superior to ECPMs[35] and may be inactivated by bile acids present in the intestinal lumen, bacterial lipases hold considerable promise for the future.[36]

Further improvements to enzyme preparations have been necessary because of the huge doses of lipase used by some patients to control symptoms. This can involve such a high capsule number that compliance has been compromised. Therefore, high-dose preparations have been developed which contain three times the usual dose of enzymes. This has resulted in decreased capsule intake and improved compliance in patients with cystic fibrosis and chronic pancreatitis.[37,38]

There have been relatively few studies looking at the treatment of pancreatic exocrine function following pancreatic resection. The type of resection can influence the efficacy of the pancreatin preparation used. In one nonrandomized study[39] the use of ECPMs >2 mm was associated with decreased efficacy in those patients who had undergone pylorus preserving pancreaticoduodenectomy compared to those who had undergone Whipple's procedure for pancreatic malignancy (TABLE 2). The use of smaller ECPMs may be indicated in those patients who have undergone pylorus or duodenal preserving surgery.

TABLE 3. Randomized controlled trial of pancreatin (Creon® 8,000) vs placebo for the treatment of pancreatic exocrine insufficiency following the Frey procedure[22]

COA (%)	Pancreatin ($n = 5$)	Placebo ($n = 6$)	$p <$
Fat	83.3 ± 2.9	52.7 ± 9.1	0.02*
Protein	84.4 ± 1.5	70.3 ± 6.1	0.2
Carbohydrate	96.2 ± 0.5	95.4 ± 0.8	0.07
Energy	88.3 ± 0.8	71.9 ± 5.2	0.02*

NOTATION: COA = coefficient of absorption; * = statistically significant difference; values are mean ± SD.

One of the few randomized studies which have been carried out, looked at a small number of patients[11] who had undergone local resection and pancreaticojejunostomy for chronic pancreatitis.[22] All patients had pancreatic exocrine insufficiency, diagnosed using 3-day stool fat measurements, with symptoms of fat malabsorption. Treatment with enzyme supplements significantly improved steatorrhea compared with the placebo group (TABLE 3). In a recent randomized, controlled double-blind cross-over study which compared the efficacy of high-dose (Creon® 25,000) and standard dose (Creon® 8,000) pancreatin in the treatment of pancreatic exocrine insufficiency following pancreatectomy for chronic pancreatitis, the pattern of steatorrhea postsurgery was examined in detail.[21] All patients were stabilized using a standard pancreatin preparation prior to entering the study. Interestingly, following this period of stabilization, 56% of patients still had steatorrhea (>7 g per day) (FIG. 3), and 38% had significant steatorrhea of >15 g/day. Direct measurement of stool fat was used to assess steatorrhea. As expected there was significant correlation between stool fat excretion and stool volume and stool frequency. Paradoxically there was a significant lack of correlation between symptoms and abdominal pain and stool fat excretion (FIG. 4), showing that in some patients with significant steatorrhea on direct testing, this did not indicate a worsening clinical situation. The majority of patients with steatorrhea were also taking regular antacid medication. Whilst on the standard therapy some patients were taking over 50 capsules a day (TABLE 4). Both standard and high-dose pancreatin preparations were equally effective, and therefore capsule number and compliance should improve with the use of

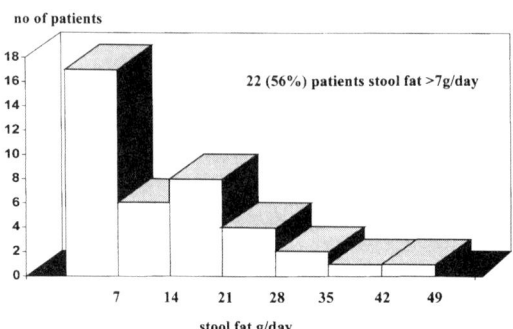

FIGURE 3. Distribution of stool fat excretion.

TABLE 4. Outcome following stabilization of pancreatic exocrine insufficiency following surgery[21a]

Criteria	
Number of patients	39
Age	52 (26–79)
steatorrhea >7g/day	22 (56%)
Daily stool (number)	1.9 (0.6–4.9)
Analgesic medication	15 (38%)
Antidiabetic medication	18 (46%)
Antacid therapy	21 (54%)
Mean number capsules taken	19.4 (9–54)
BMI estimation	23.2 (18.2–34.5)

[a]Values are mean (range); BMI = body mass index.

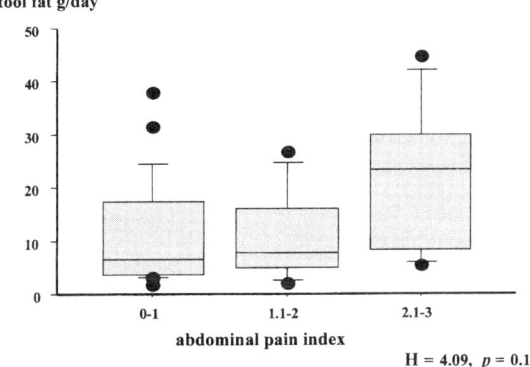

FIGURE 4. Box plot of stool fat grouped according to abdominal pain index. Low value = less severe pain, high value = severe degree of pain.

the high-dose preparation. It must be noted however that a number of patients still had significant steatorrhea whilst on high doses of effective enzyme supplements.

Improved approaches to treatment of pancreatic exocrine insufficiency are still required to eliminate steatorrhea completely. Clinical symptoms are usually used to assess efficacy of treatment in day-to-day practice, and encouragingly these do improve following treatment and good results can be seen in patients who receive high doses of effective pancreatin preparations.

REFERENCES

1. DiMagno, E.P., V.L.W. Go & W.H.J. Summerskill. 1973. Relations between pancreatic enzyme outputs and malabsorption in severe pancreatic insufficiency. N. Engl. J. Med. **288:** 813–815.

2. LAYER, P., V.L.W. GO & E.P. DiMAGNO. 1986. Fate of pancreatic enzymes during arboral small intestine transit in humans. Am. J. Physiol. **251:** G475–G480.
3. LAYER, P., J.B.M.J. JANSEN, C.B.H.W. LAMERS & H. GOEBELL. 1990. Feedback regulation of human pancreatic secretion: Effects of protease inihibition on duodenal delivery and small intestinal transit of pancreatic enzymes. Gastroenterology **98:** 1311–1319.
4. THIRUVENGADAM, R. & E.P. DiMAGNO. 1988. Inactivation of human lipase by proteases. Am. J. Physiol. **255:** G476–G481.
5. GUANNER, L., R. RODRIGUEZ, F. GUARNER & J.-R. MALAGELADA. 1993. Fate of oral enzymes in pancreatic insufficiency. Gut **34:** 708–712.
6. DiMAGNO, E.P., J.R. MALAGELADA, V.L.W. GO & C.G. MOERTEL. 1997. Fate of orally ingested enzymes in pancreatic insufficiency: comparison of two dosage schedules. N. Engl. J. Med. **296:** 1318–1322.
7. SUSUKI, A., A. MIZUMOTO, M.G. SARR & E.P. DiMAGNO. 1997. Does gastric emptying or small intestinal transit of nutrients affect intestinal absorption of nutrients in canine pancreatic exocrine insufficiency? Gastroenterology **112:** A484.
8. LAYER, P., M.R. VAN DER OHE, J.J. HOLST, J.B.M.J. JANSEN, D. GRANDT, G. HOLTMANN & H. GOEBELL. 1997. Altered post-prandial motility in chronic panceatitis: role of malabsorption. Gastroenterology **112:** 1624–1634.
9. ABRAMS, C.K., M. HAMOSH, S.K. DUTTA, V.S. HUBBARD & P. HAMOSH. 1987. Role of nonpancreatic lipolytic activity in exocrine pancreatic insufficiency. Gastroenterology **92:** 125–129.
10. BALASUBRAMANIAN, K., P.L. ZENTLER MUNRO, J.C. BATTEN & T.C. NORTHFIELD. 1992. Increased intragastric acid resistant lipase activity and lipolysis in pancreatic steatorrhea due to cystic fibrosis. Pancreas **7:** 305–310.
11. BRUNO, M.J., E.B. HAVERKORT, G.P. TIJSSEN, G.N.J. TYTGAT & D.J. VAN LEEUWEN. 1998. Placebo controlled trial of enteric coated pancreatic microsphere treatment in patients with unresectable cancer of the pancreatic head region. Gut **42:** 92–96.
12. WARSHAW, A.L., D.W. RATTNER, C. FERNANDEZ DEL CASTILLO & K. ZGRAGGEN. 1998. Middle segment pancreatectomy: a novel technique for conserving pancreatic tissue. Arch. Surg. **133:** 327–331.
13. YAGI, M., K. SHIMIZU, T. HASHIMOTO, R. IZUMI, T. NAGAKAWA, K. MIWA & I. MIYAZAKI. 1994. Pancreatic exocrine insufficiency after pancreatic surgery detected by tubeless testing. J. Clin. Biochem. Nutr. **16:** 205–209.
14. NEOPTOLEMOS, J.P., R.C.G. RUSSELL, S.R. BRAMHALL & B. THEIS. 1997. Low mortality following resection for pancreatic and periampullary tumors in 1026 patients: UK survey of specialist pancreatic units. Br. J. Surg. **84:** 1370–1376.
15. EVANS, J.D., P.G. WILSON, C. CARVER, S.R. BRAMHALL, J.A.C. BUCKELS, A.D. MAYER, P. MCMASTER & J.P. NEOPTOLEMOS. 1997. Outcome of surgery for chronic pancreatitis. Br. J. Surg. **84:** 624–629.
16. FORSSMANN, K., K. SCHIRR, M. SCMID, G. SCHWALL, D. SILBERNIK, M.V. SINGER & M. TREDE. 1997. Postoperative follow-up in patients treated by duodenopancreatectomy (Whipple's operation) in chronic pancreatitis. Z. Gastroenterol. **35:** 1071–1080.
17. BEGER, H.G., M.W. BÜCHLER & R. BITTNER. 1990. The duodenum preserving resection of the head of the pancreas (DPRHP) in patients with chronic pancreatitis and inflammatory mass in the head. An alternative surgical technique to the Whipple operation. Acta Chir. Scand. **156:** 309–315.
18. BEGER, H.G., M. BÜCHLER, R.R. BITTNER, W. OETTINGER & R. ROSCHER. 1989. Duodenum preserving resection of the head of the pancreas in severe chronic pancreatitis. Early and late results. Ann. Surg. **209:** 273–278.
19. MORROW, C.E., J. COHEN, D.E.R. SUTHERLAND & J.S. NAJORAN. 1984. Chronic pancreatitis: long-term results of pancreatic duct drainage, pancreatic resection and near total pancreatectomy and islet autotransplantation. Surgery **96:** 608–616.
20. WITTINGEN, J. & C.F. FREY. 1974. Islet concentration in the head, body, tail and uncinate process of the pancreas. Ann. Surg. **179:** 412–414.
21. NEOPTOLEMOS, J.P., S.R. BRAMHALL, R.C.G. RUSSELL, C.D. JOHNSON, R.C.N. WILLIAMSON, I.S. BENJAMIN, D. ALDERSON & J.H. KLEIBUEKER. 1997. Double-blind,

cross-over study comparing the efficacy and tolerance of Creon® 25,000 versus Creon® in patients following total or partial pancreatectomy [abstract]. Digestion **58**(Suppl. 2): 54.
22. VANHOOZEN, C.M., P.G. PEEKE, M. TAUBENECK, C.F. FREY & C.H. HALSTED. 1977. Efficacy of enzyme supplementation after surgery for chronic pancreatitis. Pancreas **14**: 174–180.
23. BOZKURT, T., D. MAROSKE & G. ADLER. 1995. Exocrine pancreatic function after recovery from necrotizing pancreatitis. Hepatogastroenterology **42**: 55–58.
24. NAKAMURA, T., T. TAKEUCHI, A. TERADA, Y. TANDO & T. SUDA. 1998. Near-infrared spectophotometry analysis of fat, neutral sterols, bile acids and short chain fatty acids in the feces of patients with pancreatic maldigestion and malabsorption. Int. J. Pancreatol. **23**: 137–143.
25. DOMNIGUEZ MUNOZ, J.E. & P. MALFERTHEINER. 1998. Optimized serum pancreolauryl test for differentiating patients with and without chronic pancreatitis. Clin. Chem. **44**: 869–875.
26. LANKISCH, P.G., I. SCHMIDT, H. KONIG, D. LEHNICK, R. KNOLLMANN, M. LÖHR & S. LIEBE. 1998. Fecal elastase 1: not helpful in diagnosing chronic pancreatitis associated with mild to moderate exocrine pancreatic insufficiency. Gastroenterology **42**: 551–554.
27. VENTRUCCI, M., A. CIPOLLA, G.M. UBALDUCCI, A. RODA & E. RODA. 1998. ^{13}C labelled cholesteryl octanoate breath test for assessing pancreatic exocrine insufficiency. Gut **42**: 81–87.
28. NANASHIMA, A., H. YAMAGUCHI, H. AYABE, T. FUKUDA & A. KURODA. 1998. Evaluation of pancreatic exocrine function using MRI imaging [abstract]. Int. J. Pancreatol. **23**: 257.
29. VECHT, J., A. MACLEE, H. GIELKENS, H. HEYERMAN & C. LAHERS. 1997. Does escalation of pancreatic enzymes decrease steatorrhea and abdominal symptoms in patients with pancreatic insufficiency? Gastroenterology **112**: A494.
30. SAUNDERS, J.H.B., J.M. CARGILL & K.G. WORMSLEY. 1978. Gastric secretion of acid in patients with pancreatic disease. Digestion **17**: 365–369.
31. MEYER, J.H., J. ELASHOFF, V. PORTER-FINK, DRESSMAN & G.L. AMIDON. 1988. Human postprandial gastric emptying of 1–3 mm spheres. Gastroenterology **94**: 1315–1325.
32. BRUNO, M.J., J.J.J. BORM, F.J. HOEK, B. DELZENNE, A.F. HOFMANN, J.J.M. DEGOEIJ, E.A. VANROYEN, D.J. VANLEEUWEN & G.N.J. TYTGAT. 1998. Gastric transit and pharmacodynamics of a two millimeter enteric-coated pancreatin microsphere preparation in patients with chronic pancreatitis. Dig. Dis. Sci. **43**: 203–213.
33. STEAD, R.J., I. SKYPALA & M.E. HODSON. 1988. Treatment of steatorrhea in cystic fibrosis: a comparison of enteric coated microspheres of pancreatic versus nonenteric coated pancreatin and adjuvant cimetidine. Aliment. Pharmacol. Ther. **2**: 471–481.
34. LANKISCH, P.G., B. LEMBCKE, B. GÖKE & W. CREUTZFELT. 1986. Therapy of pancreatogenic steatorrhea: does acid protection of pancreatic enzymes offer any advantage? Z. Gastroenterol. **24**: 753–757.
35. ZENTLER MUNRO, P.L., B.A. ASSOUFI, K. BALASUBRAMANIAN, S. CORNELL, D. BENOLIEL, T.C. NORTHFIELD & M.E. HODSON. 1992. Therapeutic potential and clinical efficacy of acid resistant fungal lipase in the treatment of pancreatic steatorrhea due to cystic fibrosis. Pancreas **7**: 311–319.
36. SUSUKI, A., A. MIZUMOTO, M.G. SARR & E.P. DIMAGNO. 1997. Bacterial lipase and high fat diets in canine exocrine pancreatic insufficiency: a new therapy of steatorrhea? Gastroenterology **112**: 2048–2055.
37. DELHAYE, M., S. MEURIS, A.C. GOHIMONT, K. BUEDTS & M. CREMER. 1996. Comparative evaluation of a high lipase pancreatic enzyme preparation and a standard pancreatic supplement for treating exocrine pancreatic insufficiency in chronic pancreatitis. Eur. J. Gastroenterol. Hepatol. **8**: 699–703.
38. GAN, K.H., H.G.M. HEIZERMAN, W.P. GEVS, W. BAKKER & C.B.H.W. LAMERS. 1994. Comparison of a high lipase pancreatic enzyme extract with a regular pancreatic

preparation in adult cystic fibrosis patients. Aliment. Pharmacol. Ther. **8:** 603–607.
39. BRUNO, M.J., J.J.J. BORM, F.J. HOEK, B. DELZENNE, A.F. HOFMANN, J.J.M. DE GOEIJ, E.A. VAN ROYEN, T.M. VAN GULIK, L. TH. DE WIT, D.J. GOUMA, D.J. VAN LEEUWEN & G.N.J. TYTGAT. 1997. Comparative effects of enteric coated pancreatic microsphere therapy after conventional and pylorus preserving pancreatoduodenectomy. Br. J. Surg. **84:** 952–956.

Genetic Prodrug Activation Therapy for Pancreatic Cancer

A.S. RIGG AND N.R. LEMOINE[a]

Imperial Cancer Research Fund Molecular Oncology Unit at Hammersmith Hospital, Imperial College School of Medicine, Du Cane Road, London W12 0NN, UK

INTRODUCTION

Ductal adenocarcinoma of the pancreas is still the fifth commonest cause of cancer death in Europe and the USA. Advances in surgery, chemotherapy and radiation therapy have made little impact on morbidity and mortality for these patients. Meanwhile there has been an increase in the knowledge of the molecular genetic profile of pancreatic tumors. In addition to facilitating accurate diagnosis this knowledge has raised the possibility of gene therapies tailored to the molecular abnormalities of a specific patient's tumor. Approaches such as replacement of tumor suppressor gene function or inactivation of oncogene expression are being attempted, in addition to numerous strategies to boost tumor immunogenicity. One example of these new gene therapies that has potential applications for pancreatic cancer is genetic prodrug activation therapy (GPAT) and will be discussed in this article. GPAT has been extensively studied *in vitro* and *in vivo*, and is now moving into the clinical arena.

GENETIC PRODRUG ACTIVATION THERAPY

Genetic prodrug activation therapy (GPAT) involves the introduction of a "suicide" gene encoding a drug-metabolizing enzyme into tumor cells followed by the administration of a prodrug that will only be converted to a cytotoxic agent in the cells producing the enzyme (i.e., the targeted tumor cells). A key element of GPAT is the ability to selectively target suicide gene transfer to tumor cells, thus avoiding the systemic toxicity associated with most chemotherapy regimens. This selective targeting can be achieved through two routes. Firstly, transductional targeting utilizes differences between target and normal cells in terms of their ability to be transduced. One example of this is the use of retroviral vectors to deliver the suicide gene, as they will only infect dividing cells. This method is particularly useful for the treatment of brain tumors that are rapidly proliferating against a background of quiescent neural tissue, but less appropriate for gastrointestinal tumors as the surrounding normal cells will also be dividing. The second route, transcriptional targeting, involves modifying the transcriptional regulatory elements (TREs) controlling expression of the suicide gene. The promoter and enhancer elements of tumor-associated genes/ protooncogenes or genes specific to the tissue the tumor is derived from can be har-

[a]Corresponding author. Phone, +44 181-383-3975; fax, +44 181-383-3258; e-mail, n.lemoine@icrf.icnet.uk

TABLE 1. Transcriptional regulatory elements potentially suitable for genetic prodrug activation therapy

Gene	Tumor or Tissue Specificity
ERBB2	Pancreatic, breast and gastric carcinomas
ERBB3	Breast and gastrointestinal carcinomas
ERBB4	Breast and gastrointestinal carcinomas
MUC1	Pancreatic and breast ductal carcinomas
α-Fetoprotein	Hepatocellular carcinoma
Carcinoembryonic antigen	Pancreatic, colorectal and gastric carcinomas
Prostate-specific antigen	Prostate carcinomas
DOPA decarboxylase	Small cell lung cancer
Bombesin	Small cell lung cancer
Tyrosinase	Melanin-producing cells
Tyrosinase related protein 1	Melanin-producing cells
Amylase	Pancreatic acinar cells
Insulin	Pancreatic β islet cells
11-β-Hydroxylase	Adrenocortical carcinoma
Thyroglobulin	Follicular carcinoma of the thyroid

nessed to drive the suicide gene (TABLE 1). Thus the suicide gene will only become transcriptionally active in cells with the correct tumor- or tissue-specificity. DeMatteo et al. investigated the use of the amylase promoter driving the reporter gene LacZ for adenovirus-mediated pancreas-specific gene regulation and found gene expression exclusively in the pancreatic acinar cells of neonatal and adult mice.[1] Similarly the promoters for the melanocyte-specific genes tyrosinase and tyrosinase-related protein-1 can be used to provide selective expression of a suicide gene in melanoma cells.[2] Tumor specificity of suicide gene function is exemplified by the use of the proximal ERBB2 promoter to drive the cytosine deaminase gene in a variety of cancer cell lines, and the level of cell killing with 5-fluorocytosine was proportional to the cellular expression of ERBB2.[3]

The engineering and combination of TREs can enhance expression of the suicide gene while maintaining strict tumor-specificity. This was demonstrated by the construction of a chimeric promoter consisting of the MUC1 enhancer element and the ERBB2 promoter and another chimera of the MUC1 promoter downstream of three AP2 transcription factor sites. These two promoters were then used to drive the suicide gene thymidine kinase. In pancreatic and breast carcinoma cell lines that were transduced by retroviruses containing these expression cassettes, only those that were MUC1-positive exhibited cell killing with the prodrug ganciclovir. If the cell line was positive for AP2 and MUC1 expression, then cell killing on administration of the prodrug was best with the AP2 and MUC1 expression cassette. After retroviral transduction, cells that were negative for MUC1 and AP2 were not sensitized to the prodrug confirming that tumor specificity had been maintained.[4]

Most GPAT systems utilize enzymes that are of nonmammalian origin or only expressed in very small quantities in normal human cells (TABLE 2). The two most commonly studied examples are thymidine kinase from herpes simplex virus or va-

TABLE 2. Enzyme-prodrug systems currently under investigation for genetic prodrug activation therapy

Enzyme	Prodrug	Cytotoxic Product
Thymidine kinase	Ganciclovir	Ganciclovir trophosphate
Cytosine deaminase	5-Fluorocytosine	5-Fluorouracil
Thymidine phosphorylase	5′-Deoxy-5-fluorouridine	5-Fluorouracil
Nitroreductase	CB1954	5-Aziridinyl-4-hydroxy-lamino-2-nitrobenzamide
Purine nucleosidase phosphorylase	6-Methylpurine-deoxyriboside	6-Methylpurine
Cytochrome P450 2B1	Cyclophosphamide	Acrolein and phosphoramide mustard
Alkaline phosphatase	Etoposide phosphate	Etoposide
Carboxypeptidase A	Methotrexate-alanine	Methotrexate
Carboxypeptidase G2	Benzoic acid mustard-glucuronide	Benzoic acid mustard
Linamarase	Amygdalin	Cyanide
Xanthine oxidase	Xanthine	Oxygen radicals

ricella zoster virus and cytosine deaminase from *E. coli*. Both systems have the advantage of involving prodrugs that have well-established human side-effect profiles. Herpes simplex virus thymidine kinase (HSVTK) catalyzes the conversion of the prodrug ganciclovir to ganciclovir monophosphate, which is then further phosphorylated by the host cell to the toxic form ganciclovir triphosphate.[5] Ganciclovir triphosphate inhibits DNA polymerase and is toxic to cells in S phase of the cell cycle.[6] The use of HSVTK for gene therapy was first described in 1986.[7] It has since been extensively used *in vitro* and *in vivo* of many cell types including pancreatic adenocarcinoma. Adenoviral and cationic lipid vectors have been used to transfer the gene HSVTK to murine disseminated intraperitoneal pancreatic tumors and pancreatic hepatic metastases with statistically significant reductions of tumor burden on administration of ganciclovir.[8–10] Yang *et al.* established pancreatic tumors by injecting human carcinoma cells directly into the pancreas of nude mice at laparotomy.[11] The mice were then treated with intraperitoneal injections of a retrovirus containing the HSVTK gene and ganciclovir. Highly significant reductions of tumor volume were observed in the treated mice compared with untreated controls.

Cytosine deaminase is present in many fungi and bacteria. It is an enzyme that is involved in the conversion of 5-fluorocytosine to 5-fluorouracil. 5-Fluorouracil inhibits thymidylate synthetase, so that DNA cannot be synthesized. Harris *et al.* showed that the ERBB2 promoter could be used to drive the cytosine deaminase gene in pancreatic and breast cancer cells that were ERBB2$^+$ resulting in cell death when 5-fluorocytosine was administered.[3] ERBB2$^-$ cells were unaffected by the prodrug.

One of the anticipated limitations of the GPAT concept was the belief that all tumor cells would need to be transduced with the suicide gene to achieve significant cell killing. Interestingly, this premise was found to be incorrect. HSVTK experiments *in vitro* suggested that if tumor cells were grown at high density, then HSVTK$^-$ as well as HSVTK$^+$ cells were killed by ganciclovir, whereas at low density HSVTK⁻ cells survived.[7] In mice inoculated with HSVTK⁺ tumor cells, on administration of ganciclovir, adjacent nontransduced tumor cells were also killed.[12] This toxic influence of transduced cells on neighboring nontransduced cells was labeled the "bystander effect." Subsequent *in vitro* experiments involved growing varying proportions of HSVTK⁺ and HSVTK⁻ tumor cells and administering ganciclovir. When only 10% of the cells were HSVTK⁺, ganciclovir caused significant cell death.[13] The bystander effect for the cytosine deaminase system has been described to be even more dramatic with only 2% of suicide gene-positive cells required to produce significant tumor reductions with 5-fluorocytosine.[14]

There are several hypotheses as to the mechanism of the *in vitro* bystander effect. For the thymidine kinase system it is probable that it occurs due to transfer of the toxic metabolite ganciclovir triphosphate via gap junctions between adjacent cells. This would also explain why the phenomenon is predominantly noted when transduced and nontransduced cells are in close proximity.[15] A second hypothesis is that the ganciclovir triphosphate remains trapped in apoptotic vesicles as the tumor cell dies and that these vesicles are then phagocytosed resulting in the death of nontransduced cells.[13] Thirdly, in the case of cytosine deaminase, 5-fluorouracil is soluble and small enough to diffuse across the cell membrane to affect adjacent cells.[14,16]

In vivo the bystander effect has been observed to cause hemorrhagic tumor necrosis (HTN) within 24 hours of inoculation of HSVTK⁺ tumor cells.[17] This has been shown for HSVTK⁺ cells injected directly into murine glioblastomas and intraperitoneally for peritoneal tumors in mice.[18,19] In both cases HTN occurred in the center of the tumors. In the experiment with intraperitoneal tumors the HSVTK⁺ cells were not injected into the tumors directly; therefore, the peripheral tumor cell death and bystander effect must have caused the central HTN indirectly, perhaps by release of a soluble cytokine such as tumor necrosis factor or an interleukin. There may well be an immunological component to the *in vivo* bystander effect. Mice with cytosine deaminase-transduced tumors that resolved with 5-fluorocytosine treatment were later rechallenged with wild-type tumor cells and exhibited resistance probably due to a T cell-mediated response.[20] There are three possible explanations for this resistance. Firstly, the dying tumor cells might induce better antigen presentation to the immune system producing inflammation. Secondly, the cytosine deaminase protein might act as a superantigen causing polyclonal activation of lymphocytes, some of which might cross-react with the tumor. Finally, successful GPAT destruction of the tumor might be the equivalent of a surgical resection producing immunity. Vile *et al.* compared the HSVTK/ganciclovir system in immunocompetent and nude mice. Experimental melanoma metastases retrovirally transduced with HSVTK were significantly reduced in the immunocompetent mice, but not in the nude mice, providing further evidence of an immune component to the bystander effect.[21] Freeman *et al.* suggested that further enhancement of this immune response with cytokines, or immunization with tumor antigens before GPAT, might improve results.[22] This has been borne out by demonstrating in a mouse pulmonary metastasis model that tumor cells producing both cytosine deaminase and interleukin-6 in the presence of 5-fluorocytosine have reduced tumorigenicity and increased immunogenicity compared with cells producing cytosine deaminase or interleukin-6 alone.[23] Wei *et al.* have demonstrated regression of chemically induced mammary tumors in rats that were injected intratumorally with retrovirus-producer cells releasing retroviruses encoding the thymidine kinase gene. In addition, distant noninjected mammary tumors were also shown to have a significant regression compared to controls. An extensive lymphocytic infiltration was seen in both injected and noninjected tumors, suggesting that an *in vivo* bystander effect had taken place and was immune mediated.[24]

GPAT has now entered the clinical arena with greater than 20 phase I trials in progress globally. The primary concern for human gene therapy is the safety of the prodrug/active drug system and the delivery vector. Prodrugs that are well used and have recognized toxicity profiles are favored over clinically untested agents; consequently, the HSVTK and cytosine deaminase systems are the main candidates to have reached clinical trial so far. Earlier this year the results of a clinical trial of HSVTK GPAT for patients with recurrent malignant brain tumors was published.[25] The 15 patients underwent intratumoral injection of retroviral vector-producer cells, followed by ganciclovir treatment i.v. for 14 days. Five of the smaller tumors showed an antitumor response. *In situ* hybridization for HSVTK confirmed the presence of mRNA, but it tended to be confined to the vector-producing cells rather than being due to gene transfer to the tumor cells. A phase I clinical trial of GPAT with transcriptional targeting has recently been completed for patients with ERBB2-positive breast cancer. Cutaneous tumor nodules were injected with plasmid DNA encoding the cytosine deaminase gene under the control of the ERBB2 promoter. The prodrug 5-fluorocytosine was then administered. Preliminary results suggest both cytosine deaminase expression and suicide enzyme functionality restricted to ERBB2-positive breast cancer cells (Pandha *et al.*, unpublished data).[26] No blood dyscrasias or auto-antibodies were detected in the patients treated.

GPAT is a gene therapy strategy that is now in the cancer clinic, although limited to clinical trials at present. Given the increasing knowledge of protooncogene and tumor-associated gene expression in pancreatic ductal adenocarcinomas, there is potential for GPAT application for this disease clinically in the near future. The most difficult aspect will be designing an effective delivery system for the suicide gene both in terms of the anatomical location of the pancreas and ensuring maximal gene transfer to the target cells. Experimental and clinical data suggest that tumor selectivity can be strictly maintained by utilizing transcriptional regulatory elements such as MUC1 or ERBB2 and that there is no significant side effect profile associated with receiving these therapies.

ACKNOWLEDGMENT

Dr. Anne Rigg is sponsored by the Mike Stone Cancer Research Fund.

REFERENCES

1. DEMATTEO, R.P. *et al.* 1997. Engineering tissue-specific expression of a recombinant adenovirus: selective transgene transcription in the pancreas using the amylase promoter. J. Surg. Res. **72:** 155–161.
2. VILE, R.G. & I.R. HART. 1993. *In vitro* and *in vivo* targeting of gene expression to melanoma cells. Cancer Res. **53:** 962–967.
3. HARRIS, J.D. *et al.* 1994. Gene therapy for cancer using tumor-specific prodrug activation. Gene Ther. **1:** 170–175.

4. RING, C.J.A. et al. 1996. Suicide gene expression induced in tumor cells transduced with recombinant adenoviral, retroviral and plasmid vectors containing the ERBB2 promoter. Gene Ther. **3:** 1094–1103.
5. HAYDEN, F.G. 1995. Antiviral agents. *In* Goodman and Gilman's The Pharmacological Basis of Therapeutics. J.G. Hardman *et al.*, Eds.: 1191–1223. McGraw-Hill. New York.
6. MAR, E.-C. *et al.* 1985. Inhibition of cellular DNA polymerase α and human cytomegalovirus-induced DNA polymerase by the triphosphates of 9-(1,3-dihydroxy-2-propoxymethyl)guanine. J. Virol. **53:** 776–780.
7. MOOLTON, F.L. 1986. Tumor chemosensitivity conferred by inserting herpes thymidine kinase genes: paradigm for a prospective cancer control strategy. Cancer Res. **46:** 5276–5281.
8. BLOCK, A. *et al.* 1997. Adenoviral-mediated herpes simplex virus thymidine kinase gene transfer: regression of hepatic metastasis of pancreatic tumors. Pancreas **15:** 25–34.
9. ROSENFELD, M.E. *et al.* 1997. Pancreatic carcinoma cell killing via adenoviral mediated delivery of the herpes simplex virus thymidine kinase gene. Ann. Surg. **225:** 609–620.
10. AOKI, K. *et al.* 1997. Gene therapy for peritoneal dissemination of pancreatic cancer by liposome-mediated transfer of herpes simplex virus thymidine kinase gene. Hum. Gene Ther. **8:** 1105–1113.
11. YANG, L. *et al.* 1996. Gene therapy of metastatic pancreas cancer with intraperitoneal injections of concentrated retroviral herpes simplex thymidine kinase vector supernatant and ganciclovir. Ann. Surg. **224:** 405–417.
12. FREEMAN, S.M. *et al.* 1992. Tumor regression when a fraction of the tumor mass contains the HSV-TK gene. J. Cell. Biochem. **16:** 47.
13. FREEMAN, S.M. *et al.* 1993. The 'bystander effect': tumor regression when a fraction of the tumor mass is genetically modified. Cancer Res. **53:** 5274–5238.
14. HUBER, B.W. *et al.* 1994. Metabolism of 5-fluorocytosine to 5-fluorouracil in human colorectal tumor cells transduced with the cytosine deaminsase gene: significant antitumor effects when only a small percentage of tumor cells express cytosine deaminase. Proc. Natl. Acad. Sci. USA **91:** 8302–8306.
15. Bi, L.B. *et al.* 1993. *In vitro* evidence that metabolic cooperation is responsible for the bystander effect observed with HSV-tk retroviral gene therapy. Hum. Gene Ther. **4:** 725–731.
16. DOMAIN, B.A. *et al.* 1993. Transport of 5-fluorouracil and uracil into human erythrocytes. Biochem. Pharmacol. **46:** 503–510.
17. FREEMAN, S.M. *et al.* 1995. Treatment of ovarian cancer using a gene-modified vaccine. Hum. Gene Ther. **6:** 927–939.
18. RAM, Z. *et al.* 1994. The effect of thymidine kinase transduction and ganciclovir therapy on tumor vasculature and growth of 9L gliomas in rats. J. Neurosurg. **81:** 256–260.
19. FREEMAN, S.M. *et al.* 1995. The role of cytokines in mediating the bystander effect using HSV-TK xenogeneic cells. Cancer Lett. **92:** 167–174.
20. MULLEN, C.A. *et al.* 1994. Tumors expressing the cytosine deaminase gene can be eliminated *in vivo* with 5-fluorocytosine and induce protective immunity to wild-type tumor. Cancer Res. **54:** 1503–1506.
21. VILE, R.G. *et al.* 1994. Systemic gene therapy for murine melanoma using tissue-specific expression of the HSVtk gene involves an immune component. Cancer Res. **54:** 6228–6234.
22. FREEMAN, S.M. *et al.* 1997. Immune system in suicide gene therapy. Lancet **349:** 2–3.
23. MULLEN, C.A. *et al.* 1996. Treatment of microscopic pulmonary metastases with recombinant autologous tumor vaccine expressing interleukin 6 and *Escherichia coli* cytosine deaminase suicide genes. Cancer Res. **56:** 1362–1366.
24. WEI, M.X. *et al.* 1998. Suicide gene therapy of chemically induced mammary tumor in rat: efficacy and distant bystander effect. Cancer Res. **58:** 3529–3532.

25. RAM, Z. *et al.* 1998. Therapy of malignant brain tumors by intratumoral injection of retroviral vector-producing cells. Nat. Med. **3:** 1354–1361.
26. PANDHA, H.S. *et al.* 1998. Phase I trial of genetic prodrug activation therapy for metastatic breast cancer. Submitted for publication.

Characterization of a Human Cell Clone Expressing Cytochrome P450 for Safe Use in Human Somatic Cell Therapy

WALTER H. GÜNZBURG,[a,c] PETER KARLE,[a] RENATE RENZ,[a,b]
BRIAN SALMONS,[b] AND MATTHIAS RENNER[a,b]

[a]*Institute of Virology, University of Veterinary Sciences, Josef-Baumanngasse 1, A-1210 Vienna, Austria*

[b]*Bavarian Nordic Research Institute, GmbH, Fraunhoferstraße 18b, D-82152 Martinsried, Germany*

ABSTRACT: We have previously demonstrated the therapeutic effect and efficacy of implantation of cells genetically modified to express cytochrome P450 2B1 in a nude mouse tumor model. The cells are encapsulated in polymerized cellulose sulphate and injected into preformed tumors. Upon administration of ifosfamide, the P450 enzyme converts the ifosfamide into antitumorigenic toxic metabolites at the site required, thereby significantly reducing tumor burden. Feline kidney epithelial cells were chosen for these studies, because they are easy to culture and can readily be transfected. However, these cells are not suitable for eventual use in human patients, since they are known to express endogenous retroviruses that are able to infect mammalian cells. They thus represent a safety risk. Here we describe the establishment of a human cell line that has been genetically modified to express the same cytochrome P450 construct and their characterization. The usefulness of mitomycin C treatment, both to protect the cells from the toxic metabolites that they produce and to incapacitate these cells from replicating, should they escape from the capsules, has also been investigated.

INTRODUCTION

The cytochrome P450 enzymes are a family of more than 200 haem-containing proteins that are involved in oxidation of compounds.[1] Certain members of the cytochrome P450 family of enzymes, such as the isoenzyme 2B1, have the ability to convert chemotherapeutic agents like ifosfamide or cyclophosphamide into toxic metabolites. These metabolites are responsible for the anti-tumorigenic effects observed after chemotherapy, as well as for the side effects of such treatment.[2] The conversion event occurs predominantly in the liver, due to the expression of CYP450 enzymes in this organ, and the resulting metabolites are distributed throughout the body by the circulatory system. The body is exposed systemically to the toxic metabolites, leading to the debilitating side effects.

[c]Corresponding author: Prof. Walter H. Günzburg, Institute of Virology, University of Veterinary Sciences, Josef-Baumanngasse 1, A-1210 Vienna, Austria. Phone, +43 1-25077-2301; fax, +43 1-25077-2390; e-mail: walter.guenzburg@vu-wien.ac.at

The ability to perform the chemotherapeutic conversion near or in the tumor, thus generating high, local concentrations of active metabolites, should have the additional benefit of alleviating the systemic side effects, particularly if lower concentrations of the chemotherapeutic are used. In such a scenario, cells that express CYP2B1 would be implanted in an immunoprotective environment at the tumor site. We have recently shown that this kind of strategy is feasible. A cell clone that has acquired and expresses the CYP2B1 transgene under the transcriptional control of the CMV promoter has been encapsulated in an immunoprotective matrix consisting of polymers of cellulose sulphate and injected into preformed tumors established on the flanks of nude mice. Subsequent treatment with ifosfamide resulted in an enhanced reduction of tumor burden and even in tumor regressions in four cases[3] (see also Löhr et al., this volume).

Here we describe the characterization of a CYP2B1 transfected and expressing cell line of human origin and suitable for implantation, after encapsulation, into patients. The treatment of these cells with mitomycin C is also examined to determine if arrested CYP2B1 expressing cells are themselves less susceptible to cell killing as a result of ifosfamide or cyclophosphamide treatment.

MATERIALS AND METHODS

Cell Culture

293 cells are of human embryonic kidney origin.[4] They were obtained from a contract research organization and grown in Dulbecco's modified Eagle's medium supplemented with 10% fetal calf serum, under Good Laboratory Practice (GLP)-like conditions.

Transfection

The cytochrome P450 expression plasmid, pc3/2B1, carrying the 2B1 isoform of cytochrome P450 under the transcriptional control of the cytomegalovirus (CMV) promoter has been previously described.[3] The plasmid was transfected into 293 cells using a Pharmacia Transfection kit, as previously described,[5] the cells were selected in G418-containing medium, and individual cell clones were isolated.

Screening of the CYP450 Cell Clones

To determine the sensitivity of the pc3/2B1 transfected cell clones to cyclophosphamide, 1×10^4 cells were plated in 6-well plates. The wells received either no cyclophosphamide or 0.17, 0.33, 0.67, 1.33 or 3.3 µg/ml cyclophosphamide, and 10 days later the cells were stained and the number of surviving cells was estimated.

Resorufin Assay

This assay was designed by Donato and co-workers[6] to detect CYP2B1 activity and is based on the ability of the enzyme to convert the substrate resorufin into a fluorescent substance, the amount of which is proportional to the amount of P450 enyzme. The assay was performed as previously described.[3] Briefly, defined num-

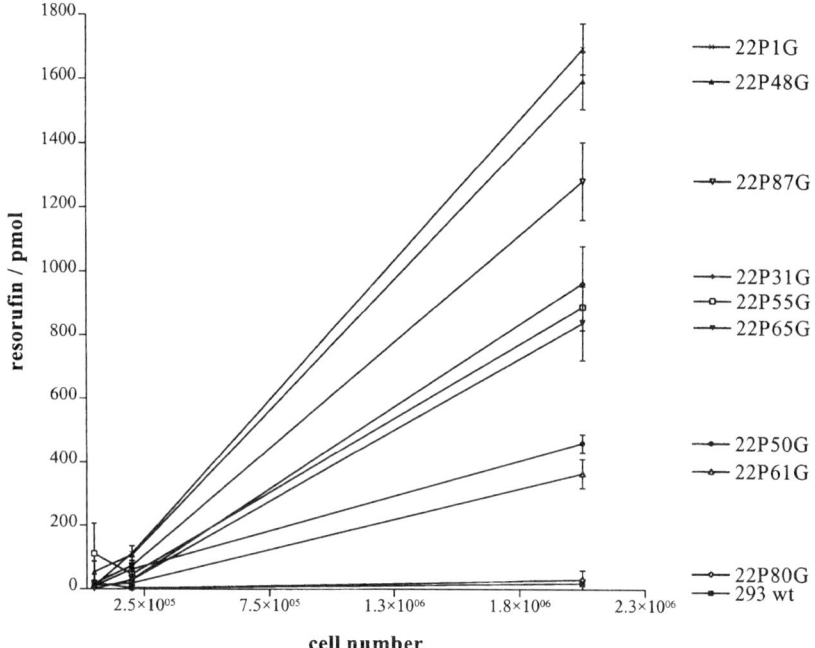

FIGURE 1. CYP2B1 activity from some of the transfected cell clones.

bers of cells (FIG. 1) were plated and one day later, after having been washed with phosphate-buffered saline (PBS), the cells were given 500 µl serum-free medium containing 15 µm 7-pentoxyresorufin (and 10 µm dicumarol, which inhibits cellular enzymes that inactivate resorufin). After incubation for 30 min at 37°C, 375 µl medium was mixed with 125 µl sodium acetate (0.1 mM) containing 75 Fishman units of β-glucuronidase per 600 Roy units of arylsulphatase to hydrolyse resorufin conjugates. After a 2-hr incubation at 37°C, the reaction was stopped by adding 1 ml of methanol, and the amount of resorufin produced was measured at 590 nm after excitation at 530 nm.

Determination of the Minimal Growth Inhibitory Concentration of Mitomycin C

The 22P1G cell clone was plated at 5×10^5 cells in T75 flasks. Two days later, 0, 0.5, 1 or 2 µg/ml mitomycin C was added to the cell culture medium, and the cells were incubated for 2 hr. After removing the mitomycin C-containing medium and washing with PBS, the cells were given fresh medium and incubated further. The number of viable cells was determined after life dead staining (Sigma) on the day of mitomycin C treatment (day 0) and on days 2, 7, 11, 16, 19, 24, 28 and 32.

TABLE 1. Analysis of some of the CYP450-transfected cell clones

Clone	Concentration of Cyclophosphamide (mM)				
	0.17	0.33	0.67	1.33	3.3
1	–	p	+	+	+
3	–	–	p	+	+
8	–	p	+	+	+
20	–	–	–	p	+
21	–	–	–	+	+
30	–	–	–	+	+
31	–	p	+	+	+
43	–	–	–	+	+
48	–	p	+	+	+
58	–	–	–	p	+
61	–	–	p	+	+
untransfected cells	–	–	–	–	+

NOTE: No obvious effect on cell growth and viability is indicated by –, whereas p indicates a partial effect and + a strong inhibition of cell viability.

RESULTS

CYP450 Expressing Cell Clones

In proof of principle experiments using a mouse model system, a CYP2B1 expressing clone of feline kidney cells was used.[3] However, such a cell line is not ideal for eventual implantation into patients for a number of reasons, including (i) the expression of one or more endogenous retroviruses[7] and (ii) susceptibility to other viral adventitious agents.[7] As well as having a qualified and well documented history, a suitable cell line should fulfill a number of criteria including being (i) readily transfectable and (ii) free of adventitious agents. The 293 cell line meets all of these requirements since the cell line has been used for adenoviral vector production for clinical trials. The cell line chosen should also show no evidence of endogenous retrovirus production and should lack the potential to cause tumors. In contrast to other mammalian cells, few if any human cells have been shown to produce endogenous retroviruses. The 293 cell line is of human origin and apparently does not produce endogenous virus. Further, 293 cells are of embryonic origin and not tumor derived as are many cell lines. Indeed, although they carry fragments of the adenovirus genome and express both E1A and E1B, 293 cells are nontumorigenic in nude mice.[8]

The CMV-CYP2B1 expression construct that was used previously[3] was introduced by transfection into 293 cells, and around 90 cell clones were isolated. These clones were screened for their ability to convert cyclophosphamide into its toxic metabolites. This activity can be assessed by analyzing cell death/survival, since cells expressing CYP2B1 essentially commit suicide upon treatment with cyclophosphamide. As can be seen in TABLE 1, many of the cell clones were sensitive to the cell-killing effects of cyclophosphamide. This is specifically due to the expression of the CYP2B1 gene, since nontransfected, parental cells were only sensitive to relatively high doses (3.3 mM) of cyclophosphamide (TABLE 1). Thus expression of CYP2B1 confers the ability to metabolize cyclophosphamide into toxic metabolites upon these cells, resulting in a suicide effect. Four of the clones (1, 8, 31 and 48) are partially killed with relatively low doses (0.33 µM) of cyclophosphamide, indicating that they may express higher levels of CYP2B1. Clone 1, hereafter referred to as 22P1G, was chosen for further studies. Polymerase chain reaction (PCR) analysis of genomic DNA isolated from this cell clone confirmed the presence of the complete CMV-CYP2B1 expression construct as expected (data not shown).

Some of these clones were also screened using the resorufin assay. This assay measures the relative levels of CYP2B1 enzyme activity. The 22P1G clone that gave good activity in the "self-killing assay" (TABLE 1) gave the best CYP2B1 activity in the resorufin test (FIG. 1). Two other clones that showed a similar suicide activity after addition of cyclophosphamide (clones 48 and 31) also showed good activity in the resorufin test (FIG. 1). Thus, the biochemical assay correlates well with self-killing activity.

Ifosfamide, like cyclophosphamide, is also converted to toxic metabolites by CYP2B1. To investigate the effects of ifosfamide on the growth of the 22P1G cell

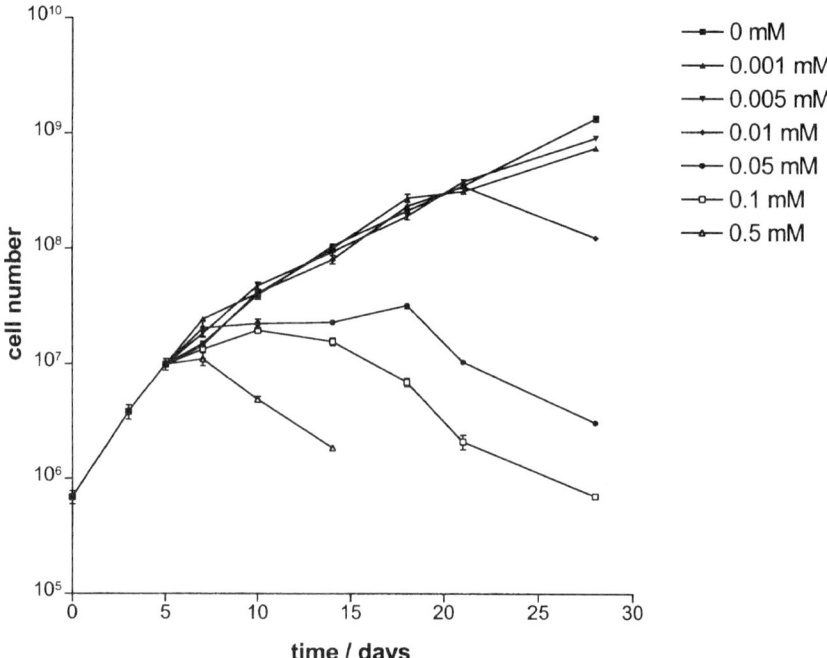

FIGURE 2. Concentration-dependent degree of cytotoxicity of ifosfamide for 22P1G cells.

clone, cells were grown either in the absence or in the presence of increasing concentrations of ifosfamide and the cell number determined over a 4-week period (FIG. 2). Very low concentrations of ifosfamide (0.001 and 0.005 mM) had no obvious effect on the growth of this cell clone, whereas 0.01 mM resulted in a weak cell-killing effect that was observable after 22 days. Higher concentrations of ifosfamide resulted in a clear killing of the cells, and the time of onset of cell death was concentration dependent (FIG. 2).

Determination of the Concentration of Mitomycin C Required for Cell Arrest

It is known that phosphoramide mustard, one of the toxic metabolites produced after conversion of ifosfamide by the CYP2B1 enzyme, alkylates DNA in a cell cycle-independent fashion. Nevertheless, DNA alkylation is not toxic for cells unless the cells undergo replication and division.[2] This suggests that if CYP2B1-expressing cells can be held in the quiescent state, they may be protected from the self-killing effect, thereby extending the window of toxic metabolite production and thus the therapeutic value. In addition, treatment of the cells with a cell-cycle inhibitory agent before encapsulation may enhance the safety profile of the cells since, should the cells escape from the capsules, they would be poorly able to divide, if at all.

In order to test whether cell cycle arrest protects the 22P1G cells from self-killing, they were treated with different concentrations of mitomycin C, an antibiotic that is known to arrest eukaryotic cells. As can be seen in FIG. 3, a concentration of 1 µg/ml caused growth arrest of the 22P1G cells over a 22-day period and was accompanied by a limited amount of cell death. A concentration of 0.5 µg/ml mitomycin C only resulted in a 10-fold reduction in the growth of the 22P1G cells. A concentration of 1 µg/ml was therefore used in subsequent experiments.

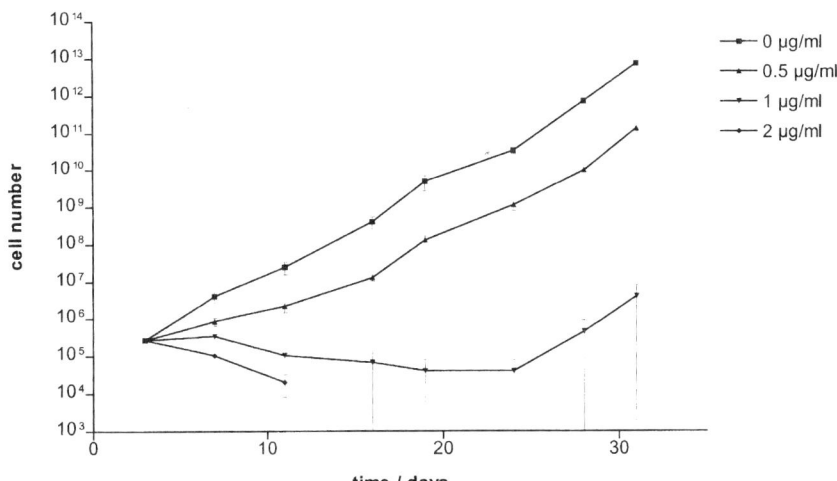

FIGURE 3. Determination of minimal growth inhibitory concentration of mitomycin C.

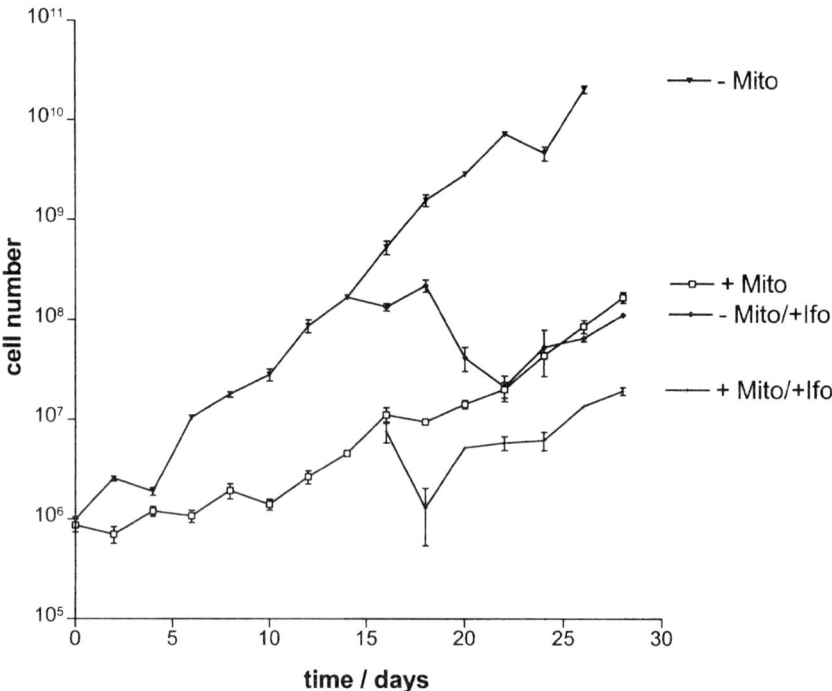

FIGURE 4. Cell growth after combined mitomycin C and ifosfamide treatment.

To determine whether mitomycin C-induced cell cycle arrest protected the cells from death due to conversion of ifosfamide to its toxic components, the 22P1G cells were treated with and without ifosfamide in combination with or without 1 µg/ml mitomycin C. Initially, one set of cells did not receive mitomycin C, whereas the other set did. The cells receiving mitomycin C grew slower than those not receiving mitomycin C (FIG. 4), but showed growth properties slightly different from those previously observed at this mitomycin C concentration (FIG. 3). This reflects a variation in the biological response to mitomycin C that we have repeatedly observed (data not shown). On day 14, some of the mitomycin C-treated and nontreated cells received 0.05 mM ifosfamide. Onset of cell death occurred two days later in the cells pretreated with mitomycin C and was only observed over a 2-day period. Thereafter, the cells recovered and remained stationary in terms of total cell number for 4 days (FIG. 4; day 20–24) before slowly beginning to proliferate. In contrast, the nonmitomycin C-treated cells showed a frank loss of cells over an 8-day period, with effects being observed immediately after ifosfamide treatment (FIG. 4; day 14). After day 22, there was a recovery in cell number that mirrored that seen in the mitomycin C-treated cells (FIG. 4).

Thus overall, the effect of ifosfamide on the nonmitomycin C-treated cells was evident immediately upon addition of the drug over an 8-day period, whereas in the mitomycin C-treated population there was a lag of 2 days before cell death was apparent, and the reduction in cell number was only seen over a 2-day period.

DISCUSSION

Although many gene therapy trials take an *ex vivo* approach, in which cells are removed from the patient, genetically modified and reintroduced into the patient, this is a very cumbersome and costly procedure. Undoubtedly, the ability to directly inject genetically modified cells or vectors into patients is much more appealing. Nevertheless, this kind of approach is fraught with problems, many of which relate to safety issues.

In our approach to solid tumor therapy, we have previously established and characterized a cytochrome P450 2B1-expressing cell line and introduced these cells into preformed tumors in a nude mouse model for human cancer of the pancreas. After we gave the clinically approved chemotherapeutic agent ifosfamide, the tumor size was reduced in all of the treated animals, with four animals showing a complete loss of discernable tumor tissue[3] (see also Löhr *et al.*, this volume). This contrasts with conventional gene therapy approaches in that it circumvents the need to use gene delivery vehicles to transfer the gene into target cells for each animal or patient and thus is safer. This is made possible by a novel encapsulation technique,[9] which protects the cells from the host immune system, but allows the toxic metabolites of ifosfamide, generated by the cytochrome P450 2B1 activity, to escape into the surrounding tumor, into which the encapsulated cells have been injected. The use of encapsulated cells also serves to physically restrain the genetically modified cells to the site where they are needed and thus also contributes to safety.

Such profound tumor responses in a preformed tumor model[3] suggests that a similar approach may be highly effective in a human trial. Even though this therapeutic strategy appeared to be safe in the model system used, a number of improvements had to be undertaken before it could be transferred to a human clinical setting. The CK cells used in the mouse model system are not suitable for use in human patients, since these cells produce endogenous retrovirus,[7] as do many other cell lines of mammalian origin. In contrast, cell lines derived from human organs do not appear to produce such endogenous retroviruses.[10] The human embryonic kidney 293 cell line was chosen as the basis for the production of a CYP2B1-expressing cell line. This cell line offers the additional advantage in that, although it carries and expresses the E1A and E1B regions of adenovirus, it is not tumorigenic in standard assays.

After transfection of a CMV promoter-driven CYP2B1-expression construct into a GMP-qualified 293 cell line, a number of clones were obtained and analyzed for biochemical (FIG. 1) and biological (FIG. 2) CYP2B1 activity. One candidate clonal cell line, 22P1G, was identified for further studies. The mechanism by which CYP2B1 mediates cytotoxicity involves the metabolic conversion of drugs such as cyclophosphamide or ifosfamide into phosphoramide mustard and acrolein. Since phosphoramide mustard alkylates DNA, resulting in DNA cross-linking, it is to be expected that the main cell-killing effect will be seen upon cell division when DNA replication is inhibited by these modifications. Thus it should be possible to protect CYP2B1-expressing cells from the main toxic effects of the system by arresting them in such a way as to ensure that they remain biochemically active (synthesizing CYP2B1) while being unable to replicate their DNA. This would allow such arrested cells to produce toxic metabolites that could diffuse to surrounding tumor cells without themselves being subjected to the toxic effects of these metabolites. Ultimately such an approach should increase the therapeutic value of the cell therapy approach described previously[3] by extending the life span of the CYP2B1-expressing cells.

Cells are commonly arrested either by treatment with γ-irradiation or mitomycin C. In our preliminary experiments, γ-irradiation was used to inhibit cell replication, but the dose required was variable (data not shown). Consequently, mitomycin C was used for further studies. Surprisingly, although it was possible to substantially inhibit cell division after treatment of the 22P1G cells with mitomycin C (FIG. 3) as well as to delay the onset of ifosfamide-mediated cell killing, indicated by loss of overall cell number, and to reduce the period of cell loss by 4-fold (FIG. 4), the overall ability of the cells to survive ifosfamide treatment was not as significantly prolonged as might have been expected (FIG. 4). This may indicate that DNA replication-independent cell killing is greater than expected, even at the relatively low (0.05 mM) ifosfamide concentrations used in our experiments. Undoubtedly, however, the lack of longterm inhibition of the growth of the 22P1G cells, at either 1 or 0.5 µg/ml mitomycin C (FIG. 3) and the variability in the results of the mitomycin C treatment that we have observed in multiple experiments (data not shown) makes it difficult to interpret these results. Further, these results underscore that mitomycin C treatment will not be easily and usefully applicable to enhance the safety and efficacy of the system.

A human clinical trial has commenced using encapsulated 22P1G cells and is now ongoing[11] (see also Löhr *et al.*, this volume). As a consequence of the results presented in this manuscript, we have elected not to treat the cells with mitomycin C, neither to increase the therapeutic window of CYP2B1 expression, nor as a safety

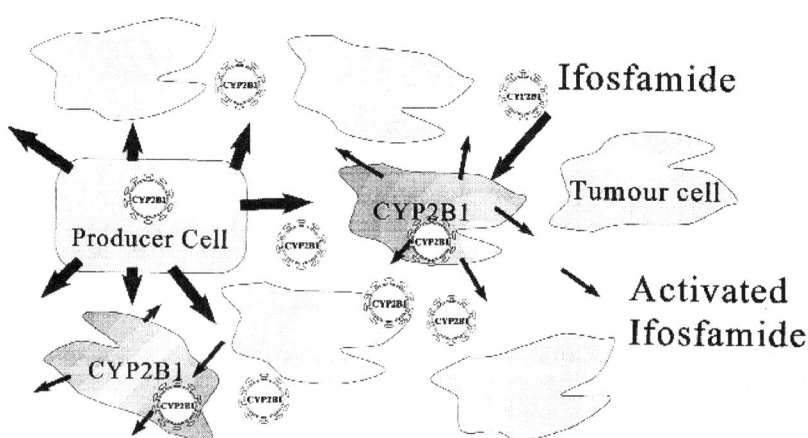

FIGURE 5. Implanted cells releasing tissue-specifically controlled CYP2B1-expressing virus infecting surrounding tumor cells.

precaution to prevent cell growth, should the cells escape from the capsules. In respect to safety, it is important to note that the cells undergo only limited cell division once encapsulated and that ifosfamide should kill any cells that may be released from the capsules. Indeed, the limited cell division after encapsulation that we have observed (data not shown) may allow us to attain the same extended therapeutic window aimed at in the mitomycin C experiments.

In the long term, it is planned to improve on the system by delivering encapsulated cells that produce a retroviral vector. It is envisaged that the retroviral vector should be of the promoter conversion type[12,13] and carry the CYP2B1 gene under the transcriptional control of pancreas-specific promoters.[14] Such a strategy should result in additional delivery of the CYP2B1 gene to the tumor cells, thereby amplifying the antitumor effect of ifosfamide as a result of its direct conversion both in the tumor cells as well as in the encapsulated cells (FIG. 5).

REFERENCES

1. GRAHAM-LORENCE, S. & J.A. PETERSON. 1996. P450s: structural similarities and functional differences. FASEB J. **10:** 206–214.
2. CHEN, L., D.J. WAXMAN, D. CHEN & D.W. KUFE. 1996. Sensitization of human breast cancer cells to cyclophosphamide and ifosfamide by transfer by a liver cytochrome P450 gene. Cancer Res. **56:** 1131–1140.
3. LÖHR, M., P. MÜLLER, P. KARLE, J. STRANGE, S. MITZNER, R. JESNOWSKI, H. NIZZE, B. NEBE, S. LIEBE, B. SALMONS & W.H. GÜNZBURG. 1998. Targeted chemotherapy by intratumor injection of encapsulated cells engineered to produce CYP2B1, an ifosfamide activating cytochrome P450. Gene Ther. **5:** 1070–1078.
4. GRAHAM, F.L., J. SMILEY, W.C. RUSSELL & R. NAIRN. 1977. Characteristics of a human cell line transformed by DNA from human adenovirus type 5. J. Gen. Virol. **36:** 59–72.
5. KARLE, P., P. MÜLLER, R. RENZ, R. JESNOWSKI, R.M. SALLER, K. VON ROMBS, H. NIZZE, S. LIEBE, W.H. GÜNZBURG, B. SALMONS & M. LÖHR. 1998. Intratumor injection of encapsulated cells producing an ifosfamide activating cytochrome P450 for targeted chemotherapy. Adv. Exp. Med. Biol. **451:** 97–106.
6. DONATO, M.T., M.J. GOMEZ-LECHON & J.V. CASTELL. 1993. A microassay for measuring cytochrome P450IA1 and P450IIB1 activities in intact human and rat hepatocytes cultured on 96-well plates. Anal. Biochem. **213:** 29–33.
7. BAUMANN, J.G., W.H. GÜNZBURG & B. SALMONS. 1998. CrFK feline kidney cells produce an RD114-like endogenous virus that can package murine leukemia virus-based vectors. J. Virol. **72:** 7685–7687.
8. MOORE, M., N. HORIKOSHI & T. SHENK. 1996. Oncogenic potential of the adenovirus E4orf6 protein. Proc. Natl. Acad. Sci. USA **93:** 11295–11301.
9. DAUTZENBERG, H., U. SCHULDT, G. GRASNICK, P. KARLE, P. MÜLLER, M. LÖHR, M. PELEGRIN, M. PIECHAZYK, K. VON ROMBS, W.H. GÜNZBURG, B. SALMONS & R.M. SALLER. 1999. Development of cellulose sulphate based polyelectrolyte complex microcapsules for medical applications. Ann. N.Y. Acad. Sci. **875:** 46–63.
10. LEIB-MÖSCH, C., R. BRACK-WERNER, T. WERNER, M. BACHMANN, O. FAFF, V. ERFLE & R. HEHLMANN. 1990. Endogenous retroviral elements in human DNA. Cancer Res. **50:** 5636s–5642s.
11. LÖHR, J.-M., Z.T. BAGO, H. BERGMEISTER, M. CEIJKA, M. FREUND, W. GELBMANN, W.H. GÜNZBURG, J. HAIN, K. HAUENSTEIN, W. HENNIGER, A. HOFFMEYER, P. KARLE, J.-C. KRÖGER, S. LIEBE, U. LOSERT, A. PROBST, M. RENNER, R. RENZ, R. SALLER, B. SALMONS, M. SCHUH, T. WAGNER & I. WALTER. 1999. Cell therapy using microencapsulated 293 cells transfected with a gene construct expressing CYP2B1, an ifosfamide converting enzyme, instilled intra-arterially in patients with advanced stage pancreatic carcinoma. J. Mol. Med. **77:** 393–398.

12. MROCHEN, S., D. KLEIN, B. SALMONS, S. NIKOL, J.R. SMITH & W.H. GÜNZBURG. 1997. Inducible expression of p21WAF-1/CIP-1/SDI-1 from a promoter-conversion retroviral vector. J. Mol. Med. **75:** 820–828.
13. SALLER, R.M., F. OZTURK, B. SALMONS & W.H. GÜNZBURG. 1998. Construction and characterization of a hybrid mouse mammary tumor virus/murine leukemia virus-based retroviral vector. J. Virol. **72:** 1699–1703.
14. GÜNZBURG, W.H., A. FLEUCHAUS, R.M. SALLER & B. SALMONS. 1996. Retroviral vector targeting for gene therapy. Cytokines Mol. Ther. **2:** 177–184.

Injection of Encapsulated Cells Producing an Ifosfamide-Activating Cytochrome P450 for Targeted Chemotherapy to Pancreatic Tumors

PETRA MÜLLER,[a,c] RALF JESNOWSKI,[a] PETER KARLE,[d] REGINA RENZ,[d] ROBERT SALLER,[c] HARTMUT STEIN,[a] KATRIN PÜSCHEL,[a,c] KERSTIN VON ROMBS,[c] HORST NIZZE,[b] STEFAN LIEBE,[a] THOMAS WAGNER,[e] WALTER H. GÜNZBURG,[d] BRIAN SALMONS,[c] AND MATTHIAS LÖHR[a,f]

[a]*Department of Medicine and* [b]*Department of Pathology, University of Rostock, Germany*
[c]*Bavarian Nordic Research Institute, Munich, Germany*
[d]*Institute of Virology, University of Veterinary Sciences, Vienna, Austria*
[e]*Department of Medicine, Medical School of Lübeck University, Germany*

> ABSTRACT: The prognosis of pancreatic cancer is poor, and current medical treatment is mostly ineffective. The aim of this study was to design a new treatment modality in an animal model system. We describe here a novel treatment strategy employing a mouse model system for pancreatic carcinoma. Embryonal kidney epithelial cells were genetically modified to express the cytochrome P450 subenzyme 2B1 under the control of a cytomegalovirus (CMV) immediate early promoter. This CYP2B1 gene converts ifosfamide to its active cytotoxic compounds, phosphoramide mustard, which alkylates DNA, and acrolein, which alkylates proteins. The cells were then encapsulated in a cellulose sulphate formulation and implanted into preestablished tumors derived from a human pancreatic tumor cell line. Intraperitoneal administration of low-dose ifosfamide to tumor bearing mice that received the encapsulated cells results in partial or even complete tumor ablation. Such an *in situ* chemotherapy strategy utilizing genetically modified cells in an immunoprotected environment may prove useful for solid tumor therapy in man.

INTRODUCTION

Although chemotherapy is used in the treatment of solid tumors, the efficacy of this approach is compromised by a number of factors. These include the accessibility of the tumor, the degree of drug sensitivity of the tumor and the local and systemic toxicity of the chemotherapeutic agent. Furthermore, tumor cells may become resistant to the toxic effects of chemotherapeutic agents. The treatment of pancreatic cancer is particularly problematic since these tumors are aggressive. Further, pancreatic adenocarcinomas have a poor prognosis and at the time of diagnosis, the tumor is

---

[f]Address for correspondence, reprints and requests: Priv.-Doz. Dr. med. Matthias Löhr, M.D., Division of Gastroenterology, Department of Medicine, University of Rostock, E. Heydemannstr. 6, D-18057 Rostock, Germany. Phone, +49 (381) 494-7497/-7349; fax, +49 (381) 494-7482; e-mail, loehr@med.uni-rostock.de

generally in an advanced stage no longer suitable for resection.[1,2] Even though recent advances have been made, for example, using agents such as 5-fluorouracil, cisplatin and gemcitabine,[3] the systemic toxicity of these agents at the concentrations required had resulted in only limited success. Local delivery of chemotherapeutic agents would circumvent these problems, but this kind of approach can also be problematic.

The compounds cyclophosphamide and ifosfamide are used for chemotherapy of a number of tumors.[4,5] These prodrugs are activated in the liver by cytochrome P450 to cytotoxic metabolites, i.e., phosphoramide mustard, which alkylates DNA, and acrolein, a protein alkylating agent.[6] The active metabolites are released into the circulation and are distributed throughout the body, resulting in toxic effects. The ability to relocate the activation step to the vicinity of the tumor should alleviate the undesirable systemic toxicity while at the same time increasing the therapeutic index of the prodrug. In order to achieve this targeting of the antitumor effect, cells genetically modified to express the liver-specific cytochrome P450 2B1 gene have been encapsulated in cellulose sulphate. The encapsulated cells have been implanted in preformed tumors derived from a human pancreatic cell line.[7,8] The cellulose sulphate capsules confine the genetically modified cells to the vicinity of the tumor and are expected to protect these cells from the host immune system.

METHODS

Cloning

The cDNA of CYP2B1[9] was cut out from the plasmid pSW1 using XhoI/XbaI and ligated into the XhoI/XbaI cut nonviral eucaryotic expression vector pcDNA3 (Invitrogen). The final construct pc3/2B1 carries the CYP2B1 cDNA under the control of the cytomegalovirus (CMV) immediate early promoter[10] (FIG. 1). The yielded DNA was proved by digest as well as sequencing.

Cell Culture

Human 293 cells used in this study were bought at ATCC (Rockville, MD). They were grown in Dulbecco's modified Eagle's medium with glutamax (DMEM (glutamax), Gibco/BRL), supplemented with 10% fetal calf serum (FCS). Every 3–4 days the cells were trypsinized and the medium was changed.

Lipofection

For transfection prepared lipofectamine (Gibco/BRL) was used. Before the day of transfection, 3×10^6 kidney cells were seeded into 100-mm dishes. On the day of transfection, 4 µg pc3/2B1 were prepared according to the instructions of the producer and added to the cell layer. After 6 hr, 1 ml DMEM (glutamax) with 10% FCS was added. The next day the cells were trypsinized, diluted and put in selection. After a fortnight the resistant clones were isolated and further investigated.

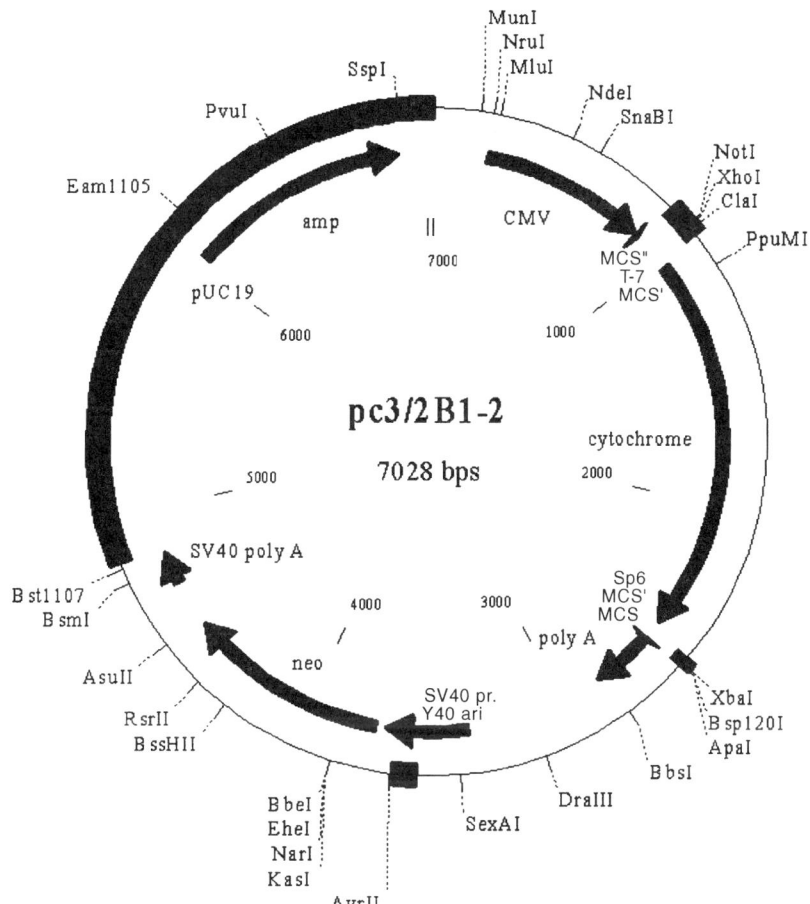

FIGURE 1. Cloning of the CYP2B1 expression vector. The cDNA for CYP2B1 was cut out from the vector pSW1 and cloned into the eucaryotic expression vector pcDNA3. The gene is now driven by the constitutivly active cytomegalo virus promoter (CMV).

Resorufin Assay and Ifosfamide Measurements

The expression of biologically active CYP2B1 in the transfectants was determined using a modified biochemical assay, which is specific for the cytochrome P450 isoforms 1A1 and 2B1.[11] The day before measurement different amounts of cells (5×10^4, 2×10^5, and 2×10^6) were seeded into a 3-cm dish. The next day the cells were washed with phosphate-buffered saline (PBS) and overlayed with 500 µl serum-free medium containing 15 µM 7-pentoxyresorufin (Sigma) and 10 µM dicumarol (Sigma). After 30 min incubation at 37°C, 375 µl of the supernatant was mixed with 125 µl 0.1 mM sodium acetate, pH 4.5 containing 75 Fishman units of β-glucuronidase/600 Roy units of arylsulfatase (Boehringer). The solution was incubated for 3 hr at 37°C, and the reaction stopped by adding 1 ml pure methanol (Sigma). Precipitated proteins were pelleted at 3000 rpm, and the amount of produced resorufin was measured with a fluorometer at 530 nm excitation and 590 nm emission.[10]

Ifosfamide was measured by flame ionization as described before.[12,13] In brief, ifosfamide was extracted into dichloromethane using the oxazaphorinone derivative trofosfamide as the internal standard. The organic layer was evaporated, and the residue was redissolved in ethyl acetate, an aliquot of which was injected onto a fused silica capillary column under isothermal conditions using N_2 as the carrier gas. Blood was drawn at the times indicated. For the comparison of tissue and serum levels, blood was drawn at 30 min, and the tumor was removed from the animal at the same time and put immediately into liquid nitrogen.

Transwell Assay

To test and quantify the bystander effect, a transwell system was used (Falcon). One (1) $\times 10^5$ pancreatic carcinoma cells PaCa-44 (ATCC)[14] were seeded into a filter insert (Falcon) of a 3-cm dish (6-well). Into the lower compartment of the dish 1×10^5 wild-type or CYP2B1-expressing 293 cells were seeded. The next day ifosfamide was added resulting in concentrations from 0 up to 2 mM. After one week the transwell filters were removed, and the remaining carcinoma cells and the CYP2B1-expressing or wild-type cells were counted.

Encapsulation

Capsules were produced as previously described.[10,15,16] Briefly, 1×10^7 cells, transfected with CYP2B1, were suspended in 1 ml PBS (pH 7) containing 2–5% cellulose sulphate and 5% FCS (Gibco/BRL). The suspension was allowed to drop freely into a precipitation bath containing 3% polydiallyldimethyl ammonium in PBS. The capsules were washed twice with normal medium (DMEM) and then either cultivated in cell culture dishes or, if empty, stored in PBS at 4°C. To assess possible toxicity of the capsule material, empty capsules were injected orthotopically into the mouse pancreas, as described,[17,18] both in nude and immunocompetent Balb/c mice (Charles River, Germany).

Cell Lines, Animals and Experimental Protocol

The human pancreatic adenocarcinoma-derived cell line PaCa-44 (ATCC), was used to establish tumors in nude mice.[7,8] PaCa-44 cells were grown in DMEM medium containing 10% FCS and supplemented with penicillin and streptomycin (Gibco/BRL). Proliferating cells were used to establish tumors in the nude mouse by injecting 1×10^6 cells subcutaneously in the flanks of nude mice (CD-1 nu/nu; Charles River, Germany). The resultant tumors were allowed to grow for 7–10 days until they reached a size of 1 cm^3. The mice were divided into a number of groups on the basis of the treatment that they received (FIG. 5): (1) controls with no treatment and no injection; controls with injection of transfected cells (2) with and (3) without encapsulation but without ifosfamide treatment, and three treatment groups encompassing (4) no injection of cells, (5) injection of naked cells and (6) injection of encapsulated cells. One (1) $\times 10^6$ cells were suspended in 100 µl DMEM, filled into a 1-ml standard syringe. The capsules were delivered through a 21G needle directly into the tumor. In a second series, the capsules were implanted 1 cm distant to the preestablished tumors by subcutaneous injection. Approximately 40 capsules were delivered per injection. Animals were treated intraperitoneally every third day for 2 weeks with 100 mg/kg body weight ifosfamide (Holoxan®, Asta Medica, Germany). At the same time, sodium 2-mercaptoethanesulphonate (MESNA/Uromitexan®, Asta Medica) was administered intravenously at the same dosage via the tail vein. Tumor tissue was harvested from anesthetized animals after three weeks. The therapeutic effect was defined as a complete response (CR), i.e., total disappearance of the tumor or a partial response (PR), indicating that more than 50% of the initial tumor mass had been eliminated.[19]

RESULTS

Characterization of Cytochrome P450 2B1 Expression in 293 Cells

Human 293 cells carrying an expression vector, in which the CYP2B1 cDNA is placed under the transcriptional control of the CMV immediate early promoter (FIG. 1), were analyzed for expression of functional CYP2B1. The specific 7-pentoxy-resorufin dealkylating activity of CYP2B1 yields the fluorescent product resorufin, which can be detected by excitation at 530 nm and emission at 590 nm.

293 cells containing the gene for CYP2B1 produced measurable amounts of flouroscenic resorufin. The resorufin-dependent flourescence correlated also with the amount of cells seeded in the assay. This demonstrates that at least the majority, if not all cells, containing the stable integrated vector pc3/2B1 express the CYP2B1 gene (FIG. 2).

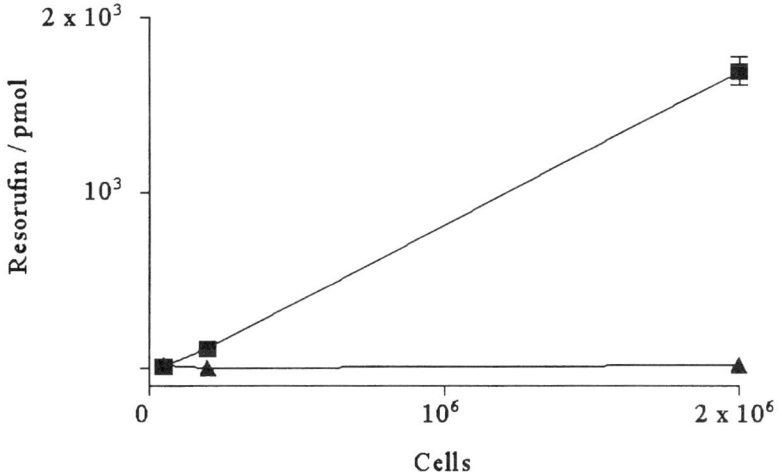

FIGURE 2. Correlation of resorufin activity with cell count. ■ indicates CYP2B1-transfected cells; ▲ indicates controls.

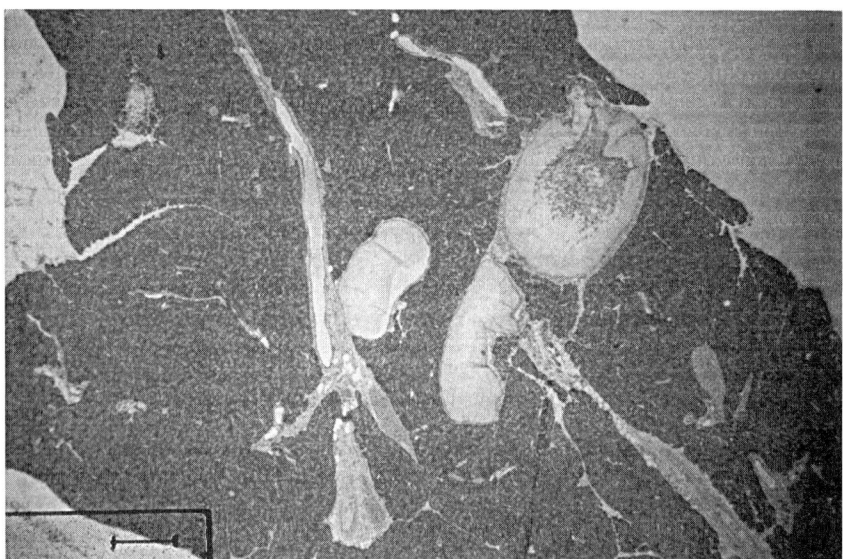

FIGURE 3. Empty cellulose sulphate capsules injected orthotopically into the nude mouse pancreas. Note the sparse inflammatory reaction surrounding the capsule. Bar equals 100 μm (×25).

Filter Assay

The activated drug phosphoramide mustard has a small molecular mass and can pass through membranes. This causes a bystander effect that is not dependent on a direct cell cell contact.[20] To show whether the released drug can also affect cocultivated 293 cells that do not express CYP2B1, a transwell system was used. In this system the cells share the same media, but are seperated by a membrane with 0.45-μm pores.

In the presence of ifosfamide the pancreatic carcinoma cells on top of the filter insert of the transwell system showed growth inhibition when cocultured with CYP2B1-expressing cells, but not when sharing the media with 293 wild-type cells. At a concentration of 0.5 mM ifosfamide the cell number was reduced by more than 50% after one week. The presence of ifosfamide alone without activating cells caused no cell growth inhibition. Thus, ifosfamide can be activated by CYP2B1, be released from the activating cell and freely diffuse in the surrounding media.

Tolerance of Empty Capsules

In order to determine the toxic potential of the capsules per se, empty capsules were injected orthotopically into the pancreas of nude and immunocompetent mice. A slight foreign-body reaction with macrophages and a few granulocytes could be detected in both animal models; however, no excessive scaring or proliferation of connective tissue was detected (FIG. 3). No signs of pancreatitis could be observed.

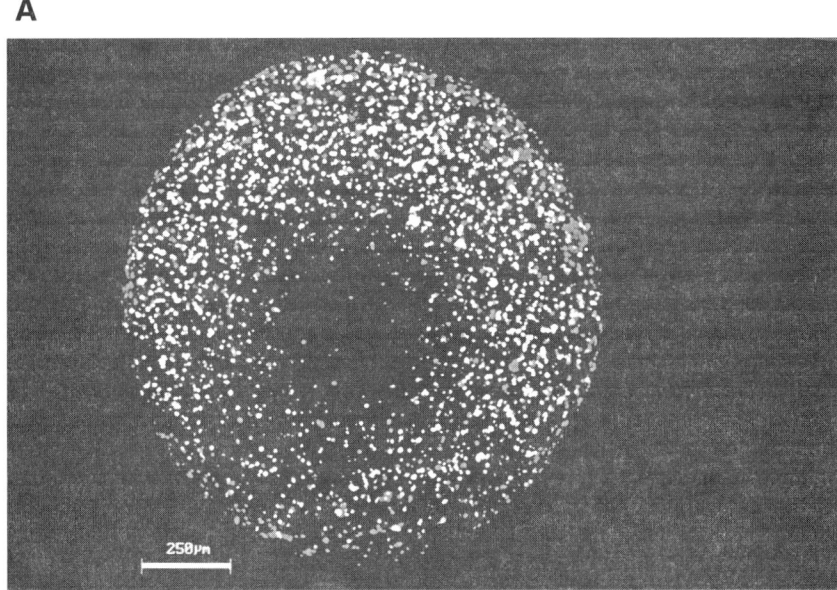

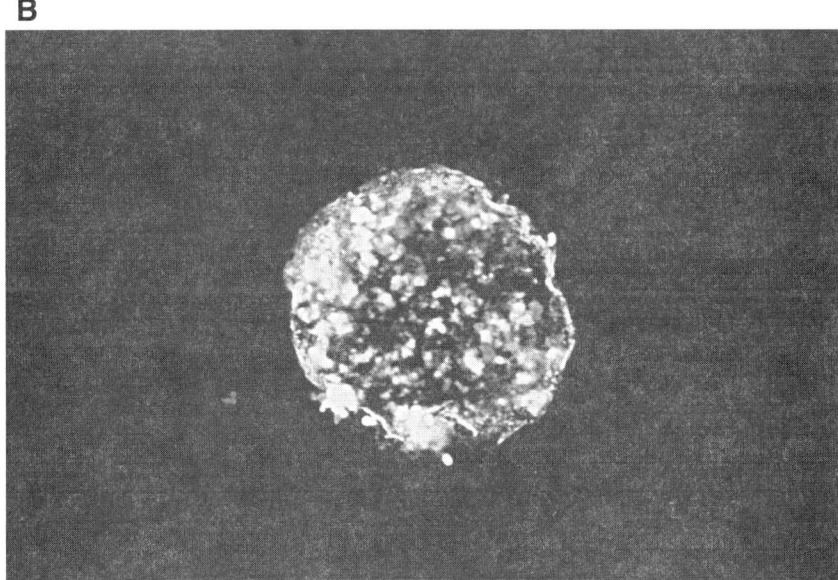

FIGURE 4. Confocal laser microscopy of encapsulated cells in a 'Life&Dead' assay. Yellow/green signal indicates living cells. (**A**) Capsules cultured for 4 weeks after encapsulation. Bar equals 100 µm. (**B**) Capsules prepared from xenotransplanted tumors after three weeks of *in vivo* treatment with ifosfamide.

Encapsulation of CYP2B1-Expressing Cells

Cells were encapsulated as described. Typically, $1-2 \times 10^5$ cells are contained by one capsule of 500 μm diameter. Enzyme activity was determined with the resorufin assay to be in the range of 0.2 pmol/L/capsule, which would be equivalent to 1×10^5 capsules since 1×10^6 cells present an enzyme activity of 2 pmol/L. After 4 weeks of continuous cultivation, viability was measured by Life&Dead assay and laser confocal microscopy. At that time, about two thirds of the cells appeared to be viable (FIG. 4).

In order to determine the therapeutic potential of CYP450-expressing cells implanted in the vicinity of a preformed pancreatic tumor, in combination with ifosfamide administration, the cells were first encapsulated in cellulose sulphate[15] to ensure that they would be confined to the tumor. The cellulose sulphate capsules carrying the CYP2B1-expressing cells had a diameter of around 400 μm, so that they could easily be injected through a 21G needle (inner diameter 0.6 mm) without damage.

Evalulation in a Pancreatic Tumor Model System

The encapsulated cells were injected into a preformed tumor grown in nude mice and derived from the human pancreatic-derived PaCa-44 cells, an established animal model for pancreatic cancer.[7,8] When injected subcutaneously into nude mice, the human pancreatic cancer derived cell line PaCa 44 forms tumors. Such preformed tumors were allowed to reach a size of about 1 cm³. Some of the tumors were then injected with either 1×10^6 CYP2B1-expressing cells or about 40 capsules carrying CYP2B1 cells. The mice were then given ifosfamide systemically. Tumor growth

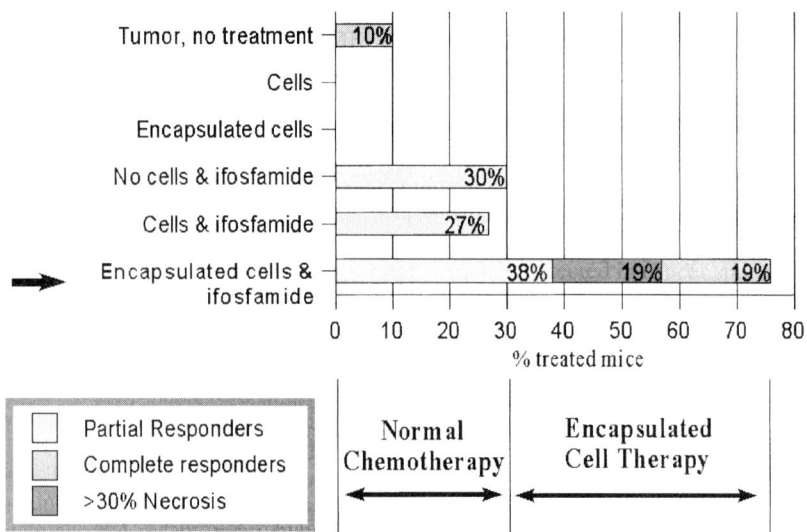

FIGURE 5. Effect of ifosfamide treatment in pancreatic tumors implanted with CYP2B1-producing, encapsulated cells and controls.

A

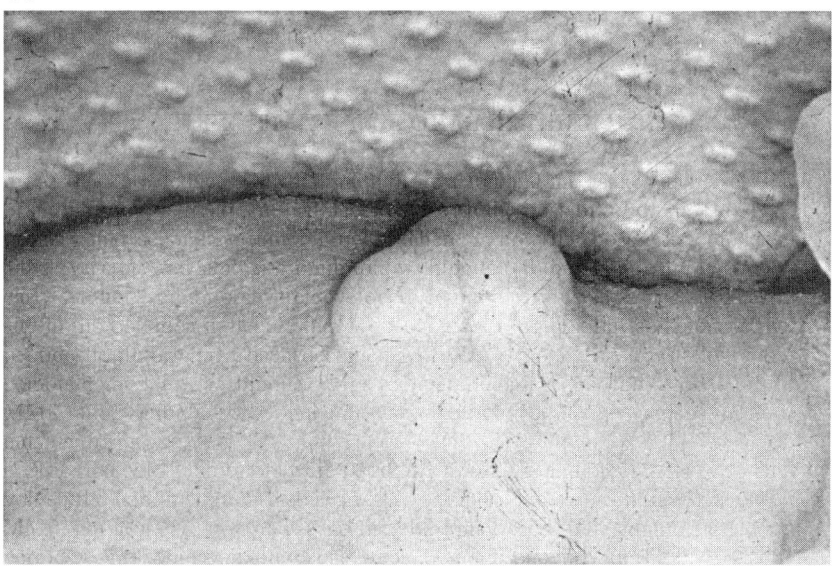

B

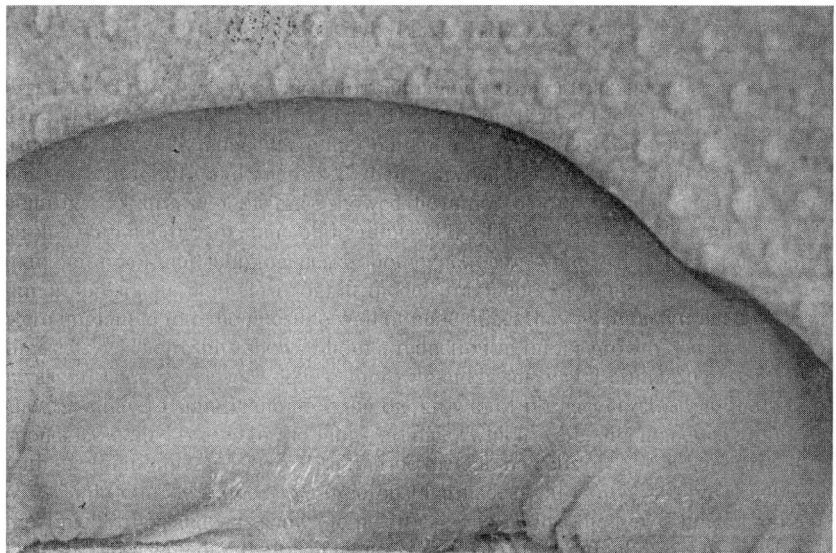

FIGURE 6. Gross appearance of a pancreatic tumor xenotransplanted to nude mice without treatment (**A,C**) and at the same time after 3 weeks of ifosfamide treatment and injection of CYP2B1-expressing, encapsulated cells (**B,D**). Direct injection of capsules (A,B) and subcutaneous implantation of capsules 1 cm apart from the tumor (C,D).

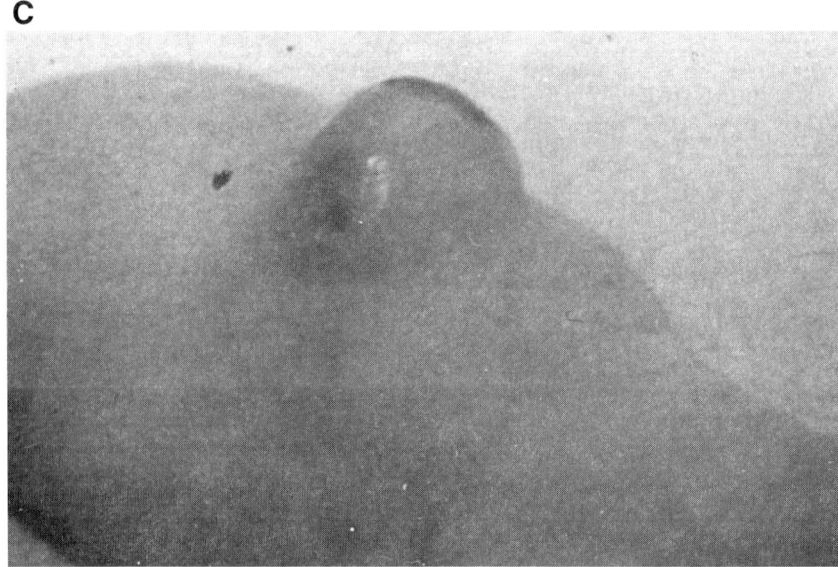

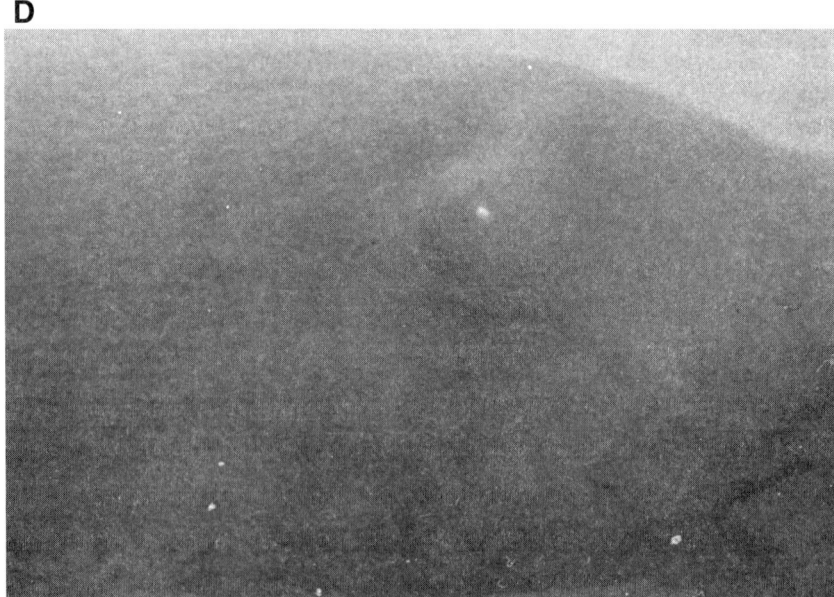

FIGURE 6. Continued.

was slightly reduced in mice that did not recieve the CYP2B1 cells (either encapsulated or not), presumably due to conversion of the ifosfamide in the livers of these mice to the toxic metabolites. However, tumor reduction was most evident in mice that received encapsulated CYP2B1-expressing cells by injection into the tumor and

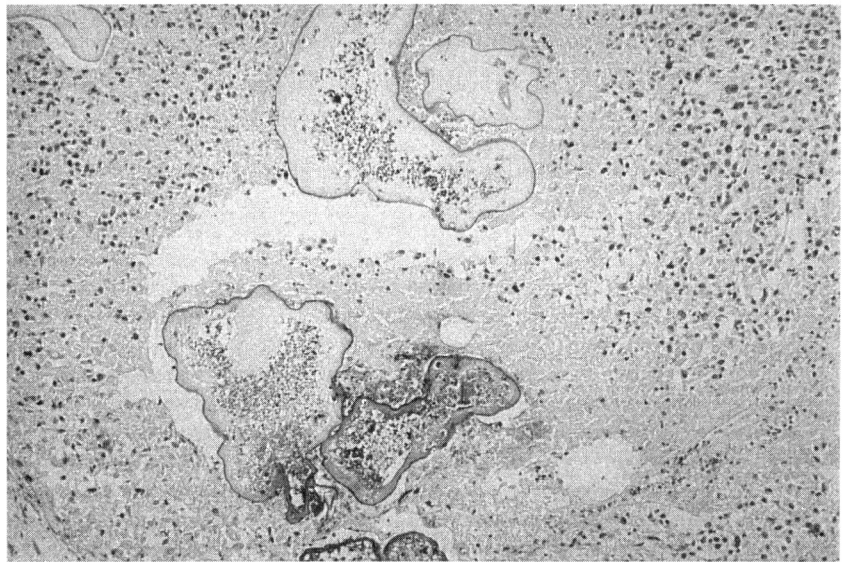

FIGURE 7. CYP2B1-expressing cells in capsules three weeks after injection into preestablished human pancreatic tumors. Note the living capsules in the intact cells and tumor cells surrounding. Magnification ×40.

subsequent treatment with ifosfamide, with 4 of the mice showing complete tumor regression (FIG. 5). Even though the ifosfamide dosage was identical in all the treated mice, animals treated with encapsulated cells also appeared healthier compared to those injected directly with CYP2B1 cells, which at best showed only a partial response (FIG. 6). A similar significant tumor reduction could also be observed if the encapsulated CYP2B1-expressing cells were implanted 1 cm apart from the preestablished tumor (FIG. 6). Upon histology, capsules appeared to be intact with viable cells surrounding the remaining tumor cells (FIG. 7). In capsules prepared from tumors removed after three weeks of treatment, a substantial number of cells remained viable after intermediate culture (FIG. 4B) and showed resorufin activity in the range of 0.16 pmol/capsule (data not shown). The serum levels of ifosfamide following a single injection of one dose (100 mg/kg BW) was comparable to results obtained earlier in the nude mose system (FIG. 8). Tissue levels reached about 50% of serum levels 30 min after injection (FIG. 8).

DISCUSSION

Ifosfamide is an approved chemotherapeutic agent that has been widely used in oncology for the treatment of solid tumors, including pancreatic cancer,[21,22] for many years. Nevertheless, the necessary local concentrations of the toxic metabolites of ifosfamide, i.e., phosphoramide mustard and acrolein, are only achieved at the expense of high systemic concentrations, since the liver is the normal site of con-

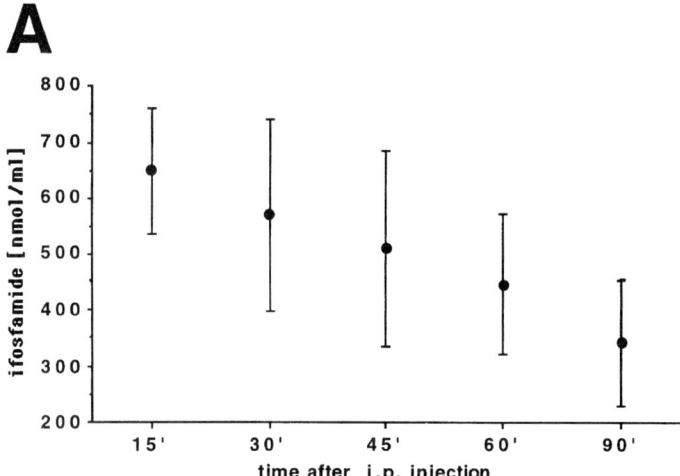

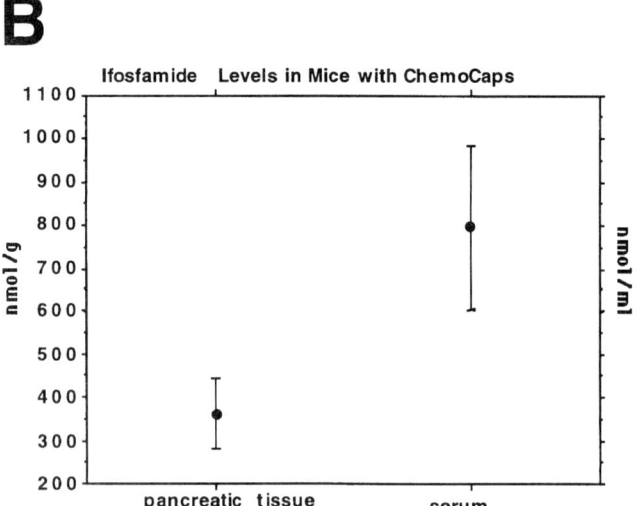

FIGURE 8. Ifosfamide levels in mice bearing pancreatic tumors injected with CYP2B1-expressing encapsulated cells. **(A)** Serum kinetics after a single intraperitoneal dose of ifosfamide (100 mg/kg BW). **(B)** Serum and tissue levels. Mean ± 1 SD.

version. High systemic concentrations lead to severe effects on nontarget organs.[12] The local delivery of either ifosfamide or the active metabolites may circumvent this problem. However, ifosfamide is only poorly activated if at all outside of the liver, and direct delivery of the activated metabolites after *in vitro* production is hampered by the short half-life (~45 min) of these compounds.[23]

In the approach described here, cells that have been genetically modified to produce CYP2B1, an enzyme that converts ifosfamide to cytotoxic metabolites, have been enclosed in capsules implanted in the vicinity of the tumor. The cells are thus physically targeted to, and confined around, the tumor. Previously we have shown that encapsulated cells injected directly into the tumor are able to activate ifosfamide, thus killing the cells.[10] More importantly, we demonstrate a bystander effect, not only in cell culture but also in mice, since in this study the encapsulated cytochrome P450-expressing cells were injected in subcutaneously, 1 cm away from the tumor, yet there was still a measurable therapeutic effect after ifosfamide administration.

The implantation of encapsulated cells as described here should allow higher local concentrations of the active metabolite to be maintained without systemic toxicity. Further, such an approach should be useful, since such encapsulated cells are protected from the host immune response.

This novel approach to targeting of chemotherapy was tested in human pancreatic tumors that had been preformed in nude mice. Treatment of mice receiving the encapsulated cells with ifosfamide resulted in a complete tumor disappearance in about 20% of the animals and a significant reduction in the tumor burden in the remaining 80%.[10] Treatment of these mice was much more successful than control mice receiving either nonencapsulated CYP2B1-expressing cells or mice that did not receive cells at all.

As demonstrated by the injection of capsules with 293 cells in the unaffected pancreas of both nude and immunocompetent mice, no tissue reaction or pancreatitis could be observed seven days after injection. In the case of the pancreas, this is an important issue, since the organ is very sensitive to manipulation and ischemia. Injection of adenovirus for gene therapy into the pancreatic duct, for instance, caused pancreatitis. Thus, the local application of such capsules seems feasible.

This novel strategy for the treatment of solid tumors combines gene/cell therapy with chemotherapy. However, since a well characterized CYP2B1-expressing cell clone is encapsulated and delivered to the tumor, no direct gene therapeutic intervention is necessary in the patient. This simplifies the treatment and enhances the safety of the system as compared to other gene therapy approaches for cancer. A prerequisite for the use of the same cell line in different patients is that the cells are not eliminated by immune responses. In a number of experiments we have not detected any obvious immune response in immunocompetent mice to encapsulated cells, in the pancreas (not shown) and in the mammary gland. Our previous study reported the use of feline kidney cells as the cell line for expression of CYP2B1. Although these cells expressed good levels of cytochrome P450, resulting in a therapeutic antitumor effect upon application of ifosfamide, such cells may not be suitable for eventual clinical use. These cells produce endogenous retroviruses, which may be released from the capsules and result in the establishment of a productive infection. The 293 cell line does not appear to produce endogenous retroviruses.[24] A further advantage to the use of cell lines of human origin may be more applicable for human clinical trials, because they are complement resistant.[25]

In summary, we have demonstrated the feasibility of a gene therapy approach to a model system of human pancreatic carcinoma. The marked response including a substantial number of complete remissions led to a phase I clinical protocol.[26]

ACKNOWLEDGMENTS

We thank Jim Halpert for the cytochrome P450 cDNA, Jörg Pohl (Asta Medica) for helpful discussions about ifosfamide, and Nora Sartori for her help in setting up the chemotherapy protocol. We would like to express our sincere thanks to Gisela Sparmann for her input and support. This work was supported by a Vaestfond grant from the Danish government to Bavarian Nordic Research Institute and EC Grant BIO4-CT-0100.

REFERENCES

1. ROSEWICZ, S. & B. WIEDENMANN. 1997. Pancreatic carcinoma. Lancet **349:** 485–489.
2. KALTHOFF, H., M. LÖHR, C. ROEDER & W. SCHMIEGEL. 1995. Das Pankreaskarzinom: Zellbiologie, Matrixproteine und Wachstumsregulation. *In* Erkrankungen des exkretorischen Pankreas. 2nd edit. G. Adler, U.R. Fölsch, J. Mössner & M.V. Singer, Eds.: 385–404. Fischer. Jena.
3. CARMICHAEL, J., U. FINK, R.C.G. RUSSELL *et al.* 1996. Phase II study of gemcitabine in patients with advanced pancreatic cancer. Br. J. Cancer **73:** 101–105.
4. KEIZER, H.J., J. OUWERKERK, K. WELVAART, C.J.H. VAN DER VELDE & F.J. CLETON. 1995. Ifosfamide treatment as a 10-day continuous intravenous infusion. J. Cancer Res. Clin. Oncol. **121:** 297–302.
5. AHLGREN, J.D. 1996. Chemotherapy for pancreatic carcinoma. Cancer **78:** 654–663.
6. DIRVEN, H.A.A.M., B. VAN OMMEN & P.J. VAN BLAEDEREN. 1996. Glutathione conjugation of alkylating cytostatic drugs with a nitrogen mustard group and the role of glutathione S-transferases. Chem. Res. Toxicol. **9:** 351–360.
7. LÖHR, M., B. TRAUTMANN, M. GÖTTLER *et al.* 1994. Human ductal adenocarcinomas of the pancreas express extracellular matrix proteins. Br. J. Cancer **69:** 144–151.
8. LÖHR, M., B. TRAUTMANN, S. PETERS *et al.* 1996. Expression and function of integrins in human pancreatic adenocarcinoma. Pancreas **12:** 248–259.
9. KEDZIE, K.M., C.A. BALFOUR, G.Y. ESCOBAR *et al.* 1991. Molecular basis for a functionally unique cytochrome P450IIB1 variant. J. Biol. Chem. **266:** 22515–22521.
10. LÖHR, M., P. MÜLLER, P. KARLE *et al.* 1998. Targeted chemotherapy by encapsulating cells engineered to deliver CYP2B1, an ifosfamide activating cytochrome P450 gene. Gene Ther. **5:** 1070–1078.
11. DONATO, M.T., M.J. GOMEZ-LECHON & J.V. CASTELL. 1993. A microassay for measuring cytochrome P450IA1 and P450IIB1 activities in intact human rat hepatocytes cultured on 96-well plates. Anal. Biochem. **213:** 29–33.
12. KUROWSKI, V. & T. WAGNER. 1993. Comparative pharmacokinetics of ifosfamide, 4-hydroxyifosfamide, chloracetaldehyde, and 2- and 3-dechloroethylifosfamide in patients on fractionated intravenous ifosfamide therapy. Cancer Chemother. Pharmacol. **33:** 36–42.
13. KUROWSKI, V. & T. WAGNER. 1997. Urinary excretion of ifosfamide, 4-hydroxyifosfamide, 3- and 2-dechloroethylifosfamide, mesna, and dimesna in patients on fractionated intravenous ifosfamide and concomitant mesna therapy. Cancer Chemother. Pharmacol. **39:** 431–439.
14. OLSEN, D., T. NAGAYOSHI, M. FAZIO *et al.* 1989. Human laminin: cloning and sequence analysis of cDNAs encoding A, B1 and B2 chains, and expression of the corresponding genes in human skin and cultured cells. Lab. Invest. **60:** 772–782.
15. STANGE, J., S. MITZNER, H. DAUTZENBERG *et al.* 1993. Prolonged biochemical and morphological stability of encapsulated liver cells—a new method. Biomat. Art. Cells Immob. Biotech. **21:** 343–352.
16. SALLER, R.M., J. STANGE, S. MITZNER, U. HEINZMANN, B. SALMONS & W.H. GÜNZBURG. 1997. Encapsulated cells producing retroviral vectors for *in vivo* gene therapy. Submitted.

17. REYES, G., A. VILLANUEVA, C. GARCIÁ et al. 1996. Orthotopic xenografts of human pancreatic carcinomas acquire genetic aberrations during dissemination in nude mice. Cancer Res. **56:** 5713–5719.
18. LÖHR, M. 1996. Zell- und Molekularbiologie der Bindegewebsreaktion bei Pankreatitis und Pankreaskarzinom. Solvay. Hannover.
19. WHO. 1979. WHO Handbook for Reporting Results of Cancer Treatment. World Health Organization (WHO). Geneva.
20. CHEN, L. & D.J. WAXMAN. 1995. Intratumoral activation and enhanced chemotherapeutic effect of oxazaphosphorines following cytochrome P-450 gene transfer: development of a combined chemotherapy/cancer gene therapy strategy. Cancer Res. **55:** 581–589.
21. CERNY, T., G. MARTINELLI, A. GOLDHIRSCH et al. 1991. Continuous 5-day infusion of ifosfamide with mesna in inoperable pancreatic cancer patients: a phase II study. J. Cancer Res. Clin. Oncol. **117**(Suppl. IV): S135–S138.
22. EINHORN, L.H. & P.J. LOEHRER. 1986. Ifosfamide chemotherapy for pancreatic carcinoma. Cancer Chemother. Pharmacol. **18**(Suppl. 2): 51–54.
23. ZHENG, J.J., K.K. CHAN & F. MUGGIA. 1994. Preclinical pharmacokinetics and stability of isophosphoramide mustard. Cancer Chemother. Pharmacol. **33:** 391–398.
24. PEAR, W.S., G.P. NOLAN, M.L. SCOTT & D. BALTIMORE. 1993. Production of high-titer helper-free retroviruses by transient transfection. Proc. Natl. Acad. Sci. USA **90:** 8392–8396.
25. TAKEUCHI, Y., C.D. PORTER, K.M. STRAHAN et al. 1996. Sensitization of cells and retroviruses to human serum by (alpha 1-3) galactosyltransferase. Nature **379:** 85–88.
26. LÖHR, M., Z.T. BAGO, H. BERGMEISTER et al. 1999. Cell therapy using microencapsulated 293 cells transfected a gene construct expressing CYP2B1, an ifosfamide converting enzyme, instilled intra-arterially in patients with advanced-stage pancreatic carcinoma. A phase I study. J. Mol. Med. **77:** 393–398.

Ablation of Tumor Cells *In Vivo* by Direct Injection of HSV-Thymidine Kinase Retroviral Vector and Ganciclovir Therapy

BRADLEY D. HOWARD,[a,c] HOLGER KALTHOFF,[a] AND TIMOTHY C. FONG[b,d]

[a]*Molecular Oncology Research Laboratory, Clinic for General Surgery, Christian Albrechts University, 24105 Kiel, Federal Republic of Germany*
[b]*Chiron Corporation, Emeryville, California 94608, USA*

ABSTRACT: The introduction of therapeutic genes into proliferating tumor cells *in vivo* by direct intralesional injection of retroviral vectors can provide an effective and valuable approach for the treatment of a variety of solid tumor types. Efficient transduction of tumor cells *in situ* by direct injection was demonstrated using a retroviral vector containing the β-galactosidase (β-gal) gene. Ablation therapy *in vivo* was demonstrated using a retroviral vector containing the *Herpes* simplex virus thymidine kinase gene (HSV-TK) to deliver the TK gene into the murine colorectal tumor cell line CT26. Ablation of CT26 tumor cells *in situ* was achieved by directly injecting high-titer HSV-TK retroviral vector preparations into the site of tumor cell inoculation followed by intraperitoneal (i.p.) delivery of ganciclovir (GCV). This gene therapy strategy demonstrated a markedly lower rate of tumor progression, with several complete regressions, compared to animals in control groups. We also demonstrated that resistance to subsequent challenges with unmodified CT26 cells and an enhanced cellular immune response is associated with tumor regression in immunocompetent animals. Our results demonstrate the feasibility of direct *in situ* administration of HSV-TK retroviral vectors for the treatment of cancer and suggest that a cellular immune response may be elicited by this therapy.

INTRODUCTION

A strategy in the gene therapy of cancer is to deliver a conditionally lethal gene to tumor cells whose gene product converts an inactive prodrug into a toxic molecule. There are several conditionally lethal or chemosensitivity genes with their corresponding prodrugs currently under investigation,[1,2] but most interest has centered upon the *Herpes* simplex thymidine kinase gene (HSV-TK). Its corresponding prodrug is ganciclovir (GCV), a nucleoside analog specifically phosphorylated by HSV-TK into an intermediate that upon further di- and tri-phosphorylation by other cellular kinases inhibits DNA synthesis.[3] An important feature of this approach is the "bystander effect," in which diffusion of phosphorylated GCV intermediates

---

[c]Corresponding author: Dr. Bradley D. Howard, Molecular Oncology Research Laboratory, Clinic for General Surgery, Christian Albrechts University, Arnold Heller Street 7, 24105 Kiel, Federal Republic of Germany. Phone, +49 431-597-1937; fax, +49 431-597-1939; e-mail, bdhoward@email.uni-kiel.de

[d]Address for correspondence: Chiron Corp., 4560 Horton Street, Emeryville, CA 94608.

through gap junctions, or uptake of apoptotic vesicles can kill nontransduced cells adjacent to the HSV-TK-transduced cell.[4–8] A possible added benefit of this approach is the transduction of proliferating endothelial cells that compose the tumor vasculature.[9] Occlusion of these vessels would result in the destruction of large portions of the tumor.

Gene transfer therapy with chemosensitivity genes and their requisite prodrug counterparts has been used for the treatment of experimental glioblastoma, meningeal carcinomatosis, bronchial mesothelioma and ovarian cancer.[7,9–19] In these studies, the principal methods of achieving HSV-TK gene transfer *in vivo* were to: i) inject a producer cell line that generated retroviral vector at the tumor site; ii) inject tumor cells expressing the HSV-TK gene by *ex vivo* transduction; or iii) inject adenoviral vector encoding HSV-TK. Injection of murine producer cell lines or the reintroduction of *ex vivo* gene-modified tumor cells back into humans raises significant safety, manufacturing, and logistical concerns.[20–22] These include health risks like adventitious agents produced by the nonhuman producer cells and undesired inflammatory responses after implantation of xenogeneic cells.

Injection of high-titer, replication-defective, recombinant retroviruses containing therapeutic genes provides a safer, more streamlined alternative to these delivery systems. An obstacle to efficient retroviral gene delivery has been the relatively low titer generated by the available producer cell lines, which result in poor transduction efficiencies *in vivo*. We have developed a producer cell line that generates high-titer retroviral vector supernatants, which delivers greater quantities of recombinant retroviruses directly to a lesion.

Animals receiving intralesional injections of high-titer HSV-TK retroviral vector and systemic GCV therapy showed extensive tumor regression. We found that this type of therapy enhanced specific antitumor immunity in these mice when compared to tumor-bearing animals. Our results show that the administration of recombinant retroviral vectors to tumor-bearing animals can result in significant tumor regression.

METHODS

Animals and Cell Lines

Eight-week-old female BALB/c and athymic *nu/nu* mice were used in these experiments and treated according to appropriate animal guidelines. CT26 (a BALB/c colorectal carcinoma cell line) was a gift of Dr. Michael Brattain, Baylor University Medical School, Houston, TX. The DA retroviral vector packaging cell line has been described.[25,26] Reagents ganciclovir sodium (GCV) was purchased from Syntex Laboratories, Inc. (Palo Alto, CA). Geneticin (G418) was obtained from Gibco/BRL (Bethesda, MD). Polybrene (hexadimethrine bromide, HDMB) and the reagents for β-galactosidase (β-gal) staining (potassium ferricyanide, potassium ferrocyanide and magnesium chloride) from Sigma Chemical Co (St. Louis, MO); and 5-bromo-4-chloro-3-indolyl-β-D-galactopyranoside (X-gal) from Gold Biotechnology (St. Louis, MO). The $Na_2^{51}CrO_4$ was obtained from Amersham, Inc. (Arlington Heights, IL).

Retroviral Vector Construct

The gene coding for thymidine kinase (ATP:thymidine 5′ phosphotransferase, EC 2.7.1.21) of *Herpes* simplex virus type 1 was generously provided by Dr. Lynn R. Enquist in the plasmid p322TK.[27,28] The coding region was isolated using polymerase chain reaction (PCR) primers to generate a 5′ Xho I site and a 3′ Cla I site. This modified gene fragment was subcloned into the Xho I and Cla I sites of an N2-based[29] vector backbone derived from the moloney murine leukemia virus (MoMLV) to generate the proviral vector plasmid, pBH-1. The ATG methionine initiator codon for MoMLV *gag* expression in pBH-1 has been mutated to ATT to inhibit *gag* expression.[30] The MoMLV long terminal repeat (LTR) controls the expression of the HSV-TK gene and an internal SV40 promoter drives the expression of the neomycin resistance marker. pBH-1 was cotransfected with an expression vector for vesicular stomatitis virus-G (VSV-G) protein[31] into an amphotropic canine packaging cell line, DA, and the VSV-G-pseudotyped vector generated was harvested 24 hr later and used to transduce fresh DA cells, and subsequently selected in G418 (800 ug/ml). Individual clones were isolated by dilution cloning and tested for $G418^R$ titer. The highest titer producer clone, DA/BH-1 #9A was selected and characterized. To make HSV-TK retroviral vector preparations, supernatants from confluent cultures containing the replication-defective HSV-TK retroviral vector were collected, filtered (pore size 0.45 mm) and stored at $-80°C$. The vector titers were determined by serial dilution and colony-forming unit (CFU) assay.[26] The DA/β-gal producer cell line has been described.[26] For some experiments, a control vector identical to the HSV-TK retroviral vector but containing the human γ-interferon (γ–IFN) cDNA[31] in place of HSV-TK cDNA, was used.

In Vitro Transduction of CT26 Cells with TK and β-gal Retroviral Vectors

CT26 cells were transduced by adding supernatants from the DA/BH-1 or DA/β-gal producer lines to 6-cm dishes containing 10^5 CT26 cells and Polybrene (4 µg/ml). The multiplicity of infection (MOI) was approximately one. Twenty-four hours later, the cells were placed under G418 selection (400 µg/ml) for 2 weeks. To maintain high-level expression of the HSV-TK or β-gal genes, the transduced cells were continually grown in G418. The transduced cell lines are referred to as CT26 TK and CT26 β-gal.

Determination of In Vivo Transduction Efficiency

Transduction efficiency of retroviral vector *in situ* was determined by injecting 200 µL of β-gal retroviral vector (1.0×10^6 CFU/ml) at the site of tumor cell inoculation. 10^5 CT26 cells were inoculated s.c. in the lower abdomen of 6-week-old female BALB/c mice, and the injection sites were marked. Two days later, these sites were injected with 0.2 ml β-gal or human γ–IFN retroviral vector with or without 4 µg/ml Polybrene every 2 days for a total of 4 injections. The MOI was estimated to be about 5 over the course of injections. Two days after the final injection, tumors were removed, disassociated, passed through a Falcon 2350 cell strainer (Becton-Dickinson, Franklin, NJ) and seeded into 10-cm dishes containing DMEM plus 10% FBS. The explanted cultures were allowed to grow *in vitro* for 7 days and harvested from the plates using trypsin/EDTA, fixed in 2% formaldehyde and then stained for β-galactosidase activity as described.[33] Eight hours later, the cells were rinsed free of the X-gal reagent, and the number of blue cells in each sample was determined using a hemacytometer.

In Vivo Therapy Experiments

To estimate the minimum level of *in vivo* transduction needed for antitumor efficacy, mice were inoculated with *ex vivo* mixtures of unmodified and TK-transduced tumor cells. After palpable tumors formed, the standard GCV treatment was given until control mice bearing 100% unmodified CT26 cells were sacrificed. Ratios of CT26:CT26/TK mixtures were 4:1, 1:1, and 1:4. The positive and negative control groups received 100% CT26/TK and 100% CT26 cells. Tumor growth was measured in three dimensions using a Vernier Caliper (Roboz Instruments, Rockville, MD). Tumor volume was estimated from the algorithm $l \times w \times h$.

Antitumor efficacy studies were performed by inoculating groups of 6-week-old female BALB/c mice with 10^5 CT26 cells s.c. on the abdomen. Control groups were inoculated with CT26/TK cells. One day after tumor cell inoculation, 4 daily injections of 0.4 ml TK or β-gal retroviral vector (10^6 CFU/ml) formulated with 4 μg/ml Polybrene were given s.c. at the tumor site. One day after the last retroviral vector injection, selected groups were treated with 2 daily injections of GCV at 62.5 mg/kg for 8 days. After that, one daily injection of GCV at 62.5 mg/kg was given for 17 days or until the control groups were sacrificed. Tumor size was measured as described.

To determine whether HSV-TK retroviral vector ablation therapy can induce an antitumor cellular immune response, T cell deficient *nu/nu* or normal mice were inoculated with 2×10^5 CT26 or CT26/TK cells, and palpable tumors were allowed to form. GCV treatment was started 7 days after inoculation and animals were monitored for tumor growth. Tumor-free, cured mice were defined as those in which no palpable tumors were observed 4 weeks after the last GCV injection. Cured mice were then challenged s.c. at a contralateral site with 2×10^5 unmodified CT26 cells to assess for protective immunity.

In Vitro Cytotoxicity Assay

The ^{51}chromium release cytotoxicity assays for murine splenic effector cells were performed as described.[25] At various intervals after complete tumor ablation with GCV, splenocytes were harvested from groups of 4 mice, pooled and incubated at a concentration of 3×10^6/ml with irradiated (100 Gy) unmodified CT26 cells (6×10^4/ml) in 25-cm^2 flasks (Corning, Corning, NY). Effector cells were harvested 5 days later and tested at several effector:target ratios in 96-well microtiter plates in a standard 4-hour assay employing Na$_2$^{51}CrO$_4$-labeled CT26 or CT26/TK target cells (10^4 cells/well in a final volume of 200 μl). Following incubation, assay culture supernatants were harvested and assayed for specific ^{51}chromium release (cpm) using a Beckman gamma spectrometer. Spontaneous release was determined as cpm from targets plus medium and was 10–20% of the maximum release. The maximum release was determined from 1M HCL-treated labeled target cells. The percent target cell lysis was calculated as: (experimental release −spontaneous release)/(maximum release −spontaneous release) × 100.

RESULTS

In Vitro and In Vivo GCV Sensitivity of TK-Transduced Tumor Cells

We have previously shown that CT26 TK cells were highly sensitive to GCV as compared to untransduced CT26 and dosing studies in mice demonstrated that CT26 TK cells were effectively eliminated with a regimen of 62.5 mg/kg GCV either once or twice daily (data not shown).

Direct In Situ Injection of Retroviral Vector Results in Significant In Vivo Transduction

The long-term goal of cancer gene therapy is to deliver a therapeutic gene to tumor cells *in situ*. To test the feasibility of this approach using retroviral vectors, BALB/c mice were first inoculated with parental CT26 tumor cells, and the site of injection was marked. Two days after tumor cell inoculation, mice were given a series of injections with either PBS with Polybrene (4 µg/ml), β-gal retroviral vector with or without Polybrene, or a human γ–IFN retroviral vector with or without Polybrene as a vector control. Each mouse received 4 injections over 8 days with a vector dose that was normalized to 2×10^5 CFU/injection. Two days after the final retroviral vector injections, tumor nodules from each of the groups of mice were removed, dissociated, and plated onto two 10-cm^2 plates in DMEM plus 10% FBS. Tumor explants were allowed to grow *in vitro* for one week. The cells were harvested, and β-galactosidase activity was determined by X-gal staining. CT26 tumors that received β-gal retroviral vector were transduced *in vivo* (TABLE 1). Injection of β-gal Retroviral vector resulted in 13% of recovered tumor cells staining positively for β-galactosidase activity. Transduction *in situ* increased to 20% with the addition of 4 µg/ml Polybrene into the retroviral preparation. The X-gal staining was specific for cells transduced with β-gal retroviral vector, since none of the explanted tumor cells injected with either PBS or the human γ–IFN retroviral vector stained blue. These results demonstrate that tumor cells may be efficiently transduced *in vivo* by a course of several direct injections of retroviral vector and that approximately 15–20% transduction efficiency can be achieved.

True levels of transduction *in vivo* may be higher, because there appears to be a gradual loss of β-gal expression *in situ* by CT26/β-gal cells over time. Approximately 70% of the G418-resistant CT26/β-gal cells stain for β-galactosidase activity *in vitro*; these same CT26/β-gal cells recovered after 12 days *in vivo* are only 32% positive. One possible explanation for the loss of β-gal expression may be the induction of an immune response against β-gal-transduced cells *in vivo*. An intracellular mechanism may also be the cause in the loss of β-gal activity. Over time, β-gal activity decreases *in vitro* even though the CT26 β-gal-expressing tumor cells were continually grown in the presence of G418. We have also observed that longer-term cultures of CT26 β-gal-expressing tumor cell lines have reduced levels of blue staining com-

TABLE 1. Determination of *in vivo* transduction efficiency after direct injection of β-gal retroviral vector

Cell Type	Injectate	Percent Positive Cells
CT26/β-gal		31.6
CT26	PBS + Polybrene	0
	γ-IFN Retroviral vector	0
	γ-IFN Retroviral vector + Polybrene	0
	β-gal Retroviral vector	13.3
	β-gal Retroviral vector + Polybrene	20.0

NOTE: Two (2) $\times 10^5$ CT26 cells were inoculated s.c. on day 1 and followed with 4 injections of the indicated retroviral vector preparation on day 2, 4, 6, and 8. Each retroviral vector injection delivered 2×10^5 colony-forming units (CFUs) in 200 µl into the site of tumor cell inoculation. Polybrene was added to a final concentration of 4 µg/ml where indicated. Tumor nodules were excised and mechanically dissociated on day 10 and stained for β-gal activity after 7 days of culture *in vitro*. A minimum of 200 cells were counted for each sample.

pared to newly transduced cell cultures. The mechanism of this loss of β-galactosidase activity is not known.

Effective Tumor Ablation Is Accomplished with 20% TK-Transduced Cells

To estimate the minimum percentage of TK-transduced cells in a tumor mass that effects complete ablation of the total tumor using GCV, several different ratios of CT26/TK cells were mixed with parental CT26 cells and inoculated as previously described. GCV treatment was initiated 7–10 days later when tumors were palpable. As few as 20% CT26/TK cells caused an overall 90% reduction in tumor size at the conclusion of the experiment (FIG. 1). A 50% mix of CT26/TK and parental CT26

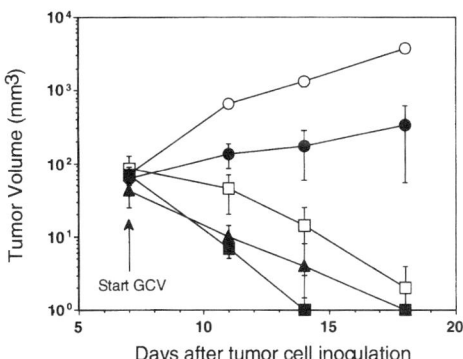

FIGURE 1. Tumor regression in mice inoculated with mixtures of CT26 and CT26/TK cells and GCV treatment. CT26/TK cells were mixed with parental CT26 cells at various ratios and inoculated s.c. into mice as previously described (*n* = 7/group); 100% CT26/TK (▲), 80% CT26/TK (■), 50% CT26/TK (□), 20% CT26/TK (●), or 100% CT26 cells (○). GCV treatment was initiated on day 7 when tumors were palpable. Tumors were measured in three dimensions and the volume is shown in $\log_{10}$ scale. Error bars represent SEM.

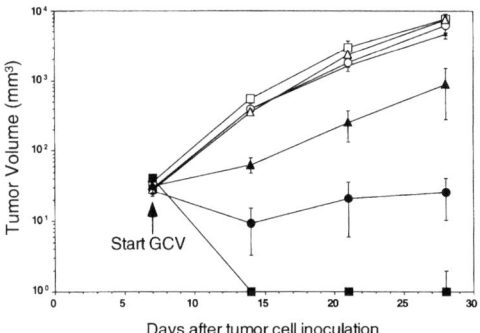

FIGURE 2. Ablation of tumor cells following direct *in vivo* injection of HSV-TK retroviral vector and GCV treatment. Mice were inoculated s.c. with 2×10^5 CT26 cells and followed with 4 injections of HSV-TK or β-gal retroviral vector one day later. A total of 4 $\times 10^5$ CFU/injection was administered. A regimen of GCV was started one day after the last retroviral vector injection in the indicated groups. The treatment groups are: untreated CT26 (✗), untreated CT26/TK (□), CT26/TK + GCV (■), CT26 injected with HSV-TK retroviral vector with GCV (●) or without GCV (○), CT26 injected with β-gal retroviral vector with GCV (▲) or without GCV (△). Tumors were measured in three dimensions, and the volume is shown in $\log_{10}$ scale. Error bars represent SEM. In mice injected with CT26 and treated with the HSV-TK vector/GCV combination, a 200-fold reduction in tumor volume was observed ($p < 0.0001$).

cells resulted in more than 1000-fold decrease in tumor volume, similar to that seen with 100% CT26/TK cells. These results show that transduction of approximately one fifth of the cells in a tumor nodule can effectively ablate the entire tumor and that the bystander effect is an important aspect of this approach to cancer therapy.

Antitumor Efficacy of Injected HSV-TK Retroviral Vector and GCV Treatment

To determine whether the direct injection of HSV-TK retroviral vector can efficiently deliver the HSV-TK gene to a sufficient number of CT26 cells *in vivo* for an antitumor effect, mice were inoculated s.c. with CT26 cells, and HSV-TK retroviral vector was injected at the tumor injection site 1 day later for 4 consecutive days. Palpable tumors were observed at the site of inoculation after day 5. One day after the last injection of HSV-TK retroviral vector, mice were given GCV twice daily for 8 days and then once daily at the same dose until the control groups had to be sacrificed on day 28 of the experiment. Tumor growth was measured for 4 weeks. Injection of HSV-TK retroviral vector without subsequent GCV treatment or injection of β-gal retroviral vector did not affect tumor growth, and large tumors formed at the inoculation site (FIG. 2). In contrast, mice inoculated with CT26 and treated with the HSV-TK retroviral vector/GCV combination, a 200-fold reduction in tumor volume was observed. Four of the mice in this group had complete responses (i.e., no palpable tumor after 2 months), and the other five mice had small tumors (<144 mm³). In control animals inoculated with CT26/TK, tumors were completely ablated after the ninth day of GCV treatment. These results demonstrate that direct injection of HSV-

TABLE 2. Systemic protection from CT26 tumor cell challenge following HSV-TK retroviral vector and GCV therapy

Mice	Tumor-Bearing Mice/Group
Naive	7/7
Cured	0/7

NOTE: Mice in which complete tumor ablation was observed following HSV-TK retroviral vector and GCV therapy, were challenged with a s.c. injection of 2×10^5 unmodified CT26 cells. Mice were considered cured of their tumor following therapy after 4 weeks in which no measurable tumor nodules were detected. Tumor cell challenges were observed and recorded in cured mice beginning 10 days after injection and followed for a minimum of 60 days. Naive mice were followed for a minimum of 21 days or until sacrificed.

TK retroviral vector can transduce sufficient CT26 tumor cells *in situ* to induce significant tumor ablation after GCV treatment.

Complete Tumor Regression Requires an Intact Cellular Immune System

Several possible mechanisms may explain the ablation of a tumor mass that is less than 100% TK positive. One possibility is that the diffusion of phosphorylated GCV intermediates through gap junctions between adjacent transduced and nontransduced cells effectively kills the nontransduced cells. This bystander effect has also been observed by several other investigators.[4–8] Another mechanism involves the generation of an antitumor cellular immune response. To evaluate the role the cellular response may have in the overall tumor ablation, mice were inoculated with CT26/TK cells and rendered tumor free by GCV treatment. These mice were then challenged with unmodified CT26 4 weeks after their initial tumor ablation. No sec-

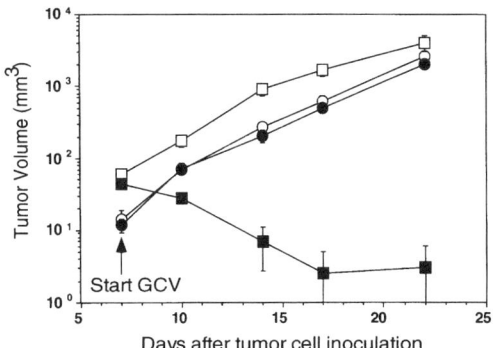

FIGURE 3. Tumor regression in nude mice inoculated with CT26 or CT26/TK cells. Nude mice were inoculated with 2×10^5 CT26 or CT26/TK cells, and palpable tumor nodules were allowed to form as previously described (n = 5/group). GCV treatment (62.5 mg/kg) was started 7 days after tumor implantation. The treatment groups are: CT26 without GCV (○), CT26 with GCV (●), CT26/TK without GCV (□), and CT26/TK with GCV (■). Tumors were measured in three dimensions, and the volume is shown in $\log_{10}$ scale. Error bars represent SEM.

ondary tumor was palpable two months post challenge on any animal whose initial CT26/TK tumor was completely ablated with GCV (TABLE 2). In contrast, naive mice injected with CT26 cells had palpable tumors after 1 week.

To further test the role the cellular immune response has in tumor regression, an experiment inoculating TK-transduced or unmodified tumor cells followed with GCV was performed in athymic *nu/nu* mice. Nude mice were inoculated with CT26 or CT26/TK cells, and a GCV regimen was started 7 days later when tumors were palpable. A control group inoculated with CT26/TK cells did not receive GCV. Tumor regression (greater than 1000-fold) was evident only in mice inoculated with CT26/TK cells and treated with GCV (FIG. 3). In this group, 3 of 5 mice had no visible tumor after 14 days of GCV treatment. One of the mice had a very small mass. No tumor ablation was seen in mice inoculated with CT26 and treated with GCV or inoculated with CT26/TK without GCV. In contrast to the results seen in immunocompetent mice, all the nude mice in the CT26/TK + GCV group showed progressively growing tumors 25 days following cessation of GCV. These results suggest that transduction with the TK gene followed by GCV treatment destroys most of the tumor cells by direct toxicity of phosphorylated GCV intermediates. However, the killing is not complete as evidenced by the reappearance of the primary tumor after stopping GCV treatment in nude mice. These data also suggest that a specific antitumor cellular response can be initiated in immunocompetent animals.

Direct Injection of HSV-TK Retroviral Vector Followed with GCV Induces a Cytotoxic Cellular Immune Response

Transduction of tumor cells with the TK gene followed with GCV treatment kills cells *in vitro*. We have shown that tumors may be ablated *in vivo* after direct injections of HSV-TK retroviral vector followed with GCV. The immune response may also help in the complete eradication of tumor cells as a secondary effect of direct TK + GCV cytotoxicity. To determine whether tumor ablation by HSV-TK retroviral vector/GCV treatment enhances antitumor CTLs, mice were inoculated with CT26/TK cells and given a course of GCV. After complete tumor ablation, the splenocytes from these mice were harvested and restimulated *in vitro* with unmodified CT26 cells for 7 days. The resulting effector cells were analyzed for their ability to lyse unmodified CT26 or CT26/TK cells in a ^{51}chromium release assay. Strong cytolytic responses against both CT26 and CT26/TK cells were observed in splenocytes obtained from mice whose CT26/TK tumors were ablated by GCV (FIG. 4). Splenocytes from CT26 or CT26/TK tumor-bearing mice exhibited marginal lytic activity. Along with the earlier results in nude mice, a likely mechanism of complete tumor ablation in TK gene therapy + GCV may be the result of direct cytotoxicity of phosphorylated GCV intermediates and the induction of a tumor-specific cytotoxic cellular immune response.

DISCUSSION

Therapeutic transfer of "suicide" genes into tumor cells using retroviral delivery systems may become an attractive strategy against various cancers. Early efforts employing intracranial implantation of murine retroviral vector-producing cell lines in

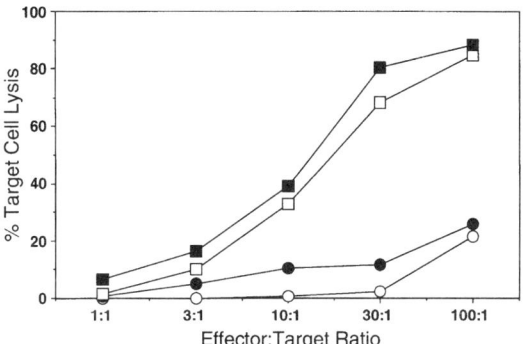

FIGURE 4. Enhanced cellular lytic activity against unmodified tumor cells in mice with complete tumor ablation. BALB/c were inoculated with 2×10^5 CT26 or CT26/TK cells, and palpable tumor nodules were allowed to form as previously described ($n = 5$/group). GCV treatment (62.5 mg/kg) was started 7 days after tumor implantation. Splenocytes were isolated, pooled and restimulated with irradiated CT26 cells for 5 days *in vitro* prior to assaying for cellular lytic activity against CT26 and CT26/TK cells in a standard ^{51}chromium release assay. Effectors from mice injected with CT26/TK and rendered tumor free by GCV treatment demonstrated higher levels of lytic activity (■, CT26 targets; □, CT26/TK targets) compared to splenocytes from mice bearing CT26 tumors (○, CT26 targets; ●, CT26/TK targets).

experimental rat glioma models has made TK gene therapy for cancer feasible in humans.[7,9–15] However, the implantation of murine vector-producing cells into humans raises concerns regarding safety and practical clinical utility. Regardless of these issues, others have initiated human clinical trials with this approach because of the limitation of low retroviral vector titers currently available.[20] In the present study, we investigated the feasibility of administering high-titer retroviral preparations directly to the tumor site. The availability of high-titer preparations of retroviral vectors may obviate the need for producer cell line implants. The recombinant retroviruses used in this study contain the HSV-TK gene as the chemosensitizing gene, are replication defective, and are free of detectable helper virus by both S + L- and cocultivation assays as previously described.[26] We have demonstrated effective *in vivo* gene delivery by direct injection of high-titered retroviral preparations resulting in complete tumor ablation in over 50% of immunocompetent animals in the CT26 model.

Tumor cells transduced with HSV-TK retroviral vector became highly sensitive to GCV. Biological activity was verified *in vivo*; BALB/c mice inoculated with CT26/TK cells and treated with GCV were rendered tumor free. Issues concerning whether sufficient numbers of tumor cells could be transduced *in vivo* were first answered by *ex vivo* mixing of CT26/TK and parental CT26 cells prior to inoculation. When mice were injected with 50% CT26/TK cells, tumor regression was similar to that seen in mice who had received 100% CT26/TK cells. Interestingly, a 90% reduction in tumor growth was seen when only 20% of the cells contain the HSV-TK gene. In fact, when mice were injected with as few as 10% CT26/TK cells and treated with GCV, a significant reduction in tumor size was evident (data not shown), suggesting that efficient tumor ablation is probably mediated by a combination of direct killing and the "bystander" effect. Once GCV is initially phosphorylated by TK, other cellular enzymes convert the monophosphate intermediate into di- and triphosphate forms, which can diffuse across gap junctions to amplify the cytotoxic effect of TK + GCV therapy to cells that neighbor the TK-transduced tumor cell.

Prior to transferring the HSV-TK gene to the site of tumor implantation, a β-gal retroviral vector was used to optimize *in vivo* transduction conditions. As much as 20% of the tumor mass could be transduced by direct administration of the β-gal retroviral vector using Polybrene (TABLE 1). The level of transduction was reduced to 13% when Polybrene was omitted from the retroviral preparation. This enhancement of transduction by Polybrene was also observed *in vitro*. It is possible that the actual level of transduction *in vivo* is higher than observed due to the unexplained decrease in *in vivo* and *in vitro* expression of β-galactosidase activity in transduced CT26 cells. In G418-selected nonclonal populations of cells transduced *in vitro* with the β-gal retroviral vector, 70% of all cells express the lacZ gene but expression gradually decreases to 30% over time. When tumors composed of 100% β-gal-expressing CT26 cells are removed from mice and stained with X-gal, less than half of the cells are positive for β-galactosidase activity (unpublished data). This finding may suggest that the β-gal protein is highly immunogenic in BALB/c mice and may induce an antitumor effect. This is supported by the general observation that β-gal-expressing CT26 tumors grow slower and were smaller than wild-type CT26 tumors in mice. The lack of β-gal expression also might be due to the relative insensitivity of X-gal staining; thus a more sensitive staining technique such as fluorescein-β1-D-(galactopyranoside) (FDG) and FACS analysis might be helpful.[36]

The level of *in vivo* transduction by direct injection was estimated by using β-galactosidase as a marker gene. In our *in vivo* studies, the β-gal and HSV-TK retroviral vectors were essentially identical, having similar titer and were injected with Polybrene. If a similar level of transduction was obtained with the HSV-TK retroviral vector as seen with the β-gal retroviral vector, then a 20% transduction level of tumor cells from direct injection can result in the inhibition of tumor growth as seen in the *ex vivo* mixing experiments. These data demonstrate that elimination of tumors *in vivo* is not dependent on every tumor cell being transduced by the retroviral vector, which may be explained by the "bystander effect." It is also possible that direct injection of HSV-TK retroviral vector transduced proliferating endothelial cells that line tumor vasculature, so that when these cells are exposed to GCV, ischemia may contribute to the overall tumor regression as well.[9]

The report describes tumor eradication *in vivo* by direct intralesional administration of high-titer amphotropic retroviral vector particles suitable for clinical applications. Vile *et al.* reported effective antitumor effects against B16F10 lung metastases using repeated intravenous injections of a murine ecotropic HSV-TK retroviral vector and GCV 2 days after inoculation.[24] The B16F10 tumor model used in those studies was designed to seed single cells in blood vessels of the lungs, and presumably single tumor cells were transduced *in vivo* by the vector. In the CT26 model described here, the tumors are nascent tumors of $1.0-2.0 \times 10^5$ cells. In our model, there is probably a greater reliance on a "bystander effect" than as noted by Vile *et al.*, and is not directly reliant on the immune system, as indicated by the transduction efficiency experiments with the β-gal retroviral vector and regressions achieved in nude mice. Although neither of these models truly mimicks the clinical situation, it is encouraging for the proposed direct administration of retroviral vectors mode of therapy that both of these very different models show significant antitumor effects. The producer cell line and retroviral vector used in these experiments were designed to qualify for human use and was based on an amphotropic packaging line (DA) that has been approved and is in use for other clinical applications.

Splenocytes from mice cured (no palpable tumor for 30 days after the last GCV treatment) of established subcutaneous CT26 tumors by treatment with HSV-TK retroviral vectors and GCV displayed potent cytotoxic activity against CT26 cells *in vitro*, and these mice were protected against rechallenge with CT26 but not other tumors. The type of T cells responsible for this activity was not identified in this study, but previous analysis of the effector cells in the CT26 system suggests that they are CD8+ and Class I restricted.[39] Preliminary data studying the kinetics of CTL induction and activity suggest that CTL activity is present early, but decreases as the tumor volume increases. Induction or augmentation of cellular immunity has also been reported in several other models, suggesting that tumor cell destruction by GCV is immunostimulatory in a way that surgical excision, chemotherapy and radiation are not.[15,24] In fact, one clear advantage of HSV-TK gene therapy is that it avoids the immunosuppressive effects of conventional treatments. The mechanism of this additional "immune effect" is unclear, but immunotherapeutic effect in HSV-TK-treated patients could have important implications for the treatment of disseminated disease.[19]

These results confirm that high-titer preparations of HSV-TK recombinant retroviral vectors were able to transfer sufficient amounts of the gene to tumor cells *in vivo* to produce marked antitumor effects. The ability of retroviral preparations to transfer gene expression obviates the need to implant retroviral producer cell lines that otherwise might create unwanted side effects in the host animal and suggests that direct administration of such a vector to tumor nodules may be a feasible therapeutic method suitable for clinical trials.

ACKNOWLEDGMENTS

The authors wish to thank Jeffrey Hunt for excellent technical assistance and Tammi Howard and Darci Knapp for vivarium support.

REFERENCES

1. MOOLTEN, F.L. 1994. Drug sensitivity ("suicide") genes for selective cancer chemotherapy. Cancer Gene Ther. **1:** 279–287.
2. MULLEN, C.A. 1994. Metabolic suicide genes in gene therapy. Pharmacol. Ther. **63:** 199–207.
3. REID, R. *et al.* 1988. Insertion and extension of acyclic, dideoxy, and ara nucleotides by Herpes viridae, human alpha and human beta polymerases. J. Biol. Chem. **263:** 3898–3904.
4. MOOLTEN, F.L. 1986. Tumor chemosensitivity conferred by inserted Herpes thymidine kinase genes: paradigm for a prospective cancer control strategy. Cancer Res. **46:** 5276–5281.

5. MOOLTEN, F.L. 1990. Mosaicism induced by gene insertion as a means of improving chemotherapeutic selectivity. Crit. Rev. Immunol. **10:** 203–233.
6. FREEMAN, S.M. *et al.* 1993. The "bystander effect": tumor regression when a fraction of the tumor mass is genetically modified. Cancer Res. **53:** 5274–5283.
7. CULVER, K.W. *et al.* 1992. *In vivo* gene transfer with retroviral vector-producer cells for treatment of experimental brain tumors. Science **256:** 1550–1552.
8. KOLBERG, R. 1992. Gene therapists test puzzling "bystander effect." J. Natl. Inst. Health Res. **4:** 68–72.
9. RAM, Z. *et al.* 1994. The effect of thymidine kinase transduction and GCV therapy on tumor vasculature and growth of 9L gliomas in rats. J. Neurosurg. **81:** 256–260.
10. RAM, Z. *et al.* 1994. Intrathecal gene therapy for malignant leptomeningeal neoplasia. Cancer Res. **54:** 2141–2145.
11. RAM, Z. *et al.* 1993. *In situ* retroviral-mediated gene transfer for the treatment of brain tumors in rats. Cancer Res. **53:** 83–88.
12. EZZEDINE, Z.T. *et al.* 1991. Selective killing of glioma cells in culture and *in vivo* by retrovirus transfer of the Herpes simplex virus thymidine kinase gene. New Biol. **3:** 608–614.
13. CHIOCCA, E.A. *et al.* 1994. Virus-mediated genetic treatment of rodent gliomas. *In* Gene Therapeutics: Methods and Applications of Direct Gene Transfer. J. A. Wolff, Ed.: 245–262.
14. BOVIATSIS, E.J. *et al.* 1994. Gene transfer into experimental brain tumors by adenovirus, Herpes simplex virus and retroviral vectors. Hum. Gene Ther. **5:** 183–191.
15. BARBA, D. *et al.* 1994. Development of antitumor immunity following thymidine kinase-mediated killing of experimental brain tumors. Proc. Natl. Acad. Sci. USA **91:** 4348–4352.
16. TAPSCOTT, S.J. *et al.* 1994. Gene therapy of rat 9L glioma tumors by transduction with selectable genes does not require drug selection. Proc. Natl. Acad. Sci. USA **91:** 8185–8189.
17. DIMAIO, J.M. *et al.* 1994. Directed enzyme pro-drug gene therapy for pancreatic cancer *in vivo*. Surgery **116**(2): 205–213.
18. SMYTHE, W.R. *et al.* 1994. Use of recombinant adenovirus to transfer the Herpes simplex virus thymidine kinase (HSV-TK) gene to thoracic neoplasms: an effective *in vitro* drug sensitization system. Cancer Res. **54:** 2055–2059.
19. FREEMAN, S.M. *et al.* 1992. Treatment of ovarian cancer using HSV-TK gene modified vaccine—regulatory issues. Hum. Gene Ther. **3:** 342–349.
20. CRYSTAL, R.G. 1995. Transfer of gene to humans: early lessons and obstacles to success. Science **270:** 404–410.
21. The FDA Points to Consider for Somatic Cell and Gene Therapy, Cell Lines Used to Produce Biologicals, Biologicals Produced by Recombinant DNA Technology and Administration of Activated Leukocytes can be obtained from the Biologics Information Staff, Office of the Director, Center for Biologics, FDA, Bethesda, MD 20205, USA.
22. Transcript of the October 25, 1993 meeting of the Vaccines Advisory Committee of the US FDA, available from the Center for Biologics, FDA, Bethesda, MD 20205, USA.
23. GEORGES, R.N. *et al.* 1993. Prevention of orthotopic human lung cancer growth by intratracheal instillation of a retroviral antisense K-ras construct. Cancer Res. **53:** 1743–1746.
24. VILE, R.G. *et al.* 1994. Systemic gene therapy of murine melanoma using tissue specific expression of the HSV-TK gene involves an immune component. Cancer Res. **54:** 6228–6234.
25. LAUBE, L.S. *et al.* 1994. Cytotoxic T lymphocyte and antibody responses generated in rhesus monkeys immunized with retroviral vector-transduced fibroblasts expressing human immunodeficiency virus type-1 IIIB env/rev proteins. Hum. Gene Ther. **5:** 853–862.
26. IRWIN, M.S. *et al.* 1994. Direct injection of a recombinant retroviral vector induces human immunodeficiency virus-specific immune responses in mice and non-human primates. J. Virol. **68**(8): 5036–5044.

27. ENQUIST, L.W. et al. 1979. Construction and characterization of a recombinant plasmid encoding the gene for the thymidine kinase of Herpes simplex type 1 virus. Gene **7**: 335–342.
28. WAGNER, M.S. et al. 1981. Nucleotide sequence of the thymidine kinase gene of Herpes simplex virus type 1. Proc. Natl. Acad. Sci. USA **78**: 1441–1445.
29. ARMENTANO, D. et al. 1987. Effect of internal viral sequences on the utility of retroviral vectors. J. Virol. **61**(5): 1647–1650.
30. CHADA, S., et al. 1993. Cross-reactive lysis of human targets infected with prototypic and clinical human immunodeficiency virus type 1 (HIV-1) strains by murine anti-HIV-1 IIIB env-specific cytotoxic T lymphocytes. J. Virol. **67**: 3409–3417.
31. BURNS, J.C. et al. 1993. Vesicular stomatitis virus G glycoprotein pseudotyped retroviral vectors: concentration to very high titer and efficient germ transfer into mammalian and non-mammalian cells. Proc. Natl. Acad. Sci. USA **90**: 8033–8037.
32. HOWARD, B. et al. 1994. Retrovirus-mediated gene transfer of the human γ-interferon gene: a therapy for cancer. In Gene Therapy for Neoplastic Diseases. B.E. Huber & J.S. Lazo, Eds. Ann. N. Y. Acad. Sci. **716**: 167–187.
33. MACGREGOR, G.R. et al. 1987. Histochemical staining of clonal mammalian cell lines expressing E. coli beta-galactosidase indicates heterogenous expression of the bacterial gene. Som. Cell Mol. Genet. **13**: 253–265.
34. LU, D. et al. 1994. Optimization of methods to achieve mRNA-mediated transfection of tumor cells in vitro and in vivo employing cationic liposome vectors. Cancer Gene Ther. **1**(4): 245–252.
35. BI, W.L. et al. 1993. In vitro evidence that metabolic cooperation is responsible for the bystander effect observed with HSV-TK retroviral gene therapy. Hum. Gene Ther. **4**: 725–731.
36. GOLUMBEK, P.T. et al. 1992. Herpes simplex-1 virus thymidine kinase gene is unable to completely eliminate live, non-immunogenic tumor cell vaccines. J. Immunother. **12**: 224–230.
37. CHEN, S.H. et al. 1995. Combination gene therapy for liver metastases of colon carcinoma in vivo. Proc. Natl. Acad. Sci. USA **92**: 2577–2581.

Enhanced Retroviral Transduction Efficiency of Pancreatic Tumor Cell Lines Using Different Envelope Glycoproteins

BRADLEY D. HOWARD,[a,c] LARS BOENICKE,[a] WULF SCHNEIDER-BRACHERT,[b] AND HOLGER KALTHOFF[a]

[a]*Molecular Oncology Research Laboratory, Clinic for General Surgery, and*
[b]*Institute of Immunology, Christian Albrechts University, 24105 Kiel, Federal Republic of Germany*

INTRODUCTION

Since the overall prognosis for pancreatic cancer remains poor, there is an urgent need to develop additional therapeutic strategies. The genetic alteration of human pancreatic tumor cells by recombinant retroviral vectors capable of delivering therapeutic genes is essential for experimental and clinical investigation. During retroviral infection, virus binding and entry into the target cell is mediated by the interaction of the viral envelope glycoprotein with specific receptors located on the cell surface.[1] Most gene therapy protocols using recombinant retroviruses employ the amphotropic murine leukemia virus (MLV) envelope glycoprotein, which binds to a phosphate transporter on the host membrane.[2] Since it has been shown by others that the expression of these transporters can be inadequate for succesful transduction, we investigated the ability of virions possessing different envelope glycoproteins to infect pancreatic tumors. We constructed a retroviral vector containing the humanized enhanced green fluorescent protein (hEGFP) gene, pseudotyped it with either the amphotropic MLV-4070A envelope, the cat endogenous virus (CEV) envelope RD114 or the rhabdovirus vesicular stomatitis virus glycoprotein (VSV-G), and used the generated virions to transduce three pancreatic tumor cell lines. Transduction efficiency was measured by fluorescence-activated cell sorter (FACS) analysis and by differences in delivered gene copy number as determined by dot blot analysis. We tested the possible influence of different media components on the transduction efficiency and gene expression of transduced cells.

MATERIALS AND METHODS

The pancreatic tumor cell lines Panc 89, PancTuI and Colo357 used in this study were grown in either Dulbecco's modified Eagle's medium (DMEM) supplemented with 10% fetal bovine serum (FBS) and nonessential amino acids (NEAA) or RPMI

[c]Corresponding author: Dr. Bradley D. Howard, Molecular Oncology Research Laboratory, Clinic for General Surgery, Christian Albrechts University, Arnold Heller Street 7, 24105 Kiel, Federal Republic of Germany. Phone, +49 431-597-1937; fax, +49 431-597-1939; e-mail, bdhoward@email.uni-kiel.de

supplemented with 10% FBS and NEAA. The FLYA13 (expressing the MLV-4070A *env*), FLYRD18 (expressing the CEV RD114 *env*) and the 293 GPG (expressing VSV-G *env*) packaging cell lines were grown in DMEM supplemented with 10% FBS and NEAA.[3,4] 293 GPG cells were cultured using 1 μg/ml tetracycline to repress the expression of the VSV-G gene. 293 GPG cells were seeded in Primaria plates (Falcon #3803) and 24 hours later were transfected with a LXIN-based retroviral backbone containing the humanized EGFP using a modified calcium phosphate method.[5,6] Forty-eight hours later, viral supernatants were harvested and used to transduce the packaging cell lines FLYA13, FLYRD18 and 293GPG, and selected in G418 (700 mg/ml). Supernatants were collected from nonclonal pools of each respective producer line, filtered through a 0.45-mm filter (Gelman Sciences Acrodisc #4184) and stored at −80°C. After titering by limited-dilution, virus supernatants were used to infect the pancreatic cell lines Panc89, PancTuI and Colo357 at a multiplicity of infection (MOI) of 10. Forty-eight and 96 hours after infection, the transduced cell lines were harvested with trypsin, washed with 1 × Hank's balanced salt solution (HBSS), fixed in 2% formaldehyde and analyzed for gene expression as measured by FACS analysis. After selection in G418, genomic DNAs were isolated and tested for delivered gene copy number by dot blot analysis.

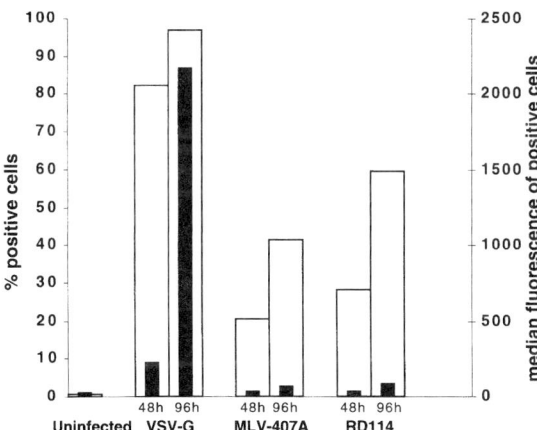

FIGURE 1. Pancreatic tumor cell line Panc89 transduced with retroviral vectors pseudotyped with either VSV-G, MLV-4070A or RD114. Pancreatic tumor cell lines Panc89, PancTuI and Colo357 were transduced with retroviral vectors pseudotyped with either VSV-G, MLV-4070A or RD114. Forty-eight and 96 hours after infection, the cells were harvested, fixed with 2% formaldehyde and analyzed by FACS using a FACS Calibur (Becton-Dickinson). The percentage of positive-transduced cells (*light columns*) and median fluorescence of the postive cells (*dark columns*) are shown in FIGURE 1 for Panc89, FIGURE 2 for PancTuI and FIGURE 3 for Colo357. Retroviral vectors pseudotyped with VSV-G infected a higher percentage of target cells and demonstrated more than 10-fold higher fluorescence levels as compared to target cells infected with retroviral vectors pseudotyped with MLV-4070A or RD 114.

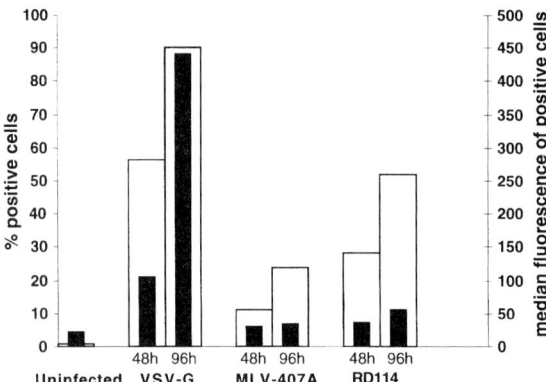

FIGURE 2. Pancreatic tumor cell line PancTuI transduced with retroviral vectors pseudotyped with either VSV-G, MLV-4070A or RD114.

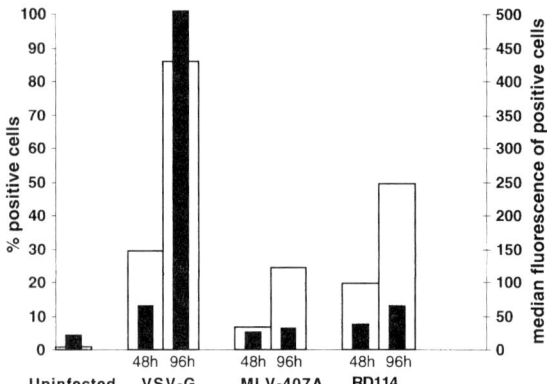

FIGURE 3. Pancreatic tumor cell line Colo357 transduced with retroviral vectors pseudotyped with either VSV-G, MLV-4070A or RD114.

RESULTS

In each of the cell lines tested, EGFP expression reached a maximum 96 hours after infection and remained strong indefinitely over extended time in culture (greater than one month). Retroviral vectors pseudotyped with VSV-G infected a higher percentage of target cells as compared to retroviral vectors pseudotyped with either MLV-4070A or RD114 (FIGS. 1–3). In addition, cells transduced with VSV-G pseudotyped virions demonstrated more than 10-fold higher fluorescence levels. Dot blot analysis of pancreatic tumor cells infected with VSV-G pseudotyped retroviral vectors showed a 10-fold increase in the number of gene copies in Panc89 and 5-fold increase in the number of gene copies in PancTuI cells as compared to Panc89 or PancTuI cells infected with MLV-4070A pseudotyped vectors (TABLE 1). We also found higher levels of EGFP expression in VSV-G-transduced pancreatic cells when

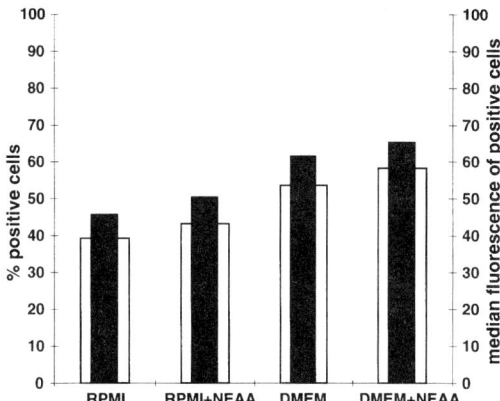

FIGURE 4. PancTuI cells transduced with VSV-G-pseudotyped retroviral vectors were grown in either RPMI medium with and without NEAA or DMEM medium with and without NEAA. The cells were harvested, fixed with 2% formaldehyde and analyzed for EGFP expression by FACS. The use of DMEM medium with the addition of NEAA increased the percentage positive cells (*light columns*) and the median fluorescence of positive cells (*dark columns*) as compared to PancTuI cells grown in RPMI with or without NEAA.

DMEM plus NEAA was used as a culture medium as compared to RPMI plus NEAA.

CONCLUSIONS

The ability to genetically modify pancreatic tumor cells *in vitro* may serve as a model for designing retroviral vectors with features that could enhance gene delivery and amplify gene expression *in vivo*. A promising approach in the gene therapy of cancer is to introduce the HSV-TK gene into pancreatic tumor cells, whose protein leads to the modification of the prodrug ganciclovir into a toxic metabolite and destroy the tumor.[7] A critical requirement for gene therapy is for a vector to deliver the HSV-TK gene and modify the highest number of cells in the targeted tumor in order to achieve a positive therapeutic outcome. We wish to improve gene delivery to human pancreatic tumors *in vivo* by identifying which of the known glycoprotein envelopes used for pseudotyping recombinant retroviral vectors can mediate the maximal transduction of human pancreatic cells *in vitro*. In this report, we used a retroviral vector containing the hEGFP gene to demonstrate that pseudotyping retroviral vectors with VSV-G glycoproteins provided the best transduction efficiency for human pancreatic tumor cells as compared to either MLV-4070A- or CEV RD114-pseudotyped retroviral vectors. The higher gene expression found in pancreatic cells transduced with VSV-G-pseudotyped retroviral vectors was due to the presence of a higher number of EGFP genes as determined by dot blot analysis. Even after G418 selection and extended growth *in vitro*, the expression of EGFP was consistently higher in VSV-G-infected cells as compared to cells infected with either MLV-4070A- or RD114-pseudotyped retroviral vectors. These data exclude the possibility

TABLE 1. Genomic DNA isolated from the various cell lines transduced with either VSV-G- or MLV-4070A-pseudotyped retroviral vectors and analyzed by dot blot

Cell Line	Panc 89		PancTuI	
DNA dilutions	1:5	1:25	1:5	1:25
VSV-G	606	124	339	101
MLV-4070A	88	10	146	12
Ratio VSV-G/MLV-4070A	6.9	12.4	2.3	8.4
Mean ratio		9.7		5.4

Note: Values were calculated by exposure to a Phospho Imager screen. Panc89 and PancTuI cells transduced with VSV-G retroviral vectors possessed 10-fold and 5-fold more gene copies, respectively, as compared to Panc 89 or PancTuI cells transduced with MLV-4070A pseudotyped retroviral vectors.

that passive antigen transfer or pseudotransduction was responsible for the enhanced expression of hEGFP.[8] In addition, we found that *in vitro* transduction efficiency and expression is affected by a variety of tissue culture media and nutritional additives. Low gene expression *in vitro* can be enhanced by using DMEM plus NEAA instead of RPMI plus NEAA. The use of richer nutritional mediums may increase the rate of division of human pancreatic cell lines and thus enhance retroviral integration. Our results suggest that the use of VSV-G glycoprotein for pseudotyping recombinant retroviruses enhances the delivery and expression of the hEGFP reporter gene in human pancreatic tumor cell lines and may be an important feature in retroviral particle design in the gene therapy of pancreatic cancer.

REFERENCES

1. MILLER, A.D. 1996. Cell surface receptors for retroviruses and implications for gene transfer. Proc. Natl. Acad. Sci. USA **93:** 11407–11413.
2. PORTER, C.D. *et al.* 1996. Comparison of efficiency of infection of human gene therapy targets cells via four different retroviral receptors. Hum. Gene Ther. **7:** 913–919.
3. COSSET, F.-L. *et al.* 1995. High titer packaging cells producing recombinant retroviruses resistant to human serum. J. Virol. **69:** 7430–7436.
4. ORY, D. *et al.* 1996. A stable human-derived packaging cell line for production of high titer retrovirus/vesicular stomatitis virus G pseudotypes. Proc. Natl. Acad. Sci. USA **93:** 11400–11406.
5. MORGAN, R.A. *et al.* 1992. Retroviral vectors containing putative internal ribosome entry sites: development of a polycistronic gene transfer system and applications to human gene therapy. Nucleic Acids Res. **20:** 1293–1299.
6. CHALFIE, M. *et al.* 1994. Green fluorescent protein as a marker for gene expression. Science **293:** 802–805.
7. MOOLTEN, F.L. 1994. Drug sensitivity ("suicide") genes for selective cancer chemotherapy. Cancer Gene Ther. **1:** 279–287.
8. GALLARDO, H.F. *et al.* 1997. Recombinant retroviruses pseudotyped with the vesicular stomatitis virus G protein mediate both stable gene transfer and pseudotransduction in human peripheral blood lymphocytes. Blood **90:** 952–957.

Construction of Recombinant Retroviruses Expressing Mutated k-ras or Mutated p53 Genes

LILIAN KADAJA,[a] RALF JESNOWSKI,[b] TOIVO MAIMETS,[a] STEFAN LIEBE,[b] AND MATTHIAS LÖHR[b,c]

[a]*Institute of Molecular and Cellular Biology, Department of Cell Biology, University of Tartu, Estonia*
[b]*Division of Gastroenterology, Department of Medicine, University of Rostock, Germany*

INTRODUCTION

Cancer of the pancreas is one of the leading causes of cancer death in the Western countries.[1] About 90% of the malignant pancreatic tumors are of ductal phenotype and presumably originate in the epithelial cells of the pancreatic ducts.

Cancer is considered to arise by the clonal evolution of cells that accumulate mutations in cellular protooncogenes and loss or inactivation of tumor suppressor genes. Within the last few years several genetic alterations associated with pancreatic carcinogenesis have been identified, namely, mutations of the ki-ras and p53[3] genes were found in most of the tumors. Mutations of the ki-ras gene were even detected in preoplastic intraductal lesions.[6] This and the high incidence implicates the ki-ras mutation as an early event in pancreatic carcinogenesis. The high frequency and wide spectrum of mutations in ras and p53 genes make them very appropriate for a descriptive molecular analysis of mammalian mutagenesis and its relationship to carcinogenesis.[4]

Though pancreatic cancer meanwhile has become one of the best characterized malignant tumors, on the other hand the molecular biology of cancer of the pancreas is still poorly understood, and little is known about the individual effect of a single genetic alteration. Cell lines derived from human pancreatic cancer have been of particular interest and have been used to study many aspects of pancreatic cancer.[2]

To investigate the effect of single genetic alterations, we tried to introduce a mutated ki-ras/p53 gene into primary pancreatic epithelial duct cells. Since these primary cells are not susceptible to common transfection methods, retroviruses with high infection efficiency were used to achieve stable and efficient transduction.

---

[c]Corresponding author: Matthias Löhr, M.D., Div. of Gastroenterology, Dept. of Medicine, University of Rostock, Ernst-Heydemann-Str. 6, 18057 Rostock, Germany. Phone, +49 (381) 494-7497; fax, +49 (381) 494-7448; e-mail: loehr@med.uni-rostock.de

MATERIALS AND METHODS

Plasmid Construction

Ki-ras cDNA (mutation at codon 12: GGT to GTT) was ligated as HpaI/StuI fragment into retroviral vector pLNCX. P53 cDNA (mutation: aa 173Val to His) was ligated as BamHI/HindIII (blunt end) fragment to vector pLXSN. Both vectors contain a selectable marker such as the neomycin phosphotransferase gene that confers the resistance to the drug G418 in eucaryotic cells. Transformation of *E. coli* and preparation of the plasmid and was performed according to standard procedures. The constructs were controlled by restriction enzyme digest and verified by sequencing (ABI Prism-System).

Cells and Transfection

The virus packaging cell line PT67 was cultured in Dulbecco's modified Eagle's medium (DMEM) supplemented with 10% fetal calf serum (FCS) at 37°C in 5% CO_2.

The cells were transfected with retroviral vectors containing p53 and ki-ras genes using CaP-transfection method by standard protocols.[7] Transfectants were selected in the presence of antibiotic G418 (500 µg/ml), and resistant clones were expanded. Virus-containing supernatants were prepared by feeding the resistant clones with 0.5 vol DMEM without G418. After 48 hr the supernatants were collected, filter sterilized (0.45 µm) and diluted 1:3 with fresh medium. After adding Polybrene (6 µg/ml final concentration), we used the supernatants for infection of primary human pancreatic epithelial cells.

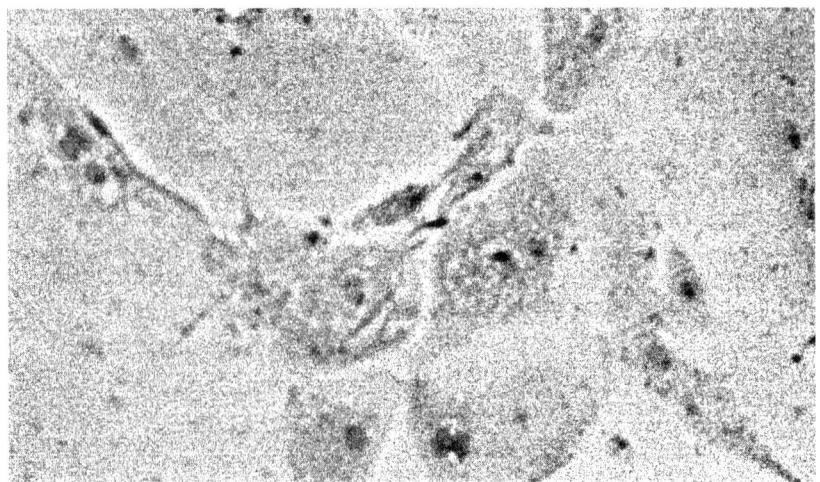

FIGURE 1. Immunocytochemistry of p53-transduced primary human pancreatic duct epithelial cells with an antibody against p53 protein.

RESULTS

As the integration of retroviral genomes only occurs actively replicating and dividing cells,[5] the transduction of primary cells is a time-consuming process. We managed to receive infected clones that are now in the phase of expansion. Detailed characterization will be carried out in the near future.

In the first preliminary assays regarding p53-transduced human primary pancreatic duct epithelial cells, the expression of the transduced p53 gene was verified using immunocytochemistry. In part the cells showed just the expected nuclear staining pattern, whereas in some cells additionally demonstrated a marked cytoplasmatic staining was visible (FIG. 1).

DISCUSSION

We have chosen this way to transfect the mutated genes directly into isolated primary duct cells rather than try to immortalize these cells first, as this immortalization would result in clones with an altered genetic background, thus disturbing the analysis of the effects induced by introducing single genetic alterations. On the other hand, it cannot be expected that the introduction of these singular defects will result in an immortalized phenotype, so that the isolation and characterization of the transfected clones will be difficult.

ACKNOWLEDGMENTS

Lilian Kadaja received an EC stipend within the Erasmus Program.

REFERENCES

1. SILVERBERG, E. & J.A. LUBERA. 1989. Cancer statistics. Cancer J. Clin. **3:** 3–39.
2. HALL, P.A. & N.R. LEMOINE. 1993. Models of pancreatic cancer. Cancer Surv. **16:** 135–154.
3. BARTON, C.M., S.L. STADDON, C.M. HUGHES et al. 1991. Abnormalities of the tumor suppressor gene p53 in human pancreatic cancer. Br. J. Cancer **64:** 1076–1082.
4. TADA, M., M. OMATA & M. OTHO. 1991. ras gene mutations in intraductal papillary neoplasms of the pancreas. Cancer **67:** 634–638.
5. MILLER, D.G., M.A. ADAM & A.D. MILLER. 1990. Gene transfer by retrovirus vectors occurs only in cells that are actively replicating at the time of infection. Mol. Cell. Biol. **10:** 4239–4242.
6. CALDAS, C., S.A. HAHN, R.H. HRUBAN, M.S. REDSTON, C.J. YEO & S.E. KERN. 1994. Detection of K-ras mutations in the stool of patients with pancreatic adenocarcinoma and pancreatic ductal hyperplasia. Cancer Res. **54:** 3568–3573.
7. AUSUBEL, F.M., R. BRENT, R.E. KINGSTON, J.G. SEIDMAN, J.A. SMITH & K. STRUHL. 1994. Current Protocols in Molecular Biology. Greene Publisher Assoc. Brooklyn, NY.

Intraarterial Instillation of Microencapsulated Cells in the Pancreatic Arteries in Pig

JENS C. KRÖGER,[a,f] HELGA BERGMEISTER,[b] ANNE HOFFMEYER,[c,d] MANFRED CEIJNA,[b] PETER KARLE,[d,e] ROBERT SALLER,[d] ILSE SCHWENDENWEIN,[b] KERSTIN VON ROMBS,[d] STEFAN LIEBE,[c] WALTER H. GÜNZBURG,[e] BRIAN SALMONS,[d] KARLHEINZ HAUENSTEIN,[a] UDO LOSERT,[b] AND MATTHIAS LÖHR[c]

[a]*Department of Diagnostic and Interventional Radiology, University of Rostock, Germany*
[b]*Center for Biomedical Research, General Hospital, University of Vienna, Austria*
[c]*Department of Medicine, University of Rostock, Germany*
[d]*Bavarian Nordic Research Institute, Munich, Germany*
[e]*Institute of Virology, University of Veterinary Sciences, Vienna, Austria*

INTRODUCTION

In pancreatic carcinoma, chemotherapy is mainly delivered systemically.[1] Recent developments include the placement of intraarterial catheters delivering the cytotoxic drugs into the celiac trunk.[2–5] On the other hand, instillation of solid microspheres for chemoembolization is a routine procedure for hepatic masses not suitable for surgery.[6–8] Our group has recently developed a model for a local chemotherapy employing genetically microencapsulated cells that produce the enzyme CYP2B1, which converts ifosfamide into its active compounds.[9] For the application in man, a supraselective intraarterial instillation in tumor-vascularizing arteries seemed a minimal invasive approach for exact placement of encapsulated cells. The aim of this investigation was to study the tolerance of the intrarterial placement into the pancreatic arteries of an animal model in order to prove the technical and biological feasibility, namely, to rule out vascular spasms and pancreatic injury.

METHODS

Animals

Adolescent pigs (mean age: 90 days, mean weight: 46 kg) were kept fasting overnight. A valid permit to perform the experiments was solicited by the authorities.

---

[f]*Corresponding author: Dr. med. Jens C. Kröger, Department of Diagnostic and Interventional Radiology, University of Rostock, E. Heydemannstr. 6, D-18057 Rostock, Germany. Phone, +49 (381) 494-9280; fax, +49 (381) 494-9272; e-mail, loehr@med.uni-rostock.de*

Microcapsules

Capsules were produced as previously described.[10–12] After encapsulation, capsules were washed and aliquoted at 100 capsules per vial and kept at 4°C until further use. A parallel sample was assessed for viability and enzyme activity as described.[9] The capsules have an average diameter of 500 µm.

Angiography

Animals were sedated and placed in a supine position on the angiography table. After placement of a central venous access, animals were intubated and ventilated. The femoral artery was exposed surgically and punctured with a 2OG angiography needle. A 4F introducer system (Terumo) was placed in by the Seldinger technique. Under fluoroscopy, the celiac trunk, splenic and common hepatic arteries were catheterized with a 4F Cobra 2 guiding catheter with an inner diameter of 0.038″ (Cordis). The initial angiography of the celiac axis was performed with Visipaque 270 (Nycomed), a dimer nonionic contrast medium, to document the special variants of vessel anatomy. Supraselective catheterization of pancreatic arteries was achieved with a coaxial 2.3F microcatheter system (Fa. Cordis). In general, pancreatic branches of the duodenal lobe were cannulated. After successful placement of the catheter in the main vessel leading into the duodenal pancreatic lobe, the second, superselective angiography was performed, and 100 capsules were instilled separately one after another to avoid occlusion of the leading vessel. At the end, control angiography documented the vascular situation after intervention. The catheter and introducing system were removed, the arterial puncture and the wound were closed surgically, and the animals were allowed to recover from anesthesia. Duration of the interventional procedure was 23–71 minutes. Animals were monitored clinically and by laboratory tests for a week. During the first 24 hours, the pigs were kept NPO but received saline infusion (500 ml/12 hours).

RESULTS

A total of 18 animals were investigated. In all animals, it was possible to cannulate both the splenic and the duodenal lobe arteries selectively (FIG. 1). In all animals, instillation of capsules was successful. Manipulation with the catheter system in small diameter vessels, injection of contrast medium and instillation of capsules resulted in 14 of 18 cases in a significant and prolonged vascular spasm that resolved spontaneously within 6–15 minutes. None of the animals developed pancreatic symptoms, but the first animal, which experienced slight tenderness of the abdomen. The amylase levels in all animal remained within normal limits.

DISCUSSION

Intraarterial instillation of microspheres via supraselective catheterization is a routine procedure in the treatment of malignant hepatic and splenic diseases.[13–15] However, the placement into vessels leading to the pancreas might be prone to in-

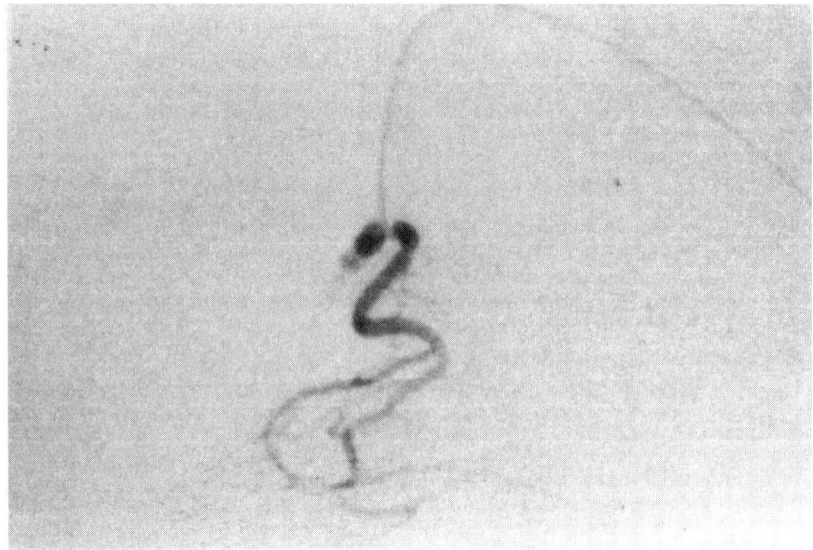

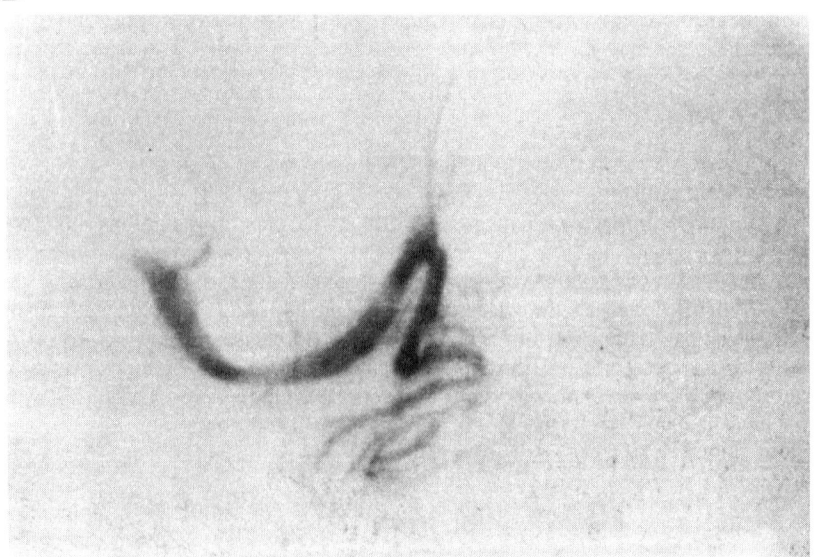

FIGURE 1. Angiography of pancreaic vessels in a pig (**A**) before and (**B**) after instillation of 100 microcapsules.

duce pancreatic injury. Furthermore, manipulation of the arteries could cause severe vascular spasm leading to irreversible damage of the vessels. In this pilot study, we have demonstrated that the instillation of capsules into pancreatic arteries in the pig is feasible technically and biologically. Furthermore, although vascular spasms occurred in most of the animals, these reactions did not lead to substantial or long-lasting effects in the animal. Based on these animal investigations, we suggest that this approach is suitable for the placement of microencapsulated cells in patients with pancreatic neoplasms.[16]

REFERENCES

1. AHLGREN, J.D. 1996. Chemotherapy for pancreatic carcinoma. Cancer **78:** 654–663.
2. ISHIKAWA, O., H. OSHIGASHI, Y. SASAKI, K. MASAO, T. KABUTO, H. FURUKAWA & S. IMAOKA. 1998. Adjuvant therapies in extended pancreatectomy for ductal adenocarcinoma of the pancreas. Hepatogastroenterology **45**(21): 644–650.
3. KAWASAKI, R., S. MORITA, Y. NODA & A. TSUJI. 1998. Arterial infusion chemotherapy of low dose 5-fluorouracil via an implantable port combined with systemic infusion of low dose cisplatin for the treatment of recurrent and advanced hepatocellular carcinoma: preliminary study. Cardiovasc. Interventional Radiol. **21**(Suppl. 1): 152.
4. MAURER, C.A., M.M. BORNER, J. LAUFFER. H. FRIESS, K. Z'GRAGGEN, J. TRILLER & M.W. BUCHLER. 1998. Celiac axis infusion chemotherapy in advanced nonresectable pancreatic cancer. Int. J. Pancreatol. **23**(3): 181–186.
5. WACKER, F.K., J. BOESE-LANDGRAF, A. WAGNER, D. ALBRECHT, K.J. WOLF & F. FOBBE. 1997. Minimally invasive catheter implantation for regional chemotherapy of the liver: a new percutaneous transsubclavian approach. Cardiovasc. Interventional Radiol. **20**(2): 128–132.
6. BERGHAMMER, P., F. PFEFFEL, F. WINKELBAUER, C. WILTSCHKE, T. SCHENK, J. LAMMER, C. MÜLLER & C. ZIELINSKI. 1998. Arterial hepatic embolization of unresectable hepatocellular carcinoma using a cyanoacrylate/lipiodol mixture. Cardiovasc. Interventional Radiol. **21**(3): 214–218.
7. FLORIO, F., M. NARDELLA, S. BALZANO, E. CATURELLI, D. SIENA & M. CAMMISSA. 1997. Treatment of hepatocellular carcinoma: a single-center study. Cardiovasc. Interventional Radiol. **20**(1): 23–28.
8. GROUPE D'ETUDE ET DE TRAITEMENT DU CARCINOMA HEPATOCELLULAIRE. 1995. A comparison of lipiodol chemoembolization and conservative treatment for unresectable hepatocellular carcinoma. N. Engl. J. Med. **332:** 1256–1261.
9. DIRVEN, H.A.A.M., B. VAN OMMEN & P.J. VAN BLAEDEREN. 1996. Glutathione conjugation of alkylating cytostatic drugs with a nitrogen mustard group and the role of glutathione S-transferases. Chem. Res. Toxicol. **9:** 351–360.
10. STANGE, J., S. MITZNER, H. DAUTZENBERG, W. RAMLOW, M. KNIPPEL, M. STEINER, B. ERNST, R. SCHMIDT & H. KLINKMANN. 1993. Prolonged biochemical and morphological stability of encapsulated liver cells—a new method. Biomater. Artif. Cells Immobilization Biotechnol. **21:** 343–352.
11. SALLER, R.M., J. STANGE, S. MITZNER, U. HEINZMANN, B. SALMONS & W.H. GÜNZBURG. 1999. Encapsulated cells producing retroviral vectors for *in vivo* gene therapy. Submitted.
12. LÖHR, M., P. MÜLLER, P. KARLE, J. STANGE, S. MITZNER, H. NIZZE, S. LIEBE, B. SALMONS & W.H. GÜNZBURG. 1998. Targeted chemotherapy by encapsulating cells engineered to deliver CYP2B1, an ifosfamide activating cytochrome P450 gene. Gene Ther. **5:** 1070–1078.
13. DE SANCTIS, S.N. GOLDBERG & P.N. MUELLER. 1998. Percutaneous treatment of hepatic neoplasms: a review of current techniques. Cardiovasc. Interventional Radiol. **21**(4): 273–296.
14. JAEGER, H.H., U.M. MEHRING, F. CASTANEDA, F. HASSE, G. BLUMHARDT, D. LOEHLEIN & K.D. MATHIAS. 1996. Sequential transarterial chemoembolization for

unresectable advances hepatocellular carcinoma. Cardiovasc. Interventional Radiol. **19**(6): 388–396.
15. NAKA, T., K. ASHIDA, S. TAKAHASHI, T. KANEKO, K. MIZUSAWA & N. KAIBARA. 1998. Effective TAE therapy using lipiodol with epirubicin for liver metastases of nonfunctioning islet cell carcinoma of the pancreas. J. Hepatobilary Pancreat. Surg. **5**(1): 108–112.
16. LÖHR, M., Z.T. BAGO, H. BERGMEISTER, M. CEIJKA, M. FREUND, W. GELBMANN, W.H. GÜNZBURG, J. HAIN, K. HAUENSTEIN, W. HENNINGER, A. HOFFMEYER, P. KARLE, J.C. KRÖGER, S. LIEBE, U. LOSERT, P. MÜLLER, A. PROBST, M. RENNER, R. RENZ, R. SALLER, B. SALMONS, K. VON ROMBS, T. WAGNER & I. WALTER. 1999. Cell therapy using microencapsulated 293 cells transfected a gene construct expressing CYP2B1, an ifosfamide converting enzyme, instilled intra-arterially in patients with advanced-stage pancreatic carcinoma. A phase I study. J. Mol. Med. **77**: 393–398.

Index of Contributors

Abbruzzese, J.L., 31–37
Abramian,, A., 31–37
Adler, G., 122–146, 219–230
Applebaum, S., 201–209
Arlt, A., 147–156

Backhaus, C., 166–170
Batra, S.K., 263–280
Beger, H.G., 281–287
Beresford, G., 263–280
Bergmeister, H., 374–378
Bernstorff, W.V., 243–251
Boenicke, L., 366–370
Booth, B.J.M., 263–280
Breslin, T., 31–37
Büchler, M.W., 110–121

Capellá, G., 103–109
Ceijna, M., 374–378
Chiao, P.J., 31–37
Colcher, D., 263–280
Cook, T., 94–102

Dionne, C.A., 252–262
Domschke, W., 157–165

Emmrich, J., 171–174, 238–242
Evans, D.B., 31–37

Farré, L., 103–109
Fleming, J., 31–37
Fong, T.C., 352–365
Frazier, M.L., 1–4
Friess, H., 110–121
Frohme, M., 122–146
Fujikawa-Adachi, K., 5–16

Gansauge, F., 281–287
Gansauge, S., 281–287
García, C., 103–109

Gebelein, B., 94–102
Geng, M., 122–146
Ghaneh, P., 288–307, 308–318
Grau, A.M., 31–37
Gress, T.M., 122–146
Günzburg, W.H., 326–336, 337–351, 374–378
Guo, X.-Z., 110–121

Harris, A., 17–30
Hauenstein, K., 374–378
Hennighausen, G., 231–237
Hoffmeyer, A., 374–378
Hoheisel, J.D., 122–146
Hollingsworth, M.A., 5–16, 38–49
Hopt, U., 171–174
Howard, B.D., 352–365, 366–370
Humphreys, M., 288–307
Hunt, K.K., 31–37

Ibrahim, S.M., 175–178

Jesnowski, R., 50–65, 166–170, 337–351, 371–373
Jonas, L., 231–237
Jones, L., 288–307

Kadaja, L., 371–373
Kalthoff, H., 83–93, 243–251, 352–365, 366–370
Karle, P., 326–336, 337–351, 374–378
Kleeff, Ö., 110–121
Klein-Szanto, A.J.P., 252–262
Klöppel, G., 66–73, 219–230
Koczan, D., 175–178
Köhler, H., 175–178
Kremer, B., 243–251
Kröger, J.C., 374–378

Lehnert, L., 83–93
Lemoine, N.R., 319–325

Lerch, M.M., 157–165
Lichter, P., 122–146
Liebe, S., 50–65, 166–170, 171–174, 175–178, 238–242, 337–351, 371–373, 374–378
Link, K.H., 281–287
Lluís, F., 103–109
Löhr, M., 50–65, 166–170, 171–174, 175–178, 238–242, 337–351, 371–373, 374–378
Longnecker, D.S., 66–73, 74–82
Losert, U., 374–378
Lowenfels, A.B., 191–200

Maimets, T., 371–373
Maisonneuve, P. 191–200
Martin, S.P., 201–209
Mayerle, J., 157–165
Merkord, J., 231–237
Micha, A., 122–146
Miknyoczki, S.J., 252–262
Müller, P., 50–65 , 238–242, 337–351
Müller-Pillasch, F., 122–146

Nan, B.-C., 110–121
Nebe, B., 238–242
Neoptolemos, J.P., 288–307, 308–318
Nishimori, I., 5–16
Nizze, H., 337–351

Onishi, S., 5–16

Pavlinkova, G., 263–280
Püschel, K., 337–351

Renner, M., 326–336
Renz, R., 326–336, 337–351
Reyes, G., 103–109
Rigg, A.S., 319–325
Ringel, B., 175–178
Ringel, J., 175–178, 238–242
Röder, C., 83–93
Ruggeri, B.A., 252–262
Rychly, J., 238–242

Saller, R., 337–351, 374–378
Salmons, B., 326–336, 337–351, 374–378
Scarpa, A., 179–190
Schäfer, H., 147–156
Schareck, W., 50–65
Schmid, A., 243–251
Schmid, R.M., 219–230
Schmidt, C., 238–242
Schmidt, W.E., 147–156
Schmiegel, W., 83–93
Schneider-Brachert, W., 366–370
Schnekenburger, J., 157–165
Schneuer, S., 166–170
Schwendenwein, I., 374–378
Simon, P., 157–165
Solinas-Toldo, S., 122–146
Sparmann, G., 171–174, 231–237
Stein, H., 337–351

Tarafa, G., 103–109
Thiesen, H.-J., 175–178
Trauzold, A., 147–156
Trost, H., 83–93

Ungefroren, H., 243–251
Urrutia, R., 94–102

Van Laethem, J.L., 210–218
Villanueva, A., 103–109
von Rombs, K., 337–351, 374–378
Voss, M., 243–251

Wagner, M., 219–230
Wagner, T., 337–351
Wallrapp, C., 122–146
Weber, H., 231–237
Wenger, C., 122–146
Whitcomb, D.C., 201–209

Zamboni, G., 179–190
Zhang, W., 31–37